+RA971 .G44 1987

RA
971
G44
1987

Georgopoulos, Basil
Spyros, 1926-

The community
general hospital

COLLEGE FOR HUMAN SERVICES
LIBRARY
345 HUDSON STREET
NEW YORK, N.Y. 10014

Continuity in Administrative Science

Ancestral Books in the Management of Organizations

A 31-volume facsimile series
reproducing classic works in the field.

Edited by
Arthur P. Brief
Graduate School of Business Administration
New York University

A Garland Series

The Community General Hospital

Basil Georgopoulos
Floyd C. Mann

Garland Publishing, Inc.
New York • London
1987

For a complete list of the titles in this series
see the final pages of this volume

This facsimile has been made from a copy
in the Yale University Library.

© The Macmillan Company 1962. Reprinted by
permission of the Macmillan Publishing Company, Inc.

Library of Congress Cataloging-in-Publication Data

Georgopoulos, Basil Spyros, 1926-
The community general hospital.

(Continuity in administrative science)
Reprint. Originally published: New York : Macmillan, 1962.
Includes index.
1. Hospitals—Administration. 2. Hospital and community.
I. Mann, Floyd Christopher, 1917- . II. Title. III. Series.
[DNLM: 1. Hospitals, Community—organization & administration.
2. Hospitals, General—organization & administration.
WX 150 G353c 1962a]
RA971.G44 1987 362.1'1 86-26933
ISBN 0-8240-8205-2 (alk. paper)

The volumes in this series are printed on
acid-free, 250-year-life paper.

Printed in the United States of America

THE COMMUNITY
GENERAL
HOSPITAL

THE COMMUNITY GENERAL HOSPITAL

BASIL S. GEORGOPOULOS
FLOYD C. MANN

*Survey Research Center and
Department of Psychology*
THE UNIVERSITY OF MICHIGAN

THE MACMILLAN COMPANY : NEW YORK
MACMILLAN NEW YORK : LONDON

© The Macmillan Company 1962

All rights reserved—no part of this book may be reproduced in any form without permission in writing from the publisher, except by a reviewer who wishes to quote brief passages in connection with a review written for inclusion in magazine or newspaper.

First printing, July 1962

Library of Congress catalog card number: 62-13440

The Macmillan Company, New York
Collier-Macmillan Canada, Ltd., Galt, Ontario
Divisions of The Crowell-Collier Publishing Company

Printed in the United States of America

PREFACE

The rapid and widespread growth of large-scale organizations is one of the most distinctive and most significant characteristics of the twentieth century. More and more, the world we live in is dominated by formal, specialized organizations. We are born into such an environment, are educated and trained for life's roles within it, and spend most of our working time and energies in one or another of its many organizational arrangements. In mid-twentieth century, organizations are indeed an ubiquitous element in everyone's life. The present work is concerned with the structure and functioning of one of the most complex of these organizations—the community general hospital. Its main objective is to add to our knowledge of the behavior and problems of this important institution.

Our book is the final research report on a study of twelve Michigan hospitals. This study, initiated in the fall of 1956, is one of the major projects of scientific inquiry into the social psychology of organizations that have been undertaken by the Organizational Behavior and Change Program of the Survey Research Center of the Institute for Social Research. Since its inception, fifteen years ago, the Program has conducted a series of studies in the area of organizational behavior, using a variety of theoretical approaches and research designs, and a variety of organizations as research sites. These have included industrial and manufacturing firms, government agencies, labor unions, voluntary and scientific associations, public utility companies, and other types of organizations. The present research extends these investigations to include the short-stay community general hospital. Our look at this essential, yet little studied, community facility adds to the Program's growing series of research, and to the research continuity envisaged, back in 1947, by Rensis Likert, Angus Campbell, and Daniel Katz in the establishment of the Program.

The overall purpose shared by most studies conducted within the Program has been to develop useful theoretical and practical knowledge about human groups and organizations, especially complex organizations like the hospital. The present study, perhaps more than any of the others which have preceded it, demonstrates the value of searching for the principles governing behavior in large-scale organizations by comparing and contrasting the properties, problems, and performance of a number of organizations simultaneously. It also demonstrates the usefulness of studying organizations as total social systems in all their complexity, and of examining comparatively problems and phenomena that have an organization-wide, or system-wide, significance, rather than dwelling upon the more limited problems of particular groups or individuals within each organization. Moreover, the results of this, our first, study of the community general hospital, apart from their factual or intrinsic value, stamp this institution as a unique and important laboratory for social scientists. This is especially true for researchers who are interested in such phenomena as those dealt with here: internal organizational coordination, leadership and supervision, intraorganizational strain, communication, organizational effectiveness, and similar other aspects of organizational behavior.

Any full-scale study of as complicated an organization as the short-stay general hospital requires the varied efforts and support of a host of people and services. In a way, the research process is analogous to the forging of a chain—it is completed piece by piece, each piece carefully handled and interlinked with those preceding and following it, the total chain proving no stronger than its weakest link. It is with real pleasure that we are able to identify many of those who have contributed to the forging of the chain represented by this volume. As is often the case, however, many individuals whose assistance has been of inestimable value to us must remain anonymous, to maintain the confidentiality of individual organizations and respondents who provided data. To all those who must go unidentified, we here express our sincere thanks.

The study was made possible financially by a PHS research grant, W-71, from the Division of Hospital and Medical Facilities of the National Institutes of Health, Public Health Service. We are very appreciative of this financial support. A number of organizations and individuals in the hospital, medical, nursing, and health fields helped us greatly at different stages of our research effort, especially at the launching and early exploratory phases, and we are indebted to all of them for their assistance. Most of these, including the Michigan Hospital Association, are specifically cited by name at the appropriate places in the text; a few will not be identified, however, in the interests of confidentiality. These outside organizations and individuals made a significant contribution to the study, even though they did not participate directly.

Our debt to the administrators, boards of trustees, medical and nursing staffs, and other personnel of the hospitals studied is obviously greater than can be expressed in the words of a preface. Two hospitals opened their doors, early in the study, to allow our research staff to conduct exploratory interviews and collect preliminary information that later proved important to the refinement of the initial conceptual framework and methodological plans of the project. Another ten hospitals participated in the research proper, providing the basic raw materials with which this volume was built. More than 1200 individuals (doctors, nurses, technicians, department heads, trustees, and

Preface

administrators) from these ten institutions furnished the essential ingredient of the research—the data. They each gave of their busy time to answer the questions that we asked. We are most thankful to all of them and wish it were possible to acknowledge them and their organizations publicly and by name.

The data were collected with the help of the Survey Research Center's Field Staff Section. A number of interviewers from the field staff, under the general supervision of Charles F. Cannell and Morris Axelrod, assisted the research staff in the collection of the data from each participating hospital. The Center's organizational apparatus for collecting, coding, and machine processing large bodies of data provided technical services and support that were necessary to carry out the research.

Informal intellectual exchange with many of our colleagues and friends at the Institute for Social Research, over a period of years, has left an indelible imprint on much of our work, including this study. In this connection, we particularly want to express our thanks and appreciation to our immediate colleagues in the Organizational Behavior and Change Program, and especially to Robert L. Kahn, Stanley E. Seashore, Arnold S. Tannenbaum, and Donald C. Pelz with whom we have had the closest work ties. The Institute itself provided the psychological climate, the physical and technical resources, and the supportive services without which this study might have never been accomplished. Rensis Likert, Director of the Institute, and Angus Campbell, Director of the Survey Research Center, must be given much of the credit for having created this stimulating research environment.

The members of the staff most directly responsible for the project deserve special mention here, even though their respective contributions are cited in specific sections of the book. In its early formative stages, the study had the help of Leo Meltzer, Ruth E. Searles, and George K. Zollschan, all of whom served as assistant study directors. The review of pertinent literature and the exploratory work in the two pilot hospitals were the responsibility of the authors and the three assistant study directors. Mrs. Helen Metzner also helped in the review of literature. With the departure of Dr. Meltzer and Mr. Zollschan for other positions, Miss Searles participated in the collection and processing of data and, then, wrote her doctoral dissertation in sociology using some of the data. During the analysis phases of the project, in which he participated actively, Paul E. Mott also joined the staff as an assistant study director. Subsequently, he too used some of the data for his doctoral dissertation in sociology. Dr. Franklin W. Neff, member of the staff of the Survey Research Center, similarly joined us, for a period of time, during the analytic stage. He organized and summarized the qualitative and descriptive data that were later incorporated in Chapter 4 in the form of individual hospital profiles. Drs. Meltzer, Mott, Neff, and Searles, all contributed importantly to the study and must share in the credit. Finally, we like to thank Mrs. Peggy

Parkman and Mrs. Paula Gebhardt, assistants in research, for having performed various computational-statistical tasks.

Behind a research team, in the office are secretaries, in the home are spouses and children. Mrs. Harriet Rose, Mrs. Sharon Radhuber, and Mrs. Margery Sanford carried the secretarial responsibilities at various stages of the project, including the typing of research instruments, working papers, project correspondence, and the transformation of rough drafts into typewritten manuscript. To them go our very special thanks. Mrs. Sanford typed the final manuscript, read galley proof and page proof, made suggestions on style, and constructed the index. At different stages, the study also had the secretarial services of Miss Ida Putansu, Mrs. Mary Long, and Mrs. Joyce Kiess. Finally, our respective wives and children made a most important contribution to the present work in their own ways, by allowing us to slight or leave undone some of our family duties and responsibilities. For their patience, help, and understanding we are grateful.

Various drafts of this volume have had a critical reading by several colleagues in our immediate or extended work environment. Dr. John P. Kirscht, Mr. George F. Wieland, and Mr. John J. Zugich read every chapter and made many useful comments and suggestions. Drs. Louis Block, Paul E. Mott, Franklin W. Neff, and Vergil N. Slee, each read and commented constructively upon certain particular chapters. And a few of the administrators whose hospitals participated in the research also made a number of suggestions on the preliminary drafts of some chapters. The book benefited a good deal as a result of these reviews.

The closing caveat is, of course, that while this research could not have been done without the valued help of many others along the way, we accept full responsibility for the final product. We are, in fact, chained to it professionally as are none of the others.

Basil S. Georgopoulos
Floyd C. Mann

Ann Arbor, Michigan
January 1962

CONTENTS

Preface v

Chapter 1. INTRODUCTION TO THE COMMUNITY
GENERAL HOSPITAL 1
The Hospital as an Organization 5
Context, Nature, and Objectives of the Research 15
The Organization of the Book 23

Chapter 2. RESEARCH DESIGN, METHOD, AND
PROCEDURE 32
Overview of the Research Design 33
The Chronology of the Research 37
The Selection of Participating Hospitals 46
The Selection of Individual Groups and Respondents from
Each Hospital 53
Research Instruments, Data Collection, Response Rates,
and Respondent Reaction 61
Forms of Description and Measurement, and Analysis
Techniques 72
Methodological Limitations 82
Summary 85

Chapter 3. THE PEOPLE AROUND THE PATIENT 89
The Personal Characteristics of Hospital Personnel 91
Sex; age; family status; formal education
Professional-Occupational Career Patterns 98
Professional-occupational training; job history; length
of association with present hospital; time on present
job and interjob shifting in the hospital
The Gross Anatomy of Work in the Hospital 106
Full-time vs. part-time work; shift work patterns;
service or divisional characteristics; turnover and

absenteeism among nursing personnel; work interaction patterns among hospital personnel
Present Job Status and Outlook 124
Work pace and pressure; skill utilization and improvement; overall satisfaction with supervision; opportunity for advancement and earnings; motivation to work and job commitment
Comparative Group Profiles of the People Around the Patient 142
The medical staff; the trustees; the administrators; the department heads; the supervisory nurses; the nonsupervisory registered nurses; the practical nurses; the aides and orderlies; the laboratory and x-ray technicians
Summary 152

Chapter 4. TEN HOSPITALS IN PROFILE: A DESCRIPTIVE OVERVIEW 156
A Sketch of the "Typical" Hospital in the Study 158
Individual Hospital Profiles 162
A Comparative Overview of the Ten Hospitals 188
Local setting and relations with the community; boards of trustees; medical staffs; relations between doctors and trustees; medical and nursing care; administration and related aspects; some additional items
Summary 196

Chapter 5. ASSESSMENT OF PATIENT CARE 198
Previously Suggested Approaches 200
The Measures of Patient Care 207
The Nursing Care Measure 209
The Medical Care Measure 223
The Measure of Overall Patient Care 242
The Comparative Measure of Overall Patient Care 249
Relationships Among the Four Measures of Patient Care 257
Summary 260

Chapter 6. ORGANIZATIONAL COORDINATION 265
Theoretical Considerations: The Concept of Organizational Coordination 269
Coordination defined; bases and means of coordination; types of coordination

Contents   xi

        Measurement of Coordination in Hospitals 279
           The measures of coordination; consistency of measures and their interrelations; further results about the consistency of measures
        Factors Expected to Affect Organizational Coordination 293
           Organizational planning; sharedness of expectations, complementarity of expectations, and cooperation among members; intraorganizational strain; problem awareness and problem solving; communication; structural features of organization
        A Technical Methodological Note 299
        Summary 302

Chapter 7. FACTORS AFFECTING COORDINATION IN HOSPITALS 305
        Results Concerning Hospital Coordination 306
           Organizational planning in relation to coordination; sharedness of expectations, complementarity of expectations, and cooperation among organizational members in relation to coordination; intraorganizational strain in relation to coordination; problem awareness and problem solving in relation to coordination; communication in relation to coordination; certain aspects of hospital structure in relation to coordination
        Coordination in the Department of Nursing 342
           Measures of nursing department coordination; nursing department coordination in relation to hospital coordination; factors affecting nursing department coordination
        The "Best" vs. the "Poorest" Coordination Hospital: Contrasting Profiles 352
        Summary and Conclusions 355

Chapter 8. FACTORS AFFECTING THE QUALITY OF PATIENT CARE 365
        Adequacy of Material Facilities and the Quality of Patient Care 366
        Financial Considerations and the Quality of Patient Care 370
        Size-Related Features of Hospital Structure and the Quality of Patient Care 376
        Composition and Distribution of Therapeutic Staff and the Quality of Patient Care 379

Absenteeism and Turnover Among Nursing Personnel and the Quality of Patient Care 383
Organizational Coordination and the Quality of Patient Care 387
Intraorganizational Strain and the Quality of Patient Care 396
Complementarity of Work-related Expectations Between Medical and Nursing Staff and the Quality of Patient Care 399
Medical Committee Behavior and the Quality of Patient Care 402
The Performance of Paramedical Departments and the Quality of Patient Care 407
Summary and Restatement 413

Chapter 9. SUPERVISORY AND ADMINISTRATIVE BEHAVIOR 422
Theoretical Considerations 425
Supervisory skills: administrative, human relations, and technical skills; the supervisory skill-mix; the relativity of "effective" supervision
Supervisory Skills, and the Relationship Among Supervisory Skills at Different Levels of Supervision 433
The measures of supervisory skills; the relationship among supervisory skills; respondent discrimination among the three supervisory skills
Supervisory Skills and the Satisfaction of Subordinates with Their Superiors at Different Levels of Supervision 444
Specific Supervisory Practices, as They Relate to Supervisory Skills and to the Satisfaction of Subordinates with Supervision at Different Organizational Levels 452
Results concerning supervision of department heads; results concerning supervision of supervisory nurses; results concerning supervision of nonsupervisory registered nurses; results concerning supervision of practical nurses and of aides; results concerning supervision of technicians; summary: the relative importance of particular supervisory practices to the satisfaction of subordinates with supervision at different levels
Supervisory Skills and Characteristics and the Quality of Patient Care 471
Supervision and organizational effectiveness; results regarding the relationship of supervisory skills and

practices to the quality of patient care in the participating hospitals
Supervisory Skills and Characteristics in Relation to Coordination 483
Summary 491

Chapter 10. THE COMMUNICATION PATTERNS OF REGISTERED NURSES IN RELATION TO NURSING ACTIVITY AND PERFORMANCE 500
Communication Among Nurses: Some Theoretical Considerations and Hypotheses 504
Methodological Considerations: Measurement of Communication and Role Performance 511
The independent variables: aspects of communication studied; the dependent variables: aspects of nursing activity and role performance
Findings 519
The importance of qualitative aspects of communication; the importance of quantitative aspects of communication; the importance of direction of communication; the importance of communication to other aspects of nursing activity
Summary and Conclusions 536

Chapter 11. COMMENTARY ON SELECTED PROBLEMS AND ISSUES 544
The External Image of the Hospital 545
The Hospital as a Place to Work 547
Problems Pertaining to the Nursing Staff 549
Issues and Problems Concerning the Medical Staff 552
The Value Orientations of the Top-Echelon Groups in the Hospital 559
The Influence of Key Groups in the Hospital 566
Organizational Change and Its Accommodation 575
Summary 586

Chapter 12. SUMMARY AND CONCLUSIONS 588
The Aims and Strategy of the Study 590
Organizational Coordination 596
Factors related to overall hospital coordination; findings concerning nursing department coordination; programed and nonprogramed coordination; preventive and promotive coordination

Patient Care 605
    Factors related to the quality of nursing care; factors related to the quality of medical care; factors related to the quality of overall patient care (noncomparative and comparative care); other findings concerning the quality of patient care

Supervision 613
    Results concerning supervisory skills and practices; results concerning satisfaction with supervision; supervision and organizational coordination; supervision and patient care

Communication 621
    Importance of the adequacy and quality of communication; importance of the quantity and frequency of communication; results involving the direction of communication; importance of the concentration of task-relevant communication in formal channels

Supplementary Data and Findings 626
Concluding Remarks 634

APPENDIX A. QUESTIONNAIRE ADMINISTERED TO NON-SUPERVISORY NURSES: A SAMPLE QUESTIONNAIRE 637

APPENDIX B. INTERVIEW WITH HOSPITAL ADMINISTRATORS: A SAMPLE INTERVIEW 671

INDEX 677

THE COMMUNITY GENERAL HOSPITAL

1 INTRODUCTION TO THE COMMUNITY GENERAL HOSPITAL

Few other institutions have a more vital significance for us all or a more far-reaching impact upon our lives than does the hospital. Few other organizations have a clearer meaning for their members and customers, or more crucial functions for the complex social order within which they operate. In our organization-oriented society, the hospital is one of the few organizations of whose purpose we are vividly aware, and with whose functioning we are unambiguously concerned. Like our family, schools, and government, the hospital ultimately touches us all, individually and collectively. Our personal physical and mental health, our community well-being, and our economic resources are all intimately affected by the work of our hospitals. In fact, seldom do we rely more dramatically or more completely on the products, or services, of an organization than we do in the case of the hospital.

The hospital is an organization which, sooner or later, we all come to know and use. And, among hospitals, the general hospital is the one with which we are most likely to be familiar. The average American now spends almost a day for each year of his life in a general hospital. This is the first social organization he encounters in life, as well as the last place with which he is likely to be in touch. Over 95 percent of all babies born in this country are delivered in hospitals, and half of us now spend our final hours in a general hospital (41). On the average, about 10 out of every 100 persons are admitted to general hospitals every year, and the adult age groups show increasingly higher admission rates. Admissions for people under 15 years of age have actually declined since the middle twenties, but admissions for the 25 to 44 age group have nearly doubled, and those for the older age groups have more than doubled (23). The average rate of admissions to short-stay hospitals during 1960 reached a new high of almost 128 admissions per 1000 population (25). Chances are that all of us will eventually encounter a short-stay general hospital as patients during our adult lifetime. In addition, many of us are likely to be working in such an organization, to have personal contacts with it, or even to have business dealings with it.

Our general and various other hospitals make up one of this nation's largest industries. In all, there are about 7000 hospitals of different kinds in the United States, employing a total of approximately 1.6 million full-time people, not counting doctors. These organizations have aggregate assets of about $17.1 billion, annual expenses of approximately $8.4 billion, and an annual payroll of about $5.6 billion. With a combined total of nearly 1.7 million beds, they handled an impressive total of 25 million patient admissions in 1960—the year to which the data cited in this paragraph refer.[1] Our hospitals, then, are a "big business," in addition to being the principal health institutions of our society. When one also considers the various educational, training, and research activities carried out by many hospitals, one can more readily grasp and appreciate the importance of these institutions for the functioning, integration, and stability of the total society.

In this hospital complex, the community general hospital occupies a central and prominent position. Of the nearly 6900 hospitals listed in the 1961 "Guide Issue" of *Hospitals* (25), about 5400 are "short-term" or short-stay institutions of different types. And approximately 5200 of these are nonfederal general hospitals, which are engaged in the care and treatment of so-called acute diseases. Of the 5200 nonfederal, short-stay general hospitals, about 2000 are either state and local government-operated institutions or proprietary organizations. The other 3200 are community, voluntary, nonprofit institutions, which together provide daily care to an average of about 330,000 patients. These are the hospitals with which the average person is likely to be in contact. Approximately one-third of these short-stay community general hospitals are church-related or affiliated institutions, the other two-thirds of them—about 2100 or so hospitals—are nondenominational institutions. The present research is concerned with hospitals of this last type, i.e., with voluntary, nonprofit, nongovernmental, nondenominational, short-stay, community general hospitals.

These hospitals are all alike in some ways, but different in others. Geographically, they are literally scattered throughout the country. Some are located in large urban communities, others in small cities or towns. Some are large-scale organizations with 500 or more beds and over a thousand employees, while many are smaller institutions with 50 or fewer beds. Some are administered by men administrators and others by women, some by lay persons and others by physicians. Many are exclusively concerned with providing patient care and treatment, while some are also engaged in the teaching of medicine and nursing, and in research activities. Some offer practically all the most elaborate and most specialized medical, surgical, and nursing services available today, others handle only the more common acute diseases and

[1] These figures are based on data reported in the 1961 "Guide Issue" of *Hospitals* (25).

Introduction to the Community General Hospital

relatively routine cases. Many serve only their immediate community, while some have patients from outside areas and other states as well. Some render better service to their patients than others, and some are more effective organizations than others. Not all these hospitals are accredited by the Joint Commission on Accreditation of Hospitals (3). Not all participate in Blue Cross–Blue Shield programs. Not all meet their financial needs in the same manner. And not all have sufficient human resources or material facilities.

In brief, the approximately 2100 voluntary, nonprofit, nongovernmental, and nondenominational, short-stay general hospitals in the nation differ from each other in many respects. They are not a homogeneous group of organizations. Even though they are all of the same general type, even though they are all concerned with the same general objective—that of providing adequate patient care effectively—even though they share a number of needs and experience certain important organizational problems in common, and even though they are similar in a number of other ways, they still constitute a very heterogeneous group of organizations. Because of this diversity, because of the unavailability of sufficient knowledge from previous research regarding the common and unique characteristics of these hospitals, because of reasons of methodological efficiency and soundness of research design, as well as for certain other reasons discussed in Chapter 2, only a small and relatively homogeneous subgroup of hospitals was actually included in our study.

Specifically, we studied a total of twelve hospitals, all of which shared the following important characteristics: (1) they were short-stay general hospitals of medium size, their size ranging between 100 and 350 beds; (2) they were neither government- nor church-operated or affiliated institutions; (3) they were community, voluntary, nonprofit organizations; (4) they were each administered by a lay, male administrator and governed by a board of trustees; (5) they were in the same state—Michigan; (6) they were located in cities having a population of at least 10,000; and (7) they were all accredited by the Joint Commission on Accreditation of Hospitals.

Two of the twelve hospitals were included only in the initial, preparatory phase of the research, for pilot study purposes. The other ten participated in the study proper and will be referred to in the book as the "participating hospitals." The selection of the hospitals involved will be fully explained in Chapter 2, where our research design and methodology will be discussed in detail. The more than 1200 persons (hospital administrators, trustees, doctors, nurses, medical technologists, department heads) who were chosen to represent the hospitals in the study as respondents will be discussed in Chapter 2 and in Chapter 3, which is concerned with a description of the various medical and nonmedical groups from which the respondents were selected. And the ten participating hospitals will be individually discussed in Chapter 4, where we shall also describe some of the major features of the "average" or "typical" hospital studied.

Based on empirical data from and about these ten hospitals, our study represents an effort toward better understanding of the structure and functioning of the community general hospital *as an organization*. With the aid of both quantitative and qualitative data, we are interested in examining and understanding the behavior of the total hospital as a complex social system; only secondarily are we interested in the special problems and characteristics of particular occupational groups or individuals in the organization. The central concern is with phenomena that have an organization-wide significance. More specifically, the objective is to investigate systematically a number of questions about hospital functioning, with special emphasis in the areas of patient care, organizational coordination and intergroup relations, supervision and administrative behavior, and communication. In these areas of primary interest, as well as in several areas of secondary interest which will be indicated later in this chapter, the research focus is on problems and issues of organizational behavior, and the theoretical emphasis is on social-psychological concepts.

The basic general question underlying both the primary and secondary interests of the study is the question of organizational effectiveness. The central aim is to identify and evaluate specific social-psychological factors that influence the quality of patient care, organizational coordination, and other aspects of hospital functioning, by comparing and contrasting the ten participating hospitals on each of a number of variables and characteristics in the several areas of research interest. Stated more generally, the aim is to find out what distinguishes the more from the less effective hospitals, and what relates to, facilitates, or hinders effective hospital functioning. This broad question of why some of the hospitals are more effective or better performing organizations than others is, of course, approached by asking and answering more specific questions regarding the quality of patient care, organizational coordination, supervision, communication, and other relevant aspects of organizational behavior. Another aim of the study is to provide descriptive information about some of the more prominent problems, needs, and characteristics of the community general hospital and of the principal groups of people working in it. A final aim is to identify current research needs in this field, and to suggest specific avenues for future investigation.

In summary, the overall purpose of this research is to contribute to our understanding of an important and complex organization—the community general hospital. The study seeks to contribute to our knowledge of certain important aspects of the structure and functioning of the hospital and, in the process, add to our knowledge of the behavior of complex organizations in general, through the investigation of the above-outlined objectives. But, before discussing the nature and objectives of the study further, it is important to consider briefly some of the key features of the community general hospital.

THE HOSPITAL AS AN ORGANIZATION

The community general hospital is an organization that mobilizes the skills and efforts of a number of widely divergent groups of professional, semi-professional, and nonprofessional personnel to provide a highly personalized service to individual patients. Like other large-scale organizations, it is established and designed to pursue certain objectives through collaborative activity. The chief objective of the hospital is, of course, to provide adequate care and treatment to its patients (within the limits of present-day technical-medical knowledge, and knowledge of organizing human activity effectively, as well as within limits that may be imposed by the relative scarcity of appropriate organizational resources or by extraorganizational forces). Its principal product is medical, surgical, and nursing service to the patient, and its central concern is the life and health of the patient. A hospital may, of course, have additional objectives, including its own maintenance and survival, organizational stability and growth, financial solvency, medical and nursing education and research, and various employee-related objectives. But, all these are subsidiary to the key objective of service to the patient, which constitutes the basic organizing principle that underlies all activities in the community general hospital.

There is little ambiguity, if any, about the main organizational objective of the community general hospital. Unlike many organizations, the hospital is able to make the role it performs in the larger community psychologically meaningful to its members. And most of its members try to give unstintingly of their energies to perform the tasks assigned to them. Many doctors and nurses look upon their profession as a sacred calling. Others find working in the hospital deeply satisfying of needs that they cannot easily express in words. They see the hospital as a nonprofit institution dedicated to works of mercy, and they sense that their mission in life is to give of themselves in order to help others. Immediate personal comfort and satisfactions, and even material rewards, are defined by most members as less important than giving good care to the patient and meeting a higher order of obligation to mankind. Serious conflicts regarding material rewards, such as those found in organizations where profit is the chief motive, are virtually nonexistent in the hospital. For all these reasons, motivating organizational members toward the objectives of the organization is much less of a problem for the hospital in comparison to other large-scale organizations. The goals of individual members and the objectives of the organization are considerably more congruent in the case of the hospital.

To do its work, the hospital relies upon an extensive division of labor among its members, upon a complex organizational structure which encompasses many different departments, staffs, offices, and positions, and upon an elaborate system of coordination of tasks, functions, and social interaction.

Work in the hospital is greatly differentiated and specialized, and of a highly interactional character. It is carried out by a large number of cooperating people whose backgrounds, education, training, skills, and functions are as diverse and heterogeneous as can be found in any of the most complex organizations in existence. And much of the work is not only specialized but also performed by highly trained professionals—the doctors—who require the collaboration, assistance, and services of many other professional and nonprofessional personnel. In addition to the medical staff, which is highly specialized and departmentalized, there is the nursing staff, which includes graduate professional nurses in various supervisory and nonsupervisory positions, practical nurses, and untrained nurse's aids. In addition to the nursing staff and the medical staff, which are the two largest groups in the community general hospital, there are the hospital administrator and a number of administrative-supervisory personnel who head various departments or services (e.g., nursing, dietary, admissions, maintenance, pharmacy, medical records, housekeeping, laundry) and are in charge of the employees in these departments. There are also a number of medical technologists and technicians who work in the laboratory and x-ray departments of the hospital, as well as a number of miscellaneous clerical and secretarial personnel. And apart from all these staffs and professional-occupational groups, there is a board of trustees which has the overall formal responsibility for the organization, and which consists of a number of prominent people from the outside community. The trustees offer their services to the hospital without remuneration and are not employees of the organization. In short, professionalization and specialization are two of the hallmarks of the hospital. (The various staffs, personnel groups, and departments of the hospital will be discussed in Chapter 2 and subsequent chapters.)

Because of this extensive division of labor and accompanying specialization of work, practically every person working in the hospital depends upon some other person or persons for the performance of his own organizational role. Specialists and professionals can perform their functions only when a considerable array of supportive personnel and auxiliary services is put at their disposal at all times. Doctors, nurses, and others in the hospital do not, and cannot, function separately or independently of one another. Their work is mutually supplementary, interlocking, and interdependent. In turn, such a high interdependence requires that the various specialized functions and activities of the many departments, groups, and individual members of the organization be sufficiently coordinated, if the organization is to function effectively and attain its objectives. Consequently, the hospital has developed a rather intricate and elaborate system of internal coordination. Without coordination, concerted effort on the part of its different members and continuity in organizational operations could not be ensured. (Organizational coordination will be discussed in detail in Chapters 6 and 7.)

It is also interesting and important to note here that, unlike industrial and other large-scale organizations, the hospital relies very heavily on the skills, motivations, and behaviors of its members for the attainment and maintenance of adequate coordination. The flow of work is too variable and irregular to permit coordination through mechanical standardization. And the product of the organization—patient care—is itself individualized rather than uniform or invariant. Because the work is neither mechanized nor uniform or standardized, and because it cannot be planned in advance with the automatic precision of an assembly line, the organization must depend a good deal upon its various members to make the day-to-day adjustments which the situation may demand, but which cannot possibly be completely detailed or prescribed by formal organizational rules and regulations. This is all the more essential, moreover, if one takes into account the fact that the patient, who is the center of all activity in the hospital, is a transient rather than a stable element in the system—in the short-stay hospital, he comes and goes very rapidly.

Fundamentally, then, the hospital is a human rather than a machine system. And even though it may possess elaborate and impressive-looking equipment, or a great variety of physical and material facilities, it has no integrated mechanical-physical systems for the handling and processing of its work. The patient is not a chunk of raw material that passively goes through an ordered progression of machines and assembly-line operators. At every stage of his short stay in the hospital, he is mainly dependent upon his interaction with the people who are entrusted with his care, and upon the skills, actions, and interactions of these different people. All of these factors necessitate heavy reliance upon the members of the organization to coordinate their activities on a voluntary, informal, and expedient basis.

Paradoxical as it may seem, however, the hospital is also a highly formal, quasi-bureaucratic organization which, like all task-oriented organizations, relies a great deal upon formal policies, formal written rules and regulations, and formal authority for controlling much of the behavior and work relationships of its members. The emphasis on formal organizational mechanisms and procedures and on directive rather than "democratic" controls, along with a number of other factors, gives the hospital its much talked about "authoritarian" character, which manifests itself in relatively sharp patterns of superordination-subordination, in expectations of strict discipline and obedience, and in distinct status differences among organizational members.

The authoritarian character of the hospital is partly the result of historical forces having their origins at a time when professionalization and specialization were at a primordial stage, and when nursing, medicine, and the hospital were all closely associated with the work of religious orders and military institutions. The absence of substantial professionalization and specialization characteristic of hospital personnel at those times, along with the emphasis of religious and military institutions on social arrangements in which the occupant of every position in the organization presumably knew "his place," and kept to his place by strictly adhering to specified rights, duties, and obligations, had much to do with the hospital's adopting a strict hierarchical and authoritarian system of work arrangements. But, the advent of professionalization and specialization, the gradual independence of hospitals from religious and military institutions, and the impact of an increasingly secular culture have greatly reduced the authoritarian character of the hospital. As Lentz (31) suggests, within the last 50 years the hospital has undergone marked changes, dropping some of its authoritarian and paternalistic characteristics and taking on those of a bureaucratic, functionally rational organization.

Today's community general hospital, however, still has some of its traditional authoritarian characteristics along with its emphasis on rational organization. Moreover, it is unlikely that it will rid itself of all authoritarianism in the near future. There are several major counterforces at work in this connection. First, there is the fact that the hospital constantly deals with critical matters of life and death—matters which place a heavy burden of both secular and moral responsibility on the organization and its members. When human life is at stake, there is little tolerance for error or negligence. And, if error and negligence can be prevented by adherence to strict formal rules and quasi-authoritarian discipline, such rules are important to have and obedience cannot very well be questioned (although blind obedience is mitigated because the hospital increasingly relies on the expertness, judgment, and ethics of professionals who, while abhorring regimentation, are presumably capable of a good deal of self-discipline). Second, there is the great concern of the hospital for maximum efficiency and predictability of performance. In the absence of mechanically regulated workflows, this concern virtually forces the organization to use many quasi-authoritarian means of control (including rigid rules and procedures, directive supervision, rigorous discipline, etc.), in the hope of: (1) attaining some uniformity in the behavior of its members, (2) regulating their interaction and checking deviance within known limits of accountability, and (3) appraising their performance. Third, there is the temptation to adhere to traditional, familiar ways of doing things which, coupled with the lack of apparently equivalent or superior alternatives that could be employed to ensure clarity of responsibility and efficiency and predictability of performance, also serves to perpetuate organizational reliance upon customary directive means of control.[2]

In brief, while historical forces might account for the origins of the au-

[2] Incidentally, the apparent unavailability of equivalent or superior organizational alternatives is partly the result of our inadequate knowledge about how best to organize and manage human activity in a situation such as that of the community general hospital, and partly the result of the inability of hospitals to utilize the findings of modern research to best advantage.

thoritarian characteristics of the hospital, it is not likely that some of these characteristics would continue to persist (especially within the context of a highly secular culture) unless they were more functional than not. And this clearly appears to be the case. In the first place, as in any organization designed to mobilize resources quickly in order to meet crises and emergencies successfully, a good deal of regimented behavior is required in the hospital. Lines of authority and responsibility have to be clearly drawn, basic acceptance of authority has to be assured, and discipline has to be maintained. In the second place, the hospital is expected to be able to provide adequate care to its patients at all times, with the precision of a machine system and with minimum error, even though it is a human rather than a machine system. It is expected to perform well continuously and to produce a machinelike response toward the patient, regardless of such things as turnover, absenteeism, and feelings of friendship or hostility among its personnel, or other organizational problems that it may be experiencing. It is also expected to be responsive to the health-related needs and demands of its community, and to meet a variety of medicolegal requirements. Because of these expectations, the hospital places high premium on being able to count upon and predict the outcome of the performances of its members. And predictability of performance can be partly attained through directive, quasi-authoritarian controls which, in the absence of apparently superior alternatives, are rather tempting to the organization.

Coupled with this great concern for predictability of performance, moreover, there is an increasing concern that the hospital operate as efficiently and economically as possible. As the hospital has become a resource for all members of the community, and not just the indigent and the impoverished, the public has come to expect of it the best medical and nursing services that can be offered. These services, however, are quite costly, as are the facilities, equipment, supplies, and medicines that are required. And while the public may be willing (though not necessarily able to afford) to pay for these essential costs of hospital care, it also expects the best care possible at reasonable cost or even at least cost. At the same time, it is neither willing to tolerate nor prepared to pay any costs that may result from inefficient operations, poor administration, duplication of services, waste, negligence, and the like. It expects its hospitals to reduce to a minimum or eliminate altogether costs of this latter type and to operate with maximum economy. The hospitals themselves are quite aware of these and other pressures for efficiency, and have come to place very high emphasis on greater efficiency. Great emphasis on economic efficiency, however, is not entirely compatible with the hospital's traditional humanitarian orientation and objective of best service to the patient; the "best" service is not always or necessarily the most economical. Furthermore, this concern for efficiency results both in progressive rationalization of hospital operations and in the institution of more rigid controls within the organization. Such controls, incidentally, serve to maintain the remaining authoritarian characteristics of the community general hospital.

But, efficiency of operations and predictability of performance in the hospital could not possibly be attained only through quasi-authoritarian and directive controls. In fact, if carried to extremes, such controls would in the long run be inimical both to efficiency and to predictability. Efficiency and predictability of performance are also, and perhaps primarily, attained through a number of other factors, which are essential to effective organizational functioning. Probably the most prominent of these factors in the case of the community general hospital are organizational coordination and professionalization.

Because of the high degrees of specialization and functional interdependence found in the hospital, coordination of skills, tasks, and activities is indispensable to effective organizational performance and its predictability. The different specialized, but interacting and interdependent, parts of the organization must fit well together; they must not work at cross purposes or in their own separate directions. If the organization is to attain its objectives, its different parts and members must function according to each other's needs and the needs and expectations of the total organization. In short, they must be well coordinated. But, as we have already pointed out, the hospital is dependent very greatly upon the motivations and voluntary, informal adjustments of its members for the attainment and maintenance of good coordination. Formal organizational plans, rules, regulations, and controls may ensure some minimum coordination but of themselves are incapable of producing adequate coordination, for only a fraction of all the coordinative activities required in this organization can be programed in advance. We shall have much more to say about organizational coordination in subsequent chapters.

The other relevant factor that we wish to consider here, in addition to coordination, is that of professionalization—professionalization being one of the major distinctive features of the community general hospital. The majority of those who hold the principal therapeutic and nontherapeutic positions in the hospital are trained as professionals. The doctors, through their training, have been schooled in certain professional obligations, ethics, and standards of appropriate behavior and have acquired a number of common attitudes, shared values, and mutual understandings about their work and work relations with others. The same is true about the registered nurses. Other groups in the organization are also on the road to professionalization: the administrators, the medical librarians, the medical technologists, the dietitians, and others in paramedical positions.

This high degree of professionalization among those entrusted with the care of the patient has developed along lines of rational, functional specialization, and has had the effect of inculcating many complementary expectations and common norms and values in the members of the principal groups of the hospital—values, expectations, and norms that are essential to the integration of

The Hospital as an Organization

the organization. These include the norms of giving good care, devotion to duty, loyalty, selflessness and altruism, discipline, and hard work. This normative structure underpins the formal rational structure of the organization, and enables the hospital to attain a level of coordination and integration that could never be accomplished through administrative edict, through hierarchical directives, or through explicitly formulated and carefully specified organizational plans and impersonal rules, regulations, and procedures. However, increased professionalization and specialization have also had the effect of sharpening some of the status differences among the people working in the hospital—and sharp status distinctions bespeak of some authoritarianism.

Among other things, increased professionalization in the hospital has helped guarantee that certain minimum levels of competence and skill will exist in the organization, thus having a direct impact upon performance and organizational effectiveness. Similarly, professionalization and specialization have contributed to greater public confidence in the hospital, and to a wider acceptance of the hospital as a resource for the health needs of all people, for high professionalization and specialization imply expertness and knowledge. Increased professionalization has undoubtedly resulted in improved patient care and, in so doing, it has also raised the expectations of the public for both high-quality care and high efficiency in hospital operations. More and more of us go to the hospital for our various health needs nowadays but, because of improved service, we stay there for a shorter and shorter period of time. In the last 30 years, the average length of stay for adult patients in general hospitals has decreased by about a third, from 12.6 to 8.6 days (24)—making it increasingly appropriate to refer to the community general hospital as the short-stay hospital.

Another of the distinctive characteristics of the community general hospital, closely related to professionalization and specialization, is the absence of a single line of authority in the organization. This feature has already been the subject of considerable discussion by Smith (51) and others, but is important enough to warrant some brief observations here. Essentially, authority in the hospital is shared (not equally) by the board of trustees, the doctors, and the administrator—the three centers of power in the organization—and, to some extent, also by the director of nursing. (We shall have much more to say about the relative influence of trustees, doctors, and administrators in Chapter 11.) In the hospital, authority does not emanate from a single source and does not flow along a single line of command as it does in most formal organizations.

A formal organizational chart of the hospital shows the board of trustees as having ultimate authority and overall responsibility for the institution. The board delegates the day-to-day management of the organization to the hospital administrator. In turn, the administrator delegates authority to the heads of the various nonmedical departments (including the director of nursing, who also wields a different kind of authority that originates in her professional expertness). The heads of these departments, in turn, have varying degrees of authority over the affairs of their respective departments and personnel. In the formal organizational chart, the medical staff, its officers, and its members are not shown as having any direct-line responsibility; they are outside of the lay-administrative line of authority. Yet, as is well known both within and outside the hospital, the doctors exercise substantial influence throughout the hospital structure at nearly all organizational levels, enjoy very high autonomy in their work, and have a good deal of professional authority over others in the organization. Over the nursing staff and over the patients, their professional authority is dominant. And although the board of trustees is in theory shown as the ultimate source of authority, the board actually has very limited *de facto* authority over the medical staff, as we will see in Chapter 11. Partly because the doctors are not employees of the hospital (they are "guests" who are granted practice privileges), partly because they enjoy high status and great prestige, partly because they have almost supreme authority in professional-medical matters, and partly for other reasons, they are subject to very little lay-organizational authority.

Professionals in staff capacities in business corporations—lawyers, doctors, accountants, and others—have little or no authority to be involved in the activities of the line; they mainly serve as consultants and advisors. But this is not so in the case of the hospital. The absence of a single line of authority in the hospital, of course, creates various administrative and operational problems, as well as psychological problems having to do with the relative power and influence on organizational functioning on the part of doctors, trustees, administrators, and others. For one thing, it makes formal organizational coordination rather difficult. For another thing, it allows for instances in which it is not clear where authority, responsibility, and accountability reside. Similarly, it allows for a situation wherein a large number of organizational members, particularly members of the nursing staff, must be responsible to and take orders not only from their supervisors but also from the doctors. The lay authority and the professional authority to which nurses are subject, of course, are not always consistent. The absence of a single line of authority also makes for difficulties in communication, difficulties in the area of discipline, and difficulties in resolving problems that must be resolved through cooperative efforts on the part of both the lay-administrative and the medical-professional sides. Frequently, the administrator, feeling that the responsibility for the overall management of the organization is his, and feeling that doctors through their power and pressures interfere in the discharge of his responsibilities, is motivated or actively attempts to circumvent the medical staff on various matters, and this too is apt to lead to problems. (The doctors, in turn, are likely to try to circumvent the administrator.) For the same reasons, the administrator is likely to be prone toward more and more bureaucratization in the hospital. And increased bureaucratization of organizational operations is likely to be fought and resented by the doctors, for it eventually means a reduction in their influence.

In general, multiple lines of authority require the maintenance of a very delicate balance of power in the organization—a balance of power that is rather precarious. On the positive side, multiple lines of authority may serve as a system of "checks and balances," which may prevent other kinds of possible problems, such as organizational inflexibility and authoritarianism, or may serve to lighten the burden of responsibility in situations where responsibility may be too great for any single group or individual to shoulder. Regardless of the advantages and disadvantages of a system of multiple lines of authority, such a system is an integral part of the community general hospital. Not only is it an integral part, moreover, but also a part that is virtually inevitable for an organization such as this. This is because much of the work in the hospital is performed by influential professionals and not by low-status workers, and because of the high degrees of both professionalization and specialization characteristic of the organization. As Parsons has aptly observed, "The multiplication of technical fields, and their differentiation from each other . . . leads to an essential element of decentralization in the organizations which must employ them" (42, p. 236). For this reason, he goes on to explain that, unlike business and military organizations, "A university cannot be organized mainly on a 'line' principle. . . ." (42, p. 236). In this respect, the community general hospital is very similar to a university. (Hospitals and universities have a number of other interesting characteristics in common, but here we are only interested in hospitals.)

In summary, the community general hospital is an extremely complex social organization that differs from business and other large-scale organizations on a number of important characteristics. Among its main distinguishing characteristics, the following are worth re-emphasizing:

1. The main objective of the organization is to render personalized service —care and treatment—to individual patients, rather than the manufacture of some uniform material object. And the economic value of the organization's products and objectives is secondary to their social and humanitarian value.

2. By comparison to industrial organizations, the hospital is much more directly dependent upon, and responsive to, its surrounding community, and its work is much more closely integrated with the needs and demands of its consumers and potential customers. To the hospital and its members, the patient's needs are always of supreme and paramount importance. Moreover, there is high agreement about the principal objective of the hospital among the members of the organization, and the personal needs and goals of the different members conflict little with the objectives of the organization.

3. The demands of much of the work at the hospital are of an emergency nature and nondeferrable. They place a heavy burden of both moral and

secular-functional responsibility upon the organization and its members. Correspondingly, the organization shows great concern for clarity of responsibility and accountability among its different members and very little tolerance for either ambiguity or error.

4. The nature and volume of work are variable and diverse, and subject to relatively little standardization. The hospital cannot lend itself to mass production techniques, to assembly-line operations, or to automated functioning. It is a human rather than a machine system, with all the attributes this entails. Both the raw materials and end products of the organization are human. And, being human, they participate actively in the production process, thus having a good deal of control over it.

5. The principal workers in the hospital—doctors and nurses—are professionals, and this entails various administrative and operational problems for the organization.

6. By comparison to industrial organizations, the hospital has relatively little control over its workload and over many of its key members. In particular, it has little direct control over the doctors and over the patients—two of its most essential components. In the short-stay hospital, the patients are not only a very heterogeneous and very transient group, but are also, mainly and ultimately, in the hands of their doctors, who are not employees of the organization.

7. The administrator has much less authority, power, and discretion than his managerial counterparts in industry, because the hospital is not and cannot very well be organized on the basis of a single line of authority. The simultaneous presence of lay, professional, and mixed lay-professional lines of authority in the hospital creates a number of administrative and other problems, which business organizations are largely spared.

8. The hospital is a formal, quasi-bureaucratic, and quasi-authoritarian organization which, like most organizations of this kind, relies greatly on conventional hierarchical work arrangements and on rather rigid impersonal rules, regulations, and procedures. But, more importantly, it is a highly departmentalized, highly professionalized, and highly specialized organization that could not possibly function effectively without relying heavily for its internal coordination on the motivations, actions, self-discipline, and voluntary, informal adjustments of its many members. Coordination of efforts and activities in the hospital is indispensable to organizational functioning, because the work is of a highly interactional character—the activities of organizational members are highly interlocking and interdependent, and the various members can perform their role only by working in close association with each other.

9. The hospital shows a very great concern for efficiency and predictability of performance among its members and for overall organizational effectiveness.

10. Finally, the community general hospital is an organization which is important to us all, and which is becoming increasingly important. Several

basic social trends tend to ensure this: the accelerating accumulation of new medical knowledge, new medical, surgical, and nursing procedures, and new drugs and medicines; rising levels of family income in the nation; increased use of the general hospital for numerous different diseases and health needs; and a growing demand by the general public for the best possible quality of medical-surgical and nursing care.

It has been the purpose of this section to introduce the reader to some of the key characteristics and organizational problems of the community general hospital. (Many of these will be examined in detail in subsequent chapters.) The characteristics and problems discussed above, along with many others to be dealt with throughout the book, show how complicated an organization the hospital is, and lead one to suspect that increased understanding of such problems and characteristics might help ease some of the management difficulties and perhaps also improve the organizational effectiveness of our hospitals.

CONTEXT, NATURE, AND OBJECTIVES OF THE RESEARCH

It is clear from the introductory paragraphs that the community general hospital is a very important institution for all of us. Yet, there is relatively little systematic research available about it. We need to know much more than we presently do about the problems and needs of the hospital, if we are to understand its operations and evaluate its weaknesses and strengths. What are the requirements of effective hospital functioning? What are the criteria of hospital effectiveness? What are the factors and conditions that facilitate or hinder the hospital's adaptation to external and internal changes or demands? What patterns or practices of administration, supervision, and communication are most appropriate for this organization? Why do some hospitals provide better patient care than others, even though they may have comparable physical and technological facilities? How does the hospital manage to articulate and channel the diverse efforts of its many different staffs, groups, departments, and individual members toward the attainment of its organizational objectives? What are the requirements and consequences of good organizational coordination? We would like to have some answers for these and many other important questions.

It is the purpose of the present work to begin to answer some of these questions and thus contribute both to our understanding of the community general hospital as an organization and to our knowledge of the behavior of complex organizations more generally. This twofold purpose indicates a basic assumption that underlies the various studies which have been undertaken during the last 15 years by the Organizational Behavior and Change Program of the Survey Research Center. The assumption is that carefully designed research projects can, through the use of the conceptual and methodological tools now available to the social and behavioral sciences, contribute simultaneously to the solution of many practical problems faced by those responsible for the administration and management of organizations, and to our scientific knowledge of the principles applicable to problems of organizing and managing human activity and resources.

The research program, organized in 1947, was designed to conduct studies of human groups and organizations, and of the behavior of individuals in different types of organizations: small and large, simple and complex, public and private, profit and nonprofit, contractual and voluntary. These studies have one fundamental objective in common: to develop knowledge about organized human behavior; to describe, understand, and explain the activities of organizations and their members. The program has completed, during the last 15 years, a number of major social-psychological studies of industrial and business organizations, commercial and service enterprises, governmental agencies, labor unions, public utilities, and professional and voluntary associations. Illustrative studies of the program (arranged here in order of recency) would include those reported by Likert (33); Mann and Hoffman (35); Tannenbaum and Kahn (55); Kahn (28); Georgopoulos and Tannenbaum (17); Georgopoulos, Mahoney, and Jones (18); Pelz (43); Kahn, Mann, and Seashore (29); Lieberman (32); Weiss (56); Morse and Reimer (40); Seashore (48); Morse (39); Jacobson, Kahn, Mann, and Morse (27); and Katz, Gurin, Maccoby, and Floor (30). The present study is one in this programmatic series of empirical research.

The particular problems and phenomena of behavior examined by the program cover a rather wide range, and they may vary from one study to another (e.g., some studies have been mainly concerned with leadership and supervision and others with productivity; some have been interested in problems of control and decision-making and in problems of organizational change; while others have dealt with worker motivation and job satisfaction, absenteeism and turnover, intraorganizational strain, and various aspects of organizational effectiveness and individual and group performance). Correspondingly, the specific concepts and variables investigated also vary from one study to another (although a certain amount of overlapping is ensured by the programmatic character of the research), depending upon the theoretical approach employed, the methodology and design of the study, the substantive objectives involved, and similar other considerations. Furthermore, while some of the studies are primarily concerned with the behavior of individuals in organizational settings, others are more interested in the behavior of groups and organizations. In the present study, the focus is not on individual persons or particular occupational groups within the hospital; it is on the total hospital as an on-going organization, and on some of the major organizational components of the hospital (e.g., the nursing department). The reasons for this are discussed throughout the book.

The study has several specific, but interrelated objectives. One objective is to provide a descriptive account of the major organizational problems and characteristics of the community general hospital, and information about the background, occupational, and work characteristics of the principal groups of people working in the hospital. Another objective is to explore a number of issues and questions that are frequently raised in the literature about hospitals and hospital functioning. A third objective is to identify important research needs in this field and to suggest possible avenues for their investigation. A fourth objective is to contribute to the methodology of studying the hospital and its problems. But, the key underlying question to which the study is addressed is the question of organizational effectiveness: What are some of the main factors that are related to, facilitate, or impede effective hospital functioning? Or, what distinguishes the more from the less effective (organizationally speaking) community general hospitals?

More particularly, in connection with this key question, the study seeks to answer a number of more specific questions about: (1) the quality of patient care in the hospitals involved; (2) organizational coordination and intergroup relations; (3) supervision and administrative behavior; and (4) communication. However, the study is especially interested in the first two of these four problem areas. These principal problem areas will be viewed both separately and in relation to one another, in an attempt to specify and evaluate some of the factors and conditions that influence the organizational effectiveness of the community general hospital. The specific concepts, variables, and questions investigated in each area will be discussed in detail in the appropriate chapters. The items listed below, however, will give the reader a sample of the kinds of questions with which we shall be concerned:

The hospital as an organization

What is the community general hospital designed to accomplish, and what kind of an organization is it? What is the nature of the division of labor within the hospital? On what does the hospital rely to get its work done? What are some of its problems, needs, weaknesses, and strengths? How do those who work in it view the hospital, and what are some of the problems they experience in their work? And, generally, what are some of the important characteristics of this organization and its members?

Patient care and hospital effectiveness

What does organizational effectiveness mean in the case of the short-stay community general hospital? What criteria of effectiveness are available, or might be developed? What is the relationship among different aspects of effectiveness? What relationships are there between the quality of patient care and such things as the composition of the medical and nursing staff, absenteeism and turnover among nursing personnel, organizational facilities, intraorganizational strain and pressures, organizational coordination, administrative and supervisory practices, etc.?

Organizational coordination and intergroup relations

What is the nature of internal coordination in the hospital? What are the different types, bases, and mechanisms of coordination? What social-psychological factors are associated with the development and maintenance of good coordination? What are some of the consequences of good and poor coordination? How important is coordination for effective hospital functioning?

Supervisory and administrative behavior

What is the role of leadership and supervision in complex organizations? What kinds of supervisory skills and practices are required in a hospital, and at different levels in this organization? What is the relationship between different supervisory practices and such things as organizational coordination, patient care, and subordinate satisfaction with supervision?

Communication

What is the organizational function of communication? How do different aspects of the communication process among professional nurses—quantity, quality, content, direction, concentration in formal channels—affect nursing activity and performance? What kinds of communication are required, and what kinds are dysfunctional?

In conjunction with the major problem areas of patient care, coordination, supervision, and communication, the study also explores certain other aspects of the hospital situation, most of which have received little or no systematic attention in previous research. Included among these areas of secondary interest are the following: intraorganizational strain, or tension and pressures in the hospital; organizational change and its accommodation; the relative influence of key groups (medical staff, nursing staff, trustees, and administrator) on hospital functioning; the value orientations of the top groups in the organization; certain problems and issues regarding the medical staff and the nursing staff; some financial aspects, and the adequacy of physical-material facilities; organizational size and size-related factors; the performance of certain medical committees and paramedical departments; certain aspects of nursing activity and performance; the composition and distribution of the therapeutic staffs (medical and nursing staffs); the relative organizational stability of different groups in the hospital; employee rewards, job satisfaction, motivation, and organizational commitment; absenteeism and turnover among nursing personnel; certain aspects of organizational planning and problem solving; and the work expectations, attitudes, and interactions of the people who make up the hospital organization. The personal and occupational characteristics and some of the work problems and needs of the principal groups in the hospital will also be examined.

It should be clear by now that the objectives of this research are partly exploratory and descriptive, and partly analytical and explanatory. On the one hand, the study explores certain "gray areas" of the hospital situation and provides descriptive information about various aspects of the structure and functioning of the hospital, as well as about the people who make up this organization. On the other hand, it is aimed at a systematic, quantitative examination of the major problem areas outlined above, in an attempt to ascertain the interrelationships among these areas and to identify some of the factors associated with the quality of patient care and organizational coordination in the hospitals studied.

Certain other important characteristics of the study should also be clear by now. First, it should be evident that the study is primarily concerned with the total hospital as an organizational system, rather than with particular individuals or groups within the system. In the main, it is interested in problems and phenomena that have system-wide significance or organization-wide implications, rather than in the more circumscribed problems and needs of particular occupational groups and individuals in the system. Accordingly, most of the concepts and variables studied are defined and measured at the organizational and not the individual level. Second, it should be noted that many of the specific areas on which the study focuses are those which administrative and executive leadership (both lay and medical) within the hospital can affect or alter, not those which are devoid of any practical implications or which are beyond the control and influence of those responsible for the affairs of the hospital. Finally, it might be well also to reiterate that the study is a comparative study of hospitals—it seeks to derive knowledge about the functioning of the community general hospital primarily by comparing and contrasting the ten hospitals which participated in the research on each of a number of variables and characteristics representing the areas of interest outlined above.

The specific methods and procedures used to accomplish the objectives of the research will be spelled out in detail in Chapter 2, where we shall discuss and explain our research strategy and design in relation to certain theoretical considerations underlying the approach followed. In anticipation of that discussion we could only add here that, apart from its substantive aspects (e.g., its concern with the area of organizational coordination, which heretofore has received little attention in empirical research), apart from its theoretical framework which attempts to view the hospital as a total organization, and apart from its emphasis on the organizational and social-psychological aspects of hospital functioning, the comparative character and overall methodology of this study distinguish it rather sharply from previous major studies in the hospital field. Many of these studies will be cited in subsequent chapters, when appropriate. However, for purposes of background, we will conclude the present section by briefly commenting on some of the more prominent of them.

Probably the first major *sociological* study of American general hospitals is that by Smith (50), reported in 1949. This was a study of three hospitals—two community general hospitals and one Veterans Administration hospital—in the Chicago area. Building on his personal experiences as an administrative officer in an army hospital during World War II, Smith studied certain sociological and organizational aspects of the three hospitals, using data from intensive interviews with hospital personnel at various levels and from personal observations. His work constitutes an excellent first study of the general hospital from a sociological standpoint and introduces the reader to some of the problems and conflicts faced by the hospital.

Smith's study was followed by another sociological study of a large general hospital in a New England city. This case study was done by Wessen (58) and was reported in 1951. Wessen investigated certain aspects of the social structure of the hospital, using both observational data and data from interviews with a sample of 75 doctors, nurses, administrative personnel, and other professional and nonprofessional employees. His approach was based on sociological theories about social institutions. This study demonstrated the need for adequate channels of communication, for agreement about institutional purposes among organizational members, and for clearly defined allocations of organizational roles and authority in the hospital. It also showed that the status system and certain imperfectly assimilated changes in the organization create barriers to free communication among hospital personnel.

In 1951, Zugich (61) completed another observational and interviewing study in five hospitals. Zugich examined the importance of interpersonal relations for hospital organization. He concluded that the "social segmentation" of the hospital structure creates a number of problems, the solution of which depends on good interpersonal relations and on effective coordination of the activities carried out by different groups and individuals in the hospital. He also pointed out that interpersonal relations are influenced in a complex manner by the whole hospital organization and, therefore, full understanding of the problems of the hospital would require studies aimed at the total hospital as a system. This study, like those preceding it, contains many insights and useful ideas and hypotheses about hospital structure and functioning, but lacks the data and methodological rigor that quantitative research could supply for testing such hypotheses.

The next major study of community general hospitals was completed in 1956 (the year our study began) by Burling, Lentz, and Wilson (10). These researchers—a psychiatrist, a sociologist, and a social psychologist—studied six general hospitals of varying size located in the eastern part of the country. Their objective was to examine and understand each hospital and each department and service as an individual case, and then to distill from their data (including data from records, interviews, and personal observations, experiences, and impressions) a meaningful picture of "the give and take in hospitals." They were particularly concerned, however, with the study of those interpersonal relations and interactions which are typical among people working in the hospital. Their methodological approach was nonquantitative, and no systematic comparisons across hospitals were made. Their framework was partly anthropological and partly social-psychological, but without any particular unifying theoretical theme. As a reviewer observed, "theoretical considerations are never in the foreground of this volume . . . primary attention is paid to demonstrating the value of sociological insight in helping hospital workers to understand and work through their human problems" (57). While it presents no quantitative evidence in support of its many insightful observations and propositions, this study provides a good simplified introduction to the hospital for a variety of readers.

Lentz's doctoral dissertation (31), also completed in 1956, is another sociological study of hospitals that should be mentioned here. This study is concerned with the institutional changes and evolution of the community general hospital over the years. Lentz discusses some of the broad developments outside the hospital which have been responsible for the tendency of this institution to move toward a more bureaucratic, more rational form of social organization. Her study contributes to our understanding of hospital changes under the impact of important social trends and introduces historical perspective as a useful dimension in this field of research.

In addition to these five studies concentrating on the social structure and functioning of the community general hospital, there are several other major empirical and nonempirical studies about various other aspects of the hospital or about hospitals. Strictly speaking, however, most of these studies (some of which are quite prominent) are neither sociological, nor organizational, nor social-psychological in nature, even though some are concerned with organizational problems among other subjects. Some of these studies deal with the hospital as seen by administration-oriented people, medical people, or business-oriented people; others deal with questions of departmentalization; some deal with attempts to change hospital practices or procedures; and others deal with problems of accounting, record keeping, and financial matters. Included in this group of studies would be: Goldwater's essays *On Hospitals* (20); Corwin's *The American Hospital* (12); MacEachern's *Hospital Organization and Management* (34); McGibony's *Principles of Hospital Administration* (37); Bailey's *Hospital Personnel Administration* (5); Davis' *Medical Care for Tomorrow* (13); Faxon's *The Hospital in Contemporary Life* (16); Backmeyer and Hartman's *The Hospital in Modern Society* (4); Southmayd and Smith's *Small Community Hospitals* (53); Wright's *Improvement of Patient Care: A Study at Harper Hospital* (60); and the recent important Michigan study of hospital medical economics by McNerney and his associates (38).

Another group of studies of a related type of institution—the mental hospital—has also contributed to our general understanding of the community general hospital. Included in this group of studies would be Stanton and Schwartz's *The Mental Hospital* (54); Belknap's *Human Problems of a State Mental Hospital* (6); Greenblatt, Levinson, and Williams' *The Patient and the Mental Hospital* (21); and Dunham and Weinberg's *The Culture of the State*

Mental Hospital (15). A careful comparative review of all the different studies in the field of hospitals would probably show that the mental hospital has been researched longer and more intensively than the short-stay community general hospital. Most studies of the mental hospital, however, like those of the general hospital, are case studies which tend to be qualitative and anthropological in their methodology, as well as quite narrow in their scope. At best, only a few of them would be actually relevant to the study of the community general hospital as an organization.

Finally, it should be noted, there are now available many special studies and surveys of particular professional or occupational groups, individual hospital departments and services, specific hospital facilities, and particular needs of the community general hospital (and of the mental hospital), as well as studies of employee morale, personnel problems and human-relations problems, and other relatively circumscribed aspects of the hospital situation. There are also several studies dealing with broader aspects of health and sickness, and with historical developments in the field of health. The large majority of studies belonging to the present category are not concerned with problems and phenomena of organizational behavior or with the study of the hospital as a social system. A limited number of them, however, are sociological, anthropological, or social-psychological studies, which are interested in particular areas of hospital functioning or in specific problems in the field of hospitals and health. Some of the more prominent of these studies are reported by Apple (1), Caudill (11), and Jaco (26). Other interesting and useful studies (not all of which are social-psychological in character) in the present category of miscellaneous research would include those of Argyris (2), Brown (7, 8), Bullock (9), Deutscher (14), Ginzberg (19), Hall (22), Matthews (36), Ponton (44), Reissman and Rohrer (45), Richardson (46), Roberts (47), Simmons and Wolff (49), Sofer (52), and Wilson (59).

In addition, of course, there are numerous other studies reported in hospital, medical, nursing, and other journals that could qualify for inclusion in the category of miscellaneous research. Some of these are very careful, systematic, and even quantitative investigations (and a number of them will be cited in appropriate parts of the book). Most of them, however, are relatively minor studies which are very limited in scope. Typically, they are qualitative, non-comparative studies which deal with very circumscribed facets of the internal and external problems of single hospitals, and which have little bearing on the study of hospitals as on-going, integrated organizational systems.

The present research was undertaken in the general context provided by those of the above studies which are relevant (as will be indicated by the specific citations in subsequent chapters) to one or more of our objectives, seeking to fill some of the more serious gaps in our knowledge of the community general hospital. The more immediate context within which our study was undertaken, however, is that provided by the research which has been conducted by the Organizational Behavior and Change Program of the Survey Research Center, as discussed earlier in this section.

THE ORGANIZATION OF THE BOOK

Following this chapter, the reader is introduced to the overall plan of the study and to the people and the hospitals involved. Chapter 2 describes the study design, methodology, and procedures used, as well as some of the limitations of the research. It shows how the hospitals were selected, how individual respondents were chosen, and how the data were collected, processed, and analyzed. A brief discussion of the chronological development of the study makes it possible for the reader not only to gain a better understanding of the research design, but also to view the unfolding of the study as a series of "live" research processes. Moreover, the discussion of methodology is deliberately couched in sufficiently nontechnical terms to permit the nonprofessional reader to understand the basic aspects of the study design (including some technical concepts that will be used throughout the book). Since many of the topics discussed here underlie most of the materials presented in later chapters, the reader could not gain a thorough understanding of the research without first reading this chapter.

Chapter 3 introduces the various people around the patient. The main purpose of this chapter is to present the personal and major job characteristics of the members of every professional-occupational and organizational group that took part in the research. Here are described our respondents' individual characteristics (sex, age, formal education, occupational training, family status) and their current work situation (full- or part-time employment, length of service, work shift, type of work schedule, absenteeism and turnover, etc.). Complementing these data is information about the job satisfaction, work pressures, opportunities for advancement, and skill utilization of different groups of respondents, information about the respondents' satisfaction with salaries or wages, and information about their commitment to the hospital. The brief profiles of the several hospital groups at the end of the chapter give the reader an overview of the *people* in the study.

Chapter 4 provides a similar descriptive overview at the *organizational* level of the hospitals studied. The reader is introduced first to the "typical" participating hospital and then to each of the ten individual hospitals as distinct (though similar) organizations, with their own unique character in their own local setting. Based on data from records and organizational documents and from personal interviews with key people in the various hospitals, an overall profile for each hospital is presented. In each profile, information is given about: the community setting of the hospital, recent significant changes in the institution, internal problems and issues facing the organization and its members, special strengths and weaknesses, patient care, the trustees, the medical and nursing staff, and the administrative staff, and their relationships. In the main, however, the profiles show the different hospitals as they are seen by their key members and other personnel who volunteered relevant information. Consequently, they do not give a complete picture of the organizations involved. The findings in the chapters which follow are all intended to provide a more complete and clearer picture. In a sense, therefore, the hospital profiles, together with the profiles of the various respondent groups in the preceding chapter, provide a descriptive backdrop against which to begin to explore and understand the relational, quantitative findings that appear in subsequent chapters.

Before it is possible to answer one of the basic questions about hospital effectiveness posed in the study—what distinguishes the "better-care" hospitals from hospitals where care is of relatively lower quality (though not necessarily "poor")—it is of course necessary to develop and choose criteria for the measurement of the quality of patient care rendered at the various hospitals. This is the task of Chapter 5, which discusses the problem of developing operations for the assessment of patient care and related issues. After reviewing different approaches to this difficult and complex problem, four principal measures that may be used to evaluate and compare the quality of patient care given by different hospitals are presented. These measures, which are relative rather than absolute measures (i.e., distinguish between better and poorer rather than between "good" and "poor" care), respectively concern the quality of nursing care, the quality of medical care, the quality of overall patient care, and the quality of overall care in a hospital *as compared to* the quality of overall care rendered in other similar hospitals, i.e, a comparative measure of the quality of overall patient care. The rationale for each measure and the manner in which it was developed are discussed in detail. The reliability and validity of each measure, and the interrelationships of the four measures, are also thoroughly explored.

Chapter 6 is concerned with the important and little understood concept of organizational coordination, which occupies a central theoretical place in the present study. The essential elements of the concept of organizational coordination are treated theoretically, and the principal bases, mechanisms, and types of coordination are discussed. Then, a number of inclusive and specific measures that can be used to study coordination in the community general hospital are presented. The importance of coordination for the functioning of complex, large-scale organizations, such as the hospital, is also discussed in this chapter. Finally, a series of social-psychological factors which are expected to affect organizational coordination are specified. These include certain aspects of organizational planning, sharedness and complementarity of work-related expectations among interacting organizational members, cooperation, intra-organizational strain, problem awareness and problem solving on the part of individuals in key organizational positions, some aspects of communication, and certain structural characteristics of organization. The empirical relationships between different measures of these factors and organizational coordination in the hospitals studied are presented in the next chapter, Chapter 7. Thus, Chapters 6 and 7 are complementary; the former lays the theoretical and methodological foundations for the latter, while the latter presents the empirical findings which test the usefulness of some of the ideas and hypotheses suggested by the former.

The findings that show what aspects of hospital structure and functioning are related to the quality of patient care in the participating hospitals are presented in Chapter 8. Here a number of different variables are examined in relation to the criterion measures of patient care developed earlier in Chapter 5, in an effort to discover some of the requirements of "good" patient care—to ascertain some of the factors that correlate with, facilitate, impede, or otherwise affect the quality of care given in the various hospitals. In short, it is in this chapter that we see what distinguishes the "better-care" from the "poorer-care" hospitals. Included among the important aspects of the hospital situation that were investigated in relation to patient care are: organizational coordination; the composition and distribution of the nursing staff and the medical staff; absenteeism and turnover among nursing personnel; certain size-related characteristics of the hospitals involved; the adequacy of material facilities and certain financial items; medical committee activity, and the performance of paramedical departments; intraorganizational strain; and complementarity of work expectations between the medical and the nursing staff.

Chapter 9 explores the role of supervision in the community general hospital. The objective of this chapter is to provide some empirical, quantitatively based answers to the general question of what kinds of supervision and administrative leadership are the most appropriate for effective hospital functioning. A theoretical approach to the study of supervision and leadership that emphasizes the relativity of "effective" supervision is outlined and partially tested. In the process, this approach is related to the existing research literature on supervision and associated phenomena (this literature also is reviewed). The principal results concerning supervision and administrative behavior in the participating hospitals are presented in the form of relationships between different supervisory skills and practices, on the one hand, and the satisfaction of subordinates with supervision, the quality of patient care, and organizational coordination, on the other. Separate analyses of the data for different supervisory-organizational levels are used to evaluate the relative importance of particular supervisory skills and practices at each level.

Chapter 10 focuses on the communication practices and patterns of professional nurses. Registered nurses in the hospital perform not only therapeutic functions, but also coordinative activities, supervisory-administrative tasks (whether formally or informally), and communication functions—all of which are important to hospital organization. For this reason and because of the central place which the nursing department occupies in the community general hospital, different aspects of the communication of professional nurses—quantity, quality, content, direction, perceived adequacy, and concentration in formal as compared to informal channels—were systematically explored. In Chapter 10, several measures of these various aspects of communication are examined in relation to certain aspects of nursing activity and performance, and in relation to such things as the commitment of nursing personnel to their work group, coordination within the nursing department, and the level of tension between nursing personnel in different classifications.

The last two chapters of the book, Chapter 11 and Chapter 12, are both integrative chapters, although they differ a great deal in their respective contents. Chapter 11 is particularly concerned with a discussion of certain topics which are considered important by both researchers and hospital people, but which, being outside the central scope of the present study, were only explored here. Many of these topics were previously touched on in Chapters 3 and 4, but some are introduced here for the first time. Practically all these topics involve problems and issues faced by the community general hospital or by major groups within the hospital—the medical staff, the administrator, the trustees, etc. Many of these problems and issues have concrete and practical implications for hospital people, while some are more theoretical in character. In either case, many of them are frequently raised in the hospital literature. The topics discussed include: the external and internal image of the hospital; certain problems pertaining to the nursing staff; a number of issues and problems concerning the medical staff; the value orientations of the top echelon groups in the organization; the relative influence of key groups on hospital functioning; certain aspects of organizational change and its accommodation; and a few other aspects of the hospital situation. The emphasis in Chapter 11 is on descriptive exposition rather than on relational analysis, however, and special attention is given to problems of the "typical" hospital studied rather than to interhospital differences.

Chapter 12, with which the volume closes, summarizes the principal findings of the study, presents a number of conclusions and suggestions, both for those concerned with the day-to-day functioning of hospitals and for researchers who might want to investigate further different aspects of hospital organization, and indicates some of the limits of our current knowledge about the structure and functioning of the community general hospital.

A Few Final Words of Caution and Optimism

It is not the purpose of this volume to tell those responsible for the administration of community general hospitals how to manage their institutions. Nor is it its purpose to recommend, much less introduce, changes in the organizational or service arrangements of the hospitals studied. The book was designed to present the results of an empirical investigation. More specifically, its

The Organization of the Book

main, if not sole, objective is to report and communicate the findings of a comparative, quantitative study of medium-size, short-stay, community general hospitals located in a midwestern state. How these findings might be applied to the solution of particular problems confronting hospitals was not an objective here. There is, of course, no question but that many of the findings have concrete implications for the management and functioning of these and other institutions. Some of the more important and more obvious practical implications have been pointed out in the various chapters as a matter of course. It is predicted that administrators, doctors, trustees, nurses, and others in the hospital field will, in the light of their experiences, be able to identify many more. It is in this sense that we expect our work to be of direct practical usefulness to many readers.

Today, the study of hospitals as organizations is undoubtedly of interest and concern to many different groups and individuals, both within and outside these particular institutions. When based on a sound theoretical orientation, carefully designed and executed empirical research can contribute both to our understanding of the structure and functioning of hospitals and to the solution of administrative and organizational difficulties encountered by hospitals and hospital people. Furthermore, it can contribute to the growing body of systematic knowledge about the behavior and problems of complex organizations in general, thus serving the interests of a rather wide audience. The possibility of simultaneous contributions to different levels of knowledge and to different audiences complicates the writing task, of course. This is particularly true if the researcher chooses to have that part of his research which is of apparent practical usefulness addressed mainly to practitioners, and that part which adds to the theory and knowledge of organizations, but which may or may not be seen as having immediate pragmatic value, addressed to researchers and scientists.

In many ways, there are wide gaps between what the hospital practitioner might want to get from a book such as this, what the social scientist or teacher of organization might find significant and stimulating, and what the scholar in the hospital field might consider of value. What the administrator, the president of trustees, the chief of the medical staff, the director of nursing, a department head, a staff nurse, or someone else working in the hospital will find interesting and useful to read will probably be different from what the student in a program of hospital administration, the sociologist concerned with large-scale organizations, or the social psychologist interested in group behavior will find worth while to study. The intelligent layman who is curious about hospitals will probably have still different needs and tastes. Some laymen and practitioners might want only the essential "hard" facts—the findings of the study stripped of qualifications and refinements, while students of hospitals would want to work through more complex formulations and detailed results. Students of organization and social scientists and researchers would certainly be concerned with the specific relationships established by the study, would expect a careful and thorough accounting of methods and procedures used, would want a theoretical justification of conclusions reached, and would like to see the empirical findings integrated with theoretical propositions.

Recognizing the multiple, and rather diverse, audiences to which our study may be relevant and notwithstanding the writing difficulties involved, we have organized and written this book with both the lay and the scientific reader in mind. A systematic effort was made to write as nontechnically as we dared, and still maintain the rigorous standards required of a book reporting the results of scientific investigation. (How successful we have been on either count remains to be seen.) To meet the lay reader's needs for quick understanding of the principal findings, a detailed summary chapter has been prepared—Chapter 12. This chapter reviews and integrates in a simplified manner the major findings discussed in all previous chapters, supplementing the already extensive summaries given at the end of each chapter. However, should the reader want to know more about the bases of the findings, he could read the chapter on research design, method, and procedure (Chapter 2) in addition. But, the entire book was actually written to accommodate the lay reader who may want to read all of it. The argument of the volume has been made as nontechnical and comprehensible as possible (at the risk of some repetition of key concepts, ideas, and results, and at the risk of detailed explanation of tabular materials and statistical terminology). Wherever statistical or other technical treatments of the data are introduced for the first time, the lay reader is given the meaning of these in his own language insofar as it is feasible.

In summary, discussions of organizational theory and concepts—those pertaining to coordination, patient care and hospital effectiveness, supervision, communication, and related organizational and social-psychological phenomena—were all developed with both the highly motivated lay reader and the scientific reader in mind, and are addressed both to researchers and students of organization and to hospital practitioners. The same applies with regard to the empirical findings and substantive conclusions of the study. While we realize that good ideas are usually simple ideas, first statements of relatively new ideas or unfamiliar concepts are frequently not easy to communicate. For this reason, some of the material in the book may seem complex on a first reading. This will, of course, be especially true for readers who have had little experience with hospitals or other organizations, and who have had little contact with organizational theory and research. Still, with a little perseverance, the ideas and results presented, as well as the manner in which the data were treated to derive particular conclusions, can all be understood by the intelligent layman who is motivated to study the book. It may be worth remembering, however, that organizational and social-psychological research in hospitals is not an old, crystallized, and well-systematized field. And, although written with several different audiences in mind, the book does report facts based on a scientific inquiry; it will not read like a novel.

REFERENCES

1. Apple, D. (ed.). *Sociological Studies of Health and Sickness.* New York: McGraw-Hill, 1961.
2. Argyris, C. *Diagnosing Human Relations in Organizations: A Case Study of a Hospital.* New Haven: Yale University Press, 1956.
3. Babcock, K. B. Accreditation. *Hospitals,* 34:43, (April) 1960.
4. Backmeyer, A. C., and Hartman, G. (eds.). *The Hospital in Modern Society.* New York: Commonwealth Fund, 1943.
5. Bailey, N. D. *Hospital Personnel Administration.* Chicago: Physicians Record Co., 1954.
6. Belknap, I. *Human Problems of a State Mental Hospital.* New York: McGraw-Hill, 1956.
7. Brown, E. L. *Nursing for the Future.* New York: Russell Sage Foundation, 1948.
8. ———— *Newer Dimensions of Patient Care.* New York: Russell Sage Foundation, 1961.
9. Bullock, R. P. *What Nurses Think of Their Profession.* Columbus, Ohio: The Ohio State University, 1954.
10. Burling, T., Lentz, E. M., and Wilson, R. N. *The Give and Take in Hospitals.* New York: Putnam, 1956.
11. Caudill, W. "Applied Anthropology in Medicine." In Kroeber, A. L. (ed.). *Anthropology Today.* Chicago: Chicago University Press, 1953.
12. Corwin, E. H. L. *The American Hospital.* New York: Commonwealth Fund, 1946.
13. Davis, M. M. *Medical Care for Tomorrow.* New York: Harper, 1955.
14. Deutscher, I. *Public Images of the Nurse.* Kansas City, Mo.: Community Studies Incorporated, 1955.
15. Dunham, W., and Weinberg, S. K. *The Culture of the State Mental Hospital.* Detroit: Wayne State University Press, 1960.
16. Faxon, N. W. *The Hospital in Contemporary Life.* Cambridge, Mass.: Harvard University Press, 1949.
17. Georgopoulos, B. S., and Tannenbaum, A. S. "A Study of Organizational Effectiveness," *Amer. Sociol. Rev.,* 22:534–40, (Oct.) 1957.
18. Georgopoulos, B. S., Mahoney, G. M., and Jones, W. N., Jr. "A Path-Goal Approach to Productivity," *J. Applied Psych.,* 41:345–53, (Oct.) 1957.
19. Ginzberg, E. *A Pattern for Hospital Care: Final Report of the New York State Hospital Study.* New York: Columbia University Press, 1949.
20. Goldwater, S. S. *On Hospitals.* New York: Macmillan, 1947.
21. Greenblatt, M., Levinson, D. J., and Williams, R. H. *The Patient and the Mental Hospital.* Glencoe, Ill.: The Free Press, 1957.
22. Hall, O. "The Informal Organization of Medical Practice in an American City." Doctoral Dissertation. University of Chicago, 1944.
23. Health Information Foundation. Trends in Use of General Hospitals. *Progress in Health Services,* Vol. VIII, No. 8, Oct. 1959.
24. Health Insurance Institute. *Source Book of Health Insurance Data.* New York: Health Insurance Institute, 1959.
25. *Hospitals.* Guide Issue. *Hospitals,* 35: Part Two, (Aug.) 1961.
26. Jaco, E. G. (ed.). *Patients, Physicians, and Illness.* Glencoe, Ill.: The Free Press, 1958.
27. Jacobson, E., Kahn, R. L., Mann, F. C., and Morse, N. C. "Human Relations Research in Large Organizations," *Journal of Social Issues,* 7: No. 3, 1951.
28. Kahn, R. L. "Human Relations on the Shop Floor." In Hugh-Jones, E. M. (ed.).

Human Relations and Modern Management. Amsterdam, Netherlands: North Holland Publishing Company, 1958.

29. Kahn, R. L., Mann, F. C., and Seashore, S. E. "Human Relations Research in Large Organizations: II," *J. Social Issues*, 12: No. 2, 1956.

30. Katz, D., Gurin, G., Maccoby, N., and Floor, L. G. *Productivity, Supervision, and Morale Among Railroad Workers.* Ann Arbor, Mich.: Institute for Social Research, 1951.

31. Lentz, E. M. "The American Voluntary Hospital as an Example of Institutional Change." Doctoral Dissertation. Cornell University, 1956.

32. Lieberman, S. "The Effects of Changes in Roles on the Attitudes of Role Occupants," *Human Relations*, 9:385–402, 1956.

33. Likert, R. *New Patterns of Management.* New York: McGraw-Hill, 1961.

34. MacEachern, M. T. *Hospital Organization and Management.* Chicago: Physicians Record Co., 1957.

35. Mann, F. C., and Hoffman, L. R. *Automation and the Worker: A Study of Social Change in Power Plants.* New York: Holt, 1960.

36. Mathews, B. P. "A Study of the Effect of Administrative Climate on the Nurse's Psychological Orientation Toward Hospital Patients." Doctoral Dissertation. Berkeley: University of California, 1960.

37. McGibony, J. R. *Principles of Hospital Administration.* New York: Putnam, 1952.

38. McNerney, W. J. "Study of Hospital Medical Economics." American Hospital Association. (*In press.*)

39. Morse, N. C. *Satisfactions in the White Collar Job.* Ann Arbor, Mich.: Institute for Social Research, 1953.

40. Morse, N. C., and Reimer, E. "The Experimental Change of a Major Organizational Variable," *J. Abnorm. & Social Psychol.*, 52:120–29, (Jan.) 1956.

41. *New England Journal of Medicine.* "Curfew," *New England J. Med.*, 264:773–74, (April) 1961.

42. Parsons, T. "Suggestions for a Sociological Approach to the Theory of Organizations: II," *Admin. Sci. Quart.*, 1:225–39, (Sept.) 1956.

43. Pelz, D. C. "Some Social Factors Related to Performance in a Research Organization," *Admin. Sci. Quart.*, 1:310–25, (Dec.) 1956.

44. Ponton, T. R. *The Medical Staff in the Hospital.* Chicago: Physicians Record Co., 1953.

45. Reissman, L., and Rohrer, J. H. *Change and Dilemma in the Nursing Profession.* New York: Putnam, 1957.

46. Richardson, H. B. *Patients Have Families.* New York: Commonwealth Fund, 1945.

47. Roberts, M. M. *American Nursing: History and Interpretation.* New York: Macmillan, 1954.

48. Seashore, S. E. *Group Cohesiveness in the Industrial Work Group.* Ann Arbor, Mich.: Institute for Social Research, 1955.

49. Simmons, L. W., and Wolff, H. G. *Social Science in Medicine.* New York: Russell Sage Foundation, 1954.

50. Smith, H. L. "The Sociological Study of Hospitals." Doctoral Dissertation. University of Chicago, 1949.

51. ——— "Two Lines of Authority One Too Many," *Mod. Hosp.*, 84:59–64, (March) 1955.

52. Sofer, C. "Reactions to Administrative Changes," *Human Relations*, 8:291–316, 1955.

53. Southmayd, H. J., and Smith, G. *Small Community Hospitals.* New York: Commonwealth Fund, 1944.

References

54. Stanton, A. H., and Schwartz, M. S. *The Mental Hospital.* New York: Basic Books, 1954.
55. Tannenbaum, A. S., and Kahn, R. L. *Participation in Union Locals.* Evanston, Ill.: Row, Peterson, 1958.
56. Weiss, R. S. *Processes of Organization.* Ann Arbor, Mich.: Institute for Social Research, 1956.
57. Wessen, A. F. Review of Burling, T., Lentz, E. M., and Wilson, R. N. "The Give and Take in Hospitals," *Admin. Sci. Quart.*, 1:536–38, (March) 1957.
58. ———— "The Social Structure of a Modern Hospital." Doctoral Dissertation. Yale University, 1951.
59. Wilson, A. T. M. "Hospital Nursing Auxiliaries: Notes on a Background Survey and Job Analysis." London: Tavistock Publications, Ltd., 1950.
60. Wright, M. G. *The Improvement of Patient Care: A Study at Harper Hospital.* New York: Putnam, 1954.
61. Zugich, J. J. "Influences on Interpersonal Relations in the Hospital Organization." Unpublished M. A. Thesis. Yale University, 1951.

2 RESEARCH DESIGN, METHOD, AND PROCEDURE

The main purpose of this chapter is to describe the overall plan and methodology of the study. The results of research in any field of endeavor are no better than the manner in which they were obtained, and one's conclusions must always be evaluated in the light of the methodological procedures on which they are based. Unless the reader knows the facts about the research processes that have preceded the printed page, he will be hard put to follow, comprehend, or evaluate what he reads. This does not mean that the reader should be burdened with unnecessary details or trivialities. However, he should not be left without knowledge of the major facts and limitations about how the researcher obtained and treated the data in order to answer the questions to which the research is addressed.

In the present case, for example, it is virtually essential for the reader to be informed about such things as how the participating hospitals were selected for study, how individual respondents from each hospital were chosen and how they reacted toward the research, how the data were collected, processed, and analyzed, and, generally, how the research progressed from its inception to its completion. We shall, therefore, attempt in this chapter to describe the main aspects of our research design and procedure, to review the chronological development of the study, and to indicate the techniques of description and the units of analysis used. The nature and measurement of the specific variables and concepts studied, however, will be discussed later in the appropriate chapters, along with the presentation of the findings. Here, we will be concerned only with the general plan of the research and those methodological aspects which underlie the content of all subsequent chapters.

First, we will present some essential characteristics of the study design to indicate the level and units of analysis with which we are concerned, and the kinds of dependent and independent variables (i.e., aspects of hospital structure and functioning) included in the research. These will be elaborated further in the subsequent sections of this chapter. Second, we will describe the manner in which the research proceeded from its beginning to its conclusion, showing the specific activities that were required at different stages in the development of the study. Following this brief chronological account, we will discuss the procedure and rationale used to select particular hospitals for study. Then, we will show how, and why, certain groups of hospital personnel were specified to represent each participating institution, as well as how individual group members were selected to take part in the study as respondents. In the next section, we will describe the main research instruments (questionnaires and interviews) used to collect data, the kinds of data collected, and the response rates attained in the study. Then, we will discuss some of the principal forms of description and measurement employed, our main techniques of analysis, and certain related aspects of statistical analysis and interpretation. In the final section of the chapter, preceding a short overall summary of the methodology of the study, we shall be concerned with the main methodological limitations of the research. The division of the chapter into the above major sections is a matter of convenience, of course, and it is not intended to imply that the different aspects of the research design can be neatly separated and treated independently of one another. There is a high degree of interrelatedness among the separately treated features of the design, which, we hope, will become very apparent to the reader.

OVERVIEW OF THE RESEARCH DESIGN: OBJECTS, UNITS, AND AREAS OF INVESTIGATION

As already indicated in the introductory chapter, this is an inquiry into certain aspects of the structure and functioning of the community, voluntary, short-stay general hospital. Accordingly, it does not purport to cover the entire hospital field, or to generalize the results to all hospitals indiscriminately, although the subject areas studied and many of the findings very probably will be relevant to several different kinds of hospitals. Mental and psychiatric institutions, specialized institutions such as children's, orthopedic, and tuberculosis hospitals, tax-supported and governmental hospitals at the federal and local levels, proprietary hospitals, long-term or chronic disease hospitals, and church-related hospitals are not included in the population, or class, from which our hospitals were selected. Furthermore, because of certain limitations which we imposed in selecting hospitals (as will be indicated in a subsequent section of this chapter), the ten hospitals which finally participated in the research cannot be considered as "representative" of all hospitals which do not belong in any of the above categories that were specifically excluded.

Of the nearly 6900 hospitals in the United States listed in the 1961 "Guide Issue" of *Hospitals* (4), about 5800 are short-stay institutions of different types. And of the latter, nearly 5200 are nonfederal general hospitals, i.e., institutions engaged in the care and treatment of acute diseases and illnesses. Of all these nonfederal, short-stay general hospitals in the nation, approximately 2000 are either state and local governmental institutions (state, county, city, city-county, or hospital district institutions) or proprietary hospitals (individual, partnership, or corporate organizations). This leaves about 3200 hospitals that are voluntary, nonprofit institutions. Another way of putting it is that, of the nearly 6900 hospitals in the United States, about 4600 are nongovernmental institutions, and of these some 3200 constitute the broad category of short-stay general hospitals that are nonprofit, voluntary, community institutions. These hospitals have a combined total of about 440,000 beds and provide daily care for an average of around 330,000 patients. They are the hospitals with which the ordinary person is likely to be most familiar or have contact as a patient or visitor.

Approximately one-third of these community general hospitals are church-related institutions. The other two-thirds, i.e., about 2100 of them, are nondenominational institutions.[1] The present research is concerned with hospitals belonging to this last category and sharing the characteristics indicated. More specific characteristics which served as criteria for including particular hospitals in the study will be presented below, in the section dealing with the selection of hospitals. In the meantime, let us briefly consider the level of abstraction and analysis at which we have operated in this research, i.e., the level at which the variables in the study were initially conceptualized, and then measured and related to one another.

It should be clear from the introduction that the present research focuses not on individual persons within the hospital, but on the total hospital as an on-going organization and on certain of its major groups and departments. The primary concern is with phenomena and variables which have a hospital-wide, or group-wide, character and significance rather than with the more circumscribed problems and activities of individual people who work in the organization or who are there as patients. Stated somewhat differently, our main unit of description and analysis is either some major department (e.g., nursing) or group (e.g., the medical staff) of the hospital or, in the majority of cases, the whole hospital as an organizational system. By the term "organizational system" we mean a complex social system which: (1) consists of many different but interlocking parts, or subunits, and interacting people; (2) possesses, and has access to, certain human and material resources and facilities; and (3) is designed to accomplish certain objectives (the primary objective in the case of the hospital being to render adequate patient care effectively), through the canalization of the varied efforts of its many members and through the proper allocation and manipulation of its resources and facilities.

[1] All figures cited above are based on data reported in the 1961 "Guide Issue" of *Hospitals* (4), and refer to the 12-month period ending September 30, 1960. The figures have been rounded to simplify presentation and reading and are, therefore, approximate rather than exact figures.

Overview of the Research Design

Most of the concepts and variables with which the study is concerned have, thus, been defined and measured at the organizational or group level, and not at the individual level, the primary interest being in the behavior of hospitals as organizations. This also means that before being used in the analysis, most of the data which were obtained from individual respondents representing the participating hospitals had to be properly combined and converted into group or organizational-hospital measures. In this connection, individual respondents from different groups within the hospital were asked not merely to provide data concerning their own personal feelings, beliefs, and actions, but also, and more importantly, to provide data containing their observations about different aspects of hospital functioning, and about the attitudes and behaviors of other people in the hospital with whom they work or interact.

Therefore, on the one hand, individual respondents were treated as *subjects* possessing certain attitudes and satisfactions or dissatisfactions, and exhibiting certain kinds of behavior or characteristics in which we were interested. On the other hand, individual respondents were selected as representatives of their organization and were treated as *observers* of the hospital situation—observers who could jointly provide us with firsthand knowledge and information on the basis of which to measure many of the concepts and variables with which we were concerned. In this latter case, the respondents representing individual hospitals were in effect used as assessors and appraisers of hospital functioning —they themselves, rather than a few outside "observers," served as measuring "instruments" in a great many cases. Carefully selected respondents (as specified below) could provide much better coverage of the areas in which we were interested than a few strategically placed outsiders, because, theoretically, these respondents are located in *all* "parts" and levels of the organization. Data from the selected respondents were supplemented, of course, by various kinds of other data, but as we will see the supplementary data also were converted into group measures, since the unit of analysis in this study is a group unit.

Generally speaking, when the research is concerned with organizational behavior, group products, or social-psychological phenomena, the proper unit of analysis is the organization or the group. When it is concerned with the characteristics of individual people, the proper unit of analysis is usually the individual. In the former case, the researcher is normally operating at the group level of behavior; in the latter, he is normally operating at the individual level of behavior. We say "normally" because sometimes, and in relation to particular problems, the researcher finds it desirable to make use of both levels to supplement his main level of analysis. (This we have also done in some of our analyses.) By saying that our main unit of analysis is the group or the organization, we simply mean that we are interested in the social and psychological problems, properties, and characteristics of the hospital and its major components, rather than in the characteristics of individual administrators, doctors, nurses, patients, etc. Thus, in the chapters that follow, we will be mostly describing, comparing, and contrasting different hospitals with one another, or different nursing departments, personnel groups, and other similar segments of the participating hospitals that involve at least two (and actually many more) persons. This also means that our statistical analyses will in most instances be based on an N, or number of cases, that is equal to the number of hospitals or groups being studied, e.g., an N of ten hospitals, ten nursing departments, or ten medical executive committees, etc. (one per hospital), and not on an N which is equal to the number of individual respondents from each hospital, from each nursing department, etc.

The level of analysis and the kinds of variables and concepts studied are dictated, of course, by the objectives of the research and by the theoretical approach employed. On the theoretical side, the present research follows a social-psychological approach. The phenomena with which it is most concerned—patient care, coordination, supervision-administration, and communication—are considered as being determined, and are expected to be best understood and accounted for, by combinations of sociological and psychological variables representing different aspects of hospital structure and functioning. From the standpoint of the research design, the phenomena which we are trying to understand and explain, and their various aspects, constitute what we refer to as the "dependent" variables of the study. The variables that we use to explain interhospital differences in the phenomena under investigation constitute the "independent" variables of the study. The results of the research show the empirical relationships (connections, or association) between the independent and the dependent variables. The details of the theoretical approach that we have used will be made clearer in later chapters. The main objectives of the research have already been discussed in the preceding chapter. However, it might be useful if we also summarized them here.

It will be recalled that the study is primarily interested in the areas of patient care and internal hospital coordination. Certain aspects of care and coordination constitute the major dependent variables in the research design. However, the study is also interested in certain other important areas of hospital operation, particularly in selected aspects of supervision and administration, communication, and group performance. It is concerned with these because we consider them as significant phenomena deserving study in their own right (i.e., as dependent variables) and, more importantly, because of their potential relevance, or relationship, to patient care and to coordination (i.e., they may be viewed as independent variables with respect to care and coordination).

In studying patient care and coordination, which constitute our major research objectives or dependent variables, we are also concerned with a variety of other variables that will help us explain the differences in patient care and coordination which may characterize the participating hospitals. These variables are called "independent" variables (or, in some cases, "intervening" or "conditioning" variables) and include: certain characteristics of the composition and skill of hospital personnel; hospital income and expenditures; the relative adequacy of material facilities available; the degree of tension and pressure prevailing among different interacting groups and departments within the hospital; measures of superior-subordinate relationships and administrative behavior; certain aspects of motivation and communication among nursing personnel; absenteeism and turnover among nursing personnel; measures of cooperation among organizational members; certain aspects of organizational planning and problem solving; and the nature of work-related expectations and understandings that organizational members have in relation to one another.

The research design calls for the measurement of these various independent variables, the measurement of the dependent variables, and an analysis which relates each of the former to each of the latter by means of correlational or other techniques which will be specified in each case. Thus, for example, we are interested in measuring the quality of patient care, including the quality of nursing, medical, and overall care that, on the aggregate, patients receive in the various hospitals, and then identifying other important aspects of the hospital situation (i.e., independent variables) which are significantly related to the quality of care, i.e., identifying factors associated with better or poorer patient care. The same may be said with respect to coordination, with one addition. We are interested not only in ascertaining social-psychological factors which affect the quality of organizational coordination in the hospital, but also in the importance of coordination for patient care. In its most general but least correct form the main question that we are trying to answer is this: What, specifically, makes for better patient care (and better coordination) in the community general hospital? Or, what are some of the crucial differences which distinguish the better-care from the poorer-care hospitals. This general question will be broken down into various more specific and more precise questions. These will be taken up in the appropriate individual chapters which follow.

THE CHRONOLOGY OF THE RESEARCH

The preceding general considerations served as the basis for initiating and carrying out the research during a four year period. The study was formally launched late in 1956, but actual collection of data did not begin until November of 1957, following the completion of certain important but preliminary activities. The first in this series of activities was to staff the project with the necessary research and supportive personnel. As soon as the staff became organized and had familiarized itself with the nature and objectives of the study, it commenced its work by setting up a tentative time schedule for the implementation of specific research activities, and by beginning a detailed review of existing literature that was relevant to the purposes of the study. The intention was to begin the study in a relatively general, exploratory way and then move as rapidly as possible toward a systematic, quantitative, and explanatory investigation.

In terms of the time schedule adopted and followed, the research was conveniently divided into three main phases, each requiring a year or more for its completion. The main objectives of the first phase were: (1) to review the pertinent literature that was available; (2) to familiarize the researchers with the hospital situation through field scouting and exploratory interviewing with relevant personnel in two "pilot" hospitals; (3) to specify in greater detail the initial objectives of the research, specify the concepts and corresponding variables that were to be studied, and formulate specific hypotheses on the basis of available theory and theory developed in the process of the research; (4) to select the particular hospitals that were to participate in the study proper, and to specify the groups of respondents that would be asked to provide necessary data; (5) to design and construct appropriate research instruments—questionnaires, interviews, and other devices—for the collection of the data that would eventually be used to describe the hospitals, measure the variables, and test our hypotheses; and (6) to make the necessary arrangements to pretest (try out) these instruments on a limited scale before finalizing them and thus "freezing" our research design.

The main objectives of the second phase of the research were: (1) to pretest the research instruments that we had developed by the end of the first phase by trying them out in an actual hospital situation; (2) to revise and finalize the instruments on the basis of the pretest experience, and then reproduce them in sufficient quantities; (3) to secure the cooperation of the individual hospitals that had been selected to participate in the study and of the major groups within each hospital whose members would be asked to provide data; (4) to obtain certain standard, advance information from each hospital on the basis of which to sample individual respondents who would represent certain groups from each organization; (5) to prepare the field staff which would collect the data from these respondents; (6) to schedule the various hospitals and respondents for data collection; (7) to collect the required data on location; and (8) to process the data mechanically, obtain preliminary tabulations, and organize these "straight-run" tabulations in special report form for distribution to the participating hospitals.

The main objectives of the third and last phase of the research were: (1) to discuss the preliminary reports with hospital administrators and other relevant individuals from each institution, in order to help them understand the reports and make the materials more meaningful to them through personal discussion; (2) to analyze the data in depth and detail; (3) to examine carefully the results of our analyses and to test specific hypotheses; (4) to organize the findings and conclusions of the research into final report form; and (5) to communicate the results of the research to others. In terms of actual time spent, the last phase of the research was the longest of the three, since it involved many months of work devoted to both extensive and intensive analyses of the data. The research, having begun late in 1956, was formally completed in 1961, with the conclusion of this third phase.

The activities listed above under each phase represent, needless to say, only the major processes preceding the conclusion of the study and do not include numerous minor activities and details involving administrative aspects, field contacts, and actual research. The more significant of the major activities indicated above will be spelled out further in subsequent special sections of this chapter. These sections will be concerned with the following important aspects of the

The Chronology of the Research

method and design of the research: (1) the selection of the ten participating hospitals; (2) the selection of the individual respondents from each hospital; (3) the research instruments and the collection of the data; (4) the mode of description and statistical analysis; and (5) the limitations of the study. The remaining activities will be summarized together at this point, according to the phase of the research within which they occurred, and beginning again with the first phase.

First Phase

Upon the initiation of the study, the research staff undertook a rather comprehensive review of available literature on hospital organization and operations. In the process, about 50 major books, monographs, and doctoral dissertations, and about 700 articles having some bearing on the subjects of the research were reviewed. These materials represented a variety of professional publication sources —journals on hospitals, hospital administration, nursing, medicine, and public health, and relevant works from sociology, psychology, and social psychology. This review enabled us to gain a basic understanding of hospital structure and functioning, as well as to ascertain what others concerned with the hospital scene have said about issues and problems in the areas on which our own research focuses. Supplementing our research experience with other types of large-scale organizations, it helped us formulate the study in terms that would be meaningful and realistic both to people in the hospital field and to others interested in the field of organizational behavior.

Two other activities were carried on concurrently with our review of the literature. First, the major professional associations whose members would be involved in the research—the Michigan Hospital Association, the Michigan Medical Society, and the Michigan Nursing Association—were contacted. The purpose and plan of the study were explained to key representatives of each association. The objective was to have all relevant professional groups fully informed about the research to prevent possible misunderstandings. No formal approval was sought from these groups, however, since we did not want the study to appear as "sponsored" by one or another of them. As a result of these contacts, the Michigan Hospital Association appointed a liaison with the project (Mr. John Zugich, Assistant Administrator of the University of Michigan Hospital).

The second major task during the first few months of the project involved establishing contacts and working relationships with two Michigan hospitals which were to serve as sites for pilot, exploratory work preceding the study proper. Based on our decision to confine the study to short-stay community general hospitals in Michigan, and in consultation with a number of people in the hospital field, we proceeded to select two hospitals for this preliminary exploration. Both hospitals shared the same major organizational characteristics as the ten institutions which later participated in the study (see appropriate section below on the selection of hospitals). One of them was located in a relatively small city in central Michigan and had 131 beds; the other was located in a suburban community of over 100,000 population and had 238 beds. (The ten hospitals which finally participated in the research proper ranged in size from 104 to 322 beds.)

In both hospitals, we first talked with the administrator through whom we gained initial access to the organization. We explained the study to him in detail, and discussed the possibility of having his hospital participate in the pilot work, without promising any direct practical gains from this exploratory venture. After the administrator was satisfied that participation would be worth while and that it would not create problems or disruptions for his organization, each decided to cooperate and help us plan the next steps in gaining acceptance of the project with important groups in the hospital. In both institutions, the process involved discussing the research with representatives of the board of trustees, the medical staff, the director of nursing, and other administrative department heads and then requesting their assistance and participation. When all groups had agreed to cooperate, we began scheduling interviews with people at all levels in the organizations, and from most professional-occupational groups and departments. In the end, 60 individuals from each of the two hospitals were interviewed during this stage of the research.

All interviews were held at the hospital. Those interviewed included the administrator, the chairman and certain members of the board of trustees, members of the medical staff, including its officers and major committee chairmen, administrative department heads, technicians in x-ray and the laboratory, and nursing personnel from all classifications. The objective was to interview "key" people in the hospital, as well as others who are primarily concerned with patient care—the hospital's product. The interviews were of the "open" type, i.e., largely unstructured and unrestricted as to content, and were conducted by members of the research staff, sometimes by one member and sometimes by two. Respondents were invited not only to answer a number of questions that we had compiled around the principal topics of the research (i.e., patient care, supervision and administration, coordination, and communication), but also to add their own suggestions and thinking about the most significant problems faced by themselves, their hospital, or hospitals in general. We were only interested in gaining insights and improving our understanding of the community general hospital, rather than in testing any preconceived notions and hypotheses during this early stage. In a sense, we wanted these people to help us formulate the study and its design as realistically and fruitfully as possible. This exploratory work in the two hospitals was carried out for a period extending over four months.

The next step in the research process included a careful examination and content analysis of our interview data, and integration of these findings with the materials which had emerged from our review of the literature, preparatory to adopting a final research design suitable to the objectives of the research. At this point, our aims were to clarify and specify further our research objectives in the light of these materials, and to begin to design questionnaires and interviews that could elicit the information required by these objectives. The process of formulating the research design in an acceptable manner, developing our theoretical and conceptual framework in sufficient detail, specifying the data required by the objectives of the study, and constructing appropriate research instruments for the collection of these data continued through the end of the first phase and into the beginning of the second phase of the research.

One important discovery made during our exploratory work in the two pilot hospitals was that doctors, trustees, and administrators talked much more openly about the problems of their hospital, about issues of concern to them, and about how things should be done than our research experience in other organizations and our review of the literature would have led us to predict. We had anticipated difficulty in obtaining information about such "sensitive" areas as the quality of patient care, tensions and problems among different groups or departments in the hospital, and differences among doctors, trustees, and administrators stemming from their differential backgrounds and experiences with organizations. To obtain data regarding these significant subjects, we had originally thought that it might be necessary to include an observational subproject in the second phase of the research. The initial plan was to make careful observations of the actual functioning and interaction of these principal groups while reviewing with them preliminary data from questionnaires and interviews. When we determined that the key people in both pilot hospitals talked freely about sensitive issues, we decided to omit the observational subproject from the study design.

Two other important tasks were also completed in the first year of the research. First, a decision was made as to what kinds of hospitals should be included in the study. It was necessary to select the hospitals that were to participate, and then to obtain their commitment to cooperate in the research, well in advance of data collection. The question of what kinds of hospitals should be covered was resolved by establishing certain criteria for selection based on the objectives of the research and the character of the emerging research design (see appropriate section below on the selection of hospitals). Second, based on the objectives and questions of the research, and on the kinds of data required to answer these questions, certain groups of respondents were specified and chosen as the relevant groups to represent each hospital and to provide the necessary data. The particular hospitals which met the criteria of inclusion in the study and were selected to participate in the second phase of the research were all contacted by the research staff during the first phase, by September of 1957.

Second Phase

By the end of the first phase of the project, we had developed and revised several tentative forms of questionnaires and interviews intended to be administered eventually to specified groups of respondents in the participating hospitals. (For the groups involved, and the manner in which individual respondents were chosen, see appropriate section below.) In addition, we had made arrangements to try out the various interviews and questionnaires in one of the two hospitals which had earlier participated in the pilot work. The second phase of the project began with a full-dress pretest of these research instruments in early October, 1957.

The pretest was designed to serve several important purposes. Included among these were: to learn what problems would be likely to arise during data collection under actual field operation conditions; to ascertain the time required of the respondents to answer our questions; and, most important of all, to provide actual data on the basis of which to improve further the various interview and questionnaire instruments. To accomplish these objectives, the pretest was carried out under circumstances that were as similar as possible to those expected to be encountered later during the collection of the data from the ten participating hospitals. Among other things, this meant that we draw a sample of respondents for the pretest in the same way that we planned to draw the final sample from each of the ten hospitals, that we use the same interviewing staff which we planned to use later in the main data collection operation, and that we generally go through all the steps necessary to have the selected respondents complete questionnaires and interviews.

The pretest was conducted in one of the two pilot hospitals—the one we had studied the most intensively during the exploratory phase. This hospital was selected for the pretest primarily because: (1) we did not want to use one of the other hospitals that had been chosen to participate in the study proper, since such a procedure would reduce the total number of potential participating hospitals by one (from ten to nine); (2) we had already established excellent working relationships with the administrator, the trustees, the doctors, and others in this hospital; and (3) we had acquired a very good knowledge and understanding of the situation in this institution from our exploratory work—an understanding which would help us greatly in appraising the results of the pretest.

Following the analysis of the pretest results, the research instruments were appropriately revised and modified once more, and then put into final form. This process involved such things as combining some of the pretested questionnaire forms into a single form and separating others, deciding to use both an interview and a questionnaire for some of the respondent groups, replacing some of the questions in the various instruments with new or more appropriate questions, deleting many specific questions that were redundant (i.e., were yielding essentially the same data as other questions), ambiguous, or too difficult for the respondents, altering the format or wording of certain questions, and the like. The objective was to sharpen our questions, and to develop as clear, relevant, and sensitive research instruments as possible. In the end, the finalized interview and questionnaire forms were mimeographed and reproduced in quantity.

A total of nine different instruments (some consisting of two parts) were finally used to collect the data from the different groups of respondents in the ten hospitals studied (see appropriate section below regarding the research instruments and data collection). In the aggregate, these various questionnaire and interview forms numbered about 270 pages, each page containing an average of five questions, but with the majority of the questions being common to all or most of the different research instruments. On the average, individual respondents were required to answer a little over 100 questions, and to spend between one and one and a half hours of their own time in so doing. Appendix A, at the end of this volume, shows the questionnaire administered to nonsupervisory registered nurses in the participating hospitals. This is the basic instrument to which all other questionnaires were keyed; i.e., most of the questions shown in Appendix A were also included, after some necessary modification, in the other questionnaire forms that we used.

Apart from finalizing the research instruments, a number of other activities had to be completed before going into the field for systematic data collection from the ten hospitals. These activities included: (1) securing the cooperation of the individual hospitals through further contacts and discussions with the administrator, trustees, medical staff, and others in each institution; (2) obtaining lists of names of relevant personnel from each hospital—doctors, nurses, trustees, depart-

The Chronology of the Research

ment heads, and others—so that we could draw samples of respondents from the various groups involved and know how to locate the respondents in advance of the visits by our field staff (for purposes of economy, we decided to select only a sample of respondents from each hospital rather than request every member of the organization to provide data); and (3) making all necessary arrangements to schedule specific hospitals for specific time periods for data collection, and to move our staff into the field for the actual collection of the data.

Data collection from individual hospitals and respondents began on November 4, 1957, and was completed on December 13, 1957, according to schedule. On the average, a full week was spent in each hospital to administer the interviews and questionnaires, but during some weeks data were collected simultaneously from two or three hospitals. During this period, we obtained data from a total of 1265 individual respondents, or about 127 different persons from each of the ten participating hospitals. Approximately 95 percent of all persons who were originally selected as respondents and who were available during the data collection period (i.e., excluding those who had been terminated or were absent for extended and indefinite periods of time) participated in the research by completing questionnaires and interviews.

Following the collection of the data, all questionnaires and interviews were taken to Ann Arbor, and the Coding Section of the Survey Research Center coded the data, i.e., converted the original data into numerical form, according to standard procedures and special instructions from the research staff, suitable for transferring onto IBM cards. Actually, a relatively small amount of time was taken by coding, since the majority of the questions had been asked in a manner that required the respondent to do most of the coding (the questionnaires were "precoded"). Coding was needed mainly for data collected through interviews rather than questionnaires, and for the few open questions included in the paper-and-pencil questionnaires. The coding process was of course preceded by a review of the completed questionnaires and interviews. This review, technically known as "editing," was carried out by the research staff to prevent any "mix-ups" or errors during coding. Immediately after coding, the Tabulating Service Section of the Center transferred (punched and verified) the data onto IBM cards, preparatory to tabulation and analysis of the data. This process was completed in February, 1958. It was followed by a number of standard and special checks, before beginning any tabulations, to eliminate any errors that could have occurred in the coding and transferring processes.

The first and simplest tabulations of the data were run in March, 1958, and continued through the spring of that year. Within a few months, straight-run tabulations became available for nearly all of the questions that had been asked of the various respondents. The objective here was to obtain frequency distributions of responses for each question in each of the several questionnaire and interview forms used, and separately for each respondent group involved. Tabulations were obtained separately for each of the ten hospitals, and for all hospitals combined. The data from these machine tabulations were then converted into percentages (showing the percentage of respondents in each case who gave a particular answer to a particular question) and put into tables. The results were reviewed table by table, and then organized according to subject matter for presentation. These preliminary findings of the study were incorporated into two special reports. *Report I* (2) and *Report II* (3), especially designed for distribution to the participating hospitals. In this manner, the hospitals studied could receive a great deal of information about their operations long before the final products of the research would be available.

The first of the two preliminary reports, *Report I*, summarizing the responses of supervisory nursing personnel, nonsupervisory registered nurses, practical nurses, aides and orderlies, and x-ray and laboratory technicians, for each individual hospital and for all ten hospitals combined, was completed and sent to the administrators in May, 1958. The second report, *Report II*, summarizing the data from trustees, doctors, administrators, and department heads, was prepared during the summer and mailed to the administrators in September, 1958. The two reports, insofar as possible, were identical in general format to facilitate comparison of data. Several copies of each report were sent to every participating hospital, one for each of the principal groups which cooperated in the research. The distribution and circulation of these reports were restricted for some time, so that relevant people in the participating institutions would have an opportunity to review the preliminary findings about their organization first. From the standpoint of timeliness, all ten hospitals received the two reports less than ten months from the time that the data were collected in each.

Some of the contents of *Report I* were presented in June, 1958, at the Annual Meetings of the Michigan Hospital Association. During these meetings, we also met with the administrators of the participating hospitals to (1) answer any questions they had about *Report I* (they had received it three weeks earlier), (2) hear their comments about the report, (3) give them information about the progress of the study and the forthcoming second report, and (4) inquire as to their plans for communicating the contents of these reports to members of their organization and for making possible use of them. While the reactions of the administrators to the report itself were very favorable, their expectations regarding possible utilization of the findings in their operations were varied. A few appeared ready to begin using some of the data immediately; two had already discussed the report with others in their hospital; and others preferred to wait to examine the second report before taking any relevant action. One or two of the administrators had not yet examined the report fully, and some raised certain questions as to the meaning of specific tables. Following our discussions, the administrators decided to meet again with the research staff in Ann Arbor, after receiving and examining the forthcoming second report, to discuss both reports together.

During the summer of 1958 we visited several of the hospitals to answer further questions about *Report I* and to request certain information from hospital records concerning such things as costs, hospital occupancy, length of patient stay, turnover and absenteeism among personnel, and similar other data we needed but had not yet obtained. We were also interested in learning whether any uses had been made of the first report. In this connection, our discussions indicated that *Report I* had been put to only a very limited use. However, most of the administrators showed considerable interest in the findings and indicated a real desire to find ways of using them. These conferences focused our attention on the problem of

The Chronology of the Research

getting the results of scientific investigation into the main streams of hospital activity. Further contacts with the hospital administrators and others from their organization served to emphasize the magnitude of this problem. As a result, certain members of the research staff decided to initiate a small follow-up study in four of the hospitals that had participated in the research for the purpose of exploring the problems faced by these institutions in attempting to utilize the data (6).

Third Phase

After *Report II* had been received and examined by the administrators, arrangements were made for the meeting between them and the research staff, as had been agreed earlier, for a one-day discussion of the two reports and related issues. The meeting was held at Ann Arbor, September 24, 1958. It was attended by six of the ten administrators whose organizations participated in the study proper, the administrator of one of the two pilot hospitals, the liaison between research staff and the Michigan Hospital Association, and the research staff.

The meeting sought to accomplish several purposes. One objective of the research staff was to help the administrators increase their ability to understand and interpret the reports, and to portray and communicate information from the reports to others in their organization. A related objective was to point out the limitations inherent in preliminary reports such as these, to show the administrators how to evaluate the results within the framework of the limitations of the data, and to warn against indiscriminate interpretations or unwarranted conclusions. It was emphasized that only tentative and limited conclusions could be reached on the basis of the two preliminary reports, and that more definitive answers would have to await lengthy and intensive analyses of the data and the final report of the research. Another objective was to learn from the administrators whether and how they had used the two reports, and of any plans that they were developing for further utilization. Finally, the conferees explored a number of problems and issues arising in relation to the utilization of the reports. The meeting ended with the research staff offering further help to individual administrators in this area. However, it was emphasized that the administrators themselves were the ones to direct the introduction of the findings to their respective hospitals, and that the extent of the utilization of the data would be a matter for the individual hospitals to decide.

Following the meeting, a brief digest of the discussions was compiled and sent to all hospitals, along with a series of illustrative charts presenting different data from the two reports. The charts were designed to be used by administrators as models for preparing and presenting information from the reports in ways that might be suitable for different topics and different audiences. After this time, except for the four institutions which later participated in the data utilization project cited above, we held no formal or common group meetings with representatives of the hospitals studied, other than occasionally corresponding with administrators on matters of mutual interest. However, we presented some additional findings at the 1959 Annual Meeting of the Michigan Hospital Association, when we again had the opportunity to meet several of the administrators informally and discuss the research with them.

Since 1959, the efforts of the research staff were primarily devoted to a thorough analysis of the data, the determination of relationships between the independent and the dependent variables studied, the testing of specific hypotheses, and the preparation of the final report of the research incorporating the findings. All detailed and complex analyses were done during this period. The results of these analyses and our interpretation of them finally culminated in the present work.

In brief, this is how the study unfolded chronologically. Let us now turn to a discussion of certain important aspects of methodology and design, beginning with the question of how the participating hospitals were selected for inclusion in the study.

THE SELECTION OF PARTICIPATING HOSPITALS

We have pointed out that the ten hospitals finally included in the research, as well as the two pilot hospitals, were selected from the broad class of short-stay general hospitals in the nation, which are nonprofit, voluntary, community institutions, and which are neither government-related nor church-affiliated institutions. This class, or population, of community general hospitals encompasses a total of approximately 2100 individual hospitals of varying size scattered throughout the United States. As we are about to see, however, the particular hospitals which were selected for study are not "representative" of all these institutions. In more technical terms, they were not selected with the intention to constitute a "probability" or "representative" sample of the population of the 2100 hospitals.

These 2100 community general hospitals make up an extremely heterogeneous population, that is, they vary greatly from one another on a number of important characteristics, even though they share the few characteristics above indicated. For one thing, some of the hospitals are extremely small, having less than 25 beds, while a few others are extremely large, having more than 500 beds each. The majority, of course, fall between these two extremes, but even a range of 25 to 500 beds is very wide. A 50-bed hospital, for example, is likely to be very different from a 450-bed hospital, and the same may be said for a 100-bed hospital in comparison to a 400-bed hospital, although the differences may be smaller in the latter case.

The differences that may be associated with the size of the hospitals virtually defy enumeration. There are differences in the size and kind of staff and personnel required by a small as against a large institution. There are differences in the number, and probably kind, of patients treated by institutions varying greatly in their size. There are differences in the environment within which larger and smaller institutions operate; a small rural community will be unlikely to be supporting a 500-bed hospital, for example. In general, with increased organizational size, there is more departmentalization, more specialization, more heterogeneity, and more complexity in organization and operations. Differences such as these undoubtedly have important (but mostly, and unfortunately, not-yet-known) implications for various aspects of the structure and functioning of hospitals, including implications for the quality of patient care, coordination, supervision,

Selection of Participating Hospitals

and communication—the very phenomena with which we are most concerned in this research.

Furthermore, the hospitals in question differ not only in size and size-related characteristics, but also on a number of other important dimensions which may be directly relevant to the objectives of the research. Included among these dimensions are: (1) the type of administrator different hospitals have—some have a lay person while others have a medical person as administrator, and some have a man while others have a woman in this position; (2) professional accreditation by the Joint Commission on Accreditation of Hospitals—while most of the hospitals are accredited, some are not (accreditation will be discussed further in Chapter 5, in relation to patient care); (3) regional-geographic location, and the type of community within which the hospitals operate—some hospitals are located in New England, some in the South, and others in the East, West, or Midwest, and, similarly, some serve huge metropolitan areas, while others serve small cities or towns. Of course, there are other dimensions on which the hospitals may vary. For our present purposes, however, the ones we have cited here are sufficient to illustrate the point that a great many significant differences—a good deal of heterogeneity or variance—characterize this population of community general hospitals.

From the standpoint of research design, the crucial problem that differences of the kind here discussed pose may be stated as follows: Unless the researcher takes cognizance of the heterogeneity of the population with which he is dealing, either by controlling many of the differences involved through his initial study design or by making sure to study the effects these differences may have upon the phenomena he proposes to investigate (i.e., upon his dependent variables), he will end up with many spurious results or "impure" findings, which he will be unable to explain. And ideally, of course, the researcher wants to be able to understand and explain the phenomena he is studying, e.g., the quality of patient care or coordination, in terms of the factors (i.e., independent variables) which he has actually measured in the study, and independently of other differences whose effects and influence upon the phenomena being studied constitute unknown and unwanted elements, i.e., differences that potentially introduce spuriousness. For an excellent exposition of the problem of spuriousness and related issues in survey research, see Hyman (5).

The problem of how to guard against spurious results due to great heterogeneity in the population of hospitals may be handled in either of two main ways. First, the researcher may restrict his inital population to a subpopulation, thus reducing much of the unwanted heterogeneity. He may impose specific restrictions and qualifications that the hospitals in the study should meet (based on what differences in the population he considers important enough to avoid, control for, or keep constant without actually measuring them), and instead of dealing with all of the 2100 hospitals, deal with a much smaller subclass of hospitals which meet certain criteria. Alternately, rather than restrict the population, he may have a large enough number of hospitals participate in the study, so as to capture (within specifiable limits) much of the heterogeneity prevailing in the whole population of the 2100 hospitals. In other words, he may increase the size of his sample, or the number of hospitals to be studied, to a number which permits him to represent reasonably well (i.e., with specifiable confidence) the entire population of hospitals by his sample.

The first of the above methods, i.e., restricting the population, will have the effect of limiting the ability of the researcher to generalize the findings of his study (which would be based on a small number of hospitals) to the entire initial population of the 2100 community general hospitals. The second method would require the inclusion in the research of a sufficiently large number of participating hospitals to yield either a probability sample that is "representative" of the total population, or at least a large enough sample to permit the institution of statistical controls. It would require, in other words, that a relatively large number of hospitals be actually studied—say 50 or more hospitals, rather than ten hospitals as is the case with the present study. In turn, this would necessitate considerably greater costs, efforts, and time than a smaller sample of hospitals.

In summary, then, restricting the population has the advantage of obtaining relatively pure rather than spurious results with relatively few hospitals participating in the study, and the limitation of generalizing the results as much as might be desired. Increasing the size of the sample, i.e., the number of hospitals to be studied, on the other hand, has the advantage of permitting greater generalization of the findings, and the disadvantage of requiring greater costs, time, efforts, and energies. Assuming limited funds, therefore, the researcher is almost inevitably forced toward restricting the population and away from a relatively large sample—something which in fact occurred in designing the present study. In this study, we ended up with a compromise wherein we restricted the initially relevant population of hospitals and, at the same time, used a number of hospitals which, though not sufficiently large to yield a "representative sample," or a sample that allows many controls, is large enough to permit the use of sound analytical techniques. (Strictly speaking, the ten hospitals which finally participated in the research constitute a "population" themselves. Theoretically, however, they may also be viewed as constituting a sample of that population of hospitals which happened to meet most of the criteria that we used to select the ten hospitals, i.e., a sample of a population of hospitals which are similar to those studied but, obviously, a population that is substantially smaller than the one comprised by the 2100 community general hospitals.)

Needless to say, the difficulties posed by the heterogeneity of the population of the 2100 community general hospitals, and by considerations of economy and feasibility, did not alone determine the selection of the particular hospitals which participated in this study. Once we decided to confine the study to a subgroup of hospitals, the number and kind of hospitals chosen for inclusion in the study were determined by a set of additional factors. Included among these determining factors were the nature of the study itself, i.e., the particular aims of the study and the questions that we hoped to answer, the character of the phenomena in which we were interested, i.e., the kind of dependent variables involved, and the willingness of the hospitals chosen for inclusion in the study to cooperate. Let us briefly comment on some of these factors, and then proceed to indicate the specific criteria which we used to select our hospitals.

The very nature of the study was an important determinant of the sample of hospitals required. Ordinarily, if the research is of an exploratory kind (e.g., like the pilot portion of the present research), aiming to yield some unavailable information, stimulate insights, or aid the formulation of hypotheses in anticipation of more systematic studies (exploratory studies in areas where little prior research has been conducted, as in the present field, are both useful and desirable), then it is not crucial for the researcher to study a large or a "representative" sample of organizations. (In fact it may not even be advisable to start out with such a sample until he knows something about the population.) The same also applies if the research is of the "case-study" type, not aiming at generalization of results or rigorous hypothesis testing, or if the research happens to be too circumscribed in its objectives as is the case with many small experimental studies. If, on the other hand, the research is of the explanatory kind (which is usually preceded by a good deal of exploratory and case-study research), aiming to test rigorously hypotheses of wide generality, or to yield results by studying a sample of the total population and then generalize these results to the whole population (i.e., to estimate the characteristics and parameters of the total population in terms of sample results and on the basis of statistical inference), then the organizations actually studied must constitute a "probability" sample that is "representative" of the whole population. However, between case studies or exploratory studies that are not concerned with problems of generalization and purely explanatory studies that are concerned with generalization, there is another, intermediate alternative: some research is in part exploratory and in part explanatory or hypothesis-testing, aiming at initially limited generalization. The present study clearly belongs to this category.

If the research is in part exploratory and descriptive and in part explanatory and analytical, designed both to develop hypotheses for further study and to test hypotheses based on already available research and theory (or test hypotheses of potentially greater generality than would be entailed by the results obtained from the particular organizations studied but without actually ascertaining or establishing the limits of this generality), then a design that restricts the population to which the results may potentially apply, but includes an adequate number of organizations in the research to permit the use of sound analysis procedures, may yield the best possible solution. Such a design provides a reasonably good alternative in place of the ideal "representative sample" design, or in place of a large sample design, which is not feasible because of considerations of costs and economy and/or because of lack of sufficient prior knowledge about the phenomena with which the research is concerned. It is this kind of design that we adopted for the present study—our first study of hospitals, and the first study of its kind (in terms of its subject areas and methodology) in this field. In terms of this design, needless to say, generalization of the findings beyond the ten hospitals studied can be attempted not on statistical grounds, but rather on the basis of logical inference from theoretical principles—and that is why theory is important here and will occupy a prominent place in several of the chapters which follow.

We have seen how the problems of spuriousness and economy, and the nature of the research affected our decision concerning the kind and number of hospitals that were eventually included in the study. This decision will be further clarified now in a discussion of the specific criteria which we employed to select the ten participating hospitals. This discussion will also show how the character of the phenomena investigated and the willingness of hospitals to cooperate entered the determination of our sample of hospitals.

Specific Criteria of Hospital Selection

The research was initiated with a proposal to study community general hospitals, i.e., the most familiar type of hospitals in the nation. Mental hospitals, government-related hospitals, and private hospitals were excluded from the beginning. However, the remaining group of hospitals was still too large and too heterogeneous to cover, and additional criteria were imposed to restrict the initial population further. One important criterion was to exclude from this first study hospitals that met all of our specific criteria but one—the criterion of religious affiliation. Denominational hospitals were not included in the study because their governing boards are different from those of other community general hospitals, and because we expected that institutional orientation to a religious denomination might have implications for other aspects of hospital functioning.

Another important criterion was length of patient stay. Long-term hospitals are different from short-stay hospitals in such important characteristics as types of illnesses treated, staff-patient ratios, services required, patient turnover, and the like, with corresponding consequences for hospital organization and functions. Accordingly, we decided to be concerned only with short-stay hospitals—hospitals for acute diseases, where average patient stay is less than 20 days and usually less than ten. Still another criterion was geographical location. Because of possible regional differences among hospitals that otherwise are of the same type, and also because of budgetary considerations, we decided to confine the study to Michigan hospitals, there being enough hospitals in Michigan that met all other criteria of selection. Even for Michigan hospitals, however, we had to institute the added criterion of community size and consider only hospitals operating in cities having at least 10,000 population, in order to minimize the potential effects of differences arising from the community environments within which the hospitals operate.

Another criterion of selection was the type of administrator present. Because, in addition to patient care and coordination, we were also interested in administrative and supervisory practices, we decided to include in the study only hospitals having a male, lay person as their administrator, thus excluding hospitals having doctors, nurses, or women as their administrators. We expected appreciable variations in administrative and supervisory behavior among hospitals having male, lay administrators and wanted to avoid possible confounding effects stemming from added variance attributable to the sex or professional status of the individuals holding the top administration post in the various hospitals. Another criterion of selection was the accreditation status of the hospitals. In this connection, we decided to study only hospitals that were accredited by the Joint Commission on Accreditation of Hospitals, such accreditation implying that these hospitals meet minimum standards of care and other requirements acceptable to the medical profession (see Chapter 5 for further details). Again, because we were interested in the quality of patient care rendered by the various hospitals, and because we expected appreciable differences in patient care quality even among accredited

Selection of Participating Hospitals

institutions, the decision was made to exclude the few nonaccredited hospitals that happened to meet all other criteria of selection. Incidentally, we might observe at this point that the reader will not fail to be impressed by the differences in both patient care and other areas that we found among the hospitals finally studied, as subsequent chapters demonstrate.

Finally, the important criterion of hospital size was also employed. Since, among other things, we were concerned with the phenomenon of organizational coordination, the objectives of the study argued in favor of selecting sufficiently complex organizations so that we would be able to investigate problems of internal coordination of activity on the part of the many groups, departments, and individual members in the participating hospitals. This meant selecting relatively large hospitals, where problems of complexity, specialization, and coordination are both more likely and more acute by comparison to small institutions. On the other hand, we did not want to tackle the largest and most complex hospital systems in our initial study in this field (e.g., hospitals having over 500 beds). Financial and professional resources would have sufficed if the study were to include only one or two such hospitals. Yet, we felt that it would be essential to include in the study as many hospitals as possible for comparative analyses, and the decision was made to adopt this alternative rather than work with only one or two large hospitals—especially in view of the fact that very little was known about the phenomena we were proposing to investigate. For these reasons, and because of an additional concern for dealing with a familiar or "typical" class of institution, we decided to study medium-size hospitals rather than larger or smaller institutions. "Medium size" was specified, upon examination of the frequency distribution of hospitals of all sizes, to include hospitals having from 100 to 350 beds.

In summary, then, the population of the particular hospitals that finally participated in the research was restricted by (1) the objectives of the research, (2) practical considerations, such as funds and resources available, and (3) characteristics of the initial population that we wished to "control" because of concern for their potential effects upon the phenomena under investigation, i.e., upon the dependent variables of the study. The restriction was accomplished by specifying certain criteria for hospital participation. According to these criteria, all hospitals selected to participate shared these characteristics: (1) they all were short-stay general hospitals of medium size (between 100 and 350 beds); (2) they all were community, voluntary, nonprofit institutions; (3) they all were nongovernmental and nondenominational institutions, administered by a lay, male administrator and governed by a board of trustees; (4) they were all accredited by the Joint Commission on Accreditation of Hospitals; and (5) they were all located in Michigan cities of over 10,000 population. (For other important characteristics shared by the participating hospitals, but not used as criteria for selecting hospitals for the study, see Chapter 4 and subsequent chapters.)

The objective of the study design was to include in the research all of the hospitals sharing all of the above criteria. A total of 15 institutions were at the end found to meet the criteria. However, two of them had already participated in the exploratory part of the research—the two pilot hospitals mentioned earlier—and had to be excluded from the study proper to avoid contaminated findings due to prior sensitization or exposure of these two organizations to the research and its objectives. During negotiations with the remaining 13 institutions aimed at securing their cooperation and participation in the research, another hospital indicated inability to participate. This institution had just changed its administrator. But even preceding and following this change, it had certain problems revolving around its relationship with the city where it operated, and it was in the process of attempting to resolve its difficulties. These problems, according to representatives of the hospital, were problems affecting the legal status and control of the institution, and not public-relations difficulties. In any event, they were sufficiently crucial to lead the hospital to withhold participation in the research, even though it viewed the research as important and worth while. We were thus left with twelve hospitals as potential candidates.

Of these twelve institutions, ten finally participated in the research and two did not. Of the latter, one had agreed to participate, but shortly before its scheduled time for data collection it developed certain internal problems involving the administrator, the board of trustees, and the medical staff, with the result that it withdrew from the study. (Actually, its problems had a longer history, but they were somewhat dormant for some time and until shortly before we were to collect the data, when certain occurrences unrelated to the study retriggered and accentuated the problems.) The other of the two hospitals also had agreed to participate, but because of inability to prepare itself for data collection on time we were forced to drop it from the study. It would have not been possible to schedule this hospital for data collection any time during the period of November 4 to December 13, 1957, when field work was carried out, because the hospital, among other things, could not provide us with necessary rosters of its members from which to sample individual respondents until late December (or, perhaps, not even then). This delay would have forced us to collect data from this one institution much later than from all the others, and we could not possibly anticipate the effects of such a delay upon the data that we would have obtained—the data would have not been completely comparable in terms of time. Rather than risk incomparability of the data, as well as added expenses from prolonging the planned data collection period, we abandoned this hospital altogether. Thus, in the end, and apart from the two pilot hospitals, a total of ten hospitals ($N = 10$) actually participated in the research proper, constituting the final "sample" of the study. The findings reported in subsequent chapters are based on data from these ten Michigan hospitals.

The ten hospitals are described individually, but without being identified, in Chapter 4 while in a sense all of the chapters in this volume describe the ten institutions collectively. The ten participating hospitals, as well as the two hospitals which took part in the exploratory phase of the study, it will be recalled, vary in their size. However, they all are medium-size hospitals, falling in the size range of 100 to 350 beds. As of the time of data collection, the actual number of beds in each of the twelve institutions, shown here in ascending order, was as follows: 104, 131, 154, 157, 160, 175, 190, 217, 230, 234, 238, and 322 beds. In accordance with the policies of the Institute for Social Research, individual hospitals, like individual respondents, shall not be identified, in the interests of

Selection of Individual Groups and Respondents

preserving the anonymity of the individual organizations and respondents and the confidentiality of the data which they kindly furnished us.

We might note, before closing this section, that the numbers assigned to particular hospitals in various parts of the book are used to facilitate the presentation of the findings and to show that we are discussing different organizations. These numbers do not follow the order implied by the size of the hospitals. However, each participating hospital always has the same distinguishing number assigned to it throughout the book in order that it may be compared and contrasted with other hospitals when appropriate. The term "participating hospitals" is always used to refer to the ten institutions which finally participated in the research proper and, consequently, excludes the two pilot hospitals.

THE SELECTION OF INDIVIDUAL GROUPS AND RESPONDENTS FROM EACH HOSPITAL

Each hospital took part in the research by (1) providing us with certain required data from its administrative and medical records, and (2) having a number of its members from different groups and positions participate in the study as individual respondents, i.e., answer the questionnaires and interviews that we had developed. The individual respondents were in all cases selected by the research staff, however, and their selection was dictated only by the objectives of the study and the nature of the research design. Shortly before data collection, the participating hospitals were requested to send us a complete roster of people in different professional-occupational groups and positions in the organization. Then, on the basis of these rosters, we selected those individuals from whom we wished to obtain data, in advance of data collection and without any knowledge on the part of the hospitals.

Even before selecting the appropriate individual respondents for each hospital, however, a decision had to be made as to which of the many groups and subgroups of hospital personnel should participate in the study in the first place, i.e., a decision as to how each hospital should be represented in the research. The final decision was to have each hospital represented by: (1) its administrator and administrative-nonmedical department heads; (2) members of its board of trustees, or its governing board; (3) members of its medical staff; (4) members of its nursing staff; and (5) technicians from its laboratory and x-ray departments. (Some groups, as we will see below, were subsequently stratified further.)

The single central idea governing the specification of these groups as respondent groups was to obtain relevant data from as many relevant groups in the hospital as would be sufficient to represent the total (or nearly the total) organizational structure—to represent and reflect, as comprehensively as feasible, the total hospital system. In this connection, it should be recalled that our main unit of analysis is the hospital as a total organization. We wanted many of our measures, especially the measures of certain dependent variables (including the quality of overall patient care and of organizational coordination), to reflect the total situation of the hospital in all its complexity. Our major concern was with phenomena involving the functioning of the whole organization as a system rather than the functioning of some of its parts only (however important and crucial individual parts might be). In other words, we wanted some of our measures to "capture" the unified response, and the end products and problem-solving characteristics of the organizational system. The problems and characteristics of specific organizational parts, administrative units, professional-occupational groups, or individual members are of secondary concern in this study; they are of concern only to the extent that they are relevant to the objectives of the research—to patient care, coordination, supervision and administration, and communication.

Since we were interested in the quality of patient care rendered at the various hospitals, it was essential that we obtain data from the medical staff and the nursing staff, and the specification of the above groups would make this possible. Similarly, since we were interested in coordination phenomena and in certain aspects of administration and supervision, it was essential that we obtain data from individuals in administrative and supervisory positions, as well as from their subordinates, e.g., from the administrator and his department heads, or from supervisory nursing personnel and their subordinates. This too would be made possible by the specification of the above groups as respondent groups. Technicians were similarly specified to be covered because of their interaction with doctors, nurses, patients, and administrative personnel, i.e., because of their relevance to our research objectives. In short, the groups selected—administrator and department heads, trustees, doctors, nurses, and technicians—were directly relevant to one or more of the major objectives of the research and could provide the specific data required by these objectives.

In addition to the preceding considerations, however, certain other important factors also entered the decision as to which groups from the hospital should be covered. In this connection, one important consideration was to obtain data about the various aspects of hospital structure and functioning in which we were interested both from the "key people" in each hospital and from other personnel, especially personnel concerned with patient care and/or coordination functions. This meant (1) collecting data from doctors, trustees, and the administrator and his department heads—the top people in the community general hospital, and (2) collecting data at least from nursing personnel in different roles and classifications, and from laboratory and x-ray technicians. Another objective was to obtain data from people at all organizational levels, from the top to the bottom of the formal hierarchical structure. This objective also could be largely fulfilled by including in the study the groups which we have specified (in the case of nursing personnel alone, for example, we have an elaborate hierarchy, from the hospital administrator and the director of nursing, through nursing supervisors, head nurses, and nonsupervisory registered nurses to practical nurses and to aides and orderlies). Still another objective was, within practical limits, to cover as many of the different professional and occupational groups in the hospital as possible, including the largest two groups in the organization—the nursing staff and the medical staff.

The final reason for specifying certain groups as respondent groups and excluding others was, of course, the matter of adopting an efficient research design, given the limited resources at our disposal (including financial and professional resources, and limitations in time and effort required). We could not possibly

Selection of Individual Groups and Respondents 55

collect data from every individual associated with every participating hospital and still include in the study all of the ten hospitals. This would have meant obtaining data from over 5000 individual persons rather than from the 1245 respondents who ultimately participated in the research. But the 5000 figure itself would have not been prohibitive to handle, if the research design had called for it. In point of fact, it was neither necessary, nor desirable, nor efficient to attempt to include in the study everyone associated with each hospital. There were at least two crucial reasons for this. First, the objectives of the research did not require data from such people as the personnel of the laundry, housekeeping, maintenance, and dietary departments of the hospital (other than from the department head in each case), for these people could have hardly provided meaningful data about such things as the quality of patient care or coordination (in this connection, see our discussion in Chapter 3). Second, and more important, statistical and sampling techniques are available that enable the researcher to "represent" relatively large groups of people by actually including in his study only a sample, or a portion, of the total membership of the groups involved—something which we did in the case of the nursing staff and medical staff.

Specification of Individual Respondents

The first determinant of the selection of individual respondents from each participating organization was the above decision, and the underlying rationale, to have the hospitals represented in the study by certain groups—their administrative staff, trustees, medical staff, nursing staff, and laboratory and x-ray technicians. The second determinant was the relative size of these respondent groups. Some of the groups were too large to be completely covered, i.e., they contained too many members, and it would have been both unnecessary and difficult to administer questionnaires and interviews to all their members. In view of the feasibility of employing sampling techniques to represent the entire group by only a proportion of its members, it was more economical, easier, less time consuming, and generally more desirable, as well as potentially less disruptive to the normal functioning of the organizations involved, to use sampling in the case of the largest respondent groups. Another related determinant was the composition of each group involved. For example, the nursing staff contains a number of subgroups and classifications of personnel—personnel having strikingly different characteristics (see Chapter 3). Accordingly, this group had to be stratified further, and individual respondents had to be sampled from each of its various classifications in order to represent the entire group. A similar procedure was also used in the case of the medical staff. Another determinant as to how many and which individuals from each group should be selected was relevance. This criterion was applied in the case of doctors and trustees in the manner and for the reasons indicated below.

A final, and very crucial, determinant was the nature of the research design. Specifically, since the design called for sampling within hospital groups, we wanted to have enough respondents selected from each group and subgroup involved (and, ultimately, enough respondents from each hospital) to obtain stable measures and to satisfy certain statistical requirements (without which it would not be possible either to represent the entire group by only a sample of group members or to appraise the significance of the data). In other words, each sample had to be of sufficient size (contain enough individual respondents) to permit us to make precise statistical statements of significance concerning the data, and to use data from the sample to represent the entire group from which the sample was drawn. At the same time, however, the sample should not be too large because it would defeat some of its very objectives, e.g., the objectives of economy, efficiency, time, etc. This latter consideration, among other things, necessitated that, since each group sampled consisted of considerably more individuals in some of the hospitals than in others (depending on the size of the hospitals and other factors, a particular hospital might have 150 nonsupervisory registered nurses, while another might have only 50), we use different sampling rates for the different hospitals. More concretely, this meant, for example, that in some hospitals we select every other practical nurse to be included in the sample, while in others we select every third or every fourth one.[2] When the groups involved were relatively small, however, as in the case of department heads, then there was no problem because every member could be selected to participate as respondent—this being equivalent to "sampling" at a 1:1 ratio, or 100 percent rate, in such a case.

Taking all of the above considerations into account, the following people were finally selected from each of the ten participating hospitals as respondents to represent their respective groups and hospitals:

1. The hospital administrator (i.e., the administrator, director, or superintendent of the hospital) from each institution.

2. All nonmedical, administrative department heads of each institution. This highly heterogeneous group includes the directors of all nonmedical departments —nursing, dietary, records, housekeeping, maintenance, admissions, personnel, etc.

3. All members of the executive committee of the board of trustees of each hospital, including the chairman of this committee and the president of the board of trustees (if different persons), and the officers of the board.

4. All technicians (persons formally designated as such) from the laboratory and from the x-ray department of each hospital.

5. All "key members" of the medical staff of each hospital. This group includes doctors holding the following offices, positions, or administrative responsibilities: the chief of staff or his equivalent (e.g., president of the staff); the chairman of the executive committee of the medical staff and the members of this committee, who are usually the officers of the staff and/or the chiefs of major medical services; the chairmen of the tissue, audit, medical records, education, and credentials committees, i.e., the major committees of the staff; the chief pathologist, or director of the laboratory; and the chief radiologist, or director of the x-ray department of each hospital. This group of "key members" of the medical staff is actually a small group because the same doctor often holds more than one of the above positions in the hospital. Henceforth, we shall refer to this group of key doctors as the "selected medical staff" group.

6. A representative sample of the remaining medical staff members of each

---

[2] In turn, of course, the use of differential sampling rates required that, in computing some measures which involved data from several groups of respondents, we weight the data by the sampling rate with which the respondents providing them had been chosen.

Selection of Individual Groups and Respondents 57

hospital, i.e., attending doctors who are either "active" or "associate" members of the medical staff, but who hold none of the above specified key positions. Henceforth, we shall refer to this group of doctors as the "general medical staff" group to distinguish it from the "selected medical staff" group.

7. All full-time and part-time persons in supervisory nursing positions (e.g., floor supervisors, night shift supervisor, other nursing supervisors, the associate director of nursing, if one, head nurses), from "head nurse" on up through the director of nursing.

8. A representative sample of the nonsupervisory registered nurses of each hospital, including both full-time and part-time nurses. Persons in "assistant head nurse" positions were included in this stratum, for their duties and functions are much more like those of nonsupervisory registered nurses than those of head nurses or other supervisory nursing personnel.

9. A representative sample of the practical nurses (whether "licensed" or not) in each hospital.

10. A representative sample of full-time aides (in most hospitals called "nurse's aides," and in a few "nurse assistants"). Because aides constitute the largest group within the nursing staff in most hospitals, and because a relatively small proportion of them are likely to be working on a part-time basis, only full-time aides were included in the study. (To this sample of aides, we subsequently added the few full-time orderlies from each hospital. Orderlies are equivalent to male nurse's aides.)

It will be noted that sampling is involved in only four of the above ten groups or strata; namely, the sixth group and the last three groups (groups 6, 8, 9, and 10). In all other cases, every person belonging to the specified group was automatically requested to participate in the study as a respondent—to fill out a questionnaire or be interviewed. In other words, hypothetically, in the case of groups 1, 2, 3, 4, 5, and 7, we "sampled" at 100 percent rate. In the case of the four groups where actual sampling was used, of course, not every group member was requested to participate; some members were selected as respondents while others were not. Before indicating how individuals were selected into the sample in the case of these four groups, however, we should like to comment briefly on the above mentioned criterion of "relevance" that was applied in the case of doctors and the case of trustees.

According to the above list of respondents, it is clear that only the members of the executive committee of the board of trustees were included in the study and not all the members of the board. The reason for doing this is that the total board of trustees meets as a whole only a few times a year, with most of its members being unfamiliar with the day-to-day functioning of the hospital (in this connection, see pertinent data in Chapter 3 and Chapter 4). Thus, except for the members of the executive committee, the other trustees could not provide the data we wanted—they were not a relevant group in this sense. The issue of relevance was also involved in the case of the medical staff, but in a somewhat different form. First, we wanted to make sure to obtain data from the key doctors in each hospital, i.e., from the "selected medical staff," because of their special positions in the organization and their specialized knowledge in a number of areas of medical practice and hospital functioning. The selected medical staff was a group of high relevance to the research objectives. At the same time, however, we also wanted to obtain data from the "general medical staff" group, which might see things from a different perspective than the selected medical staff. The selected staff group interacts more frequently with nonmedical members of the organization, particularly the administrator and the trustees, in addition to being the locus of "power" for the total medical staff, and may or may not be in agreement with the general staff in its evaluation of the situation. For these reasons, we decided to separate the two groups of doctors and, later, to combine them if we found no differences in the data obtained from the two groups. Finally, in connection with our sample of doctors from the general medical staff group, we excluded from the study so-called "courtesy" members of the medical staff. These are doctors who practice in the hospital only infrequently, bring to the hospital only a few of their patients, and have limited privileges there. They are an irrelevant group in the sense that they are not sufficiently familiar with the situation in the hospitals where they practice on a courtesy basis.

Let us now return to answer the question of how individual persons were selected into the sample in the case of the four groups that we have indicated—the general medical staff, nonsupervisory registered nurses, practical nurses, and nurse's aides. When the participating hospitals sent us their personnel rosters, we found that the size of each of these four groups was large enough to suggest that we employ sampling and select only some rather than all of the members of the group as respondents. Furthermore, we found that the size of each of the four groups varied considerably from one hospital to another, and this suggested that we use differential sampling ratios for the same group in the different hospitals, i.e., select a different proportion of group members in different hospitals to obtain samples of adequate yet manageable size. The criterion as to what sampling ratio should be used in each case was determined by the size of the total group and the goal of having enough group members in the sample so as to obtain stable data, as economically as possible, and satisfy statistical requirements for handling the data. In more concrete terms, this meant that the sample we drew for each of the four groups, in each of the ten participating hospitals, should contain roughly and on the average 15 to 25 individual persons (the precise size of the sample, of course, would ultimately depend on the size of the group being sampled and on the sampling rate used). This rule of thumb determined the particular sampling rates that were used.

Once the particular sampling rate for each group and each hospital was decided upon, we proceeded to draw the samples. For each group to be sampled, separately for each hospital, we had a complete, alphabetically ordered list of its members, i.e., a list containing the names of all persons belonging to the group. Each alphabetical list was numbered serially, beginning with number one. Then, using the appropriate sampling rate and a table of random numbers, we began the sampling procedure by choosing as the first person into the sample that person whose position in the alphabetical-numbered list was the same as the first random number we drew that was contained within the sampling interval used, i.e., a number being smaller than or equal to the sampling rate used. If, for example, the sampling rate for the practical nurses group of a given hospital was four,

Selection of Individual Groups and Respondents

meaning that every fourth person from this group should be selected in the sample, the first random number we drew that was between one and four determined who would be the first person from our list of names to be included in the sample. If, in the present example, the number we drew was three, for instance, then the third person on the list would be the one to be chosen as the first individual in the sample. Once the first individual to be included in the sample was determined in this manner, we continued selecting the other individuals systematically by applying the appropriate sampling rate, i.e., using a sampling interval equal to the sampling rate involved. In the above case where the sampling rate was four, for example, we continued to include in the sample every fourth name from the list following the first randomly chosen name, until the entire list was exhausted.

Samples drawn according to the above procedure are technically known as systematic random samples. In effect, these samples give every group member an equal and known chance, or probability, of being selected into the sample, and the set of individuals selected into the sample may be properly used to represent the entire group from which they were selected. The probability of being selected into the sample, in each case, is equal to the sampling ratio used. The sampling ratio itself is computed by dividing one by the sampling rate used, e.g., if the sampling rate is three, then the sampling ratio is one to three. Table 1, below, shows the sampling ratios used to sample individual persons from each of the four groups that were subjected to sampling—general medical staff, nonsupervisory registered nurses, practical nurses, and nurse's aides—and separately for each of the ten participating hospitals.

Table 1 tells us, for example, that in the case of Hospital #0 every fourth member of the general medical staff was selected into the sample, while in the case of Hospital #3 every second member of the same group was selected. Similarly, the table shows that every third practical nurse in the case of Hospital #4 was selected into our sample of practical nurses from that hospital, and so on. Incidentally, as footnoted in Table 1, in sampling from the nonsupervisory registered nurses group, we applied the same sampling ratio to both full-time and part-time R.N.'s in each participating hospital. However, the sampling itself was done on the basis of separate lists for full-time and part-time R.N.'s (for all hospitals combined, about 55 percent of all R.N.'s were working full-time, and 45 percent part-time). In the case of the practical nurses group, the sampling ratios shown were applied to full-time P.N.'s (full-time personnel in this category, for all hospitals combined, accounts for about 95 percent of the total personnel), with the few part-time P.N.'s from each hospital subsequently added to the sample. In the case of aides, the sampling ratios shown were applied only to full-time personnel, since no part-time aides were included in the study. To our samples of aides we then added the few orderlies from each hospital. The orderlies group of respondents, for all ten hospitals combined, amounts to about one-fourth of all aides and orderlies participating in the research.

In summary, then, for some of the specified respondent groups we required every group member to participate in the study as a respondent. These groups, being the same for every participating hospital, are: all members of the executive committee of the board of trustees of each institution; the selected medical staff group, consisting of doctors in key positions in each hospital, as described above; the administrator of the hospital; all administrative, nonmedical department heads; all nursing personnel in supervisory roles, from head nurse on up through the director of the nursing department; and all technicians from the laboratory and the x-ray department of the hospital. For certain other groups, however, we required only a representative sample of group members to participate in the study as respondents. These groups, also being the same for each of the ten participating hospitals, are: the general medical staff group, as described above; the nonsupervisory registered nurses group, including representative samples of both full-time and part-time R.N.'s; the practical nurses group, including the few part-time P.N.'s from each hospital; and the nurse's aides group, including only full-time aides (to which group we later added the few orderlies from each hospital). The major background characteristics of each participating respondent group are described in Chapter 3.

TABLE 1. The Sampling Ratios Used to Select Individual Respondents from Each of Four Organizational Groups in Each Participating Hospital

Participating Hospital	General Medical Staff	Nonsupervisory Registered Nurses *	Practical Nurses (full-time) †	Nurse's Aides (full-time)
#0	1:4	1:3	1:4	1:4
1	1:3	1:3	1:1	1:4
2	1:2	1:2	1:2	1:3
3	1:2	1:2	1:2	1:2
4	1:2	1:3	1:3	1:3
5	1:2	1:2	1:2	1:5
6	1:2	1:3	1:3	1:5
7	1:3	1:3	1:3	1:4
8	1:3	1:3	1:3	1:2
9	1:2	1:3	1:3	1:3

* In each hospital, the same sampling ratio was applied to both full-time and part-time R.N.'s, but full-time nurses were sampled separately from part-time nurses. For all hospitals combined, 55 percent of all nonsupervisory nurses were working full-time, and 45 percent part-time.

† For this group we sampled only among full-time P.N.'s who, for all hospitals combined, constituted about 95 percent of the entire population of P.N.'s. The few part-time P.N.'s were then added to the sample. In terms of numbers, of a grand total of 147 P.N.'s initially selected to participate in the study, 131 were full-time and only 16 were working part-time.

Number of Individuals Initially Selected as Respondents from Each Respondent Group and Each Participating Hospital

The processes of selection discussed above ultimately resulted in selecting, from all hospitals and all respondent groups involved, a grand total of 1396 individual persons from whom we wished to obtain data by means of questionnaires and interviews. Table 2 shows the exact distribution of all these individuals by hospital

Research Instruments and Data Collection 61

and by respondent group. As we will see in the next section of this chapter, questionnaires and interviews were finally administered to and completed by a little over 90 percent of the initially selected respondents (1265 of the 1396 persons) shown in Table 2. (The effective response rate was even higher, however, because some of the initially selected respondents had left the hospital permanently by the time of data collection.)

TABLE 2. Number of Individuals Selected from Each Specified Group in Each Hospital to Participate in the Study as Respondents

Respondent Group	#0	1	2	3	4	5	6	7	8	9	Group Total (All Hospitals)
Selected medical staff	19	14	11	11	10	11	11	13	15	10	125
General medical staff	20	21	14	17	14	15	13	22	16	17	169
Supervisory nursing staff *	26	18	20	18	19	13	37	4	15	14	184
Nonsupervisory registered nurses	26	26	29	18	28	23	21	21	26	22	240
Practical nurses †	19	12	13	16	19	11	9	14	21	13	147
Aides and orderlies ‡	25	30	22	14	23	24	27	21	23	12	221
Laboratory and x-ray technicians	24	25	8	9	12	13	15	11	19	9	145
Administrative department heads	10	9	8	10	10	10	13	11	11	11	103
Trustees	4	4	4	4	5	4	9	4	7	7	52
Hospital administrators	1	1	1	1	1	1	1	1	1	1	10
TOTALS:	174	160	130	118	141	125	156	122	154	116	1396

* In this table, the director of nursing, who is both a supervisory nursing person and an administrative department head, has been included with the department heads group and is, therefore, not counted with the supervisory nursing staff. (Incidentally, in Hospital #7 only 4 persons, in addition to the director of nursing were formally designated as holding nursing supervisory positions, while in Hospital #6 the number was 37.)

† Of the 147 practical nurses from the ten hospitals, 131 were full-time nurses and 16 were part-time nurses.

‡ Of the 221 individuals in this group, 167 were aides and 54 were orderlies.

RESEARCH INSTRUMENTS, DATA COLLECTION, RESPONSE RATES, AND RESPONDENT REACTION

The bulk of required data was obtained from the respondents specified in the preceding section by means of standardized paper-and-pencil questionnaires and personal interviews. These data were then supplemented by certain other data from organizational documents and the administrative and medical records of each hospital, and by a special rating of the quality of medical care in each hospital that was performed by a group of doctors who were familiar with the hospitals studied but who were not on the staff of any of the participating hospitals. The rating of medical care by outside doctors is presented and discussed in Chapter 5. The data from hospital records are presented and discussed in several subsequent chapters, especially in Chapters 3, 4, and 5. Therefore, in this section, we shall confine discussion to the questionnaire and interview instruments.

The several questionnaire and interview forms used to collect the necessary data were finalized and reproduced in quantity following several preliminary drafts and a final draft after the full-dress pretest. The main purpose of both the questionnaires and the interviews, of course, was to elicit relevant data for the measurement of the different concepts and related dependent and independent variables with which the study is concerned. A second purpose of the research instruments was to provide some data about the characteristics of the different respondents. A third purpose was to use research instruments that would allow the respondents to offer any other information they wished whether directly relevant to the study or not, in the hope of (1) helping us better understand and evaluate their answers to our own questions, and (2) furnishing us with data that might be relevant to some important aspect of hospital operations which, in the eyes of the respondents, was not being tapped by our questions. Finally, the research instruments were structured so as to maximize their probability of being answered by the respondents frankly and completely which, among other things, meant that the instruments should not be unduly long, and the questions should be clear, meaningful, and concise.

Because of differences in the background characteristics of the different groups of respondents involved (such as formal education, professional training, and the like), because of differences in the positions different respondents held in the hospital, because of differences in the familiarity of respondents with particular areas of hospital functioning, because most individual respondents could not possibly provide answers to all of the questions in which we were interested, and because of reasons of economy and convenience, several different (but overlapping and complementary) forms of questionnaires and interviews were designed to satisfy the above objectives. These were administered, in each participating hospital, to the groups of respondents that we have specified as follows:

Form 1, Questionnaire: for nurse's aides and orderlies.
Form 2, Questionnaire: for nonsupervisory registered nurses, and for practical nurses.
Form 3, Questionnaire: for supervisory nursing personnel, except the director of nursing who completed Form 5 and Form 5a.
Form 4, Questionnaire: for laboratory and x-ray technicians.
Form 5, Questionnaire: for administrative, nonmedical department heads, including the director of nursing, who also completed Form 5a—a special shortened version of Form 3.
Form 6, Questionnaire: for the general medical staff group of respondents.
Form 7, Part A–Interview, and Part B–Questionnaire: for the selected (key) medical staff group of respondents.
Form 8, Part A–Interview, and Part B–Questionnaire: for trustees.
Form 9, Part A–Interview, and Part B–Questionnaire: for the hospital administrators.

Thus, different groups of respondents were required to complete different forms of questionnaires and, in the case of the selected medical staff, trustees, and administrator, different forms of interviews as well. In all the ten participating hospitals, however, the members of each particular respondent group were required to complete identical research instruments to ensure comparability of the data across hospitals. The different questionnaire forms were all of the paper-and-pencil type, consisting mainly of multiple-choice or check-list questions with fixed response alternatives following each question. The main purpose of using questions of this type is standardization; every individual belonging to a particular group of respondents is exposed to the same stimulus. That is, respondents from the same group are presented with, and requested to answer, the same identical questions by choosing one of a number of specified alternative answers for each question. (Respondents were asked to choose the alternative best describing their position in each case, but were also told to write in their answer in their own way if they so preferred; of course, they were also free not to answer a particular question if they felt that they could not answer it.) Standardization is an important consideration in all quantitative research. A few of the questions in some of the questionnaire forms used (questionnaire *Forms 3, 4, 5,* and *6*), however, were of the open-ended type, to allow respondents complete freedom in answering. The main purpose of these questions was to give respondents the opportunity to expand or elaborate their position in connection with certain issues or subjects that were best answerable in a free, unstructured manner.

Unlike the questionnaire forms, the three interview forms consisted mainly of open-ended questions and were intended to supplement the standardized-type questions contained in the questionnaire forms. All the previously specified groups of respondents, it will be noted, filled out a questionnaire form. In addition, however, the administrator, the trustees, and the selected medical staff group of respondents from each hospital, were personally interviewed by members of our field staff, partly to secure additional information that could be more readily obtained through interviews and partly because of the high status of these respondents. Of the several forms of questionnaires listed above, questionnaire *Form 2* was the basic or key instrument in the sense of containing most of the questions that we wanted answered by most, if not all, of the several groups of respondents from each participating hospital. A great many of the specific questions in the other questionnaire forms were identical, parallel, or nearly identical (i.e., properly modified to fit the organizational position of the respondents) with most of the questions appearing in *Form 2,* and only a number of questions in the other forms were new or different questions. For these reasons, we have reproduced *Form 2* in its entirety, in Appendix A. Similarly, of the three interview forms used in the study, interview *Form 9A* (the interview for administrators) was the basic instrument to which the interviews for doctors and for trustees were keyed. Therefore, we have also reproduced this interview form in its entirety in Appendix B.

Appendix A and Appendix B together show most of the questions asked of respondents belonging to the various groups which participated in the study. Other questions that were asked in the case of particular respondent groups, but do not appear in the two appendixes, will be presented and discussed in the various chapters which follow, along with corresponding findings, as will the data which we obtained from other sources. In fact, the questions and data used to measure specific concepts and variables, as well as the measures themselves, will be presented and discussed in the appropriate individual chapters rather than here. We might only add at this point that all of the questionnaire and interview forms employed in the study, as listed above, amount to an aggregate total of about 270 mimeographed pages of questions, each page containing an average of five different questions. However, as already noted, there is considerable overlapping in the questions appearing in the different questionnaire and interview forms so that, in effect, the average individual person was asked to answer only a little more than 100 questions, requiring an average time of about one hour (the time varied, depending upon the instruments and the respondents involved, from about 45 minutes to about two hours). By comparison to *Form 2*, which is shown in Appendix A, questionnaire *Forms 1, 4, 5a, 6, 7B*, and *8B* were shorter in total length, questionnaire *Forms 3* and *5* were of approximately equal length, and questionnaire *Form 9B* was longer (this questionnaire, filled out by the hospital administrators, was the longest instrument). The interview forms administered to doctors and to trustees were shorter in total length than interview *Form 9A*, which was given to the administrators, and which is reproduced in Appendix B.

Data Collection

The process of data collection in each hospital has in part been described in an earlier section. Here, we shall continue and complete this description. The data were collected by administering the above described questionnaire and interview instruments to the groups of respondents that we have specified. In addition to the members of the research staff, a group of six professional interviewers was used to carry out the data collection operation—the same interviewers employed earlier in connection with the pretest of the research instruments in one of the two pilot hospitals. The interviewers had been trained by the Field Section of the Survey Research Center, by which they are employed, and had participated in many previous surveys. In addition, they were given special training by the research staff for the present study. With the assistance of these interviewers, data collection began on November 4, 1957, and was completed by December 13, 1957, with the exception of a few late returns of questionnaires that were mailed directly to us by a few respondents from each hospital who were absent during field work. The completion of a field operation of the present magnitude in such a short time would have been impossible without considerable preparatory work by both the research staff and the participating hospitals, and without the efforts and excellent cooperation of our interviewers and our many respondents.

The data were collected in the fall of 1957, a period of "normal" hospital functioning (after summer vacations for hospital personnel, after relatively low summer patient loads, and before the Christmas period). Each participating hospital was scheduled for a full week, during which members of the research staff and of the field staff were present at the hospital to collect the data. During some weeks, however, data collection was carried out simultaneously in two or three hospitals. Certain arrangements designed to alert hospital personnel to the field operation had, of course, preceded our arrival at the hospital on the designated date.

When we arrived at the hospital, we had complete lists of the individual persons from the various respondent groups to whom we wished to administer questionnaires and interviews. These lists contained the names and positions of the respondents, the service in which respondents were working, and their work shift, when applicable. For those of the respondents who were to fill out questionnaires only, we had placed appropriate questionnaires in individual Manila envelopes. Neither the questionnaires nor the envelopes had any identification marks, however, since all respondents without exception were promised complete anonymity and strict confidentiality for their answers. The envelopes containing the questionnaires were distributed directly to the individual respondents by members of our own staff as soon as the respondents were located, and the names of persons to whom questionnaires were distributed were checked off our lists of names. The respondents were given their questionnaire, were asked to complete it at their convenience within the next day or two, and then bring it back in the envelope we had provided directly to a member of our staff at a predesignated location in the hospital. Respondents were asked to complete their questionnaire on their own, and without any discussion with anyone else. As soon as a respondent returned with his completed questionnaire, he was asked to drop it in a box which contained other completed questionnaires, and then he was asked to tell us his name in order that we might indicate on our list (in the presence of the respondent) receipt of his questionnaire.

At the same time that we were passing out questionnaires, we began contacting respondents who were to be personally interviewed in addition to filling out a questionnaire (the selected medical staff, the trustees, and the administrator) to find a convenient time for a personal interview. Our interviewer had both the interview form and the questionnaire form for each designated respondent. Then, at the scheduled time, the interviewer would visit the respondent at the designated place and proceed to administer the interview form first, and then the questionnaire. The interview contained the most general questions to be asked of the respondent, thus enabling the interviewer to establish good rapport with the respondent. The interviewers recorded the answers of the respondents verbatim on the interview schedule, while the respondent was answering the questions. When the interview was completed, if the respondent still had time available he was handed the questionnaire form and was asked to complete it, while the interviewer was there, and then hand it back to the interviewer. (While the respondent was filling out the questionnaire, the interviewer was editing the interview just completed with the respondent.) If the respondent did not have sufficient time, he was asked to take the questionnaire with him, complete it, and then return it to a member of our staff, or the interviewer would go to pick it up personally.

Most of the individuals interviewed were interviewed in the hospital. A few of the trustees and a certain number of doctors, however, were interviewed at their private office or at their home, depending upon their wishes. All interviews were conducted in strict privacy, with only the interviewer and the interviewee present. Many of the interviews were conducted in the evening. The questionnaires were processed during the day, in the evening, and late at night, as many of the respondents were working on the afternoon and night shifts. The questionnaires were usually passed out and collected at the beginning of each shift.

Throughout the process of distributing and collecting questionnaires and interviewing, scrupulous care was taken to preserve the anonymity of our respondents and the confidentiality of their answers. Anonymity and confidentiality were promised verbally and in the instructions contained in the cover page of the questionnaire (see Appendix A). No person from the hospital was allowed in the immediate area where interviews and questionnaires were being handled by our staff, and completed instruments were at all times under the personal care of a member of the staff. Similarly, no person from the hospital was ever allowed to see any of the completed questionnaires or interviews, or the answers of any respondent. In fact, anonymity and confidentiality were always emphasized and strictly maintained from the beginning of data collection, during data collection, and afterward through the reporting of the findings. When field work was completed in each hospital, the completed instruments were taken directly to Ann Arbor by the research staff for processing.

Data were collected in each hospital during the scheduled period from the large majority of the respondents. Between 5 and 10 percent of all designated respondents from each hospital, however, were absent during the data collection operation, being on vacation, on leave, sick, or out of town. In these cases, appropriate questionnaires were left for the respondents with their respective department head. The questionnaires were placed in stamped envelopes bearing the address of the Survey Research Center (again no identifying information was contained in the questionnaires or on the envelopes) and showing only the name of the hospital where originating. The department head in each case was asked to hand out the envelopes to the designated respondents, conveying to them our request to fill out the questionnaire at their convenience and then mail it directly to us without signing their name. In this manner we could only count the number of mailed questionnaires from each respondent group and each hospital and thus compute a return rate, without being able to identify individuals who mailed in questionnaires.

The large majority of these respondents mailed their completed questionnaires to us. However, a deadline for accepting such questionnaires was set to maintain time comparability between questionnaires completed on location and mailed questionnaires. The deadline was three weeks from the completion of the data collection operation in each hospital. (A total of three questionnaires were actually returned after the deadline and were not included in the tabulations.) Finally, in the case of the few respondents who were absent during data collection but whom we wished to interview personally, we returned to some of the hospitals shortly after the field work was completed and conducted the interviews when possible.

In general, the data-collection operation was carried out as successfully as one might possibly hope, without any serious problem with individual respondents and without disrupting the normal functioning of the organizations involved. The success of the field operation exceeded our best expectations—representing a tribute to the interest and cooperation of our many respondents and a measure

Research Instruments and Data Collection

of the preparatory work and cooperation between the hospitals and our staff. We are indeed deeply grateful to the hundreds of people who helped us, and who participated in the research as respondents by giving one to two hours of their own busy time, without any remuneration, to complete our questionnaires and interviews. As the response rates discussed below indicate, the cooperation of doctors, trustees, administrators, department heads, nurses, and technicians from all hospitals was excellent, as was the cooperation of our interviewers.

Response Rates and Nonresponse

Of the grand total of 1396 initially selected individuals from the ten hospitals to participate in the study as respondents (see Table 1 in preceding section), 26 individuals (nearly 2 percent of the total) had left their respective hospitals permanently by the time of data collection. Of these 26 individuals, 10 were nonsupervisory registered nurses, 6 were aides, 4 were technicians, 3 were doctors, 2 were supervisory nurses, and 1 was a practical nurse—these figures corresponding remarkably well with the relative organizational stability and turnover characteristic of the various respondent groups, as discussed in Chapter 3. The number of potential respondents who had permanently left the organization, for any and all possible reasons, varied from hospital to hospital, ranging between 0 and 9, with an average of 2.6 persons per hospital. No substitute replacements were made for these 26 individuals who had gone, however, since they were no longer members of the organizations studied. Therefore, excluding these people, the actual number of possible respondents from the ten participating hospitals was 1370.

Questionnaires and interviews were eventually handed out or administered to 1319 of the 1370 possible respondents, i.e., to 96.3 percent of all designated potential respondents. In other words, we failed to reach a total of only 51 persons, or an average of 5 individuals per hospital. (This number varied across individual hospitals from a low of 2 to a high of 10 persons.) Of these 51 individuals, 41 would have only taken questionnaires and 10 would have been interviewed in addition. Of the 51 unreachable respondents, 13 were doctors, 9 were technicians, 9 were nonsupervisory nurses, 7 were supervisory nurses, 6 were trustees, 6 were aides, and 1 was a department head. The reasons for not reaching these people were many and varied: some individuals were part-time members who were working in the hospital only occasionally; some were indefinitely absent because of illness or leave; some were on extended vacation or extended travel; and some were not planning to return to the hospital, even though they had not been officially terminated. The important point is that neither questionnaires nor interviews were administered to these individuals, and no questionnaires were left for them to complete and mail to us later. For all practical purposes, this was an unavailable and unreachable group of potential respondents.

Thus, the total number of available respondents from all ten hospitals combined turned out to be 1319. All these individuals were given the opportunity to complete a questionnaire or both an interview and a questionnaire either at the time of data collection or, in a number of cases, by completing questionnaires which we left for them at the hospital. (This latter was a group of individuals who, for various reasons, were absent from the hospital during data collection but who were expected to return shortly thereafter.) Of the 1319 available respondents,

TABLE 3. Attained Gross and Net Response Rates for all Respondent Groups Combined, but Separately for Each Participating Hospital *

Participating Hospital	All Respondent Groups Combined			
	Gross Response Rate (percent)	N's Involved	Net Response Rate (percent)	N's Involved
#0	91	(157/172)	94	(157/167)
1	91	(137/151)	97	(137/141)
2	93	(117/126)	95	(117/123)
3	94	(108/115)	100	(108/108)
4	94	(131/140)	96	(131/136)
5	91	(110/121)	95	(110/116)
6	92	(144/156)	98	(144/147)
7	92	(112/122)	93	(112/120)
8	95	(145/152)	97	(145/149)
9	90	(104/115)	93	(104/112)
All Hospitals Combined:	92.3	(1265/1370)	95.9	(1265/1319)

* The gross response rate is always smaller than the net response rate. The former is computed by dividing the number of respondents who finally provided the data requested of them by the total number of possible respondents. The latter is computed by dividing the number of respondents who finally provided the data requested of them by the total number of available respondents. The total number of available respondents is somewhat smaller than the total number of possible respondents because it does not include a few individuals (a total of 51 persons from the ten hospitals) who were absent for extended periods and could not be reached to be given questionnaires or interviews. The rates are computed on the basis of the numbers of individuals shown in the parentheses.

1265 finally completed their questionnaires and interviews, making the overall net response rate attained by the study 96 percent. (The gross response rate was 92 percent. This is computed by dividing 1265 by 1370, i.e., the number of respondents who finally provided data by the total number of possible respondents regardless of their availability.)

Stated differently, of the 1319 available potential respondents only 54 did not finally complete their questionnaires as intended, although they were given the opportunity to do so. This group of 54 "nonrespondents" averages 5.4 persons per hospital, the number varying across hospital between 0 and 10 individuals but with nine of the hospitals contributing three or more nonrespondents each. The nonrespondents were: 26 doctors, 11 nonsupervisory nurses, 7 technicians, 6 aides and orderlies, 3 supervisory nurses, and 1 department head. All 54 persons were supposed to have completed questionnaires only, i.e., none were individuals scheduled for interviewing.

The reasons accounting for the failure of these 54 individuals to provide us with the requested data varied widely. Some of these people belonged to the group of respondents for whom we had left questionnaires at the hospital, but they failed to mail their questionnaires to us or, in the case of the three individuals mentioned earlier, they returned their questionnaires too late. Some others filled only a small

Research Instruments and Data Collection

TABLE 4. Average Gross and Net Response Rates for Each Group of Respondents, For All Participating Hospitals Combined *

Respondent Group	Average Gross Response Rate (percent)	N's Involved	Average Net Response Rate (percent)	N's Involved
Hospital administrators	100	(10/10)	100	(10/10)
Trustees	88	(46/52)	100	(46/46)
Doctors †	87	(252/291)	91	(252/278)
Department heads ‡	98	(101/103)	99	(101/102)
Supervisory nurses	95	(172/182)	98	(172/175)
Nonsupervisory nurses § (registered and practical)	95	(356/376)	97	(356/367)
Aides and orderlies ‖	90	(203/215)	97	(203/209)
Laboratory and x-ray technicians #	89	(125/141)	95	(125/132)
All Respondent Groups:	92.3	(1265/1370)	95.9	(1265/1319)

* The gross response rate is in most instances smaller than the net response rate, and is computed by dividing the number of respondents who finally provided data by the total number of possible respondents in each case. The net response rate is computed by dividing the total number of respondents who finally provided data by the total number of available-reachable respondents. The rates are based on the numbers of individuals shown in the parentheses.

† This group of 252 final doctor respondents, from the ten hospitals, consists of 121 members of the selected medical staff group (as previously defined) and 131 members of the general medical staff group (as previously defined).

‡ This group includes the ten directors of nursing, who have not been included with the supervisory nurses group in this table.

§ This group of 356 final nurse respondents consists of 196 registered nurses, 140 practical nurses, and 20 nurses who failed to indicate their classification (registered or practical).

‖ This group of 203 aides and orderlies consists of 153 aides and 50 orderlies.

This group of 125 technicians consists of 78 laboratory technicians and 47 x-ray technicians from the ten hospitals.

part of their questionnaire and for this reason they were classified as nonrespondents. A few others returned their questionnaires without filling them out, i.e., completely blank (some returned them blank at the hospital during data collection, while others mailed them blank later). Finally, a few individuals refused to participate outright for personal reasons. These refusals accounted for about 5 percent of all the nonrespondents. (Of the some 1300 individuals from the ten hospitals only 54 were finally classified as nonrespondents, and of these only 3 individuals refused to participate in the study in any manner.)

In summary, then, a grand total of 1265 individual respondents from the ten participating hospitals out of a maximum possible total of 1370 respondents provided requested data, yielding an overall gross response rate of 92 percent. And of a grand total of 1319 available (as defined above) respondents, 1265 returned completed questionnaires and interviews, yielding an overall net response rate of 96 percent. The response rate attained in the study is, thus, very satisfactory by comparison to studies of a similar research design. It clearly eliminates the possibility of bias due to no response and provides one indication of the extent of cooperation and interest of the respondents. Equally important, in this connection, is the fact that the response rates attained are high in each and every hospital, for each and every respondent group involved—something due, in large measure, to the sensitivity and painstaking efforts of the field staff toward both attaining a maximum response rate and avoiding the possibility of having any particular respondent group contribute disproportionately to the final nonresponse rate.

Tables 3 and 4, pp. 68, 69, summarize the attained response rates in each participating hospital and for each group of respondents. Table 3 shows the gross response rate and net response rate for all respondent groups combined, but separately for each hospital. Table 4 shows the average gross response rate and the average net response rate for all ten hospitals combined, but separately for each major group of respondents.

Distribution of Final Respondents by Respondent Group and Hospital, and the Reaction of Respondents to the Questionnaire They Completed

The response rates discussed above were computed on the basis of the final number of individual persons from the ten hospitals who participated in the study by completing questionnaires, or both questionnaires and personal interviews. A total of 1265 individuals, or an average of about 127 persons per hospital, make up this group of final respondents. Table 5, below, shows how these respondents are distributed across the ten participating hospitals, and among the different groups of hospital personnel which were included in the research. As shown in this table, each hospital was finally represented in the study by at least 100 individual respondents, the total number of final individual respondents from each hospital ranging from a low of 104 to a high of 157. (The reader may wish to compare Table 5 with Table 2, presented earlier, which showed the number of initially selected individuals from each group and each participating hospital.) In summary, the ten hospitals together are represented in the study by the following respondents, who provided the data requested of them: 10 hospital administrators; 46 trustees; 252 doctors; 101 department heads (including the 10 directors of nursing); 172 supervisory nurses (excluding the directors of nursing); 196 nonsupervisory registered nurses; 140 practical nurses; 203 aides and orderlies; 125 laboratory and x-ray technicians; plus another 20 nurses who failed to indicate whether they were registered or practical nurses. The majority of the findings presented in subsequent chapters are based on the data which these respondents provided. For the major background characteristics of the different respondents, as well as for additional information concerning their organizational characteristics and positions in the hospital, see Chapter 3.

At this point, the question might be raised as to how the respondents reacted toward the research. In addition to being interesting, this is a rather important question, for its answer tells us something about the quality of the data that we were able to obtain from the respondents—on which data most of our findings are based. Judging by a number of different things, and apart from our personal

Research Instruments and Data Collection

TABLE 5. Final Number of Respondents from Each Respondent Group and Each Participating Hospital

Respondent Group	#0	1	2	3	4	5	6	7	8	9	Group Total (All Hospitals)
Selected medical staff	19	11	11	11	9	11	11	13	15	10	121
General medical staff	16	16	10	15	11	11	11	16	13	12	131
Supervisory nurses *	25	17	19	17	20	13	36	5	16	14	182
Nonsupervisory registered nurses	20	19	22	15	27	18	14	20	23	18	196
Practical nurses	17	10	13	14	19	11	8	14	21	13	140
Aides and orderlies	25	26	18	12	20	22	26	20	22	12	203
Laboratory and x-ray technicians	21	18	8	8	10	10	15	11	16	8	125
Administrative department heads †	9	8	7	8	9	9	12	9	10	10	91
Trustees	4	4	4	4	4	4	7	3	6	6	46
Hospital administrators	1	1	1	1	1	1	1	1	1	1	10
Hospital Totals:	157	130	113	105	130	110	141	112	143	104	1245 ‡

* Includes the director of nursing in each hospital, and all nurses in supervisory positions from head nurse on up.

† Does not include the director of nursing, who is also a department head but who has been included with the supervisory nurses in this table.

‡ In addition to this total of 1245 final respondents, another 20 nurse respondents from the various hospitals completed questionnaires, but because they failed to indicate their particular nursing classification (i.e., whether they were registered or practical nurses) they are excluded from this table. The final grand total of individual respondents in the study is, of course, 1265 persons (1245 + 20).

impressions, it is possible to provide an answer to this question. As the following evidence indicates, the answer is that the respondents reacted with considerable interest, very favorably, and very cooperatively. First, the gross and net response rates attained by the study attest to the high interest of the respondents and to the cooperation they accorded us. The actual degree of interest and cooperation on the part of the respondents is probably even higher than the response rates suggest, moreover, if we take into account: (1) the fact that only 3 out of more than 1300 individuals from the ten hospitals refused to cooperate in the research, (2) the fact that the entire process of data collection was carried out extremely smoothly, rapidly, and without any unpleasant incidents or disruptions to the normal functioning of the hospitals, and (3) the fact that respondent interest and cooperation were high in each and every hospital, and on the part of each and every group of respondents involved.

Second, the degree of interest and cooperation of the respondents may be inferred from the fact that the vast majority of them answered all, or virtually all, of the many questions contained in their questionnaires and interviews—with a good number of respondents volunteering additional information in the form

TABLE 6. Respondent Reaction to the Questionnaire Forms Used in the Study, as Indicated by the Percentage of Respondents from Each Group Who Gave Certain Answers to the Question: "Now That You Have Filled It out, How Do You Feel about This Questionnaire?" *

Percentage of Group Members, for All Hospitals Combined, Who Felt That Their Particular Questionnaire Was:

Respondent Group	"Excellent," or "Very Good" ("it covers everything" or "almost everything that I feel is important")	"Good" ("it covers most things that I feel are important")	"Fair" ("it covers some important things, but misses others")	"Poor" ("it misses the things that I feel are important")	N
General medical staff †	46	36	15	3	120
Supervisory nurses (excluding directors of nursing)	52	37	10	1	167
Nonsupervisory registered nurses	47	33	17	3	190
Practical nurses	61	26	12	1	131
Aides and orderlies	65	26	8	1	186
Laboratory and x-ray technicians	51	39	10	0	110
Administrative department heads (including directors of nursing)	68	27	4	1	98
Trustees	83	17	0	0	46
Hospital administrators	90	10	0	0	10
All Respondent Groups Combined ‡	57	31	11	1	1058

* The data shown are from respondents who filled out questionnaires, and pertain to the particular questionnaire forms that were administered to each respondent group, as earlier specified.

† The selected medical staff group of 121 respondents, as earlier specified, is not included here. Respondents from the selected medical staff completed a different questionnaire in addition to being personally interviewed, but they were not asked the present question in their questionnaire.

‡ A grand total of 1058 individuals answered the present question, and 604 of them, or 57 percent, indicated that their questionnaire was "excellent" or "very good." Of those who said that their questionnaire was excellent or very good, 34 percent said excellent and 66 percent said very good.

of writing in comments on their questionnaires. The instances where a particular question was not answered by at least 90 percent of the specified respondents are indeed very rare. When data from the few questions that were not answered by more than 90 percent of the respondents involved are discussed in later chapters, special mention of the response rate will be made.

Forms of Description, Measurement, and Analysis 73

A third piece of evidence for the high interest and cooperation of our respondents is the attainment of high response rates regardless of the facts that: (1) practically all respondents were very busy people, (2) participation in the study was completely voluntary for all respondents, and (3) participation meant that the average respondent give free between one and two hours of his time in order to complete the research instrument(s) specified for him.

Finally, the preceding, and more or less inferential, evidence concerning the interest and involvement of the respondents in the research is further corroborated and reinforced by the respondents' own appraisal of the questionnaires which they were asked to complete voluntarily, anonymously, and confidentially. Specifically, the very last question appearing in each questionnaire form used in the study (except for the form completed by the selected medical staff group of respondents) was especially designed to provide direct information on how the respondents felt about their questionnaires. The question was:

Now that you have filled it out, how do you feel about this questionnaire? (Check one.)

_____(1) Excellent; it covers everything that I feel is important.
_____(2) Very good; it covers almost (about) everything that I feel is important.
_____(3) Good; it covers most things that I feel are important.
_____(4) Fair; it covers some important things, but misses others.
_____(5) Poor; it misses the things that I feel are important.

The data from this question, summarized in Table 6, provide strong support for the conclusion that the respondents reacted with great interest and very favorably toward the research. Of all those who answered the question, Table 6 shows 57 percent considered their questionnaire as "excellent" or "very good"—as covering all, or nearly all, things that the respondents themselves felt are important. An additional 31 percent of the respondents considered their questionnaire as "good" —as covering most things that they felt are important. By contrast, only the remaining 12 percent of the respondents considered their questionnaire as less than good: 11 percent considered it as "fair" (covers some important things, but misses others), and only 1 percent considered it as "poor." For a more detailed picture of how respondents belonging to particular respondent groups answered the above question and for the numbers of respondents involved, see Table 6.

FORMS OF DESCRIPTION AND MEASUREMENT, AND ANALYSIS TECHNIQUES

The data obtained from the respondents, as well as from the other sources used, constitute the basic materials for the discussion and findings contained in all subsequent chapters, where the primary purpose is to describe the results of the research. The objective of this section is to familiarize the reader with certain aspects of this description process. How are the data treated and summarized? How are the measures for the concepts and variables of the study derived from the data? How are relationships between independent and dependent variables ascertained? How are such relationships interpreted? And, generally, how are the data treated and analyzed? These are the questions which we will try to answer here in a brief and rather nontechnical manner. More details will be presented, when appropriate, in the various individual chapters. Nonessential technicalities will be avoided, however, and, as far as possible, an attempt will be made to present data and results that are similar in a consistently uniform manner.

The first of the above questions on how the data are summarized is relatively simple and easy to answer. Some of the data are presented in the form of qualitative descriptions concerning different aspects of hospital structure and functioning. Our earlier discussion about what hospitals and groups of respondents were selected for study, including many of the criteria of selection, or about the kinds of data we collected, for example, illustrates the qualitative mode of description. Similarly, most of the data in Chapter 4, which contains a brief profile for each participating hospital based on organizational documents, interview excerpts, and volunteered comments by a number of respondents from each institution, are summarized and presented in the form of qualitative-descriptive statements. Information contained in such statements as "all of the hospital administrators in the study are male," "nursing personnel from all shifts and all classifications participated in the study," "the problems of greatest concern to the medical staff are . . . ," "all hospitals are located in Michigan cities," and "Hospital X is not a Blue Cross hospital" also represents the qualitative form of description.

However, most of the data and findings will be summarized and reported in a quantitative form, which presupposes such measurement processes as those of counting, ordering, summation, multiplication, etc., and which involves the use of numbers, percentages, proportions, averages, or other scores. In other words, the quantitative mode of description requires some mathematical manipulation of the data. Although most of the data will be converted into numerical form and presented in a quantitative manner, most of the measuring devices that will be used are rather simple and require no special mathematical knowledge on the part of the reader. This will become clear in the next few paragraphs. In addition, of course, quantitative expressions will in most instances be accompanied by qualitative, interpretative, or explanatory comments.

The familiar percentage figures constitute one of the quantitative forms of measurement and presentation that we will use. Table 6 in the preceding section illustrates the use of percentages. Examining Table 6, for example, we see that 46 percent of all doctors from the general medical staff group of respondents considered the questionnaire which they completed excellent or very good, while another 36 percent of them considered it good. We also see that 52 percent of all supervisory nurses from all participating hospitals combined considered their questionnaire excellent or very good, etc. In other cases, instead of percentages, we will use proportions—another familiar tool. Statements such as "one out of every five supervisory nurses believes . . . ," "department heads devote .35 of their total working time to . . . ," and "three-fourths of the nonsupervisory registered nurses in the study feel . . . ," for example, illustrate the use of proportions.

Frequently, we will use rank-orders to present the data. For example, we will order or arrange the ten participating hospitals with reference to a particular characteristic or variable, such as size, to show their relative position with one

Forms of Description, Measurement, and Analysis 75

another. To rank-order the ten hospitals according to their size, for instance, we will begin with the largest (or smallest) institution and assign to it the number 1. Next, we will assign number 2 to the second-largest (or second-smallest) hospital, and continue to complete the rank-order by assigning the number 10 to the smallest (or largest) of the ten institutions. We may, of course, use rank-orders not only with reference to hospital size, but also with reference to other variables representing quantitative or qualitative characteristics of the hospital situation—provided that, in each case, the ten hospitals can be arranged in relation to one another from the highest (or lowest) scoring hospital through the lowest (or highest) scoring hospital. The hospital with the highest or most favorable score on a particular variable can be assigned the number 1, or first place, the hospital with the second highest or second most favorable score can be assigned the number 2, etc., until the ordering is completed with the lowest or least favorably scoring hospital being assigned the number 10. In general, it is possible to rank-order the ten hospitals on the basis of percentages, proportions, means (or averages), or some other score.

In a great many cases, we will use arithmetic means, popularly referred to as "averages," on the basis of which to rank-order the hospitals, before pursuing particular analyses further. Means are especially useful because, very often, they can best summarize and represent the answers to a particular question given by a group of respondents (or by several groups of respondents). When we want to represent the answers of an entire group of individuals, and we are not merely interested in the answer given by a single person, by certain particular persons, or by a fraction of the total group membership, the arithmetic mean is likely to prove very useful. Mean scores, unlike proportions and percentage figures, make this representation possible while, at the same time, they take into account the nature of the answer given by each and every group member involved. A single percentage figure, or proportion, cannot ordinarily summarize all of the data from a particular question that was asked of a group of respondents, while a single mean score can (provided, of course, that it is possible to compute it from the data). Means have certain additional technical advantages over proportions and percentages (e.g., when dealing with relatively few cases, say ten cases, mean scores are likely to be more stable measures than percentage figures; under certain conditions, means can themselves be averaged, while percentages cannot; etc.), but these need not concern us here. What is of importance is that means can be used to depict the responses, position, and characteristics of an entire group of respondents, or of several such groups combined. When we recall from our earlier discussion that the main unit of analysis and hypothesis-testing in this study is the group, or the organization (i.e., the hospital), rather than the individual, it is easy to see why the use of means will occupy a prominent place in this volume.

How means are derived from the data is a technical question that goes beyond the scope of the present section. However, for the benefit of some of our readers, we might use a simple illustration at this point. Let us once more refer to Table 6, in the preceding section, and to some of the data reported in it, specifically the data from the practical nurses group. In Table 6, we find that 131 practical nurses (of a possible 140) from the ten participating hospitals answered the question "Now that you have filled it out, how do you feel about this questionnaire?" Of the 131 who answered this question, 61 percent indicated that their questionnaire was excellent or very good (not shown in the table, 25 percent said excellent and another 36 percent said very good), 26 percent indicated that their questionnaire was good, 12 percent indicated that their questionnaire was fair, and the remaining 1 percent indicated that their questionnaire was poor. Now, instead of using all these figures, to represent the attitude of practical nurses toward their questionnaire, we could compute the arithmetic mean, i.e., a single score, from the original data. To obtain the mean, we need (1) to know how many of the practical nurses gave each of the various answers possible—how many said excellent, very good, good, fair, or poor (that is, we must know the frequency distribution of all the responses), and (2) we need to assign a different value to each of the five possible answers.

In the present illustration, the frequency distribution of the answers practical nurses gave to the above question is as follows: 33 nurses considered their questionnaire as excellent, 47 considered it as very good, 34 considered it as good, 16 considered it as fair, and 1 considered it as poor. Next, looking back at the question from which the data were obtained, and examining the response alternatives listed under the question, as presented earlier, we find that each of the five alternatives is preceded by a number, in the following manner: (1) excellent, (2) very good, (3) good, (4) fair, and (5) poor. The numbers preceding the five alternatives are the values that we need to assign to the corresponding answers given by the practical nurses in order to compute the mean. The next step is to multiply the number of nurses who gave each particular answer with the value assigned to that answer, add the products, and then divide the total sum by the total number of nurses involved.

This last step can be expressed as follows: 33 × 1, plus 47 × 2, plus 34 × 3, plus 16 × 4, plus 1 × 5 divided by 131; or, 33 plus 94 plus 102 plus 64 plus 5 divided by 131; or, 298 divided by 131, which yields a score of 2.27. This last score is the arithmetic mean that we wanted computed. In the present case, i.e., with reference to the particular question and response alternatives involved, a mean score of 2.27 corresponds closely to the value that had been assigned to one of the five response alternatives, namely to the alternative "very good," which has a value of exactly 2.00. We can, then, say that the obtained mean shows that, as a group, practical nurses considered the questionnaire which they filled out as "very good." Incidentally, we may also point out here that the five response alternatives offered by the above question form what is known as a five-point scale. Theoretically, when means are computed on the basis of five-point scales, such as the above, they can vary between 1.00 and 5.00. In the present case, of course, the obtained mean happened to be 2.27. (Most of the questions shown in Appendix A were specifically designed to elicit answers in terms of a five-point scale in each case.)

Means can, of course, be computed not only for the practical nurses group of respondents, but also for each of the other respondent groups which participated in the study. In fact, with reference to a particular questionnaire item, means can be obtained separately for each group of respondents from each individual hospital, for a given group of respondents from the ten hospitals combined, and for two or more groups of respondents from the same hospital or from all hospitals

Forms of Description, Measurement, and Analysis

—provided that the questionnaire item was answered in terms of a five-point scale (or some other scale), and was answered by all of the respondent groups which we wish to include in computing the desired means. Henceforth, when using a mean which is based on the answers of several groups of respondents representing a hospital, we shall refer to that mean as a "hospital mean." From a technical standpoint, the computation of a hospital mean is somewhat more complex than the preceding illustration. Generally, it requires that we first compute the mean separately for each of the respondent groups involved (remember different groups of respondents had been selected on the basis of different sampling rates), and then properly combine and average these several group means to obtain the hospital mean. This combining and averaging process necessitates that each group mean be weighted by the sampling rate with which the members of the group had been chosen to participate in the study as respondents—a procedure which we have used very extensively, since we were mainly interested in obtaining measures which reflect the total hospital situation (e.g., in obtaining hospital means) rather than in the characteristics of specific respondent groups or individuals.

Further Considerations on Measurement and Analysis

The different concepts and variables with which the study is concerned will be measured by converting the original relevant data into one or more of the different kinds of scores we have just discussed—percentages, proportions, rank-orders, simple arithmetic means, and weighted means or hospital means—and then assigning to each hospital its respective score on each of the variables involved. In certain cases, when we will be dealing with multifaceted concepts such as the concept of organizational coordination rather than with simple variables, more complex measurement procedures will be used. In these cases, the procedure employed will be described and explained at the appropriate place. In fact, the particular data and measures used in connection with each concept and variable studied and reported will in every case be indicated, before engaging in the testing of specific hypotheses or in analyses aimed to show how a given variable relates to another. Consequently, we need not go into further detail about the problems of measurement at this point. It would be worth while, however, to say something about the more frequent techniques of analysis that we will be using and about the interpretation of the results.

The main purpose of analysis is to show how, and to what extent, the concepts and variables (or their corresponding measures) with which the study deals are interrelated. For each pair of variables studied, we first want to know whether or not the two variables are related, i.e., whether they are associated or they are independent of each other. For example, is coordination related to the quality of patient care in the various hospitals? Second, if two variables are found to be interrelated, we want to know the degree (high or low) of the relationship between them, or how closely they are related. Third, in addition to the degree of the relationship, we want to know the direction of the relationship. Is the relationship between the two variables a positive one or a negative one? (The relationship would be positive if an increase in the value of one variable is accompanied by an increase in the value of the other, or if a decrease in value of one variable is accompanied by a decrease in the value of the other; the relationship would be negative if an increase in the value of one variable is accompanied by a decrease in the value of the other.) Fourth, in addition to ascertaining the presence of a relationship between two variables, the magnitude of the relationship, and the direction of the relationship, we want to know how much confidence we can place in the obtained relationship. In other words, we want to know whether we are dealing with a "real" relationship—a relationship which is likely to recur, or whether the obtained relationship could be attributed to mere chance or coincidence rather than to the nature of the variables.

In most cases, the above objectives can be satisfied by using a standard correlational technique as the statistical tool of analysis and hypothesis-testing. For this reason, in most of our analyses we have used the correlational technique. More specifically, we have typically used rank-order correlations. The conventional rank-order correlation is the most appropriate technique for a number of reasons: (1) Since the unit of analysis in this study is the hospital and not individual respondents, the number of cases with which we are dealing is relatively small, namely ten hospitals; and for an N of 10 the rank-order correlation is more suitable than the product-moment correlation. (2) The rank-order correlation makes fewer statistical-mathematical assumptions about the nature of the available data and measures than the product-moment correlation, and the assumptions which it makes are met by our data. (In technical terms, because of the ordinal nature of many of our measures, a nonparametric correlation technique, such as the rank-order correlation, should be used.) And (3) the rank-order correlation is simpler, more familiar, more preferable, and generally more appropriate for our purposes than other correlational techniques available (e.g., tau-correlations, biserial correlations, etc.).

The procedure of computing the rank-order correlation between two variables, e.g., between some aspect of organizational coordination and the quality of nursing care in the participating hospitals, is relatively simple. First, hospital means (or other scores) are obtained from the data as the measures of the variables involved. In the example cited here, one set of ten hospital means, or other scores instead of means (one mean for each hospital), is required to measure the variable of coordination, and another set of ten means is required to measure the variable of nursing care. Then, the hospitals are rank-ordered, from one through ten, according to the magnitude of their respective mean, or score, on (1) the variable of coordination (which is represented by the first of the above two sets of means), and (2) the variable of nursing care (which is represented by the second set of means). Having rank-ordered the ten hospitals with respect to the coordination variable and the nursing care variable, we can proceed to compute the rank-order correlation between the two variables, using the conventional rank-order correlation formula. The same procedure may, of course, be applied to any pair of variables other than the pair we have chosen here to illustrate the procedure. The formula and the mechanics of computing the correlation take us beyond the scope of the present discussion. And, since they can be found in any general text of statistics, we shall dispense with any further details regarding computations at this point.

In any event, the end result of computing the correlation between two variables is expressed in numerical form and is referred to as the correlation coefficient,

Forms of Description, Measurement, and Analysis

or simply as the correlation. (Most of the tables in most subsequent chapters will show correlation coefficients.) Correlation coefficients can vary in size from a minimum of 0.00 to a maximum of ±1.00. A correlation of zero simply means that the two variables are not related; they are totally unrelated and completely independent of each other. A correlation of ±1.00, which in practice occurs very rarely, means that the two variables are perfectly related; for all practical purposes, the two variables are identical (which means that we are likely to be dealing with only one variable instead of two as we had thought), so that knowing the value of one variable you also know the exact value of the other variable. The sign, plus or minus, preceding the coefficient indicates the direction of the correlation, i.e., whether the two variables are related positively or negatively. (Usually, however, the plus sign is omitted when presenting positive correlation coefficients.)

The vast majority of correlations obtained in this study, or any other study for that matter, are neither zero nor perfect, i.e., ±1.00; they fall between these two extremes. The more closely a particular correlation approaches the maximum value of ±1.00, the higher, or the greater, the relationship which it signifies. Conversely, the more closely a correlation approaches zero, the smaller the relationship between the variables involved. The question then arises as to how high a particular correlation coefficient has to be in order that we may be confident that it is unlikely to represent a relationship attributable to mere chance or coincidence rather than to the nature of the variables involved. In other words, what are the odds that a correlation of a given size is or is not significant (i.e., is or is not significantly different from zero)—what are the odds that it really represents, or does not represent, an actual relationship or connection between the two variables involved?

Available statistical tools provide an answer to this question. In its general form, the answer is that, whether or not a particular correlation is significantly different from zero (or, simply, significant) depends upon: (1) the size of the correlation; (2) the number of cases involved, or the N on the basis of which the correlation was computed (in the present study, and for most cases, $N = 10$, or the number of cases is equal to the number of hospitals for which we have data); (3) the kind of correlational technique used which, in the present study, is the rank-order correlation technique; and (4) on certain other statistical considerations. If we know these things, we can then make a precise statement indicating the odds that the correlation is or is not significant.

More concretely, assuming an N of 10 (as is the case for most of the correlations that we will present), which is equal to the number of participating hospitals, and assuming that a rank-order correlation technique was used, we can then say that for a correlation to be significant (or significantly different from zero) at the .05 level it must be as great as ±.56 (actually, ±.564) or higher, and to be statistically significant at the .01 level it must be as great as ±.75 (actually, ±.746) or greater. What matters here is the size of the correlation not its sign —whether the correlation is positive or negative is irrelevant from the standpoint of its statistical significance. The values of ±.56, for the .05 level of confidence, and ±.75, for the .01 level of confidence, are known as the critical values of the rank-order correlation coefficient and are computed on the basis of statistical-mathematical considerations rather than arbitrarily. However, these critical values remain the same as long as we are dealing with rank-order correlations based on an N of 10 cases.

The only remaining point to be explained here is the meaning of the statement that a correlation of $\pm.56$ is significant at the .05 level, or that a correlation of $\pm.75$ is significant at the .01 level. Saying that a correlation of $\pm.56$ is significant at the .05 level means that a correlation of this particular size, or of higher size, could be due to chance, or could have been obtained by pure chance, only 5 percent of the time; the odds are only 1 in 20 that a correlation as large or larger than $\pm.56$ would not be significantly different from zero, and 19 to 20 that it would be significantly different from zero. In other words, we can be confident that, in 95 instances out of every 100 instances, a correlation as large as $\pm.56$ could not be the result of chance and, consequently, the probability is high that the variables involved are actually correlated. Similarly, saying that a correlation of $\pm.75$ is statistically significant at the .01 level means that a correlation of this particular size, or of greater size, could be attributed to chance only 1 percent of the time, or once in every hundred instances.

Thus, when later in the tables, we see correlations as large as $\pm.56$ or higher, we can be confident that such correlations are significant—that these represent relationships which are very unlikely to be due to chance (provided, of course that the correlations are based on an N of 10 cases, or hospitals in our case). More precisely, we can be confident of their significance "at the .05 level." When dealing with correlations that are significant at the .05 level or better (e.g., the .01 level), i.e., with correlations as large as $\pm.56$ or larger, we shall refer to them as significant, and to the relationships which they represent as significant relationships. In the case where a correlation approaches $\pm.56$ rather closely (technically, when it is significant at the .10 level, or between the .10 and the .05 level, but not quite at the .05 level), we shall call it suggestive rather than significant. When a correlation is not close to .56 (e.g., for correlations having a size falling between 0.00 and $\pm.40$), we shall call it nonsignficant, for such a correlation is not significantly different from zero (at least at the .10 level) and it could be due, therefore, to chance 10 or more times in 100 times. (Frequently, knowing that a particular correlation, or relationship, is statistically significant at a particular level of confidence is not sufficient to prove or negate a given hypothesis. The researcher must examine the total pattern of all available correlations that are relevant to the hypothesis in order to arrive at the proper conclusion. Such an examination will be made in connection with many of the hypotheses of the study.)

Now, the analysis does not cease when we have determined that the correlations we have obtained, or the relationships between the variables represented by these correlations, are statistically significant. We also want to be able to account for the obtained relationships, i.e., to understand the relationships, as much as possible. This takes us into the province of interpretation and explanation. Interpretation and explanation link the obtained empirical relationships (e.g., the correlational findings) to the theory, the concepts, and the hypotheses that have led the researcher, in the first place, to investigate and measure the relationship between the variables with which he is dealing. In addition, of course, interpretation and explanation provide the basis for the conclusions that one can draw from the

Forms of Description, Measurement, and Analysis

results of the analysis. In practice, analysis and interpretation and explanation are often overlapping and, sometimes, inseparable processes. They are all coordinated and integrated with the theoretical framework and hypotheses on which the research has been built. Stated differently, one major purpose of analysis and interpretation is to determine how well (or how poorly) the empirical findings and relationships fit the hypotheses of the study. If the results of the analysis are on the whole consistent with the initial hypotheses and theory, then the theory itself accounts for the results. But, if the results are not as expected, or as predicted by the theory, then further explanation and interpretation are essential in order to understand the findings. (These statements, of course, apply much more to what we have termed as explanatory studies earlier in this chapter than to research of the exploratory kind; in the latter case we usually have little theory and few, if any, hypotheses to go by.)

Interpretation and explanation, however, do not only involve finding out whether the obtained empirical results are consistent with the initial underlying theory or whether they support the hypotheses investigated. Certainly, this is one crucial objective. Another important objective is to try to find out how pure and unambiguous the obtained relationships are, apart from the question of their statistical significance which, presumably, has been answered in the affirmative at this stage. For example, it is often important to find out if there are any limiting conditions that surround an obtained relationship, and whether corresponding qualifications should be made on the basis of available knowledge.

Similarly, it is often important, especially in suspect cases, to determine whether an obtained relationship is more apparent than real—whether it is spurious rather than genuine. A relationship between two variables is likely to be spurious if it is due to, or caused by, the intervention of some third variable, whether this outside variable is known (or measured) or not. A relationship between two variables may, of course, be either totally or partly spurious, depending on how much of it is attributable to a foreign variable. Along the same lines, it is also important to guard against contaminated or confounded findings. Sometimes, an obtained relationship, even though statistically significant, may actually be due not to the nature of the variables involved, but to the fact that the measures used for the variables are somehow faulty (e.g., when, in technical terms, the measures of the independent and the dependent variable lack operational independence). In cases of this kind, the obtained relationship will, in whole or in part, have resulted from the contamination involved in our measures of the variables and cannot be said to represent social reality. This discussion should give the reader some idea of what is involved in the analytical and interpretative stages of research. For a more comprehensive discussion of analysis problems encountered in survey research, see Hyman (5). In general, good theory and good methodology, apart from reason, experience, and common sense, are the requirements for obtaining useful and clear-cut results from a research project.

We have discussed the problems of analysis and interpretation that are more frequently encountered when using correlational techniques to sensitize the reader about methodological matters that are relevant to most of the findings presented in the various chapters. Some of the findings, however, are not based on correlational analysis. In certain cases, we have used different techniques. For example, to test some hypotheses, it was necessary to compare or contrast the situation prevailing in the individual participating hospitals, using means, percentages, or rank-orders rather than correlations. Similarly, in connection with certain data, it was necessary to use a statistical technique which permits a test of the significance of the difference between mean scores. In another case, it was necessary to use a rather complex analysis technique known as factor-analysis. In the cases where we used some analysis technique other than the correlational technique, we attempted to discuss the meaning of the results in sufficient detail and in a rather nontechnical manner. The objective was to avoid burdening the reader with further technical matters, while treating the material in a manner understandable to him.

METHODOLOGICAL LIMITATIONS

Perhaps the most serious limitation, but also the greatest advantage, of the research design described in the preceding pages, is the deliberate restriction of the population of hospitals studied. In this connection, it will be recalled that, early in the research, the decision was made to confine the study to a particular group (population or universe) of hospitals. This was done to avoid a great many methodological and theoretical difficulties that would have been introduced as a result of the many differences (the great variance) characterizing the broader population of hospitals of which the hospitals studied constitute a subpopulation. Of course, there were other reasons arguing in favor of delimiting the population of hospitals to be covered, not the least of which was the relative paucity of prior research in the hospital field relevant to the objectives of the present study, coupled with the accompanying necessity for structuring the study in a partly exploratory and partly explanatory way. In any event, the net advantage of restricting the population covered is that serious pitfalls in interpreting and explaining the findings could be avoided, because the variance across hospitals with respect to such characteristics as might have a bearing upon the phenomena being studied was reduced by design. This means, in effect, that, as a consequence of the restriction of the population, the results of the study are much more "pure" and unambiguous than they would otherwise be.

Unfortunately, however, restricting the population also means that the results cannot be extrapolated and generalized with confidence to all or most community general hospitals in the nation on a statistical basis. In the strictest sense possible, and from a purely statistical standpoint, the obtained findings apply only to the group of hospitals that was actually studied. Further generalization of the results may be made with caution (and is made in the various chapters) only according to theoretical considerations and in terms of the confirmation of particular hypotheses derived from the theoretical framework of the research. To generalize all of the findings from the present research to all community general hospitals would require further empirical work—empirical work based on a research design that would eliminate the restriction of the population effected by the design of the present study. The relative inability to generalize the findings with statistical assurance to as many hospitals as we would like, or to a broader but specified population than the one actually studied, obviously constitutes a rather important limitation—a limitation that can be removed through further research. To gen-

Methodological Limitations

eralize the findings to community general hospitals other than those studied, we must know how similar, or different, the hospitals to which we wish to generalize are.[3]

A second, and closely related, limitation stems from the fact that the number of hospitals studied is relatively small ($N = 10$). The fact that, in most analyses, we are dealing with only ten participating organizations does not permit as many comparisons or cross-breaks as we would have liked to be able to make in order to pursue the analysis as far as might be theoretically desirable in certain particular cases. Similarly, for certain analyses more refined statistical techniques would have been used if we had a larger number of hospitals with which to work. For example, with an N of 10, one cannot properly employ standard partial and multiple correlation techniques other than the partial tau-correlation, which we have used in Chapter 9 (not without some misgivings), and for which no statistical significance test exists. In general, and other things being equal, a larger N is preferable to a smaller one from a methodological point of view.

A third, and less serious, limitation stems from the fact that, while many different groups of hospital personnel provided required data regarding patient care, patients were not included in the study as respondents. Accordingly, although we know a good deal about patient care in the participating hospitals from the available data, we do not know directly how patients feel about their care and their hospital, or whether and to what extent the attitudes and evaluations of patients are congruent with what doctors, nurses, and other members of the hospital have to say about patient care and hospital functioning. Indirectly, however, we know something even in this area on the basis of certain data about patient feelings and reactions toward patient care and the hospital that we obtained from medical, nursing, and administrative people in each hospital. (In this case, these people served as "observers" of patient reaction.)

Patients were not included in the study primarily because: (1) excepting the area of patient care, they could not provide pertinent data on the basis of first-hand knowledge and experience about the areas in which we were interested; (2) even with reference to patient care, it is doubtful and debatable that patients could provide valid data—see our discussion in Chapter 5 regarding this point; and (3) certain practical considerations, including the limited professional and financial resources at our disposal, and a number of difficulties that would have had to be overcome in order to draw an acceptable sample of patients from each hospital (and do so not without some risk of disrupting normal organizational functioning), also argued against including patients in the study as respondents. Excluding patients would be a more serious omission in studying long-term hospitals, such as mental institutions and hospitals for chronic diseases, where the patient remains in the

---

[3] In this connection, Block's (1) "prototype study" of the 200-bed short-stay general hospital in the United States provides some useful data, which suggest that the hospitals studied by Block are in many ways quite similar to the group of hospitals included in our study (which it may be recalled are hospitals of medium size, their size ranging from a low of 104 beds to a high of 322 beds). To the extent that a particular group of hospitals is similar to the group of hospitals we have studied, to that extent the findings of the present study may be generalized to that particular group of hospitals. For further discussion of this point see Chapter 4, where Block's study is discussed in relation to a sketch of the "average" hospital in our own study.

hospital long enough to familiarize himself with the situation and to become a, more or less, "socialized" member of the organization. In community, short-stay general hospitals, patient stay is so short, and patient turnover is so rapid, that it is doubtful whether patients could be theoretically and fruitfully considered as members of the organization, in spite of the fact that hospital functioning centers about the patient.

A final general methodological limitation is closely related to the stage of present-day theory concerning organizations, and to the current state of social-psychological knowledge about the phenomena with which the study is concerned. In general, and other things being equal, when adequate theoretical knowledge is available about a particular phenomenon, the researcher can employ a more perfect methodology than he is able to employ with respect to phenomena about which little is known. In other words, the concepts in the study can be more perfectly specified, operationalized, measured, and understood, the more theory one has about them. And the same is true regarding the use of measuring and analytical techniques. The better the theoretical knowledge available, the more powerful, more sensitive, and more refined the measures and tools of analysis at the disposal of the scientist. Consequently, the methodology that we have used is better in relation to some of the areas and topics investigated than to others, depending upon the theoretical foundations of each area. The average reader will have little difficulty in locating weaknesses in the method that may be directly attributed to the nature of the theory available, especially since we have tried to appraise the theory in each case.

Apart from a number of rather specific methodological difficulties that we have encountered in different parts of the study and have attempted to make explicit at the appropriate place in each case, the above general limitations are what we consider to be the most serious general limitations of our methodology about which we must caution the reader. (Incidentally, the "timeliness" of the data, i.e., the fact that the data were collected several years ago, does not constitute a methodological problem, for the research is much more concerned with the study of underlying relationships among the data rather than with providing up-to-date practical information regarding specific aspects of the situation of specific hospitals.) While it is not possible to gauge the net effect of the above limitations upon particular findings obtained in the study, it is our belief that the nature of specific results and conclusions of the study would not be substantially altered upon removal of the limitations in question. The methodological limitations involved affect much more the total knowledge that we were able to acquire through the research, and the generality of this knowledge, rather than the nature and validity of specific findings. The specific results are relatively clear-cut and unambiguous in the majority of cases.

The statement that the specific results of the study are "relatively clear-cut and unambiguous in the majority of cases" is partly intended to indicate that in some cases the results are not as clear-cut as we would like them to be. The main reason for this lack of clarity for some of the results—a reason that corresponds to a general methodological limitation of a different kind than the kind discussed above—is that the direction of causation in relational findings (i.e., which factor, or variable, causes which) cannot be ascertained conclusively in field studies of the survey type or, for that matter, in any nonexperimental studies. This means that, while we know that certain concepts and variables are related to certain other concepts and variables, that the relationship is of a certain magnitude, that we can have a certain amount of statistical confidence in the relationship, and that the relationship is or is not as predicted by the theory, we still may not know which of the two variables in each relationship is the cause and which is the effect. Only through controlled experimentation is it possible to establish cause and effect conclusively. In nonexperimental studies, such as the present one, the direction of causation cannot be empirically established—we can infer from the theory, and then only in some cases and not in others, or speculate as to which of two related variables is the cause and which is the effect. Accordingly, the nonexperimental nature of the study entails this additional general difficulty.

In this section we have deliberately emphasized the limitations of the research in an effort to show the main methodological weaknesses of the study and, hopefully, to prevent possible misunderstanding or misuse of the findings on the part of some well-meaning but, conceivably, methodologically naïve readers. For the expert reader, of course, we anticipate no difficulty in this connection, and the average reader should not find it too hard to appreciate the methodological problems discussed in this section or in other parts of the book. Concerning the merits of the research design and the advantages of the methodology of the study, or the importance and usefulness of the findings, we need say nothing at this point.

SUMMARY

This study of the short-stay community general hospital focuses on the total hospital as an on-going organizational system. Patient care, organizational coordination, superior-subordinate relationships and administrative problems, communication practices among nursing personnel, and certain other aspects of organizational structure and functioning constitute the main areas of interest. In all cases, the emphasis is on organizational and group phenomena rather than on the more circumscribed problems and characteristics of specific personnel or individuals in the organization. In other words, we are interested in factors affecting the functioning and performance of the hospital as a whole, or of major subunits within the hospital, and not in the behavior of individuals. As a consequence, the unit of measurement, analysis, and hypothesis-testing is the total hospital or some major segment of the hospital. Basically, the research design involves the comparison and contrast of the various participating hospitals with one another on each of the variables, or characteristics, with which the research is concerned, and the examination of relationships among these variables through correlational analyses. It has been the purpose of this chapter to provide a thorough understanding of the research design, and of the methods and procedures used in carrying out the design.

Twelve Michigan hospitals were selected to participate in the study. Two of these served as sites for a considerable amount of exploratory work, preceding the research proper. The remaining ten hospitals participated in the main research, comprising the "sample" of the study. In selecting the hospitals an attempt was made, insofar as possible, to "control" through the research design a variety of important factors which may have a direct bearing, or influence, upon the phenomena under investigation, but which, being of no special interest to the research, were not themselves measured in the study. Control was attained by establishing certain criteria for hospital selection. Specifically, all of the participating institutions met all of the following criteria:

1. Type of service rendered: short-stay general hospitals
2. Size: between 100 and 350 beds, or "medium" size
3. Ownership, and institutional control and affiliation: community, voluntary, nonprofit institutions; nongovernmental and nondenominational
4. Administration: administered by a lay, male administrator, under a board of trustees
5. Status: fully accredited by the Joint Commission on Accreditation of Hospitals
6. Region and geographic location: located in Michigan
7. Community size: larger than 10,000 population

Data for the measurement of the dependent and independent variables representing specific aspects of hospital structure and functioning that are relevant to the objectives of the research were obtained from various sources. Standardized paper-and-pencil questionnaires and personal interviews administered to certain people in each hospital constitute the main source of the data. Organizational documents, and administrative and medical records constitute a second source. A group of doctors who were familiar with the situation in the participating hospitals, but who were not on the staff of any of these hospitals, constitute the last source of data. These outside doctors provided data about the quality of medical care in the hospitals studied.

The questionnaires and interviews were administered in each hospital to over 100 individuals, who were selected to represent their respective hospitals and to furnish required data. These individuals were: the hospital administrator; the members of the executive committee of the board of trustees; members of the medical staff; administrative, nonmedical department heads; nursing personnel in different classifications; and technicians from the laboratory and x-ray department of each institution. For some of these groups, all of the members of the group were asked to provide data; for other groups, only a sample of the total group membership was asked to participate. When groups were sampled, every member of the group was given an equal and known chance of being selected into the sample (in technical terms, systematic random sampling procedures were employed). Most of the respondents were required to complete paper-and-pencil questionnaires, but certain respondents were required to complete a personal interview in addition. In either case, respondents were treated both as "subjects" (provided data about their own feelings, attitudes, etc.) and as "observers" (provided data containing their observations about various aspects of hospital functioning).

Prior to data collection, 1396 individuals were selected from the ten hospitals to participate in the study as respondents. By the time of data collection, however, 26 of these individuals had left their respective hospitals permanently, thus reducing the total number of potential respondents to 1370. Of these, another 51 individuals could not be reached, within a specified period, to provide data—these were people who were absent from the hospital for indefinite but extended periods of time for various reasons, including illness, extended travel, etc. Thus, the total number of potentially available respondents turned out to be 1319. At the end, 1265 of these individuals, or 96 percent, provided the data requested of them. Thus, on the average, each participating hospital is represented in the study by 127 persons, who are roughly distributed as follows: 1 administrator, 5 trustees, 25 doctors, 10 department heads, 18 supervisory nurses, 20 nonsupervisory registered nurses, 14 practical nurses, 20 aides and orderlies, and 13 technicians.

The principal measures of dependent and independent variables derived from the data are in the form of arithmetic means, percentages or proportions, and rank-orders. The principal technique of analysis used is the correlational technique. Accordingly, the bulk of the findings will be reported in the form of correlations showing the relationship between particular variables. Apart from any specific shortcomings which may characterize our various measures of patient care, organizational coordination, and other phenomena, the principal methodological limitation of the study stems from a deliberate decision to restrict the population of hospitals covered to a particular class of hospitals, as indicated above. This decision (which in effect limits the statistical generalization of the findings) was necessary due to the fact that too little was known, theoretically or empirically, about the objectives with which the research is concerned to argue in favor of a broader coverage of hospitals. In view of the paucity of prior relevant research, the present study itself represents partly an exploratory and partly an explanatory effort.

REFERENCES

1. Block, L. "Prototype Study: 200 Bed Hospital," *Mod. Hosp.*, **82**:76–80, (Jan.) 1954.

2. Georgopoulos, B. S., Mann, F. C., and Searles, R. E. "A Study of Ten Community General Hospitals in Michigan. *Report I:* A Report for Participating Hospitals on Various Aspects of Hospital Structure and Functioning, as Seen by Nursing Personnel and Technicians." Ann Arbor, Mich.: Institute for Social Research, 1958.

3. ———— "A Study of Ten Community General Hospitals in Michigan. *Report II:* A Report for Participating Hospitals on Various Aspects of Their Operation, as Seen by People in Upper Organizational Levels." Ann Arbor, Mich.: Institute for Social Research, 1958.

4. *Hospitals.* Guide Issue. *Hospitals,* 35: Part Two, (Aug.) 1961.
5. Hyman, H. H. *Survey Design and Analysis.* Glencoe, Ill.: The Free Press, 1955.
6. Mann, F. C., and Georgopoulos, B. S. "Two Interlocking Studies of the Community General Hospital." In *Conference on the Techniques of Research.* Saint Louis, Mo.: Health Organization Research Program, Saint Louis University, 1960.

3 THE PEOPLE AROUND THE PATIENT

In a broad sense, one may certainly consider all those working in or for the hospital as "the people around the patient," for almost everyone associated with a community general hospital serves the patient, directly or indirectly, even though the functions of some personnel may be less crucial to the organization and the patient. In a stricter sense, however, when speaking of the people around the patient in this volume, we refer to those professional and nonprofessional groups and subgroups of hospital members which participated in the study. These include people who are directly responsible for the treatment and care of the patient, as well as people who hold important positions in the hospital but who have no therapeutic functions or direct personal contact with patients. The more than 1200 respondents from the ten hospitals in the study, who provided data relevant to some aspect of the research, were chosen to represent both their respective institutions and all key groups of people working in the hosiptal.

As indicated in the preceding chapter, each hospital is represented in the research by members of its medical staff, members of its nursing staff, laboratory and x-ray technicians, nonmedical administrative department heads, the administrator, and members of its board of trustees. These are referred to here, collectively, as the people around the patient. Although every organizational and occupational group contributes to the objective of patient care, these are the people who run both the hospital and the patient, in addition to running the various groups of personnel not included in the research.[1]

Our main purpose in this chapter is to discuss the background and major job characteristics of the members of every group which took part in the re-

[1] Except for the department head in each case, personnel from the dietary, housekeeping, and maintenance departments, from the front office, the switchboard, the laundry, and miscellaneous clerical-secretarial positions have not been included in the study. On the aggregate, these people constitute about 40 percent of all personnel employed and paid by the typical hospital, but only about one-quarter of all people working in the hospital. For good descriptions of several of these groups, in hospitals similar to those participating in this research, the reader may refer to the work of Burling, Lentz, and Wilson (5).

search. Although this is a study of hospital functioning and patient care, and not a study of particular professional-occupational groups within the hospital, it is still important to know what the different people around the patient look like. An individual's personal characteristics such as sex and age, his formal education and occupational training, his past work experience, the position he currently occupies in the organization, his job satisfactions and dissatisfactions, and similar other background factors often influence his attitudes and opinions about the organizational situation of which he is a part, and his role performance in the organization. Because the members of a given occupational or organizational group also tend to be more alike with one another than with outsiders with respect to such characteristics as these, moreover, different groups may view the same situation from a different perspective.

Familiarity with the major characteristics of each organizational group is therefore a valuable aid to our understanding of the group itself and (more importantly for our purposes) of its relationships with other groups and with the total organization. Many intergroup differences in attitudes, outlook, and behavior often become more meaningful if viewed in the context of the background of the members of the groups involved. Knowledge of the attributes and characteristics of the members of a particular group, moreover, helps the researcher decide how to handle many of the data supplied by the members of the group. In a study such as the present one, for example, while it would be inappropriate to expect the aides from the nursing department to provide an acceptable appraisal of the quality of patient care rendered at their hospital (as the data on the formal education and occupational training of this group will show), it would be entirely proper to have them tell how they feel about their job or the hospital. The reader who is more conversant with the characteristics of the various groups in the study, after reading this chapter, will generally find himself better equipped both to evaluate our data and to assimilate the findings therefrom.

For these reasons, and in anticipation of the analyses which are to follow in later chapters, we shall here describe the main characteristics of every group participating in the study. Special attention will be given to the background and job characteristics of nonmedical personnel, however, both because we have more information about these people, in this area, and also because of the relatively high homogeneity of medical staff members. The information to be presented derives from a number of questions that were asked of the various respondents in the participating hospitals. These questions were designed to yield data about the respondents' own personal characteristics, about their job and organizational position, and about their work situation in general. Information will be presented separately for each respondent group, but for all hospitals combined. The groups involved are: the selected medical staff; the general medical staff; the supervisory nursing staff; the nonsupervisory registered nurses; the practical nurses; the aides and orderlies; the

Personal Characteristics of Hospital Personnel

laboratory and x-ray technicians; the nonmedical administrative department heads; the administrators of the various hospitals; and the members of the executive committee of the board of trustees of each institution studied. The composition and size of each group and the manner in which its members were chosen from the ten hospitals for inclusion in the research were described in the preceding chapter.

The contents of the present chapter have been organized into five major sections, with an additional brief summary. In the first section, we will describe the personal demographic characteristics of the members of each group, including sex, age, family status, and formal education. In the second section, we will be concerned with the professional-occupational career patterns of the respondents. In the third section, we will discuss certain aspects of the work situation in the hospital, as related to the different groups, including full-time vs. part-time employment, shift-work patterns, turnover and absenteeism, and interaction among different personnel. In the fourth section, we will be concerned with the present job status and outlook of nonmedical employees as reflected in such things as job satisfaction, opportunities for advancement within the organization, actual earnings and satisfaction with earnings, motivation to work and job commitment, and the like. In the fifth, and last major section, we will summarize and compare the main characteristics of the various respondent groups, providing a short profile for each group.

THE PERSONAL CHARACTERISTICS OF HOSPITAL PERSONNEL

The influence of such relatively invariant personal attributes as age, sex, formal education, and family status on the attitudes and role performance of individuals is in some cases well known and, in others, rapidly coming under scrutiny. The studies by Stouffer and his associates (16) of the American soldier during World War II, for example, indicate that older, married, and better educated soldiers had the highest combat effectiveness ratings. And although our study was not designed to investigate the importance of the personal characteristics of the people around the patient in relation to their role performance, it would be useful to know how the respondents are distributed with respect to such characteristics.

Sex

Excepting the medical staff, the top lay personnel, and the patients, the world within the hospital is largely feminine. The nursing staff, for instance, which constitutes the largest single organizational group in the community general hospital—the medical staff being the next largest—has but a few male members. Of a total of some 700 respondents representing the different classifications of nursing personnel in the ten hospitals studied, only a handful were men. Among the 182 persons who occupy the supervisory nursing positions in the various institutions only 7 were male, including, interestingly enough, 2 of the 10 directors of nursing involved.[2] Among the 196 nonsupervisory registered nurses in the study, not a single one was male, and among the 140 practical nurses only 2 individuals were men. Among the 203 aides and orderlies, however, 50 were male; but all of the men in this group were orderlies, the aides being all women.

Similarly, of the 125 technicians in the study (78 laboratory and 47 x-ray technicians), only 23 percent were male. Even in the case of the 101 nonmedical administrative department heads (including again the directors of nursing), less than half (42 percent) were men. The high percentage of female members in this group is not too surprising, since the heads of maintenance, housekeeping, admissions, medical records, dietetics, and nursing belong to this group. From the standpoint of a formal, hierarchical organization having the majority of its top administrative jobs filled by women, however, the hospital is relatively unique among large-scale organizations.

All preceding groups have a predominantly female membership, and the same holds true for hospital personnel not covered by the study (e.g., people in the dietary, medical records, and housekeeping departments, front office personnel, and the various clerical-secretarial personnel), except for the staff of the maintenance department where the reverse is true. Even so, the community general hospital can hardly be thought of as a woman's world. When it comes to the very top organizational echelon, group membership is predominantly male. One finds few women on the medical staff, the board of trustees, or among hospital administrators. Of a total of 252 doctors in the study, representing the active-attending medical staff of the ten hospitals, only 3 were women. And of the 46 trustees in the study only 5 were women. The administrator of each participating hospital was a lay, male person, since only hospitals having such an administrator (among other things) were studied. Many hospitals have, of course, a female administrator, but most hospitals which are not church-related, particularly the medium- and large-size institutions, are likely to have a male administrator. Thus, while the overall work force in the community general hospital is largely feminine, it is still under masculine dominance, since the most influential groups in the organization—doctors, trustees, and administrators—have a predominantly male membership.

Age

The first two tables, below, present the age distribution of the members of the various groups of respondents. In part, the age distribution of the

[2] In this connection, a variety of data from the two hospitals having male directors of nursing show that respondents from one hospital generally evaluated the male director of nursing as better than "average," while in the other hospital the male director of nursing was evaluated as poorer than average.

Personal Characteristics of Hospital Personnel

people around the patient reflects some of the work force dynamics of the contemporary hospital scene. For example, the data in Table 7 show that three out of every four supervisory nurses are between 30 and 50 years old. Supervisory nurses clearly constitute the middle-age nursing group in the community general hospital. The members of this group are, of course, partly drawn from registered nurses who have some seniority in the organization, and partly from that portion of registered nurses who have withstood the vicissitudes of migration and marriage. Table 7 also shows that, of the four nursing groups, practical nurses have the highest proportion of their members in the 50-or-over age bracket (22 percent), and the second highest proportion in the middle-age bracket (52 percent). Practical nurses constitute the older-age group within the nursing staff. Having not had the required training to become registered nurses when relatively younger (over one-third of them lacking even a complete high-school education), but having been able to acquire some nursing training when relatively older (often after having worked in the hospital as aides), these women tend to fall in the middle- and older-age categories.

TABLE 7. The Age Distribution of Nursing Personnel and Technicians for All Hospitals Combined

Respondent Group	30 Years Old or Under 30	Between 30 and 50	50 Years Old or Over	N
Supervisory nursing staff, excluding directors of nursing	21	75	4	172
Nonsupervisory registered nurses	44	45	11	196
Practical nurses	26	52	22	140
Aides and orderlies	44	45	11	203
Laboratory and x-ray technicians	56	38	6	125

The age characteristics of nonsupervisory registered nurses and of the aides and orderlies are identical, but for different reasons. In both cases, 44 percent of group members are 30 years old or younger, 45 percent are between 30 and 50, and the remaining are older. Registered nurses are predominantly young partly because of a good deal of turnover in their ranks, which very frequently results from marriage, family responsibilities, and spatial mobility—these factors tending to shorten, and often end, the professional career of the registered nurse. The prevalence of low salaries and comparatively few rewards for registered nurses in hospitals (as we will see in this chapter) also serve to mitigate against long-term hospital careers for these people. Another relevant element, which is also worth noting in this connection, is the fact that among all nursing groups the nonsupervisory registered nurses staff contains the highest proportion of part-time members (45 percent). The aides are also a young group in the hospital. As in the case of registered nurses, there is a good deal of turnover among aides, and this is congruent with the age distribution of this group. But more importantly, and unlike the case of registered nurses, the aides are drawn from young girls and women in the labor force, who lack even the little nursing training of practical nurses, and the majority of whom (55 percent) have been unable to complete high school. Because of the shortage of trained nursing staff, and because they can easily hire almost two aides with the salary of one registered nurse, however, hospitals generally tend to have a relatively large number of aides, regardless of turnover or occupational training.

TABLE 8. The Age Distribution of Medical, Administrative, and Trustee Groups for All Hospitals Combined

Respondent Group	40 Years Old or Under 40	Between 40 and 50	50 Years Old or Over	N
Selected medical staff	26	48	26	121
General medical staff	41	25	34	131
Hospital administrators	30	30	40	10
Nonmedical administrative department heads, including directors of nursing	31	29	40	101
Members of the executive committee of the board of trustees	4	29	67	46

The laboratory and x-ray technicians, about three-fourths of whom are women, are the youngest of all the groups in the study. The majority (56 percent) are not yet in their thirties, and only 6 percent of them are at least 50 years old. Increasing specialization and advances in the general area of medical technology have contributed to the development of this group, which has a very recent origin and which has not as yet established itself firmly as a recognized "professional" group in the hospital field. The professional youth of this group serves to account for the personal youth of its members.

The age distribution of doctors, trustees, administrators, and administrative department heads is shown in Table 8. The trustees group has the highest proportion of 50-years-old or older members (67 percent), trustees usually being well-established members of the hospital's community who, among other things, are able to offer their services to the hospital without remuneration. The members of the selected medical staff constitute primarily a middle-age group; 48 percent are between 40 and 50 years old, with the remaining distributed equally between the younger and the older age brackets. Age-wise, the selected medical staff group resembles the supervisory nurses group. The members of the general medical staff are a younger group, 41 percent being 40 or under, and another 25 percent being between 40 and 50 (although if we consider only the proportion of doctors who are 50 or over, the general medical staff has somewhat more people in this category than the selected medical staff). The hospital administrators and the nonmedical administrative department heads, who are their immediate subordinates, exhibit almost identical age patterns. In each case, about 30 percent are 40 years old or younger, another 30 percent are between 40 and 50, with the remaining 40 percent being at least in their fifties. On the whole, the doctors are younger than trustees, administrators, and department heads, but older than nurses and technicians.

Family Status

The marital and parental status of doctors, trustees, and hospital administrators is essentially the same. Ninety-six percent of all doctors in the study are married, and less than 2 percent are single. Of the trustees, 93 percent are married, and none is single. All ten hospital administrators are married. Moreover, at least nine out of every ten members of these three groups have children—96 percent of the trustees, 91 percent of the doctors, and 90 percent of the administrators have one or more children. Therefore, the family status of people in these top groups is practically identical; but it is significantly different from that of administrative department heads. Of the members of this latter group, only 66 percent are married and only 62 percent have children; almost one-fourth (23 percent) are single. The marital status of department heads is very similar to that of supervisory nurses, while their parental status is very similar to that of aides and orderlies.

Considering the nursing groups, we find that 63 percent of the supervisory nurses, 74 percent of the nonsupervisory registered nurses, and 62 percent of the practical nurses, as well as of the aides and orderlies, are married. Another 25 percent of supervisory nurses, 17 percent of nonsupervisory nurses, 14 percent of practical nurses, and 22 percent of aides and orderlies are single. With respect to parental status, 52 percent of supervisory nurses, 66 percent of nonsupervisory registered nurses, 71 percent of practical nurses, and 62 percent of the aides and orderlies have children.

Thus, among nurses holding the supervisory positions in the various hospitals, only six out of every ten are likely to be married, and only one in two are likely to have children. By contrast, three out of every four nonsupervisory registered nurses are likely to be married, and two out of every three are likely to have children. Among all nursing personnel, the nonsupervisory nurses are the group with the highest proportion of their members married, and the supervisory nurses are the group with the highest proportion of their members single. Among both nursing and other personnel in the hospital, practical nurses are the group with the highest proportion of divorced and separated or widowed members—24 percent. The corresponding percentages for supervisory nurses, nonsupervisory nurses, and aides and orderlies, are 12, 9, and 16 percent respectively. It is also interesting to note that, while a significantly higher proportion of nonsupervisory registered nurses are married than practical nurses, a somewhat smaller proportion of the former have children compared to the latter. This apparent incongruity is readily resolved by the fact that practical nurses both tend to have a higher average age and a higher divorce-separation rate than do registered nurses.

The laboratory and x-ray technicians, which happen to be the youngest of all groups included in the study, are also, not surprisingly, most likely of all groups to be single (38 percent), and least likely to be married (54 percent) or have children (41 percent). Next to the technicians, the supervisory nurses, among all of the respondent groups, are least likely to have children (52 percent).

Formal Education

Compared to most large-scale organizations, the hospital exhibits somewhat of an anomaly in that its action structure requires frequent interaction among large numbers of people with widely different educational backgrounds. In response to a question concerning their formal education, the various nonmedical personnel supplied the information which is summarized in Table 9. The doctors were not asked this question, since all of them have attended college, all have graduated from medical school, and many have received even further formal professional education. Needless to say that, as a group, the doctors constitute the most highly educated group in the hospital. The other groups in the study vary a great deal, both from the medical staff and from one another, in formal education, according to the data.

If one were to rank the nonmedical groups according to the proportion of their members who have at least had some college education, based on the figures in Table 9, he would obtain the following order: hospital administrators; trustees on the executive committee; administrative department heads, including directors of nursing; laboratory and x-ray technicians; nonsupervisory registered nurses; supervisory nursing staff; practical nurses; and, finally, aides and orderlies. The range in formal education level is very great; while all administrators have attended college, only 15 percent of the aides and orderlies have.

The administrators constitute the highest formal-education group, 70 percent of them having completed college. The trustees group is the next most highly educated group, 58 percent having completed college. The administrative department heads, being an extremely heterogeneous group, exhibit an interesting educational pattern: 41 percent have finished college, but another 19 percent have less than a complete high-school education. The laboratory and

TABLE 9. Percentage of Members of Nonmedical Respondent Groups Giving Certain Answers to the Question: "How Much Formal Education Have You Had?"

Respondent Group	Completed College	Some College	Completed High School	Some High School	Grade School Only
Aides and orderlies (N = 200)	1	14	30	43	12
Practical nurses (N = 136)	3	18	42	28	9
Nonsupervisory registered nurses (N = 184)	10	41	47	2	0
Supervisory nursing staff (N = 169)	14	31	50	5	0
Laboratory and x-ray technicians (N = 125)	24	34	35	5	2
Administrative department heads (N = 100)	41	25	15	14	5
Executive trustees (N = 45)	58	22	18	2	0
Hospital administrators * (N = 10)	70	30	0	0	0

Percentage of Members, in All Hospitals Combined, Who Had:

* Of the seven administrators in the study who had completed college, two had also attended graduate school.

x-ray technicians group is most similar to the professional nurses group education-wise. The aides and orderlies, of course, constitute the least educated of all groups in the study—55 percent have less than a complete high-school education, with 12 percent having had only grade school, and only 15 percent (mostly orderlies) having had any college. The practical nurses group is the next least educated group, with 37 percent of its members having less than a complete high-school education. We may also note at this point that, in most of our later analyses, we will be using only a few data from practical nurses and aides and orderlies, as a result of the low formal-education level of these personnel. Data from the administrative department heads will likewise not appear in some chapters because of the extremely heterogeneous composition of this group (actually, the administrative department heads constitute an organizational "category" rather than a real group) in terms of professional, occupational, educational, and other characteristics rather than because of low formal-education level.

The formal-education patterns of the professional nursing staff and of the technicians are also interesting. The data show that a substantial percentage of the members of these groups have attended college. Almost one-fourth of the technicians have completed college, and an additional one-third have had some college education. In the case of the supervisory nurses group, 14 percent have completed college, and another 31 percent have had some college. And, of the nonsupervisory registered nurses, 10 percent have completed college (most of these are probably nurses who have graduated from four-year collegiate schools of nursing) and—perhaps even more surprising—another 41 percent have attended college, apparently in addition to nursing school. The overall college attendance of supervisory nurses (45 percent) is probably not too unexpected because hospitals often require college degrees for persons in some of their supervisory nursing jobs. In the case of nonsupervisory registered nurses, however, the college attendance figure of 51 percent is somewhat surprising, both because no college degree requirements are set by hospitals for this particular role, and also because the figure here is even slightly higher than for the supervisory nurses group (51 vs. 45 percent).

Having discussed the sex, age, marital, parental, and educational characteristics of the respondents, we will now turn to a similar description of their professional-occupational career patterns.

PROFESSIONAL-OCCUPATIONAL CAREER PATTERNS

In this section, we will discuss some of the professional, or occupational, characteristics of the people around the patient. These include professional-occupational training, previous job history, length of association with the hospital, and time on present job in the present hospital. The emphasis will again be on the characteristics of nonmedical personnel, particularly on the characteristics of nursing personnel in the different classifications. Very few questions were asked of doctors, trustees, and administrators in this area.

Professional-Occupational Training

In addition to the data on formal education, information was obtained about the training of the majority of our respondents by asking the members of the various groups the following question: "How much *professional schooling* have you had?" Of the four nursing groups in the study, the aides and orderlies were not asked this question because, with very few exceptions, these people lack any formal occupational training. Doctors were not asked this question, since they are the most highly professionalized, most highly trained, and most specialized people in the entire hospital organization.[3] The trustees, likewise,

[3] One indication of their professional training, however, can be obtained by considering the relative proportion of medical staff members in the various hospitals who are "board men," i.e., who have specialized in certain areas and have been certified as specialists by established medical boards—such certification presupposing more training and higher competence for the certified doctor over his noncertified colleagues. In this connection, data from hospital records show that an average of 38 percent of all active-attending medical staff members in the ten hospitals studied are board men, this figure

TABLE 10. Percentage of Members of Certain Respondent Groups Indicating That They Have Had Certain Years of "Professional Schooling" or Training

Respondent Group	At Least Four Years	Three Years	Two Years	One Year	Less Than One Year
Supervisory nursing staff ($N = 171$)	14	83	3	0	0
Nonsupervisory registered nurses ($N = 196$)	11	87	2	0	0
Practical nurses ($N = 135$)	0	3	15	62	20
Laboratory and x-ray technicians ($N = 113$)	14	7	21	42	16
Administrative department heads ($N = 87$)	25	18	14	17	26
Hospital administrators ($N = 8$)	0	0	24	38	38

Percentage of Members, in All Hospitals Combined Who Had the Indicated Years of Training

were not asked the question about training, for their professional and occupational origins and characteristics are very heterogeneous. When asked to indicate their occupation, 46 percent of all trustees classified themselves as executives, managers, or directors of manufacturing and business organizations, another 13 percent classified themselves as bankers or investors, and the remaining 41 percent indicated a variety of other professions and occupations, including those of salesman, attorney, insurance man, housewife, publisher, and several others.

The data concerning the professional-occupational training of the remaining respondents are summarized in Table 10. As might be expected, almost 100 percent of the supervisory and nonsupervisory registered nurses have had at least three years of professional schooling, with 14 percent of the former and 11 percent of the latter having had at least four years of professional training (these are mostly nurses from four-year collegiate schools of nursing). Of the practical nurses, 62 percent have had one year of occupational training, 15 percent have had two years, and fully 20 percent have had less than a year. The aides and orderlies (not shown on the table) did not even have one year of formal occupational training. It may also be recalled in this connection, moreover, that aides and orderlies and the practical nurses constitute the two lowest formal education groups among all respondents. Yet, among all groups in the hospital, it is these two groups whose members in-

---

ranging across individual hospitals from a low of 27 percent to a high of 53 percent. (Additional data show that an average of 29 percent of the doctors in the ten hospitals are "general practitioners," this figure varying across hospitals from a low of 19 to a high of 41 percent.)

teract most frequently and spend the greatest amount of time with the patient. (In fact, the volume and length of interaction between patients and medical-nursing staff vary inversely with the professional training and formal education of the various groups which make up the therapeutic staff.)

The data about the occupational training of laboratory and x-ray technicians are very interesting. Of the 125 technicians in the study only 113 answered the question about professional schooling, showing a nonresponse rate of 10 percent. This nonresponse rate is among the highest in the present study (regardless of questionnaire item or respondent group involved), apparently suggesting that the technicians group has not yet completely crystallized professionally, at least in the area of training. In any event, of those who answered the question, 21 percent said that they have had at least three years of professional schooling (compared to almost 100 percent of the registered nurses). Another 21 percent had two years of training, 42 percent had one year, and the remaining 16 percent had less than one year's professional schooling. As we will see in a later part of this chapter, these figures on professional training are sharply incongruous when viewed in the context of salaries paid to the technicians in relation to salaries paid to professional nurses.

Of the nonmedical, administrative department heads in the ten participating hospitals, 14 percent did not answer the question about professional schooling, reflecting the great diversity of occupational origins and characteristics of those belonging to this group. Of those who responded (a total of 87 individuals, including the 10 directors of nursing), however, 25 percent indicated that they have had at least four years of professional schooling, and another 18 percent have had three years. At the other extreme, 26 percent have had less than one year's training. Of the remaining, 17 percent have had one year, and 14 percent have had two years of professional-occupational schooling. These data are, of course, not surprising, if we remember the extremely heterogeneous composition of the present group. Finally, of the ten hospital administrators, eight provided us with information about their professional-occupational schooling. Of the eight, two said that they have had two years of professional training (these two had attended a hospital administration program), three have had one year, and the remaining three have had less than a year of professional training.

Most respondents were asked not only to indicate the amount of their occupational training, but also to indicate how satisfied they are with the training which they have received. Regarding satisfaction with training, the data show that, while the majority of respondents from each group involved express varying degrees of satisfaction with their training, a certain proportion of them express dissatisfaction. Specifically, 18 percent of the technicians, 12 percent of the department heads, 11 percent of supervisory nurses, 11 percent of practical nurses, and 6 percent of nonsupervisory registered nurses felt at least "somewhat dissatisfied" with the training they have had. The proportion of respondents who felt "completely satisfied" with their training, on the other hand, is as follows: for the technicians, 21 percent; for the department heads, 13 percent; for supervisory nurses, 13 percent; for practical nurses, 26 percent; and for the nonsupervisory registered nurses, 23 percent. Of the ten hospital administrators in the study, one felt "very dissatisfied," two felt "fairly satisfied," and the other seven felt "very well satisfied" with the training they have had for their present job.

In general, these data show that people in the administrative and supervisory positions in the hospital tend to feel somewhat less satisfied with their training than people having no administrative or supervisory responsibilities. This hypothesis should be partially qualified, however, since the technicians express more than average dissatisfaction with their training, when this group is compared with the rest. In this connection, we might also add that, in the case of supervisory nurses and department heads, dissatisfaction with training has probably no reference to the technical aspects of their job; in all probability, it pertains to their training to supervise those under them. In the case of technicians, however, dissatisfaction with training very likely refers to the technical aspects of their job, for very few of the technicians have supervisory roles.

Job History

Table 11 presents information concerning the previous work experience of the members of the various nonmedical groups in the study. For each group, it shows (1) the proportion of members who previously held the same or a similar job at another hospital, (2) the proportion who previously held a different job, but a job in the general field of health, (3) the proportion who held a previous job totally unrelated to hospital work, and (4) the proportion who had no previous regular job at all. These data are based on the answers of nonmedical personnel to this question: "Did you have a regular job before you joined this hospital?"

Prior to their present job in their respective hospitals, almost exactly half of the supervisory nurses, registered nurses, practical nurses, technicians, and administrative department heads had a job either at another hospital or in the field of health. Of the other half, some had no previous regular job whatever, while others held a job entirely unrelated to their present one. Of the aides and orderlies, only 38 percent had a previous job related to hospital work, while an additional one-third of them had a job not related to hospital work, suggesting lack of professional status for these people. Other data in Table 11 show that about three out of every ten department heads, two out of every ten technicians and practical nurses, one out of every ten supervisory nurses, and less than one in ten nonsupervisory registered nurses had a previous job totally unrelated to their present job. It is also interesting to find that 43 percent of the nonsupervisory registered nurses and 39 percent of the supervisory nurses in the ten hospitals report no previous regular job at all (compared to between 15 and 29 percent of the members of the other nonmedical groups). The fact that so many nonsupervisory registered nurses had no previous regular job indicates that a good many of them are entering the profession, and the hospital, for the first time, apparently having just finished nursing school—something which is consonant with the relative youth of this particular hospital group, as earlier commented.

TABLE 11. Percentage of Members of Certain Respondent Groups Giving Certain Answers to the Question: "Did You Have a Regular Job Before You Joined This Hospital?"

Respondent Group	Had Same or Similar Job in Another Hospital	Had a Different Job, but in Field of Health	Had a Different Job Unrelated to Present	Had No Previous Regular Job at All
Supervisory nursing staff ($N = 165$)	24	26	11	39
Nonsupervisory registered nurses ($N = 190$)	28	22	7	43
Practical nurses ($N = 137$)	34	15	22	29
Aides and orderlies ($N = 199$)	26	12	33	29
Laboratory and x-ray technicians ($N = 123$)	38	13	22	27
Administrative department heads ($N = 97$)	33	20	32	15

Further examination of the data in Table 11 reveals something about the interhospital mobility characteristic of the various groups. Specifically, we find that 38 percent of the technicians, 34 percent of the practical nurses, and 33 percent of the department heads held the same or a similar job in another hospital before joining the present hospital. Apparently, a good deal of interhospital recruitment (if not "raiding") occurs in the case of these groups, especially in the case of technicians. The corresponding figures for the remaining groups are 24 percent for supervisory nurses, 28 percent for nonsupervisory registered nurses, and 26 percent for aides and orderlies. Of all the groups involved, technicians are most likely, and supervisory nurses are least likely, to have experienced interhospital mobility. The vast majority of supervisory nurses have obviously been promoted to their present jobs from the ranks within the same organization.

The fact that only 24 percent of the supervisory nurses and 28 percent of the nonsupervisory registered nurses previously held the same or a similar job in another hospital, coupled with the fact that 39 percent of the former and 43 percent of the latter had no previous regular job at all, strongly indicates that the hope of hospitals for coping with professional nurse shortages lies primarily in the recruitment of young nurses just fresh from nursing school, and in minimizing turnover. In the light of this implication, the necessity for training more and more professional nurses to begin with—especially in view of continuous population increases, continuous nurse shortages, and relatively high turnover rates among registered nurses—becomes clearly evident, at least if future hospital needs in Michigan are to be met.[4] This necessity, in turn, suggests still another one, namely, the need for interesting and attracting more and more individuals to the nursing profession.

Length of Association with Present Hospital

Table 12 shows, for every group participating in the study, the percentage of its members who have been associated with their present hospital (not necessarily their present job in their particular hospital) for specified periods of time. These data about one's total length of association with one's institution provide a good indication of the relative organizational stability of the various groups in the hospital.

TABLE 12. Percentage of Respondents from Each Participating Group, for All Hospitals Combined, Who Have Been Associated with Their Particular Hospital for Given Lengths of Time *

Respondent Group	One Year or Less	Between One and Five Years	Five Years or More	N *
Selected medical staff	0	18	82	117
General medical staff	8	25	67	131
Supervisory nursing staff	9	30	61	172
Nonsupervisory registered nurses	28	42	30	195
Practical nurses	16	38	46	140
Aides and orderlies	36	46	18	202
Laboratory and x-ray technicians	21	41	38	125
Administrative department heads	12	28	60	101
Members of the executive committee of the board of trustees	4	32	64	46
Hospital administrators	10	30	60	10

* If, for a given group, the percentage figures appearing in this table, or in any other tables, do not add exactly to 100 percent (e.g., some may total 99 percent and others 101 percent), this is due to rounding off decimals and not to computational errors.

[4] For a related discussion of specific future nursing needs in the Detroit metropolitan area, see Murray, "Nursing Needs and Resources for 4½ Million People" (12).

In terms of length of institutional association, or from the standpoint of organizational stability, doctors constitute the most stable group in the community general hospital, according to the data. Of the members of the selected medical staff, 82 percent have been associated with their present hospital for at least five years; and, of the members of the general medical staff, 67 percent have been affiliated with their present hospital for the same length of time. Trustees constitute the next most stable group, 64 percent of them having been associated with their present hospital for five or more years. This fact, incidentally, is often viewed unfavorably in hospital circles, on the ground that there should be greater turnover among trustees because trustees tend to self-perpetuate themselves "unduly" and because they tend to be "too conservative" in attitude and outlook. The implication, in this connection, is that the relatively high organizational stability of trustees somehow makes for organizational rigidity and, to an extent, this is probably true. On the other hand, of course, organizational continuity is also important and frequently advantageous.

After doctors and trustees, the hospital administrators and the department heads are the next most stable groups in the hospitals studied, with 60 percent of their members having been with the hospital for five or more years. The supervisory nurses, as we will see, are also as stable as the department heads in this respect. In general, then, the very top groups in the hospital organization are also the groups with the most stable membership. In each case, the majority of group members have been with the hospital for at least five years. Only 12 percent of the department heads, 10 percent of the administrators, and less than 10 percent of the doctors and trustees have been with their present hospital for one year or less.

Among nursing personnel and technicians, supervisory nurses are the most stable group, organizationally speaking, 61 percent of them having been with the hospital for at least five years. Table 12 shows that the organizational stability pattern of supervisory nurses is practically identical with the pattern exhibited by hospital administrators and by administrative department heads. Practical nurses constitute the next most stable group, 46 percent having been with the hospital for five or more years, and only 16 percent having been with the hospital for one year or less. The most unstable of all groups studied is the aides and orderlies group. Of the members of this group, only one in every five has been with the hospital for as long as five years, while twice as many have been with the hospital for one year or less. Nonsupervisory registered nurses constitute the second least stable group in the hospital. Only three out of every ten registered nurses have been with their present hospital for at least five years, while almost as many have been with the hospital for one year or less. Finally, of the laboratory and x-ray technicians, 38 percent have been with the hospital for five or more years, while another 21 percent have been with the hospital for one year or less. Technicians constitute the third least stable group among all groups in the study.

In general, as might be expected, the above data on length of institutional affiliation are consistent with the earlier data about the job history and age distribution of the various people around the patient. Those who have been with their present hospital for shorter periods of time also tend to be younger and to have had a shorter professional-occupational career in the hospital field. The converse is generally true for those who have been associated with their present hospital for relatively longer periods of time. One final point should be made about institutional association. While doctors, among all groups, have the highest proportion of members associated with the present hospital for five or more years, it should not be assumed that they have been exclusively associated with that hospital. Fully 83 percent of all doctor respondents in the study indicated that, at the time of data collection, they were also on the staff of at least one additional hospital.

Time on Present Job and Interjob Shifting in the Hospital

In addition to the information about total length of association with the hospital, in the case of nursing personnel and technicians, data were also obtained about the length of time these personnel have been on the same job in the present hospital. The latter data provide us with an indication of on-the-job experience and, when compared with the former, with an indication of interjob shifts within the organization. What do the data show? For one thing, they show that a substantial number of nursing personnel and of technicians have been doing their present job in the present hospital for a relatively short period of time. This undoubtedly creates some difficulties in integrating, or trying to integrate, people and jobs. For another thing, the data show a good deal of interjob shifting within the hospital for all nursing personnel, except aides and orderlies.

First, we find that while only 9 percent of supervisory nurses have been with the hospital for one year or less (see Table 12, above), the proportion who have been at their present job in the hospital for one year or less is much higher—24 percent. The corresponding figures for nonsupervisory registered nurses are 28 and 39 percent, respectively. Those for practical nurses are 16 and 28 percent, and those for aides and orderlies are 36 and 42 percent, respectively. The corresponding figures for laboratory and x-ray technicians are 21 and 26 percent, respectively. Second, and conversely, we find that while 61 percent of supervisory nurses have been associated with the hospital for at least five years, only 21 percent of them have been at their present job in the hospital for at least five years. The corresponding figures for registered nurses are 30 and 17 percent, respectively; for practical nurses, they are 46 and 34 percent; for aides and orderlies, they are 18 and 15 percent; and for technicians, they are 38 percent and 32 percent, respectively.

Obviously, the supervisory nursing staff has experienced a rather great amount of interjob shifting within the hospital. Apparently, the main reason for this is promotion to a supervisory role from a nonsupervisory position. Thus, interjob shifting in this case implies promotional mobility. The nonsupervisory registered nurses group has also experienced some job shifting, but to a much lesser degree than supervisory nurses. In the case of this group, interjob shifting is probably due mainly to movement from student nurse status to full professional nurse status within the hospital (and, accordingly, in hospitals which themselves do not have schools of nursing, the amount of interjob shifting for nonsupervisory nurses who do not move to supervisory nursing positions should be practically zero). The practical nurses group has also experienced some interjob shifting, roughly equal in amount to that experienced by nonsupervisory registered nurses. In the case of this group, job shifting can be largely accounted for by the fact that many practical nurses work in the hospital as aides prior to receiving some training and becoming practical nurses. The aides and orderlies group has experienced practically no interjob shifting within the same hospital, and nearly the same holds true for the technicians group. Members of these last two groups are apparently being recruited almost exclusively from outside the organization.

THE GROSS ANATOMY OF WORK IN THE HOSPITAL

Some personnel in the hospital hold a full-time job, while others work only part-time. Some work in one section, or medical service, and others work in other sections, with greater or lesser regularity. And, since hospitals operate on a 24-hour basis and with three shifts, some personnel work in one shift while others work in another, again with greater or lesser regularity. Similarly, some groups in the hospital are more stable than others from the standpoint of absenteeism and turnover among their membership. And, finally, some groups tend to work more closely with certain groups than others, with greater or lesser ease, exhibiting particular interaction patterns. It is these aspects of work that will occupy our attention in this section. Once more, the emphasis will be on the characteristics of nursing personnel.

Full-time vs. Part-time Work

As might be expected, the majority of the people around the patient, none of whom was unionized at the time of data collection, are working full-time in the hospital. Doctors and trustees, however, are not. The trustees, with an occasional exception, spend only a few hours of their time per week at the hospital, or on hospital-related affairs. Generally, they have their own jobs in the community, and volunteer their services to the hospital on a part-time basis, without remuneration. The trustees are not employees of the hospital. The doctors cannot be said to be "working" full-time because of three main reasons: (1) The members of the medical staff are not employed by the hospital; they only have staff privileges to bring their patients to the hospital and to treat them there. (2) Most doctors have their own offices in the community, devoting a great deal of their time to their office patients. (3) As we have already seen, 83 percent of the doctors in the study indicated that they were also on the staff of at least one additional hospital; accordingly, they must spend some time in these other hospitals.

Apart from the doctors and trustees, the majority of all other personnel are full-time employees of the hospital. The administrators, of course, work more than full-time on their hospital job. With only rare exceptions, the same is true in the case of the nonmedical, administrative department heads. Of the laboratory and x-ray technicians, 92 percent indicate that they are working full-time. Among nursing personnel, the proportion of those working full-time varies, to an extent, from one classification to another.

Of all the supervisory nurses in the various hospitals (excluding directors of nursing), 93 percent said that they are working full-time. Of the practical nurses in the study, 88 percent said that they are working full-time—this figure being almost identical with what the complete personnel rosters of the various hospitals show. (Of the grand total of 403 practical nurses in the ten hospitals, only 53 were part-time workers at the time of data collection.) The aides and orderlies were not asked to indicate whether they were working full-time or part-time, because only full-time members from this group were included in the research as respondents. However, according to the nursing personnel rosters of participating hospitals, we find that only 9 percent of the aides (59 out of a grand total of 671 aides) and 17 percent of the orderlies (13 out of a total of 78 orderlies) in the ten hospitals are part-time workers. Thus, considering aides and orderlies together, about nine out of every ten (or more) of the members of each nursing classification, excepting nonsupervisory registered nurses, are full-time employees.

The case of nonsupervisory registered nurses, however, is sharply different. We find that of the 196 nonsupervisory registered nurses in the study, only an average of 55 percent indicated that they are working full-time in their respective hospitals (this ranges from a low of 42 percent in one of the hospitals, to a high of 67 percent in another). This percentage figure, which, incidentally, is almost the same with what the personnel rosters of the various hospitals show for the present nursing group (of a grand total of 659 nonsupervisory registered nurses in the ten hospitals, only 358 were listed as full-time employees), reflects very clearly the problems of professional nurse shortages and turnover generally experienced by hospitals. It is a rather alarmingly low figure, for it suggests great difficulty on the part of hospitals to provide their patients with much attention by professional nurses. (We have already seen that it is the aides, followed by practical nurses, who have the most frequent and lengthiest contact with the patients.) Because of the fact that so many of the nonsupervisory registered nurses in the various hospitals are part-time workers, because of the relatively small number of registered nurses by comparison to the nonprofessional nursing staff,[5] and because registered nurses carry out many coordinative and quasi-supervisory activities, in addition to therapeutic functions, the professional nurses find less and less time to spend on actual bedside care. In a later chapter (Chapter 8), we shall also have occasion to show how the composition of the nursing staff, in terms of the proportion of professional and nonprofessional staff members in each hospital, affects the quality of patient care.

In numerical terms, of all nursing staff members in the participating hospitals, about 18 percent are part-time employees. But, in full-time equivalents, part-time nursing personnel account for only about 10 percent of the total nursing work force in the ten institutions. However, of all part-time nursing personnel in the ten hospitals (a total of 425 individuals), only three out of every ten are not professional registered nurses. Seventy-one percent of all part-time nursing staff members are registered nurses, 12 percent are practical nurses, 14 percent are aides, and 3 percent are orderlies. By contrast, of all full-time nursing personnel in the ten hospitals (a total of 1558 individuals), excluding directors of nursing, 34 percent are registered nurses, both supervisory and nonsupervisory, 23 percent are practical nurses, 39 percent are aides, and 4 percent are orderlies. It is also worth noting here, moreover, that we find no tendency on the part of those hospitals which have proportionately fewer full-time registered nurses to compensate with proportionately more part-time nurses. Considering the nonsupervisory registered nurses group, which accounts for the large majority of part-time nursing staff, we find no relationship whatsoever between the proportion of full-time nursing personnel in the various hospitals who are registered nurses and the proportion of part-time nursing personnel who are registered nurses. The rank-order correlation between these two proportions is .07, which, based on an N of 10 hospitals, is not statistically significant from zero; in fact, for all practical purposes, it is zero.

Shift Work Patterns

The members of the four nursing groups participating in the research were asked to indicate the shift on which they were working during data collection and also to indicate the regularity with which they were working on that

---

[5] In terms of full-time equivalent figures, only 42 percent of the total work force in the ten hospitals are professional nurses, and this includes supervisory nurses. If supervisory nurses are excluded, only 36 percent of the total remaining nursing staff in these hospitals are registered nurses.

Gross Anatomy of Work in the Hospital

TABLE 13. The Distribution of Nursing Personnel According to Shift, for All Hospitals Combined

Respondent Group	Percentage of Group Members on:		
	Day Shift	Afternoon Shift	Night Shift
Supervisory nursing staff ($N = 170$)	70	17	13
Nonsupervisory registered nurses ($N = 193$)	38	32	30
Practical nurses ($N = 140$)	55	30	15
Aides and orderlies ($N = 203$)	42	35	23

shift. The information which they furnished is summarized in Table 13 and Table 14, below. The other groups in the study are all day-shift groups, although physicians make afternoon and night rounds, and administrative personnel often work into the late afternoon and, on occasion, at night also.

As may be expected, for each of the four nursing subgroups, the day shift is the most populous of the three shifts, while the night shift is the least populous. On the aggregate, only about one-third of the total nursing force works at the hospital during the afternoon shift, and not more than one-fourth works during the night shift. About half of the total nursing staff work during the day shift. The most evenly distributed group across the three shifts is the nonsupervisory registered nurses group. Of all members in this group, 38 percent work on the day shift, 32 percent work on the afternoon shift, and the remaining 30 percent work on the night shift. Apparently, both because they have to coordinate the work of others, and because professional nursing service to the patient cannot be cut below some minimum level at any time, about three out of every ten registered nurses have to work on the afternoon shift, and nearly as many have to work on the night shift. The large majority of supervisory nurses (70 percent), on the other hand, work on the day shift, and of the practical nurses, again a majority (55 percent) work on the day shift. Of the aides and orderlies, 42 percent work on the day shift and 35 percent work on the afternoon shift.

According to the data in Table 14, there is very little intershift rotation of nursing personnel in the hospitals studied. For each of the four nursing groups, we find that at least two out of every three individuals who indicate that they work on a given shift also say that they "always" work on that particular shift. Shift-wise, supervisory nurses constitute the most stable nursing group—82 percent "always" work on the same shift, with an additional 12 percent working on the same shift "most of the time." The aides and orderlies group is almost equally stable. By comparison, however, of the practical nurses 69 percent work on the same shift always, and only 67 percent of the nonsupervisory registered nurses work always on the same shift. The nonsupervisory registered nurses group is apparently the most "unstable" group, organizationally speaking, both in regard to shift work and in many other respects, as we have already pointed out in our preceding discussion of the other characteristics of this group.

TABLE 14. The Distribution of Nursing Personnel According to How Regularly They Work on Present Shift, for All Hospitals Combined

Respondent Group	Percentage of Group Members Indicating That They Work on Present Shift:		
	Always	Most of the Time	Less Frequently
Supervisory nursing staff ($N = 170$)	82	12	6
Nonsupervisory registered nurses ($N = 193$)	67	23	10
Practical nurses ($N = 140$)	69	20	11
Aides and orderlies ($N = 203$)	81	7	12

Service or Divisional Characteristics

Doctors and nurses—the two groups in the hospital which perform therapeutic functions, and which are the two largest groups in the institution—are organized along service or division lines. Each of the ten hospitals in the study has four major medical services plus several minor specialized services. The major services are surgery, medicine, obstetrics and gynecology, and pediatrics. Most medical staff members tend to work exclusively in one of these four services or divisions, and the same is true about the nursing staff. Upon entering the employment of a hospital, nursing personnel are usually assigned to a particular shift, as well as to a particular medical service.

The distribution of the medical and nursing staffs according to medical service is shown in Table 15. Of the four major services, surgery has the largest complement of medical staff, while pediatrics has the smallest. Of all doctors participating in the research, 28 percent indicated that they are working in surgery, 20 percent indicated that they are working in medicine, 14 percent indicated that they are working in obstetrics and gynecology, and 10 percent indicated that they are working in pediatrics, the remaining 28 percent being distributed among a number of other specialized areas.[6] The

---

[6] In response to a related question about their "major field of interest," 22 percent of the doctors in the study mentioned surgery as their field, 14 percent mentioned medicine, 11 percent mentioned obstetrics and gynecology, and 9 percent mentioned pediatrics. Another 9 percent indicated pathology or radiology as their main field of interest, and 19 percent indicated various specialties such as urology, ophthalmology, orthopedics, and otolaryngology. The remaining, about 16 percent of all doctors, mentioned "general practice" as their main field of interest. This last figure, however, is an underestimate of the proportion of doctors in the various hospitals who are general practitioners, due to the fact that it is based on both the general and the selected medical staff subgroups

Gross Anatomy of Work in the Hospital

order suggested by these percentages parallels very closely the distribution of hospital beds among the four medical services. Usually, surgery has more beds than medicine, which has more beds than obstetrics and gynecology, which has more beds than pediatrics, as we will see in the next chapter. The distribution of the nonsupervisory nursing staff across the four services, moreover, is not very different from the distribution of the medical staff.

TABLE 15. The Distribution of Medical and Nursing Staff Members According to the Major Service in Which They Work, for All Hospitals Combined

Respondent Group	Surgery *	Medicine	Medicine & Surgery Combined †	Obstetrics & Gynecology	Pediatrics	All Other ‡
Total medical staff ($N = 237$)	28	20	—	14	10	28
Supervisory nursing staff ($N = 168$)	19	9	12	16	8	36
Nonsupervisory registered nurses ($N = 192$)	27	12	14	20	11	16
Practical nurses ($N = 139$)	19	13	14	22	14	18
Aides and orderlies ($N = 197$)	20	14	12	14	14	26

* In the case of nursing groups, this category includes individuals working either in a surgical section or in the operating room.

† This category includes only nursing personnel who work in "mixed" sections, i.e., sections having both surgical and medical patients, rather than in separate divisions. Some hospitals have such mixed sections.

‡ For medical staff members, this category largely represents various specialties such as pathology, radiology, orthopedics, urology, etc. For nursing staff members, it represents various sections such as the central supply room, emergency, nursing office, and others, also including "floating" persons.

Considering the nursing groups, for all hospitals combined, we find a similar pattern. Of the supervisory nurses, 19 percent work in surgery, 9 percent in medicine, and another 12 percent in mixed medical-surgical sections; an additional 16 percent work in obstetrics and gynecology, and 8 percent in pediatrics. The remaining supervisory nurses are either assigned overall supervisory responsibilities, such as those of night or afternoon nursing supervisor, relief supervisor, and floor supervisor, or work in the nursing office rather than in any of the four major medical services. Of the nonsupervisory

---

participating in the study—the latter subgroup has fewer general practitioners than the entire medical staff. In this connection, other data from hospital records show that, in the ten hospitals, an average total of 29 percent of all active-attending medical staff members are classed as "general practitioners." Across individual hospitals, this figure ranges from a low of 19 percent to a high of 41 percent.

registered nurses, 53 percent work in surgery and medicine (compared to 40 percent of the supervisory nurses), the remaining being distributed among all other services, as specified in Table 15. And, of the practical nurses, as well as of the aides and orderlies, 46 percent work in surgery and medicine. In general, surgery has more nursing personnel from every classification than does medicine and, among the four major services, pediatrics has the smallest complement.

Any implication from the above data, however, that the different services have a more or less permanent nursing staff of their own, over a period of time, or that the nursing work force in the hospital is static, would be incorrect. Nursing personnel do move a great deal from one service to another. In response to the question "Have you ever worked in some other division (service) of this hospital other than your present division?" 71 percent of supervisory nurses, 65 percent of nonsupervisory registered nurses, 79 percent of practical nurses, and 62 percent of aides and orderlies answered "yes." Thus, the great majority of the members of each nursing group have experienced interdivisional transfers, either on their own request or by assignment. Such transfers, however, are apparently less frequent in the case of aides and orderlies, and in the case of nonsupervisory nurses, than for the remaining nursing staff.

The data concerning interdivisional movement for each nursing group are completely consistent with other data concerning the length of time members of each group have been working in their present service or division. Proportionately more aides and orderlies (53 percent), and more nonsupervisory registered nurses (45 percent) than practical nurses (30 percent) and supervisory nurses (20 percent) indicated that they have been working in their present division for up to one year only. Conversely, proportionately more supervisory nurses (33 percent) and more practical nurses (28 percent) than aides and orderlies (10 percent) and nonsupervisory registered nurses (14 percent) indicated that they have been working in their present division for at least five years.

Finally, based on the above and on earlier presented data, it is also interesting to point out that for each nursing group, except supervisory nurses, a relatively higher proportion of group members have worked in their present job than in their present division for a period of five or more years. Of the aides and orderlies, for example, 15 percent have worked in their present job in the hospital for at least five years, but only 10 percent have worked in their present division that long. The corresponding figures for practical nurses are 34 percent and 28 percent, respectively; and for nonsupervisory registered nurses, they are 17 and 14 percent, respectively. By contrast, the figures for supervisory nurses are in a reverse direction, being 21 and 33 percent, respectively.

Gross Anatomy of Work in the Hospital 113

Turnover and Absenteeism Among Nursing Personnel

The organizational stability of a given personnel group may in part also be gauged by examining the turnover and absenteeism which occur in the group. Because of the intrinsic interest of these two phenomena, and because we also wanted to study their consequences for the quality of patient care (see Chapter 8), an effort was made to obtain measures for each. Specifically, we had the nursing departments of the various hospitals examine their records for the last quarter of 1957 (the period during which data were collected from participating respondents, which is also the period for which most nursing departments could supply the most complete and most accurate information), and provide us with certain data about absences and turnover among nursing personnel. The required data were generally available for full-time personnel working in the hospitals during the specified period, but no data were obtained for supervisory nurses due to their relatively high organizational stability. In the end, with respect to absenteeism, we were able to secure the required data for full-time nonsupervisory registered nurses, practical nurses, and aides (orderlies were excluded because of the relatively small size of this group) from nine of the ten participating institutions. With respect to turnover, we were able to obtain sufficient data for nonsupervisory registered nurses and for aides from eight of the ten hospitals.

Turnover was primarily measured on the basis of personnel terminations, but also on the basis of work force stability within each nursing classification involved. Our main measure of turnover is represented by this ratio: total number of individuals in a given classification who, regardless of reason, were terminated during the last quarter of 1957, divided by the average total number of all individuals in that classification during the same period. A supplementary, but similar, measure was obtained by determining what percentage of the individuals in a given classification who were on the hospital payroll as of October 1, 1957, were also on the payroll as of December 31, 1957. This percentage figure, of course, represents personnel stability rather than turnover, but its complement (i.e., its difference from 100 percent) represents maximum turnover. For registered nurses, the turnover measure correlates $-.75$ with the stability measure; for aides, turnover correlates $-.68$ with stability. Complete turnover data were available in eight of the ten participating hospitals.

Examination of the turnover data shows the following results: (1) Of all full-time nonsupervisory registered nurses working in the eight hospitals during the last quarter of 1957, an average total of 10.5 percent had been terminated for various reasons as of December 31, 1957. Across individual hospitals, however, this turnover figure ranges from a low of only 2 percent, in one case, to a high of 14 percent, in another. (2) The comparable turnover figure for full-time aides is 5.7 percent, ranging across hospitals from a low of 3 percent to a high of exactly 10 percent. Apparently, the average turnover rate for registered nurses (10.5 percent) is twice as high as that for aides (5.7 percent), once more attesting to the relatively high organizational instability of the nonsupervisory registered nursing staff. Interestingly enough, moreover, we find no significant association (no significant correlation) between registered nurse turnover and aide turnover rates in the eight hospitals for which data are available. That is, a hospital with a high (or low) turnover rate among its registered nurses is just as likely to have a high turnover rate among its aides as it is to have a low or a medium rate, and vice versa.

The results obtained when using the personnel stability measure are entirely consistent with the above results. More specifically, we find: (1) Of all full-time registered nurses on the hospital payroll on October 1, 1957, a total of 87 percent were still on the payroll as of December 31, 1957—suggesting an average maximum turnover rate of 13 percent. The percentage still on the payroll as of December 31, 1957, ranges across the various hospitals from a high of 100 percent in one case to a low of 73 percent in another. (2) In the case of aides, of all those on the payroll as of the first of October, 93 percent were still on the payroll as of the last of December; this figure suggests an average maximum turnover rate of 7 percent and ranges across hospitals from a high of 97 to a low of 85 percent. Again, aides are likely to have about half the turnover rate of nonsupervisory registered nurses. All preceding findings about turnover, it must be remembered, refer to the last quarter of 1957.

Absenteeism was measured by the number of times each person from each classification involved was absent from work during the last quarter of 1957, regardless of specific reasons, and regardless of how many days the individual stayed away from the job. The data were obtained by counting the number of times each person in each nursing classification was regularly scheduled to work a particular shift but did not work that shift, "with the result that a substitute had to be found or the job remained uncovered." In short, the present measure concerns what may be thought of as "unexcused" absenteeism. The data on absenteeism are both more interesting and more complete than the data about turnover. Here, we have information from nine of the ten participating hospitals, and for all three of the nonsupervisory nursing groups in the study.

Our data show that the incidence of absenteeism (i.e., being absent at least once as against not being absent at all) is relatively widespread in all nursing groups, but the rates of absenteeism (i.e., being absent a certain specified number of times, but more than once) vary considerably from one nursing group to another, as well as among hospitals. Concerning the incidence of absenteeism, we find that only an average of 35 percent of practical nurses, 41 percent of aides, and 43 percent of nonsupervisory registered nurses in the various hospitals were not absent from work at least once during the last quarter of 1957. The majority of group members in each case were absent at least one time with the consequence that either a substitute had to be found or the job remained unfilled. The specific proportion of group members absent at least once during the indicated period (and, by exclusion, also the proportion never absent), however, varies a great deal among hospitals. For practical nurses, it ranges between a low of 20 percent in one of the hospitals to a high of 93 percent in another. For aides, it ranges from a low of 26 to a high of 86 percent. And, for nonsupervisory registered nurses, it ranges from a low of 41 percent to a high of 77 percent.

Thus, in general, the incidence of absenteeism in the community general hospital is most likely among practical nurses and least likely among nonsupervisory registered nurses, with the aides occupying an intermediate position, but one closer to that of registered nurses. It is also important to know in this connection, however, that the mere incidence of absenteeism in any one of the three nursing groups involved does not correlate significantly with the incidence of absenteeism in any of the other two groups (using the hospital as the unit of analysis)—a finding replicating the one concerning turnover rates among registered nurses and among aides. On the other hand, we are about to see that absenteeism rates (i.e., being absent two, three, or more times) within a particular nursing group correlate positively with absenteeism rates within each of the other nursing groups in the hospitals studied. Apparently, the incidence of absenteeism constitutes what appears to be primarily an individual level phenomenon, while absenteeism rates seem to constitute an organizational level phenomenon, i.e., they appear to be largely determined by group or organizational forces rather than by the characteristics of individual persons.

What, precisely, do the data show with respect to absenteeism rates? First, we find that the proportion of group members absent twice or more often between the first of October and the last of December 1957, averages 35 percent for nonsupervisory registered nurses, 39 percent for aides, and 43 percent for practical nurses, again being lowest among registered nurses and highest among practical nurses. Second, across hospitals, the proportion of group members absent at least twice ranges between a low of 11 percent and a high of 60 percent for registered nurses, between 14 and 57 percent for aides, and between 0 and 68 percent for practical nurses. Third, we find that those hospitals which have a relatively high proportion of registered nurses absent at least twice are also significantly more likely than other hospitals to have a high proportion of aides absent to the same extent. The rank-order correlation between these two proportions is .62, which, for an N of 9 hospitals, is statistically significant at the .05 level. A comparable finding is obtained, moreover, when we consider the proportion of practical nurses absent twice or more often in relation to the corresponding proportion of aides; here the correlation is .58, being practically significant at the .05 level. The corresponding correlation between the proportion of registered nurses and the proportion of practical nurses absent twice or more often, in the various hospitals, however, is not significant, although it too is positive, being .20.

When we consider the proportion of group members absent from regularly scheduled work three times or more often (rather than twice or more often) during the last quarter of 1957—which obviously includes all those individuals who are, more or less, "chronic" absentees—the results are essentially similar to the above, but yield much higher correlations. The average proportion of registered nurses who were absent at least three times is 20 percent, ranging across hospitals from 0 to 48 percent. The comparable proportion for aides is 26 percent, ranging between 8 percent and 50 percent. And the comparable proportion for practical nurses is 26 percent, i.e., the same as for aides, ranging across hospitals from 0 to a high of 60 percent. Concerning the interrelationship among these proportions, we find that the proportion of registered nurses absent three or more times correlates .73 with the proportion of practical nurses absent to the same extent, and .78 with the comparable proportion of aides, while the latter two correlate .83. Based on an N of 9 hospitals, these correlations are all statistically significant at better than the .05 level. Thus, hospitals having relatively many (or few) absentees of the, more or less, "chronic" kind (in the present case absent at least three times during the last quarter of 1957) within a particular nursing group, or level, are also significantly more likely than other hospitals to have many (or few) absentees of the same kind within their other nursing groups, or levels. High absenteeism rates among nursing personnel in the different classifications are very closely interrelated. Therefore, any attack against absenteeism rates on an individual basis would be fruitless. An effective attack should take into account the entire nursing organization—it should be made on a group basis.

On the basis of the preceding results, it may be concluded that an appreciable amount of turnover and absenteeism occurs among nursing personnel in the various hospitals, some of the hospitals being more vulnerable in this respect than others. One obvious consequence of turnover and absenteeism for the hospital is the difficulty of maintaining an adequate and stable staff at all times. A related difficulty is the fact that both absenteeism and turnover tend to aggravate the problem of nurse shortages. The effects of absenteeism and turnover among nursing personnel upon the quality of patient care, particularly the quality of nursing care, in the participating hospitals will be discussed in Chapter 8. Before concluding the present discussion, however, let us raise and answer two other pertinent questions. First, is there any relationship between turnover and absenteeism for a given group in the various hospitals? Second, is there any relationship between incidence of absenteeism and absenteeism rates for each group involved?

To answer the first question, we related our measure of turnover to our measures of absenteeism (using the hospital rather than individual persons as the unit of analysis). This analysis was carried out separately for nonsupervisory registered nurses and for aides—the two groups for which both absenteeism and turnover data were available—from the eight hospitals which supplied data. The results show that none of the obtained correlations is statistically significant, although all are in a positive direction. The specific correlations between turnover and incidence of absenteeism, as well as absenteeism rates, are generally small, ranging between .10 and .50. Since they are based on an N of 8 hospitals, these correlations are not significantly different from zero. At most, they suggest the possibility for only a slight tendency for turnover and absenteeism to be associated. For all practical purposes, however, it seems that those hospitals which have a relatively high rate of turnover among registered nurses (or among aides) are not necessarily more likely than other hospitals to have also a wider incidence of absenteeism, or high absenteeism rates, among their registered nurses (or among aides). Accordingly, the first of the above questions must be answered in the negative. In this study, we find no relationship between turnover and absenteeism among nursing personnel in the various hospitals.

To answer the second of the two questions raised above (using again the hospital as the unit of analysis), we intercorrelated incidence and rates of absenteeism separately for registered nurses, for practical nurses, and for aides from the nine hospitals for which data were available. The results may be summarized as follows:

1. The hospitals with higher proportions of their aides absent at least once, i.e., with high incidence of absenteeism, are also significantly more likely than other hospitals to have a higher proportion of aides absent twice or more often. They also tend to have a higher proportion of aides absent three or more times. The rank-order correlation between the proportion absent at least once and the proportion absent twice or more often is .72, and that between the proportion absent at least once and the proportion absent three or more times is .52. Similarly, the proportion of aides absent twice or more often correlates .63 with the proportion absent three or more times. Based on an N of 9 hospitals, the first and third of these correlations are significant at the .05 level, but the second does not reach statistical significance at this level.

2. Concerning practical nurses, the results are essentially the same as those for aides. The proportion of practical nurses absent at least once correlates .60 with the proportion absent twice or more often, and .44 with the proportion absent three or more times, while the proportion absent twice or more often correlates .76 with the proportion absent three or more times.

3. Concerning registered nurses, however, the results yield a partly different pattern. First, there is no relationship whatever between the proportion of registered nurses absent at least once, on the one hand, and either the proportion absent twice or more often, or the proportion absent three or more

times, on the other. In the former instance, the obtained correlation is only .16, and in the latter it is only —.15, for all practical purposes being both equivalent to zero. This means that hospitals having a relatively high proportion of registered nurses absent at least once are neither more nor less likely than other hospitals to have also a high proportion of registered nurses absent twice or more often, or absent three times or more. When we consider the proportion absent twice or more often in relation to the proportion absent three or more times, however, the results are sharply different, for these two proportions correlate very highly, .80, and significantly.

Thus, those hospitals with a high proportion of their registered nurses absent at least twice are also significantly more likely than other hospitals to have a high proportion of their registered nurses absent three times or more often (during the last quarter of 1957). And, as the above results show, the same holds true with respect to both practical nurses and aides. These findings are especially interesting, moreover, in view of the fact that the hospitals studied vary a great deal from one another in their respective absenteeism rates among their nursing staff. One implication which emerges from the results concerning absenteeism is that while being absent at least once (or, conversely, not being absent at all) may be a phenomenon largely accounted for in terms of the individual-personal characteristics of the various nursing personnel, having relatively high absenteeism rates (in the present case, being absent at least twice, and being absent three or more times, during the last quarter of 1957) among the members of each nursing group in the hospital is apparently an organizational phenomenon, i.e., a phenomenon which depends upon the particular hospitals themselves, rather than a phenomenon which can be explained by the absence behavior of individual employees. In future studies with a larger number of organizations than the present one, it would be worth while to pursue this hypothesis further.

Work Interaction Patterns Among Hospital Personnel

In subsequent chapters, different aspects of the nature of interaction among the various people around the patient will be discussed in detail. For example, one chapter will be almost exclusively concerned with communication among nursing personnel, two chapters will deal with coordination phenomena, and another chapter will be concerned with superior-subordinate relationships. Such specific aspects of interaction as intergroup tensions, and the question of mutual understanding of one another's problems and needs on the part of different groups in the hospital, will likewise be examined in some detail in the chapters which follow. In this section, however, by way of background information, we would like at least to sketch out the web of interaction among different personnel groups. In broad terms, what is the work interaction like in the community general hospital?

Gross Anatomy of Work in the Hospital

First, as may be expected, by virtue of their size and by virtue of the high mutual interdependence in their work, the medical staff and the nursing staff interact more frequently among themselves, and between themselves and the patients, than any other pair of groups in the hospital. Second, the nursing staff constitutes the one single group in the hospital with which most other groups have their greatest interaction. In addition to its therapeutic functions, and unlike the medical staff, which is not employed by the hospital, the nursing staff carries out a good deal of coordinative functions with other groups and departments in the organization. Third, in general, apart from their mutual interaction and their contact with patients, both the medical staff and the nursing staff have most of their interaction with the various medical and paramedical services of the hospital, having fewer dealings with the nonmedical services such as housekeeping, maintenance, front office, laundry, and the like. But, let us be more specific.

Most of the respondents in the study were asked two check-list type questions about overall interaction. The first question was designed to provide some information about the relative amount of contact with others. The second was designed to provide some information about the nature of interaction with others. Regarding the volume of contacts, data were obtained from the general medical staff, from supervisory nurses, from nonsupervisory registered nurses, from practical nurses, and from the administrative department heads. Regarding the nature of interaction, data were obtained from the same groups and, in addition, from aides. First, we will present the results concerning interaction volume.

The members of the general medical staff from the various hospitals were asked the following question about their interaction with other hospital members:

On the following list, please check the *three* departments with which you usually have most contacts in connection with your work:
_____(1) Nursing
_____(2) Dietetics
_____(3) Maintenance
_____(4) Housekeeping
_____(5) X-ray
_____(6) Laboratory
_____(7) Business Office
_____(8) Records
_____(9) Admissions
_____(0) Pharmacy

For all hospitals combined, the five most frequently chosen departments by the general medical staff, ordered here according to the frequency with which they were mentioned, are: nursing; x-ray; laboratory; records; and admissions, in fifth place. Personnel from the first three of these departments, it will be recalled, have been included in the study as respondents.

Nursing personnel from the various hospitals were asked the same question about interaction as the medical staff, with the exception that the list of departments used in this case did not include the medical staff. Our early exploratory work had already established the fact that the nursing staff interacts most frequently with the medical staff, among all hospital groups (and the above data from the doctors also confirm this fact). Nursing, being the respondents' own department, was likewise omitted from the list. Excluding the medical staff, which would place first among the various groups, the interaction data obtained from nursing personnel may be summarized as follows: (1) the three most frequently chosen departments by supervisory nurses, by nonsupervisory registered nurses, and by practical nurses, as the departments with which each group has most of its contacts are the laboratory, the pharmacy, and the dietary department; (2) the x-ray department and admissions are the fourth and fifth most frequently chosen departments by the same respondents, except that supervisory nurses chose the front office (or business office) in fifth place, with x-ray placing sixth; and (3) the remaining departments on the list (housekeeping, maintenance, and records) are the lowest interaction departments for the nursing staff.

The nonmedical, administrative department heads were asked the same question as the nursing staff, except that the list of departments in this case included nursing in place of the (medical) records department. The data show that the five most frequently chosen departments by the department heads, as the departments with which these respondents have most contact, are according to frequency as follows: nursing; front office; maintenance; housekeeping; and dietetics, in fifth place.

Regarding the nature of their interaction, all of the respondent groups which answered the question about contact with others, and the aides group in addition, were asked the following: "On the following list, please check the *two* departments that you find most difficult (least easy) to work with or deal with: . . ." For each respondent group, the list of departments was identical with the list involved in the previous question concerning amount of contact with others (for the aides group it was identical with that used for the other nursing groups). The data show that, on the whole, the "most difficult to deal with" departments, for all respondents from all ten hospitals combined, are the dietary, the laboratory, and housekeeping, in that order. But, the department heads most frequently mentioned nursing as the most difficult to deal with of all departments. Nursing was also chosen by doctors as the third most difficult to deal with department.

In order of the frequency with which they were chosen in each case, the four most difficult to deal with departments for each of the respondent groups involved are as follows:

Gross Anatomy of Work in the Hospital

1. For the medical staff respondents, they are: dietetics, laboratory, nursing, and business office (front office).
2. For the department heads, they are: nursing, maintenance, laboratory, and x-ray.
3. For the supervisory nurses, they are: housekeeping, dietetics, laboratory, and x-ray and maintenance tied in fourth place. It should also be reiterated in this connection, however, that the medical staff was not included on the list from which supervisory and nonsupervisory nursing personnel chose the most difficult to deal with groups.
4. For nonsupervisory registered nurses, they are: dietetics, laboratory, housekeeping, and pharmacy.
5. For practical nurses, they are: dietetics, housekeeping, x-ray, and pharmacy.
6. And, for aides, they are: dietetics, pharmacy, laboratory, and maintenance.

The interaction patterns discussed above are, of course, based on data from all ten hospitals in the study. It is needless to say, therefore, that a particular hospital may not conform to one or more of the specific patterns, for differences among individual hospitals also exist. Nevertheless, the interaction patterns shown for each respondent group provide us with a good indication about who interacts with whom, and how much, among the people around the patient, as well as with an indication of where interaction problems are likely to arise most frequently within the community general hospital. In this connection, it is also interesting to note that concerning interaction among the top three groups in the hospital (doctors, trustees, and administrator) other data from the present study show that the doctors, the trustees, and the administrators from the participating hospitals agree in reporting more tension between doctors and other doctors in the hospital than between doctors and the hospital administrator, and in reporting least tension between doctors and trustees.

Concerning tension between doctors and other hospital groups, data supplied by both medical and nonmedical respondents generally show less tension between doctors and trustees, between doctors and administrator, or between doctors and x-ray *than* between doctors and other doctors, doctors and nurses, or doctors and the records department; tension between doctors and the laboratory, and between doctors and admissions approximates the same level as tension between doctors and the records department. Concerning tension within the nursing staff, data from nursing personnel indicate more tension among nursing staff in the different shifts than among nursing staff in the different classifications (levels), than among nursing staff in the different sections or services of the hospital. Perhaps the most interesting of the results about tension among hospital groups are: (1) the fact that we find more tension between doctors and other doctors than between doctors and any other major group in the hospital; (2) the fact that we find less tension between doctors and trustees than between doctors and any other major group in the hospital; (3) the existence of a good deal of tension between doctors and nurses; and (4) the fact that there is less tension among nursing personnel in different classifications (e.g., between registered and practical nurses) than between nursing personnel in the different shifts. Our specific measures of tension, as well as additional findings about intergroup tension, will be discussed in subsequent chapters.

Much of the tension prevailing among hospital groups undoubtedly stems from the nature of the work structure in hospitals. That work in the hospital is generally of a highly interactional character, or that most personnel do their work in association and close interdependence with other personnel, requires no special comment. Patient care, the main organizational product of the hospital, demands concerted efforts on the part of many different individuals, groups, staffs, and departments. The vast majority of the people around the patient have to cooperate with one another, to a greater or lesser extent, as part of the technical or task requirements of their job. In the process, apart from the fact that tensions and problems are likely to arise, the work of these different people has to be adequately coordinated, moreover, and coordination itself involves further interaction among some of the personnel, over and above the interaction necessitated by the purely technical aspects of their work.

Much of this coordination in the community general hospital is carried out by the administrative department heads and by the nursing staff, particularly the supervisory and nonsupervisory registered nurses, the nursing staff being the one single group in the hospital with which most other groups have most of their contacts as we have already seen. The department heads have to coordinate the activities of the different departments of the hospital, as well as the work of their respective personnel within their own department. Before concluding the present section, therefore, let us also present some data which demonstrate the fact that the role of department heads and of supervisory nurses entails a great many coordinative functions.

The relevant data were obtained in response to a question which was asked of supervisory nurses and of department heads in the various hospitals. The question was: "To what extent does your job involve each of the following?" The term "following" referred to five specific items listed under the question. The respondents were requested to indicate the extent to which their job involved each of the items, on a scale ranging from "To a very great extent" to "Not at all." The five items, in the order of their listing under the question, were:

> Trying to fit different jobs or activities into one another—to coordinate the work of various people or departments.
>
> Getting people to work together to accomplish a common purpose.
>
> Trying to iron out unnecessary duplications or overlappings that arise in the working relationships of people in different jobs.
>
> Trying to reconcile differing interests of various personnel or departments.
>
> Trying to reduce conflicts, waste, and other disruptive interferences in the process of achieving hospital goals.

Gross Anatomy of Work in the Hospital

Table 16 shows the percentage of supervisory nurses (SNS) and of administrative department heads (ADH), from all hospitals in the study, who indicated that their job involves each of the above five activities to specified degrees.

TABLE 16. Percentage of Supervisory Nurses (SNS) and of Administrative Department Heads (ADH), from All Hospitals Combined, Giving Certain Responses to the Question: "To What Extent Does Your Job Involve Each of the Following Items?"

Item Involved:	Respondents	"To a Very Great Extent"	"To a Great Extent"	"To Some Extent"	"To a Small Extent" or "Not at All"	N
		(percent)				
Getting people to work together to accomplish a common purpose	SNS:	44	29	16	11	167
	ADH:	38	28	16	18	100
Trying to reduce conflicts, waste, and other disruptive interferences in the process of achieving hospital goals	SNS:	37	24	24	15	167
	ADH:	34	27	17	22	99
Trying to fit different jobs or activities into one another—to coordinate the work of various people or departments	SNS:	30	20	25	25	166
	ADH:	29	25	21	25	98
Trying to reconcile differing interests of various personnel or departments	SNS:	15	16	27	42	163
	ADH:	15	14	23	48	97
Trying to iron out unnecessary duplications or overlappings that arise in the working relationships of people in different jobs	SNS:	12	11	30	47	167
	ADH:	11	20	23	46	96

The results in Table 16 clearly show that, as anticipated, the roles of supervisory nurses and administrative department heads in the community general hospital, to a large degree, involve coordinative functions. Interestingly enough, moreover, the pattern of responses from supervisory nurses is practically the same as that from the department heads, even though the latter group is a highly heterogeneous group by comparison to the former. For example, we find that a substantial majority of both supervisory nurses

(73 percent) and department heads (66 percent) indicate that their job involves "getting people to work together to accomplish a common purpose" to a very great extent or to a considerable extent. Only about one out of every ten respondents in each case say that their job involves this activity to a small extent or not at all. The results concerning the item "trying to reduce conflicts . . ." are very similar. Again, the majority of supervisory nurses (61 percent) and of department heads (61 percent) indicate that their job involves this activity to a very great extent or to a considerable extent. The results concerning the item "trying to fit different jobs or activities into one another . . ." are also similar, with about half of the respondents saying that their job involves this function to a very great extent or to a considerable extent.

It should be noted that all three of the activities to which the above data refer are essentially coordinative activities. The same is also true of the remaining two items about which data are shown in Table 16. In connection with these latter two items ("trying to reconcile different interests . . ." and "trying to iron out unnecessary duplications . . ."), however, the proportion of respondents who say that their job involves each item to a very great extent or to a considerable extent is much smaller than for each of the three items already discussed. Apparently, both the supervisory nurses and the department heads spend a good deal of their time on the previous three activities and less time on the last two. In all probability, moreover, there was no great need in the various hospitals studied for the respondents to try "to reconcile differing interests . . ." or to try "to reduce conflicts . . ." at the time when the data were collected.

PRESENT JOB STATUS AND OUTLOOK

Thus far, we have discussed the personal characteristics of the people around the patient, their professional and occupational career patterns, and certain aspects of their work at the hospital. In this section, we shall be concerned with some of the most fundamental aspects of the job itself: What are the general patterns of effort, reward, satisfaction, and motivation which characterize the people who hold most of the nonmedical jobs in the hospital, and how do the different personnel groups compare with one another on these patterns?

Do people feel free to set their work pace?
Do they feel under pressure at work?
Does their job in the hospital enhance their self-confidence?
How satisfied are they with their supervisors?
How satisfied are they with their chances for advancement?
What are their earnings like, and how satisfied are they with them?

Present Job Status and Outlook 125

What are the main reasons which keep them at work in the hospital?
How strongly identified do they feel with their profession, their work group, the hospital, and the community?
What do they think of the hospital as a place to work, and how long would they like to stay there?
Do the key people in the institution make them feel an important part of "the team"?

These are the questions that we shall try to answer in this section with reference to the nonmedical personnel, especially the nursing staff, in the hospital. Their importance for the individuals involved, as well as for their respective organizations, should require no particular comment here.

Work Pace and Pressure

Administrative department heads, nursing personnel, and laboratory and x-ray technicians from each hospital were asked two questions that provide us some information about the nature of their respective jobs. The questions were: "On the job, how free do you feel to set your own work pace?" And, "On the job, do you feel any pressure for better performance over and above what you think is reasonable?" The former question provided five response alternatives, ranging from "I feel completely free to set my own work pace" to "I have no freedom at all to set my work pace." The latter offered six response alternatives, ranging from "I feel a great deal of pressure . . ." to "I feel no pressure at all over and above what is reasonable."

On the whole, the data show that for most groups involved the majority of members feel "completely free" to set their pace of work, but, at the same time, the majority experience at least some pressure for better performance over and above what they consider as reasonable pressure. As might be expected, however, in both instances, there are considerable differences both among personnel groups and among individual hospitals. Apart from these differences, the general tendency is for personnel whose job entails administrative or supervisory responsibilities to feel more free than others with respect to regulating their work pace, but also to experience more "unreasonable" pressure than others.

We find that, on the average, less than 10 percent of the members of each respondent group feel "little" or no freedom to set their work pace, while a substantial proportion in each case feel complete freedom. Yet, differences among groups exist, and the same is true for hospitals, only much more so. Of all department heads in the ten hospitals, 61 percent indicate that they feel completely free to set their work pace, but, across hospitals, this figure ranges from as low as 20 percent in one institution to as high as 82 percent in another. For supervisory nurses, the corresponding average is 60 percent, with an interhospital range between 31 and 88 percent. For nonsupervisory registered nurses, it is 51 percent, with a range between 41 and 65 percent. For practical nurses, it is 51 percent, with a range between 25 and 60 percent. For aides and orderlies, it is 49 percent, with a range between 25 and 59 percent. And for the technicians, it is only 35 percent, with a range between 20 and 50 percent. Technicians are, therefore, least likely of all personnel to feel free to regulate their work pace, while department heads and supervisory nurses are most likely of all the groups involved.

The results concerning pressure for better performance show that, while only a small proportion of the members of each group feel "considerable" pressure or "a great deal" of pressure over and above what they think is reasonable (an average of between 2 percent in the case of practical nurses to 13 percent in the case of supervisory nurses, depending on which group we consider), a majority in each case, except for practical nurses, state that they experience at least some unreasonable pressure. Practical nurses constitute the least pressured group, while department heads and supervisory nurses constitute the most pressured groups, being closely followed by the technicians. Of the nonsupervisory groups, the technicans feel least free to set their work pace and most unreasonable pressure for better performance.

In terms of specific figures, we find that of all administrative department heads in the study only 28 percent state that they feel "no pressure at all" for better performance over what is reasonable, this figure ranging across hospitals from a low of 15 percent to a high of 50 percent. The corresponding average figure for all supervisory nurses in the study is 32 percent, ranging across hospitals from 0 to 65 percent. Of the technicians, an average of 37 percent feel no pressure at all, the range among hospitals being between 13 and 73 percent. The corresponding average figure for nonsupervisory registered nurses is 48 percent, and ranges between 23 and 65 percent; for aides and orderlies, it is 47 percent, and ranges between 23 and 67 percent; and for practical nurses —the least pressured group—it is 63 percent, and ranges between 36 and 84 percent across individual hospitals.

Apart from the obvious differences which characterize the various groups of personnel with respect to pressure, as well as pace of work, at this point we need only draw attention to the rather impressive interhospital differences indicated by the range of the above data—something which holds true for the great bulk of other results obtained in the present study and reported in subsequent chapters.

Before concluding the present discussion, we may also raise the question as to the origins of unreasonable pressure experienced by the different groups of personnel. In this connection, those of the respondents from each group who indicated that they felt at least some pressure were asked to indicate the main source of the pressure on a list containing the following possible sources: "the people I usually work with" (or "the people I supervise"); "the kind of work I do"; "my superiors"; "people from other departments"; "the patients";

"patients' relatives or visitors"; "myself"; "the doctors"; "something else, other than the preceding." The most frequently indicated sources of pressure are shown below, separately for each group, together with the percentage of group members who named each source. The percentage figures are of course based on the total number of group members in each case who felt at least some pressure; those feeling no pressure at all are not included.

The main sources of "unreasonable" pressure are as follows:

1. For administrative department heads ($N = 65$): the kind of work I do (43 percent), myself (17 percent), people from other departments (8 percent), and all other sources combined (32 percent).
2. For supervisory nurses ($N = 107$): the people I supervise (20 percent), the kind of work I do (18 percent), my superiors (17 percent), myself (12 percent), and all other sources (33 percent).
3. For nonsupervisory registered nurses ($N = 92$): my superiors (18 percent), the kind of work I do (15 percent), myself (15 percent), people from other departments (11 percent), the doctors (10 percent), and all other sources (31 percent).
4. For practical nurses ($N = 48$): the people I work with (23 percent), my superiors (15 percent), the kind of work I do (10 percent), myself (10 percent), people from other departments (8 percent), and all other sources (34 percent).
5. For aides and orderlies ($N = 93$): the people I work with (34 percent), my superiors (15 percent), the kind of work I do (11 percent), myself (11 percent), and all other sources (29 percent).
6. For the technicians ($N = 74$): the doctors (20 percent), the people I work with (19 percent), the kind of work I do (19 percent), my superiors (18 percent), and all other sources (24 percent).

In general, then, consistent with the highly interactional character of hospital work, "the kind of work I do," "my superiors," "myself," "the people I work with (or I supervise)," and "people from other departments," including doctors, are the main sources of "unreasonable pressure" for better performance for the nonmedical staff in the community general hospital. It is interesting to observe, moreover, that the origins of pressure tend to be least diffuse, or most concentrated, for the department heads, the aides and orderlies, and the technicians. Of similar interest is also the fact that not a single one of the groups involved considers the patients as the main source of pressure, while "myself" constitutes one of the main sources of pressure for every group except the technicians. At least one in ten of the group members in each case reports "unreasonable" internalized pressure for better performance.

Skill Utilization and Improvement

Organizational utilization of the skill supply in the community general hospital seems to be good, but it is better for personnel holding supervisory and administrative jobs and for technicians than for people in nonsupervisory nursing jobs. For every hospital in the study, at least four out of every ten department heads, supervisory nurses, and technicians feel that their job gives them a very good chance to do the things "they are best at." In fact, in response to the question "How much does your job give you a chance to do the things you are best at?", an average of 73 percent of all department heads, 65 percent of all technicians, and 54 percent of all supervisory nurses indicated that their job gives them a "very good" or an "excellent" chance. At the same time, no more than 3 percent of the members of each of these groups felt that their job gives them only a little or no chance; the remaining members in each case indicated "a good chance" or "a fair chance." Across individual hospitals, the percentage of those indicating a very good chance or an excellent chance ranges between 42 and 90 percent for department heads, 40 and 100 percent for supervisory nurses, and between 38 and 80 percent for technicians.

Considering the nonsupervisory nursing personnel, we find that an average of 46 percent of all registered nurses, 47 percent of all practical nurses, and 45 percent of all aides and orderlies felt that their job gives them a very good chance or an excellent chance to do the things they are best at—these percentages being appreciably smaller than those for the preceding groups. Conversely, less than 10 percent of the members of each of the three nonsupervisory nursing groups felt that their job gives them only a little chance or no chance to do the things they are best at. With respect to interhospital differences, we find that the percentage of group members who indicated a very good or an excellent chance varies between 24 and 61 percent for registered nurses, between 15 and 73 percent for practical nurses, and between 26 and 67 percent for aides and orderlies. As in most other instances, some of the hospitals fare considerably better, and others considerably worse, than the average figures for all ten hospitals combined indicate.

The three nonsupervisory nursing groups were also asked two additional items which have some bearing on the question of enhancing personnel skills through the job. These items were: "To what extent does your work here help you learn more about your profession or occupation?" and "To what extent does your work here help you develop more confidence in yourself?"

Of all nonsupervisory registered nurses in the study, 53 percent felt that their work helps them to a "great extent" or a "very great extent" to learn more about their profession (with a range across hospitals between 33 and 75 percent), and 61 percent felt that their work helps them as much to increase their self-confidence (the interhospital range being from 48 to 79 percent). The corresponding figures for practical nurses are 67 percent (with a range between 43 and 91 percent), and 73 percent (with a range between 57 and 100 percent), respectively. Similarly, of the aides and orderlies 65 percent (with a range between 48 and 92 percent) felt that their work in the hospital helps them to a great or very great extent to learn more about their occupation, and 69 percent (with a range between 46 and 89 percent) felt that their work

Present Job Status and Outlook

helps them to the same extent with respect to developing more confidence in themselves. If anything, therefore, their job seems to enhance the skills of nonsupervisory nursing personnel.

Thus, on the whole, the situation in the community general hospital, with respect to skill utilization and skill improvement, as reflected in the above items, appears to be a satisfactory and rewarding one for most members of most groups. But, interhospital differences must again be kept in mind, as must the differences among personnel groups shown by the data.

Overall Satisfaction with Supervision

In the chapter on superior-subordinate relations, we shall examine in detail many aspects of the relationship between people in supervisory positions and their subordinates. At this point, by way of background information, we will present data only about the general attitude of employees toward their supervisors, as assessed by their responses to the following question: "Taking all things into consideration, how satisfied are you with your immediate superior?"

The data from this question show that an average of from six to more than nine out of every ten members of the several groups which we have been discussing feel "completely satisfied" or "very well satisfied" with their immediate superiors. Of the six nonmedical groups involved, the administrative department heads are most satisfied with their immediate superior, while the laboratory and x-ray technicians are least satisfied. Ninety-one percent of all department heads from all hospitals in the study said that they are completely or very well satisfied with their immediate superior, in comparison to 60 percent of the technicians. Of the nursing groups, aides and orderlies are most satisfied, and nonsupervisory registered nurses are least satisfied, with their immediate superiors—89 percent of the former compared to 72 percent of the latter indicated that they are completely or very well satisfied. Of the remaining two groups, the supervisory nurses are similar to the registered nurses, and the practical nurses are similar to the aides and orderlies in overall satisfaction with supervision. Seventy-four percent of supervisory nurses, and 82 percent of practical nurses, are completely or very well satisfied with their immediate superiors.

Since, on the average, the great majority of the members of each group express high satisfaction with supervision, one would expect little interhospital range on this variable. The interesting thing is, nevertheless, that in most cases a fairly wide range actually characterizes the ten hospitals in the study. For administrative department heads, whose immediate superior in most cases is the hospital administrator, the percentage indicating complete or very good satisfaction with their immediate superior ranges across individual hospitals from a low of 70 to a high of 100 percent. For supervisory nurses, whose immediate superior in most cases is the director of nursing, it ranges between 47 and 100 percent. For nonsupervisory registered nurses, whose immediate superior in most cases is a supervisory nurse, it ranges between 55 and 84 percent. For practical nurses, whose immediate superiors are supervisory and nonsupervisory registered nurses, it ranges between 69 and 100 percent. For aides and orderlies, whose immediate superiors are members of the other nursing groups, it ranges between 82 and 100 percent. And for technicians, whose immediate superior is usually a head technician or a doctor, it ranges between 36 and 90 percent—the largest interhospital range of all groups involved. Disregarding the differences among hospitals, however, the data clearly show that most nonmedical employees are very well satisfied with their immediate superior, "taking all things into consideration."

When taking specific things into consideration, however, as we will see in our chapter on superior-subordinate relations, things are not always as rosy in the area of supervision as one might infer from the above data. In this connection, we need only mention here, for example, that regardless of which of the above six groups is examined we find less than half of its members feeling that their immediate superior expresses to them appreciation for their work "very often" or "always." At the same time, depending upon the group examined, an average of between 10 and 22 percent of group members say that their immediate superior "seldom or never" expresses appreciation for their work. But, let us defer the discussion of specific aspects of superior-subordinate relations, for it takes us beyond the scope of the present chapter.

Opportunity for Advancement and Earnings

Employee satisfaction with what may be called the "hard," or most tangible organizational rewards in the hospital, unlike satisfaction with supervision and other social-psychological aspects of the job, is rather low by comparison. In this area, we asked department heads, nursing personnel in the several classifications, and technicians to answer two specific questions. The first question was: "How satisfied do you feel about your chances for advancement or for promotion in this hospital?" The question provided seven response alternatives, ranging from "completely dissatisfied" to "completely satisfied." The second question was: "How satisfied are you with your present salary or wages?" It too offered seven response alternatives—in fact the same alternatives as the first question, but in reverse order—ranging from "completely satisfied" to "completely dissatisfied." Additional data about actual salaries were secured from hospital records.

Both questions yielded rather disquieting results and, as we will see, not without good reason. First, we will discuss the results about advancement. In this connection, excepting personnel in administrative and supervisory positions, we find that only an average of between 34 and 44 percent of the members of each group involved feel "very well" or "completely satisfied" with their chances for advancement or promotion in their respective hospitals. Conversely, an average of between 18 and 38 percent of group members—depending on which group is examined—feel at least "somewhat dissatisfied." Of all groups providing information, the administrative department heads express the highest satisfaction with their chances for advancement in the hospital. Only 11 percent of them express some dissatisfaction, while another 62 percent feel very well or completely satisfied (the remaining express lower degrees of satisfaction). Across hospitals, the percentage expressing high satisfaction ("very well" or "completely satisfied") ranges between 25 and 100 percent, the average of course being 62 percent. Supervisory nurses constitute the second best-satisfied group: 55 percent feel very well satisfied or completely satisfied (with an interhospital range of between 32 and 92 percent), and 14 percent express at least some dissatisfaction with their chances for advancement. For all other groups, we find less satisfaction and, correspondingly, more dissatisfaction in this area.

Technicians constitute the least satisfied group with respect to opportunity for advancement. Only one out of every three technicians (34 percent) feels very well satisfied or completely satisfied (the range across hospitals being from 10 to 56 percent), while another one in three (32 percent) feels at least "somewhat dissatisfied" (the range in this case being from 0 to 64 percent); the remaining one-third of technicians feel just "fairly satisfied" or only "a little satisfied." The data in fact show that, for five of the ten hospitals in the study, the proportion of technicians who express some dissatisfaction exceeds the proportion who feel very well or completely satisfied. The results for the three nonsupervisory nursing groups, with the interhospital range enclosed in parentheses, are as follows: Of the registered nurses, 37 percent (24 to 50 percent) feel very well satisfied or completely satisfied, with an additional 18 percent (5 to 38 percent) expressing at least some dissatisfaction. Of the practical nurses, 44 percent (15 to 70 percent) are similarly satisfied, with another 26 percent (0 to 54 percent) being similarly dissatisfied. And of the aides and orderlies, 38 percent (26 to 64 percent) are comparably satisfied, with an additional 31 percent (18 to 43 percent) being comparably dissatisfied with their chances for advancement in the hospital.

Most dissatisfaction on the part of technicians and nonsupervisory nursing personnel concerning chances for advancement probably stems from the fact that, for the vast majority of group members in each case, both upward mobility and interoccupational mobility are very limited in the hospital situation. It seems to be generally true, for example, that "once a technician always a technician," and "once a practical nurse always a practical nurse," save for those leaving the hospital. On the other hand, some aides eventually become practical nurses; but, the majority do not. Similarly, although some nonsupervisory registered nurses may be given supervisory-administrative roles, the large majority neither are offered such roles nor are they prone to seek them. (Many registered nurses would have nothing to do with supervisory duties which tend to take them away from the patient.) Promotions to a higher job within the hospital being very limited, and movement to a better profession or occupation also being very limited, for most personnel advancement comes to mean simply a change in pay scales. But, as the data about salaries and satisfaction with salary will next show, most people do not have a realistic chance for much advancement in this connection—at least for the time being. To some individuals, advancement could conceivably also mean moving from a less desirable section or service in the hospital to a more desirable one, without any other connotations, but we doubt that many of the respondents answered the question about advancement with this frame of reference in mind.

Regarding employee earnings, it is rather common knowledge that nonmedical personnel in hospitals are generally paid low salaries and wages, although it is not too widely known how low actually salaries are for specific personnel classifications. It is also fairly widely known that, in hospitals such as those in this study, payroll expenses roughly account for nearly two-thirds of the total expenses of the institution, and that most hospital income goes into payroll. What is not well known, however, is that both hospital income and total expenses have in recent years risen somewhat disproportionately higher than the average earnings of hospital personnel.

For the year ending September 30, 1955, for example, the aggregate total expenses of the ten hospitals in the study amounted to 13.85 million dollars (total income exceeding this figure slightly), of which 65 percent went to payroll. The average (mean) annual salary per full-time (or full-time equivalent), hospital-paid employee—counting all employees, in all positions, in all ten hospitals—that same year amounted to $2767. By comparison, for the year ending September 1958, aggregate hospital expenses amounted to 18.23 million dollars, representing a cumulative increase of 31 percent over 1955, or an average annual increase of about 10 percent. Of these expenses, 62.5 percent, or 2½ percent less than for 1955, went to payroll. The average annual salary per full-time employee in 1958 was $3093. It had increased, cumulatively, only by about 11 percent over 1955, or a little less than 4 percent per year (and, if one takes into account the increases in cost of living during that three-year period, hospital employee earnings remained practically unchanged). In short, total hospital expenses increased at a faster rate than did the average earnings of nonmedical hospital personnel (total income, moreover, having increased proportionately to total expenses, the former slightly exceeding the latter for the ten hospitals combined).

For the year ending September 1959, total expenses in the ten hospitals amounted to 18.43 million dollars, and total payroll amounted to 12.35 million. Payroll represented almost 67 percent of total expenses. The average annual salary per full-time paid employee was $3207. In dollar figures, since September 1955, total hospital expenses had increased by 33 percent, while payroll expenses had increased by about half this rate, 15.9 percent.[7] At the

[7] In the following chapter, as well as in the chapter on factors affecting patient care, additional data will be presented about some of the financial aspects of hospital functioning.

same time, the total number of beds in the ten hospitals had remained practically constant (1962 beds in 1955 compared to 1970 beds in 1959), and the same is true of the average number of full-time paid employees per hospital (380 employees in 1955 compared to 385 in 1959).

The implication of the above data, when viewed in conjunction with the fact that hospital personnel are admittedly underpaid, is anything but encouraging, both from the standpoint of attracting, hiring, and maintaining competent personnel (especially in a period of shortages), and from the point of view of the hundreds of people in each hospital who serve the increasingly demanding patient 24 hours a day, including Sundays and holidays. Under prevailing circumstances, as sketched above, one would hardly expect hospital personnel to feel euphoric about their salaries and wages. And, the data actually show a good deal of discontent in this area on the part of hospital employees—generally showing more dissatisfaction than in the area of opportunity for advancement. What seems surprising, however, is the absence of more dissatisfaction rather than the presence of a relatively low level of satisfaction with earnings indicated by the data. Before discussing the extent to which different groups of employees express satisfaction or dissatisfaction with their earnings, however, let us see what their actual salaries were in the last quarter of 1957—the period during which data were collected from the respondents. Table 17 presents this information.

The actual salary data in Table 17 speak for themselves, although they may not speak out loud enough. Let the reader draw his own conclusions, however. We will only draw attention to a few points which highlight the situation. Of the 14 categories of personnel shown, considering all participating hospitals together, only 3 (department heads in all cases) averaged an annual salary exceeding $4500 as of the end of 1957, while 5 personnel categories averaged a salary between $3700 (nonsupervisory registered nurses) and $1800 (unskilled kitchen help). The highest salary, for any group in any hospital, was $9300, in the case of one director of nursing, and the lowest was $1350 for the maids in housekeeping in two of the hospitals; the second-highest salary was $8800, again for one director of nursing, and the second-lowest was $1400 for the unskilled kitchen help in one hospital. Not shown in Table 17, moreover, excepting department heads, the overall annual average salary for all full-time, hospital-paid employees belonging to the groups shown in the table was $3184 in the ten hospitals, as of the end of 1957. And, as this book goes to press, judging from past experience, it is very doubtful that this figure has reached more than $3500, or that average salary increases have exceeded a cumulative 10 percent since the beginning of 1958. (For the year ending September 30, 1959, the average annual earnings of all paid employees, both those included and those not included in the study, in the ten hospitals amounted to $3207 per full-time employee.)

The 4 lowest paid groups of the 14 shown in Table 17 are unskilled kitchen help, maids, aides, and orderlies, in that order. If one were to select the two groups which seem "overpaid" by comparison to the rest, these would probably be the laboratory technicians, and the x-ray technicians, respectively averaging an annual salary of $4450 and $4400, as of the end of 1957. Certainly, when compared with the professional nurses groups, on the basis of such things as professional training, formal education, and other characteristics discussed in this chapter, the technicians are very well paid. They earn about $700 more per year than nonsupervisory registered nurses and about $400 more per year than head nurses, averaging an annual salary equal to that of the remaining supervisory nursing staff, excepting the directors of nursing. One of the most underpaid groups, if not indeed the most underpaid, using similar

TABLE 17. The Average (Mean) Annual Earnings of Various Nonmedical Personnel from All Ten Hospitals Combined, and the Corresponding Range of Average Earnings Across Hospitals, Based on Salary Rates Prevailing in the Last Quarter of 1957 *

Personnel Category †	Total Annual Salary, Averaged for the Employees in the Ten Hospitals	The Range of Average Annual Salary, Across Individual Hospitals ‡
	(dollars)	
Directors of nursing	7000	5400 to 9300
Heads of maintenance	6100	4100 to 8600
Heads of dietetics	5300	3000 to 6500
Heads of housekeeping	4000	3000 to 6000
Registered laboratory technicians	4450	3000 to 5500
Registered x-ray technicians	4400	3300 to 5400
Supervisory nurses, excluding directors of nursing and head nurses	4500	3800 to 5150
Head nurses	4050	3500 to 4800
Nonsupervisory registered nurses	3700	3300 to 4200
Practical nurses	2650	2400 to 3000
Aides	2150	1800 to 2700
Orderlies	2600	2200 to 3150
Maids in housekeeping	1850	1350 to 2300
Unskilled kitchen help	1800	1400 to 2100

* Figures are for full-time personnel in all cases.
† The figures for the first four categories of personnel have been rounded to the nearest 100 dollars, and for all other categories to the nearest 50 dollars.
‡ In each case, the range represents the lowest-paying and the highest-paying hospital among the ten institutions in the study.

Present Job Status and Outlook

standards of comparison as the above, is probably the nonsupervisory registered nurses group. The members of this group averaged $3700 per year in the ten hospitals, during the last quarter of 1957, averaging as low as $3300 in one hospital and only as high as $4200 in just one of the participating institutions. Viewed in the light of continuous shortages for professional nurses, and in the light of the relatively high organizational instability of this group, commented upon repeatedly in previous pages, this situation is anything but comforting.

Apart from their salaries, and the hospital's contribution to social security, the vast majority of employees receive no other compensation from the hospital. However, employees receive a certain number of days of vacation and sick leave per year. For example, nonsupervisory registered nurses who have worked in the hospital for three years, full-time, usually receive ten to twelve days of paid vacation per year. (In one hospital, however, they receive only six days, while in a second hospital they receive 21 days—this being both the maximum for the hospitals studied, and somewhat unusual in that the next highest figure for any hospital is 16 days.) In addition, they are entitled to between ten and twelve days of sick leave per year, but these are not always fully paid days, for in at least two hospitals we are told that registered nurses are entitled to twelve days of sick leave per year at half pay. Similarly, full-time practical nurses having worked for the hospital for three years also average between ten and twelve vacation days, and the same number of sick-leave days per year. The aides average about ten days of vacation, and the same number of days for sick leave. The exact number of vacation and sick-leave days varies somewhat across hospitals, but not as considerably as salaries tend to vary for different personnel.

Returning now from this short digression to the question of employee earnings, the meaning of the dollar figures presented in Table 17 may become clearer, when viewed through the eyes of the various people to whom the figures refer. The psychological meaning of earnings need not correspond closely with what the figures themselves may imply. Let us, therefore, also find out how the various groups of nonmedical respondents participating in the research feel about their salaries. As was earlier indicated, the department heads, the nursing groups, and the technicians were asked the question, "How satisfied are you with your present salary or wages?" (It should also be reiterated at this point that the salaries shown in Table 17 are applicable to the same time period as the data obtained from the present question.) What do the relevant data show?

With the exception of administrative department heads, a substantial proportion of the members of each group involved indicated that they feel at least "somewhat dissatisfied" in response to the above question. And, in the case of aides and orderlies, as well as the case of practical nurses, the proportion expressing some dissatisfaction well exceeds the proportion expressing relatively high satisfaction. Even in the case of department heads, who constitute the most satisfied (and least dissatisfied) of all groups, we find that only 50 percent of all department heads in all ten hospitals feel "very well" or "completely" satisfied with their salaries, with an additional 9 percent feeling at least "somewhat dissatisfied"; the remaining 41 percent indicate that they are "fairly satisfied" or only "a little satisfied." The proportion of department heads who are very well or completely satisfied ranges across hospitals from as low as 13 percent to as high as 82 percent, the average being exactly 50 percent. The proportion who express at least some dissatisfaction ranges from 0 to 33 percent across individual hospitals.

Of all supervisory nurses in the study (excluding directors of nursing, but including head nurses), 33 percent are very well satisfied or completely satisfied with their salary; this varies across hospitals between 20 and 40 percent. Another 24 percent are somewhat to very dissatisfied; this varies across hospitals from 0 to 47 percent. The corresponding figures for the other groups, with the interhospital range shown in parentheses, are as follows: Of all nonsupervisory registered nurses 35 percent (13 to 59 percent) are very well or completely satisfied, and another 21 percent (6 to 42 percent) express at least some dissatisfaction with their salaries. Of all practical nurses, 23 percent (0 to 55 percent) are comparably satisfied, and another 33 percent (18 to 50 percent) are comparably dissatisfied. Of the aides and orderlies, only 17 percent (0 to 33 percent) are similarly satisfied, while another 44 percent (25 to 60 percent) are similarly dissatisfied. In five of the ten hospitals in the case of practical nurses, and in eight of the ten hospitals in the case of aides and orderlies, moreover, the proportion who are "very well satisfied" or "completely satisfied" with their salary is considerably smaller than the proportion who are at least "somewhat dissatisfied." Finally, of all laboratory and x-ray technicians in the study, 29 percent (9 to 75 percent) are very well satisfied or completely satisfied with their salary, while another 22 percent (14 to 37 percent) are at least somewhat dissatisfied.

It is clear from these data that the most dissatisfied (and also least satisfied) of all groups here discussed are the aides and orderlies and the practical nurses —the two groups which also average the lowest annual salary, as shown in Table 17. It is also clear that department heads, of all groups, are the most satisfied and least dissatisfied with their salaries. As can be seen in Table 17, the members of this group, as a whole, average the highest salaries among nonmedical hospital personnel, excepting of course the hospital administrators for whom we have no data. Thus far, the results are not surprising. When it comes to the nonsupervisory registered nurses group and to the technicians group, however, the results are somewhat surprising.

In the case of registered nurses, who averaged a salary of only $3700 at the time when the data concerning satisfaction with salary were collected, the surprise lies in the absence of more dissatisfaction (and the presence of less

Present Job Status and Outlook 137

satisfaction) than is actually the case, as depicted by the pertinent figures presented above. In the case of technicians, the reverse applies. The surprise here lies in the absence of more satisfaction than the figures regarding satisfaction with salary indicate—especially if technicians are compared with registered nurses, for the latter averaged a salary of $700 less per year than the former (in spite of the fact that, in terms of professional training, formal education, and the like, the nonsupervisory registered nurses show equally as good, if not better, overall qualifications than the technicians, according to the data). The fact that the technicians are even less satisfied with their salaries than registered nurses are with theirs, though enjoying a much higher average salary, obviously cannot be explained in terms of the actual salaries of the two groups. Nor can it be accounted for in terms of male-female differentials, in this connection, for over three out of every four technicians are also women. It can only be explained in psychological terms. Apparently, the psychological rewards derived from their work in the hospital are much greater for the nurses than for the technicians. In fact, they are probably high enough to compensate to a substantial degree for the obviously low salaries that the nonsupervisory registered nurses are paid in the community general hospital.

Motivation to Work and Job Commitment

Why do people work, and how committed are they to their work at the hospital? Ideally, this question would deserve a specific study on its own right but, obviously, in the present research it could not be given that much attention, for our objectives here are to study patient care, internal organizational coordination, and other aspects of hospital functioning rather than the motivations of the different people around the patient. Nevertheless, because of its importance, the question of work-related motivation could not be left completely unanswered and, consequently, some relevant information had to be obtained. This information was obtained from nursing staff members and from technicians in the various hospitals. These respondents were asked two main questions in this area, one about their reasons for working in the hospital, the other about commitment to their job and the hospital. The first question was:

Of the following, which one would you say is your main reason for working here? (Check *only* one.)
_____(1) To be financially independent
_____(2) To maintain myself temporarily until I get married or get another job
_____(3) It is my career—my profession
_____(4) To supplement my family's income
_____(5) I just like my job and want to keep it
_____(6) I live here
_____(7) Other reasons

The results from this question are summarized in Table 18. In general, eight or more out of every ten respondents from each group involved indicated that the main reason for working in the hospital was either career commitment, or to supplement their family's income, or simple job liking. Supervisory nurses most frequently (44 percent) gave career or profession as their main reason, and the same is true of practical nurses (32 percent), and of technicians (47 percent). Nonsupervisory registered nurses, on the other hand, most frequently (44 percent) chose "to supplement my family's income" as the main reason, although a substantial proportion of them (30 percent) did give career as the main reason. The aides and orderlies most frequently (38 percent) chose job liking as their main reason for working in the hospital. Supervisory nurses and technicians are obviously the most profession- and career-oriented groups, while aides and orderlies are the least career-oriented group.

TABLE 18. Percentage of Group Members, among Nursing Personnel and Technicians from All Hospitals in the Study, Who Chose Each of Certain Reasons as Their Main Reason for Working in the Hospital

Respondent Group	"It is my career—my profession"	"To supplement my family's income"	"I just like my job and want to keep it"	All Other Reasons *
	(percent)			
Supervisory nurses, not including directors of nursing ($N = 171$)	44	24	16	16
Nonsupervisory registered nurses ($N = 194$)	30	44	14	12
Practical nurses ($N = 134$)	32	27	26	15
Aides and orderlies ($N = 198$)	15	26	38	21
Laboratory and x-ray technicians ($N = 123$)	47	15	21	17

* This category includes such specific reasons as "to be financially independent," "to maintain myself temporarily, until I get married or get another job," and "I live here," plus other reasons given by respondents, but which are different from the reasons stated here or specified in the table.

Of all possible reasons, according to the data, career commitment and supplementing one's family income provide the primary motivation to work for almost seven out of every ten supervisory nurses, three out of every four nonsupervisory registered nurses, three out of every five practical nurses, three out of every five technicians, and two out of every five aides and orderlies. These results assume added significance, when juxtaposed with some of the findings about salary and satisfaction with salary, as discussed in the preceding

Present Job Status and Outlook 139

subsection. The fact that income is the most potent stimulus for work in the case of nonsupervisory registered nurses, for example, viewed in the light of low salaries and only moderate satisfaction with salaries and opportunity for advancement, perhaps accounts for no small part of the organizational instability of this group in the community general hospital—a characteristic already demonstrated by ample evidence. Higher salaries (among other things) for registered nurses are indicated, if the continuous shortage and fairly high turnover of this hospital group is to be alleviated—certainly, if shortages and turnover are to be reduced. This conclusion is further reinforced by other data which show rather low organizational and career commitment on the part of nurses.

Data concerning job and organizational commitment were obtained from the nonsupervisory nursing staff and from the technicians in the various hospitals, in response to the following question:

> How strongly identified do you feel (how much do you feel that you *really belong*) with each of the following? Or, how committed do you feel you are to each of the following?

The question was in tabular form. It offered four response alternatives, ranging from "very strongly" to "a little" (some minimal identification was assumed in all cases), and the respondents were to answer by indicating the degree of their identification with each of five separate referents. The particular referents were listed immediately under the question, in this sequence: "My immediate work group;" "This hospital and its goals;" "My profession or occupation;" "The team that treats the patient;" and "The community outside." The last two items, however, were not included in the questionnaire which the aides and orderlies filled out.

The findings about organizational and job commitment are summarized in Table 19, which shows the percentage of the members of each group who indicated that they feel "very strongly" identified with, or committed to, each of the five referent objects of identification. In reviewing this table, the reader should note that the percentage figures shown for any given group exceed the sum of 100 percent. This is due to the fact that many individuals in each case indicated that they feel very strongly identified with more than one of the referent items. Thus, for instance, 56 percent of all practical nurses felt very strongly identified with their profession, or occupation, but, at the same time, 51 percent also felt very strongly identified with the team that treats the patients, and 45 percent felt identified to the same degree with their immediate work group.

The results in Table 19 show that, as may be expected, the majority of registered nurses (59 percent), practical nurses (56 percent), and technicians (54 percent) feel very strongly committed to their profession-occupation. Of the five objects of identification involved, one's profession-occupation is the object of highest commitment, or the object with which respondents feel "very strongly" identified most frequently. The next highest-commitment object for both practical and registered nurses is "the team that treats the patients," followed closely by one's immediate work group. In the case of technicians this order is reversed, apparently because technicians do not have as much direct contact with the patients as do nurses. Of the aides and orderlies, exactly the same proportion (42 percent) feel very strongly identified with their occupation and with their immediate work group. (Data concerning the team that treats the patients are not available for this group.)

TABLE 19. Percentage of Group Members, among Nonsupervisory Nursing Personnel and Technicians in the Various Hospitals, Who Indicated That They Feel "Very Strongly" Identified with (or Committed to) Each of Five Referent Items *

Respondent Group	"My profession or occupation"	"The team that treats the patients"	"My immediate work group"	"This hospital and its goals"	"The community outside"
Nonsupervisory registered nurses (average N = 190) †	59	49	48	25	24
Practical nurses (average N = 131)	56	51	45	28	28
Aides and orderlies (average N = 192)	42	NA	42	36	NA
Laboratory and x-ray technicians (average N = 121)	54	32	48	27	28

* The sum of percentages across referent items for each group of respondents exceeds 100 percent, because many group members felt very strongly identified with two or more referent items rather than just one.

† The total number of respondents fluctuates slightly from one referent item to another and, for this reason, we are indicating here the average number of respondents. The fluctuation is so small, however, that it may be completely disregarded.

Of greater interest, and perhaps surprising, are the results regarding identification with the hospital and the larger community which it serves. We find that only 25 percent of the registered nurses, 28 percent of the practical nurses, and 27 percent of the technicians feel very strongly identified with their respective hospital and its goals. The organizational commitment of the members of these groups obviously leaves much to be desired, especially by comparison to their professional and work group commitment. And, the same applies with respect to how strongly identified these people feel with their community outside the hospital. For nurses, as well as for technicians, the proportion feeling very strongly identified with the community is almost identical with the proportion feeling very strongly identified with the hospital. The hospital and the community constitute the lowest-commitment objects among the five objects about which we have data.

Differences among individual hospitals naturally exist, both with respect to the specific reasons given by group members in each case as their main reason for working in the hospital, and with respect to the identification patterns of group members here discussed. Notwithstanding these differences, however, the data are very telling in both instances. Supplementary findings about the organizational commitment of nursing personnel and technicians, moreover, are consistent with the above results. When asked to indicate how long they would like to stay with their respective hospitals, an average of only 48 percent of supervisory nurses (ranging across hospitals from 18 to 75 percent), 50 percent of nonsupervisory registered nurses (ranging between 32 and 58 percent), 52 percent of practical nurses (ranging between 13 and 78 percent), and 31 percent of technicians (ranging between 13 and 55 percent) said that they would like to stay for "as long as I can work." Of the aides and orderlies, however, an average of 59 percent (ranging across hospitals between 48 and 83 percent) said that they would like to stay for as long as they can work, in spite of their rather high organizational instability and relative dissatisfaction with wages and advancement shown by previous data. The explanation for the aides' desire to stay with the hospital more so than any of the other groups probably lies in the absence of high realistic aspirations for occupational advancement, which often requires mobility from one organization to another.

The absence of higher organizational commitment on the part of nurses and technicians, however, should not be interpreted as implying any widespread dislike for working in their respective hospitals. On the contrary, other data show that the majority of these people like the hospital very much. In response to the question "On the whole, what do you think of this hospital as a place to work?" about six out of every ten professional nurses, eight out of every ten practical nurses, seven out of every ten aides and orderlies, and nearly six out of every ten technicians evaluate their hospital as an "excellent" or a "very good" place to work, with the remaining group members in each case being somewhat less favorable, but not particularly critical in their evaluation. On the other hand, these evaluative data refer to the hospital as a whole, "all things considered." They must not be interpreted, therefore, as implying equally favorable evaluations of different specific aspects of the hospital or the job. As previous results have demonstrated, there are many job-related things about which a substantial proportion of nursing personnel and technicians have expressed reservations and, sometimes, dissatisfaction, and these things undoubtedly account for a large part of the lack of higher organizational commitment on the part of these people.

Finally, it should be obvious that organizational commitment could be strengthened in various ways, and such ways have been suggested, more or less explicitly, in our discussion in the preceding pages of this chapter. We might conclude this section, however, with one more suggestion which emerges from some additional data bearing on the issue at point. Among the many questions asked of nursing personnel in the different classifications, and of laboratory and x-ray technicians, was this one: "On the whole, to what extent do the *key people* in this hospital make an effort to make you feel that you are an important part of the team?" The respondents could answer along a five-point scale, whose alternatives ranged from "to a very great extent" to "not at all." What are the results?

Of all nonsupervisory nurses in the study, an average of 46 percent (this ranges from 18 to 80 percent across hospitals) believe that the key people in their hospital make an effort to a "very great" or "great" extent to make them feel that they are "an important part of the team." Another 16 percent, however, feel that the key people make an effort only to "a small extent" or "not at all." The results are quite similar, moreover, for the remaining groups which answered the above question. Specifically, 53 percent of the practical nurses, 48 percent of the aides and orderlies, and 45 percent of the technicians indicate that the key people in their hospital make a great or a very great effort to make them feel an important part of the hospital team. But, another 22 percent of practical nurses, 14 percent of aides and orderlies, and 19 percent of technicians indicate that the key people in their organizations make little if any effort to make them feel an important part of the team. Particular hospitals, of course, differ from these averages. On the whole, the data suggest some room for improvement, although they cannot be viewed as unfavorable.

COMPARATIVE GROUP PROFILES OF THE PEOPLE AROUND THE PATIENT

Although the data in the preceding sections were presented in a manner that allows one either to follow a particular personnel group through the various areas and items which were discussed or, if one wishes, to compare the different groups with reference to a particular area or item, we shall use this section both to summarize some of the demographic and other characteristics of each group and to compare and contrast each group with others on some of the variables. In the short profiles which follow, as in previous sections of this chapter, greater emphasis will be placed upon the similarities and differences which were found to characterize the four nursing groups, the technicians, and the administrative department heads, since we have more information about these groups in the areas covered by the chapter.

Details will be disregarded in the profiles, however. For a more thorough picture of what a group looks like, one must refer to the preceding pages, where the data were discussed in detail, and where the implications of many specific findings for the hospital, as well as for the various people who work there, were pointed out. Our discussion here will likewise dispense with the question of interhospital differences indicated in previous sections, although the same group of personnel often exhibits significantly different patterns from one hospital to another in its various characteristics than the "average" patterns shown by its profile below, which is based on data from all ten hospitals combined. In other words, the individual hospitals differ, sometimes considerably, both from one another and from the average, on many of the items reported in this chapter. With these observations in mind, let us now consider each participating group separately, beginning with the top groups of the community general hospital.

The Medical Staff $N = 252$

The medical staffs of the ten participating hospitals are represented in this study by two subgroups—a sample of the active-attending members of the staff who hold neither staff offices nor major committe or administrative responsibilities in their respective hospitals, and all doctors from each hospital who hold such offices or positions. The former are referred to here as "the general medical staff," and the latter as "the selected medical staff."

The data show that, in terms of their demographic and background characteristics, the two medical subgroups differ significantly on only two items—age distribution and length of institutional association. The members of the selected medical staff from the ten hospitals are predominantly middle aged, 48 percent being between 40 and 50 years old, with the remaining equally divided between the younger and older age brackets. Of the members of the general medical staff, 41 percent are 40 or under, 25 percent are between 40 and 50, and the remaining are older. On the average, the members of the selected medical staff have been associated with their present hospital longer than the members of the general medical staff. Eighty-two percent of the former, compared to 67 percent of the latter, have been associated with the hospital for at least five years (as of the time of data collection). Excepting age and length of institutional affiliation, the two medical subgroups are very similar and will henceforth be treated as one group.

Virtually all 252 doctors in the study are male, only three being women. Over 95 percent of the doctors are married, and approximately nine out of every ten have at least one child. In terms of their distribution among the major services in the hospital, surgery has a higher proportion of doctors than medicine, medicine has a higher proportion than obstetrics and gynecology, and the latter has a somewhat higher proportion than pediatrics. Seventy-two percent of all doctors work in these four services, all other specialties and services accounting for the remaining 28 percent. Of all doctors, 38 percent are "board-certified men," i.e., they are recognized specialists in particular areas and certified as such by established medical specialty boards. Another 29 percent are "general practitioners." Finally, it is also of interest to know that more than eight out of every ten of the doctors in the study were on the staff of at least one additional hospital than the hospital they represented during data collection.

The Trustees

Of the 46 trustees on the executive committees of the boards of trustees of participating institutions, 64 percent have been associated with the hospital for five or more years. Trustees are the oldest group in the hospital, with 67 percent of them being at least in their fifties. Only about 10 percent of the executive trustees are women. About nine out of every ten are married and have children. In terms of formal education, eight out of every ten had at least some college, with six in ten having completed college. Trustees are usually well-established members of the hospital's community, who offer their part-time services to the hospital without remuneration. Of all executive trustees in the ten hospitals studied, only two were doctors (both from the same institution). Occupationally, 46 percent of the trustees are managers, directors, or executives of business and manufacturing firms, another 13 percent are bankers or investors, and the rest are salesmen, attorneys, insurance men, housewives, publishers, etc.

The Administrators

All ten hospital administrators in the study are male, lay individuals, by specification of the research design. Three of the ten are 40 years old or younger, and another four are 50 or older. All ten are married, and all but one have children. Six of the administrators have been with the present hospital for at least five years. Seven have completed college, with two of these having also done some graduate work in hospital administration. Half of the administrators, moreover, indicate that they have had one or two years of "professional schooling." On the average, compared to the doctors, the administrators have been with their respective hospital for a shorter period of time, and the same is true when compared to trustees. In general, the administrators are similar to the trustees and the department heads in their attitudes and evaluations of hospital functioning.

The Department Heads

The administrative (nonmedical) department heads from the various hospitals constitute the most heterogeneous of all groups in the study, followed by the trustees in second place. Statistically speaking, they are undoubtedly an anomalous group because of the diversity of their backgrounds, professional and occupational characteristics, and organizational roles and responsibilities in the hospital. Yet, they are all heads of departments, and for this reason one may treat them as a group. Compared to the other upper echelon groups in the hospital, fewer department heads are male (42 percent), fewer are married (66 percent), and fewer have children (62 percent). Approximately the same proportion are 40 years old or under (31 percent) and between 40 and 50 (28 percent), the remaining being at least in their fifties. Like the administrators, six out of every ten department heads have been associated with their present hospital for five or more years. The department heads, like the administrators, but unlike doctors and trustees, are employees of the hospital.

About one-third of the 101 department heads from the ten hospitals (including the directors of nursing) have had the same or a similar job at another hospital prior to joining their present institution. Among the top groups, they are the least educated group, only two-thirds having had some college education, and only four in ten having completed college. About three out of every ten indicate that they have had one or two years of professional schooling, with another four in ten claiming three or more years of professional schooling. Actually, these figures on formal education and professional training, however, are more a reflection of the wide assortment of skills encompassed under the relatively amorphous title of department head rather than a reflection of inadequate education, or professional preparation, for the job. The title includes such diverse people as directors of nursing, heads of maintenance, dietetics, records, and housekeeping, and even, on occasion, heads of switchboard operations.

Seventy-three percent of the department heads from the ten hospitals feel that their job gives them a very good or an excellent chance to do the things they are best at, and over half of them are completely satisfied or very well satisfied with the training they have had for their present job. Exactly half of the department heads are very well satisfied or completely satisfied with their salaries, and about six in ten are quite optimistic about their chances for advancement or promotion in the hospital. In general, as a group, department heads tend to be more satisfied and less critical of different aspects of their job, of the work situation, and of organizational operations, than the medical staff, the nursing groups, or the laboratory and x-ray technicians in the study. For example, department heads are considerably more satisfied with their salaries and chances for advancement in the hospital than either supervisory nursing personnel or nonsupervisory registered nurses, and the same is true concerning the extent to which they are satisfied with their immediate superiors. Exceptions to the general trend also occur, however. For instance, department heads feel more pressure for better performance, over and above what they consider as reasonable, than the members of the various nursing groups. Department heads still tend to be more optimistic and to evaluate different aspects of hospital functioning more favorably than these other groups, however. In this respect, the department heads share the general outlook and resemble very closely the views of the hospital administrators and of the trustees (while doctors, professional nurses, and technicians resemble one another fairly closely, all being more critical than the former).

The Supervisory Nurses

Let us now consider the nursing groups, beginning with the supervisory staff (all nurses in supervisory positions from head nurse on up, except for directors of nursing who were included with department heads in this discussion). The data show that 61 percent of all supervisory nurses, from all hospitals combined, have worked in their present hospital for at least five years, and one in three have worked in their present hospital division that long. All but five of the 172 supervisory nurses in the ten hospitals are women. Three out of every four are between 30 and 50 years old, and about six in ten are married, one in four is single, and about half (52 percent) have children. Practically all have completed high school, and close to half of them (45 percent) have had some college education in addition. Regarding their professional training, virtually all have had at least three years of training, with 14 percent having had four or more years. About one-fourth of all supervisory nurses had the same or a similar job at another hospital prior to joining their present organization. Supervisory nurses work predominantly on the day shift (70 percent), and the large majority of them (76 percent) have been doing their present job in the hospital for at least one year. Their organizational role, among other things, entails a great many coordinative functions.

Compared to other nursing personnel, nursing supervisors tend to fall predominantly in the middle age brackets, three-fourths of them being between 30 and 50, while nonsupervisory registered nurses tend to be younger and practical nurses tend to be older. Among all nursing groups, supervisory nurses are most likely to be single and least likely to have children. They have worked in the present hospital, and present division, longer than any other nursing group. Of all groups, they are least likely to have had the same or a similar job at another hospital, suggesting that they have been advanced to a supervisory position from the ranks within their respective institutions.

While the majority of the supervisory nurses are well satisfied with the training they have had for their job, about one in ten express some dissatisfaction with their training. Moreover, over one-half of them feel that their job gives them a very good or excellent chance to do the things they are best at, and the majority are very well satisfied with their chances for advancement or promotion in their respective hospitals. Regarding salary, while one in three are very well satisfied, or completely satisfied, one in four express varying degrees of dissatisfaction.

Compared to the other nursing groups, supervisory nurses are more likely to consider their profession or career as the main reason for working in the hospital. They are more apt to report that they feel very free to set their own work pace. Similarly, they are more likely to be satisfied with their

Group Profiles of People Around the Patient

chances for advancement, and more likely to feel that their job affords them a good opportunity to do the things in which they excel. On the other hand, they are less likely than the members of other nursing groups to express high satisfaction with their training, less likely to feel no unreasonable pressure for better performance, and less likely to feel that they would like to stay in their present hospital for as long as they can work. We see the nursing supervisor as a person who finds a good deal of satisfaction in the responsibilities and perquisites of her job, but who sometimes feels unprepared for the demands made of her. With relatively high professional commitment, she does not seem averse to leaving the hospital, should a better opportunity arise elsewhere.

The Nonsupervisory Registered Nurses

All 196 nonsupervisory registered nurses in the study are women. Forty-four percent of them are 30 years old or younger, and another 45 percent are between 30 and 50. Three-fourths of all registered nurses are married, and two-thirds have children. Practically all have completed high school, and half of them have some college education, in addition. Virtually all have had at least three years of professional training, and about one in ten have had four or more years. Two-thirds of the registered nurses are very well satisfied with the training they have had for their job, but only about half (46 percent) feel that their job gives them a very good chance to do the things they are best at. Furthermore, they are not particularly optimistic about their chances for advancement in the hospital. Only 37 percent feel very well satisfied in this connection, with another 18 percent expressing varying degrees of dissatisfaction. With respect to their salary, 35 percent are very well satisfied, while another 21 percent express at least some dissatisfaction, the remaining being only moderately satisfied.

In terms of their organizational characteristics, the nonsupervisory registered nurses constitute one of the most unstable—if not the most unstable—groups in the hospital. Significantly, this group is the most part-time group in the hospital, with only 55 percent of its members working full-time. This group is also characterized by a relatively high turnover rate, having twice the turnover rate of aides and orderlies who, in turn, have a higher rate than practical nurses. On the other hand, registered nurses have the smallest incidence and lowest rates of "unexcused" absenteeism of all nonsupervisory nursing personnel (practical nurses have the highest). More than any other group, registered nurses are likely to have had no previous regular job at all (43 percent), and more than any other professional group in the hospital they are likely to have been in their present job in the present hospital for one year or less (39 percent). And, although seven out of every ten registered nurses have been working in their present hospital for over a year, only 45 percent have been working in their present division that long. Of all nursing groups, the nonsupervisory registered nurses are least likely to be always working on the same shift, but most likely to be evenly distributed across the three shifts.

Other comparisons show that, as a group, nonsupervisory registered nurses tend to be younger than either supervisory nurses or practical nurses. Among all nursing groups, they are most likely to be married, and more likely than any other nursing group, except practical nurses, to have children. In terms of training and formal education, they are almost identical with the supervisory nurses, these two groups having had considerably superior schooling to that of practical nurses and aides. Registered nurses are more likely than any other nursing group and technicians to indicate that supplementing their family's income is their main reason for working in the hospital. In general, they are somewhat better satisfied with their salary than other nursing groups, but they are less likely to view the hospital as an excellent or very good place to work. On the whole, the nonsupervisory registered nurses are more critical than any other nursing group, or administrative group, in the hospital in their evaluations of numerous aspects of hospital functioning.[8]

The Practical Nurses

Of the 140 practical nurses representing the hospitals studied, only two were men. In terms of age, half of the practical nurses are between 30 and 50 years old, with another two out of every ten being at least 50 years old. In terms of family status, six out of every ten are married, one in four are divorced, separated, or widowed, and the remaining are single. Seven out of every ten practical nurses have children. In terms of education, 37 percent have had less than a complete high-school education, with another 42 percent having completed high school. The majority (62 percent) have had one year of occupational training; of the remaining, half have had less and the other half have had more than one year's training.

> For a fuller account of the characteristics of registered nurses in the present study, and to ascertain how they compare with other nursing and hospital groups, see the previous sections of this chapter. For other studies dealing with the professional and organizational characteristics of nonsupervisory and supervisory nurses in hospitals, or with the particular functions and tasks of hospital nurses—a topic with which we have not been concerned in our own research—see such studies as those by Argyris (3), Bullock (4), Burling, Lentz, and Wilson (5), Deutscher, *et al.* (6), Ford and Stephenson (7), Gordon (8), Hanson and Stecklein (9), and Stewart (15). For general statistical information about nurses and nursing in the United States, see the annual publication, *Facts About Nursing*, of the American Nurse's Association (1). For a historical account of nursing in the United States, see *American Nursing: History and Interpretation*, by M. M. Roberts (13). For brief bibliographical accounts of recent and current studies of various specific aspects of nursing, see *Nurses Invest in Patient Care* (2), and the annual publication, *An Inventory of Social and Economic Research in Health*, of the Health Information Foundation (10). The various journals in the fields of nursing, hospitals, and health, of course provide additional sources of contemporary accounts of research in nursing.

Compared to the other nursing groups, practical nurses are on the whole older, less likely to be single, and more likely to have children. These characteristics mitigate against the mobility potential of this group, and many of the data presented in previous sections attest to the relatively high organizational stability of practical nurses in the hospitals studied. Practical nurses are more likely than any other group, except supervisory nurses, to have worked in their present hospital for at least five years (46 percent), even though they are also more likely to have had the same or a similar job at another hospital prior to coming to the present institution. Of all nursing groups, they are most likely to have been doing their present job in the hospital for five or more years, and to have worked in different divisions of the hospital.

Practical nurses are least likely of any other nursing group, or technicians, to express feelings of unreasonable pressure on the job, and most likely to express satisfaction with the hospital as a place to work. Excepting aides and orderlies, moreover, they are also most likely to indicate that they would like to stay in the present hospital for as long as they can work. Consistent with these data is also the fact that practical nurses, as a group, show less turnover than aides and orderlies or registered nurses. However, absenteeism is somewhat higher among practical nurses than among either of these other two groups. Of the various nursing groups and the technicians, but excepting supervisory nurses, practical nurses are most likely to feel very well satisfied or completely satisfied (44 percent) with their chances for advancement in the hospital. On the other hand, next to the aides and orderlies, practical nurses are the least satisfied (or most dissatisfied) group with respect to their salaries. Only 23 percent feel very well or completely satisfied with their salary, while another 33 percent express varying degrees of dissatisfaction. Yet, on the whole, practical nurses, together with the aides and orderlies, are the least critical of all nursing groups and technicians in their attitudes and evaluations of the many aspects of the hospital situation covered in the research.

The Aides and Orderlies

Of the 203 aides and orderlies in the study, 50 were male, these being the orderlies (who are essentially "male aides"). Here we will summarize some of the main characteristics of aides and orderlies combined, although previously we have sometimes treated the two subgroups separately. Only full-time aides and orderlies were included in the study, for the proportion of part-time workers among them is negligible (not quite 10 percent). In terms of their age distribution, aides and orderlies are similar to the nonsupervisory registered nurses group, 44 percent being 30 or under, and only 11 percent being 50 or over. With regard to marital status, aides and orderlies are most comparable to supervisory nurses, both groups having about a quarter of their members single, and a little over 60 percent married. But, aides and orderlies are more likely than supervisory nurses to have children (62 percent vs.

52 percent). The aides and orderlies constitute the least educated and least trained of all groups participating in the study. The majority (55 percent) have had less than a complete high-school education and, except for brief in-service training and on-the-job experience, virtually all of them lack any formal occupational training. In one of the ten hospitals studied, however, the aides are called "nurse assistants," and are required to attend certain formal training sessions.

Aides and orderlies are more likely than any other group to have held a previous job elsewhere, that is, totally unrelated to their hospital work (33 percent). They are most likely of all groups to have worked in their present hospital for less than one year (36 percent), and least likely to have worked for five or more years (18 percent). Similarly, they are most likely to have been doing their present job in the present hospital for less than a year (42 percent), and least likely to have been doing it for five or more years (15 percent). And, the same is true about their having worked in their present division in the hospital. Like the nonsupervisory registered nurses, therefore, the aides and orderlies constitute one of the most unstable groups in the hospital, from an organizational standpoint.

Among nursing personnel and technicians, the aides and orderlies are least likely to mention occupational career as their main reason for working in the hospital, and most likely to mention "I just like my job and want to keep it" as the main reason. By contrast, a higher proportion of the members of this group than of any other would like to stay with the hospital for as long as they can work, and a higher proportion view their respective hospital as an excellent or a very good place to work. At the same time, the aides and orderlies constitute by far the least satisfied of all participating groups with regard to earnings. Only 17 percent feel very well or completely satisfied with their wages, while more than twice this proportion (44 percent) express varying degrees of dissatisfaction (from "somewhat" to "completely dissatisfied"); the remaining 39 percent feel "fairly satisfied" or only "a little satisfied." In most areas about which we have data, however, the aides and orderlies, as a group, tend to express very favorable feelings and attitudes. In this respect, they are very similar to the practical nurses group.

The Laboratory and X-ray Technicians

The laboratory and x-ray technicians are the only remaining group of the several groups which participated in the research. Technicians, especially those in x-ray, are also one of the least studied personnel groups in hospitals.[9]

For some comparable and additional information about the characteristics of technicians, particularly laboratory technicians, as well as for descriptive data concerning the tasks and functions of technicians in hospitals and medical laboratories, see the studies of Burling, Lentz, and Wilson (5), Heinemann, Bauer, and Kundsen (11), Sister Mary Carmelita (14), and Thruelson (17)—among the few available studies.

Group Profiles of People Around the Patient

Slightly more than three-fourths of the 125 technicians in the study (a total of 78 laboratory and 47 x-ray technicians) are women. Of all respondent groups, technicians are the youngest, 56 percent of them being 30 or under. Of all groups, moreover, they are least likely to be married (54 percent), or to have children (41 percent). Compared to the nursing groups, technicians are more likely to have had the same or a similar job in another hospital (38 percent), and less likely to have had no previous regular job at all (27 percent).

Nearly four out of every ten technicians have worked in their present hospital for five or more years, but another two in ten have worked there for one year or less. With respect to length of time on the present job, they most closely resemble practical nurses. Thirty-two percent have been doing the same job in the present hospital for at least five years, with another 26 percent having been doing the same job for one year or less. In terms of formal education, about one-fourth of all technicians have completed college, and nearly six out of every ten have attended college; only 7 percent have not completed high school. Concerning training, we find that 16 percent of the technicians have had less than one year of professional-occupational training, 42 percent have had one year, 21 percent have had two years, and the remaining 21 percent have had three or more years of professional training. Like most other groups, the majority of technicians express varying degrees of satisfaction with their training, but only 21 percent are "completely satisfied," while another 18 percent are at least somewhat dissatisfied with the training they have had for their job.

Compared to the four nursing groups in the study, proportionately more technicians feel that their job gives them a very good chance to do the things they are best at, and more indicate that profession or career is their main reason for working in the hospital. Of the nonmedical groups of hospital employees, technicians are least likely to feel free to set their own work pace, however. Similarly, compared to the nursing groups, they are least likely to indicate that they would like to stay in the hospital for as long as they can work, or to view their respective hospital as an excellent or a very good place to work. In addition, they are less likely to be satisfied with their chances for advancement or promotion in the hospital, also tending to be less satisfied than any of the nursing groups with the training they have received. In passing, we may also mention here that our findings about the technicians contradict rather than support the comparable results of Burling, Lentz, and Wilson, who, in a recent study of hospitals (5), found that technicians in the laboratories were, on the whole, quite satisfied.

Regarding salaries, technicians are somewhat more satisfied than either practical nurses or aides and orderlies, but less satisfied than either supervisory nurses or nonsupervisory registered nurses. This is an especially interesting finding, for technicians average an annual salary which is $700 higher than the average salary of all nonsupervisory registered nurses—whom they resemble very closely in a great many respects—in the ten participating hospitals (based on the salary rates prevailing in the various hospitals during the last quarter of 1957). The average annual salary of both laboratory and x-ray technicians in the various hospitals is also about $400 greater than that of all the head nurses in the same hospitals, being almost equal to that of the remaining supervisory nursing staff, excluding of course the directors of nursing. Finally, the technicians, like the nonsupervisory registered nurses, are generally more critical than the remaining groups in the study (including doctors) in their attitudes, and their evaluations of different aspects of hospital functioning.

SUMMARY

The main purpose of this chapter was to present the background and major job characteristics of the people around the patient and, in the process, to compare the several occupational and organizational groups which participated in the research. More specifically, our objective was to discuss: (1) the personal characteristics of the respondents, such as age and sex distribution, formal education, and family status; (2) the professional-occupational career patterns of the various hospital personnel, including training, job history, and service in the present organization; (3) some of the more important aspects of the current work situation in the hospital, as they relate to the different personnel groups, including shift-work patterns, full-time vs. part-time employment, turnover, and absenteeism; and (4) certain job-related variables, such as skill utilization, opportunities for advancement, salaries and satisfaction with salaries, motivation to work, and organizational commitment —variables which depict the present job status and outlook of the members of the several groups representing the hospitals studied. An additional aim was to compare and contrast the several groups of respondents, in each of the above areas, and to provide a short overall profile for each participating group, summarizing the background characteristics of its members.

Relevant information was presented for each of the following groups: doctors; trustees; administrators; nonmedical, administrative department heads; supervisory nurses; nonsupervisory registered nurses; practical nurses; aides and orderlies; and laboratory and x-ray technicians from the ten hospitals studied. However, particular attention was given to the characteristics and situation of nursing personnel in the different classifications. The data were analyzed separately for each group, but for all hospitals combined; e.g., findings were summarized for all supervisory nurses from all ten hospitals together. That is, differences among the hospitals themselves were generally disregarded here, for our concern was with particular occupational groups in the hospital rather than with hospitals. Nevertheless, for the majority of the items that were discussed the interhospital range was also shown to indicate the

Summary

variation which prevails among hospitals. The findings were presented in a manner that allows the reader both to follow a particular personnel group through the various topics and items covered in the chapter, and to compare the various groups with one another on the same topic or the same item about which data are available. In either case, the objective was to familiarize the reader with the hospital people who furnished most of the data for the present volume.

Although our research focuses on the community general hospital as a total organization, rather than on particular groups within the hospital or their individual members, it is still important to have some clear understanding of the background and outlook of the people who make up the organization and who serve the patient. The purpose of our discussion in this chapter was to provide this understanding, for such understanding, among other things, facilitates the task of appraising the results of subsequent analyses in the chapters that follow. In the next chapter, we shall engage in a parallel discussion of some of the major characteristics of the hospitals themselves, since the people around the patient work and interact within specific and well-defined organizational settings rather than merely as individuals or as members of particular professional-occupational groups. Our findings about patient care, organizational coordination, superior-subordinate relationships, and other important aspects of the structure and functioning of the community general hospital will, of course, be taken up in later chapters, after we have had the opportunity to familiarize ourselves adequately both with the hospitals in the study and with the different groups of people who keep these hospitals going.

Many of the findings presented in this chapter carry a number of practical and theoretical implications for hospital action, for research, and for the members of the different groups to which they refer. The more important of these implications have been dealt with in previous sections of this chapter, however, and need not be repeated here. Similarly, no attempt need be made here to summarize the major characteristics of each participating group, for such a summary was presented in the last section of this chapter. Before concluding the chapter, however, a few general observations might be made in order to re-emphasize some of the more interesting results which emerge from a review of the preceding discussion.

First, as might be expected, the data show a great many differences, in the areas covered, among the various personnel groups involved. On the whole, however, we find more pronounced differences among the nonmedical-nonsupervisory groups rather than among the nonmedical-supervisory and administrative groups. For example, the administrative department heads are often very similar to the supervisory nurses on such things as organizational stability, satisfaction with different aspects of the job, and the like, while the practical nurses differ very considerably from the nonsupervisory registered nurses and from the technicians. Apart from differences among personnel groups, however, we find even more striking differences among individual hospitals on nearly every single evaluative item discussed in the chapter, notwithstanding the fact that the ten hospitals in the study share a number of important organizational characteristics in common. Variation among hospitals was, of course, expected (in fact, the element of variation was one of the most crucial reasons for using the hospital as the unit of analysis in this study), but not to the extent indicated by the results of this chapter, or the results of subsequent chapters.

One of the more interesting conclusions to be drawn from the contents of the present chapter concerns the relative organizational stability of different hospital personnel. In this connection, data about length of service with the hospital, job history, occupational characteristics, turnover, organizational commitment, and other items all point to the interesting and important conclusion that, organizationally speaking, the nonsupervisory registered nurses constitute the most unstable of all groups studied. Finally, not unrelated to the question of organizational stability, the results concerning opportunity for advancement in the hospital, actual personnel earnings, and satisfaction with salary and other aspects of the job are full of practical implications. When viewed in the light of the educational, training, and other career attributes of the members of the different nonmedical groups, and in the context of hospital efforts to attract, hire, and maintain an adequate staff (especially professional nurses) at all times, these results are very instructive.

REFERENCES

1. American Nurses' Association. *Facts About Nursing.* New York: Annual publication of the American Nurses' Association.
2. ——— *Nurses Invest in Patient Care: A Preliminary Report.* New York: American Nurses' Association, 1956.
3. Argyris, C. *Diagnosing Human Relations in Organizations: A Case Study of a Hospital.* New Haven: Yale University Press, 1956.
4. Bullock, R. P. *What Do Nurses Think of Their Profession?* Ohio State University, 1954.
5. Burling, T., Lentz, E. M., and Wilson, R. N. *The Give and Take in Hospitals.* New York: Putnam, 1956.
6. Deutscher, I., et al. *A Survey of the Social and Occupational Characteristics of a Metropolitan Nurse Complement.* Kansas City, Mo.: Community Studies, Inc., 1956.
7. Ford, T. R., and Stephenson, D. D. *Institutional Nurses: Roles, Relationships, and Attitudes in Three Alabama Hospitals.* University of Alabama Press, 1954.
8. Gordon, H. P. "Who Does What: The Report of a Nursing Activities Study," *Am. J. Nursing,* 53:564–66, (May) 1953.
9. Hanson, H. C., and Stecklein, J. E. *Nursing Functions in General Hospitals in the State of Minnesota.* University of Minnesota, 1955.
10. Health Information Foundation. *An Inventory of Social and Economic Research in Health.* New York: Annual publication of the Health Information Foundation.
11. Heinemann, R. I., Bauer, H., and Kundsen, H. L. "Design for Development of

References

Medical Laboratories: Personnel and Practices," *Am. J. M. Technol.*, 25:145–65, (May–June) 1959.

12. Murray, M. "Nursing Needs and Resources for 4½ Million People." Detroit and Tri-County League of Nursing, 1959.

13. Roberts, M. M. *American Nursing: History and Interpretation.* New York: Macmillan, 1954.

14. Sister Mary Carmelita. "The Medical Technician Figures in Good Human Relations," *Hospitals,* 28:102–4, (March) 1954.

15. Stewart, D. D. *Source Book for the Function of the General Duty Nurse in Ten Arkansas Hospitals.* University of Arkansas, 1955.

16. Stouffer, S. A., et al. *The American Soldier: Combat and Its Aftermath* (Volume II). Princeton, N.J.: Princeton University Press, 1949.

17. Thruelson, R. "Lab Technicians," *Saturday Evening Post,* 221:34–35, 120, 122, 124–25, Feb. 19, 1949.

4 TEN HOSPITALS IN PROFILE: A DESCRIPTIVE OVERVIEW

The preceding chapter dealt with a discussion of the background characteristics of the people around the patient. There the focus was on different professional and occupational roles across all participating hospitals combined, and the objective was to provide an answer to the question of what kind of people our respondents are. This chapter seeks to provide a similar answer to the parallel question of what kind of organizations the hospitals in the study are, describing the hospitals themselves. Here the objective is to introduce the reader to each hospital as an individual organization with its own unique character, weaknesses, and strengths, and to all ten hospitals as a group of similar organizations.

First, we shall describe very briefly the "average" or the "typical" participating hospital, to supply an introductory frame of reference against which the individual hospitals may be viewed. Then, we shall look at each of the ten hospitals separately, showing the general features of each institution, in the form of a short profile. Finally, we will bring together various common themes from these different vignettes to provide a background against which the findings in subsequent chapters could be viewed.

Our sketch of the average hospital in the study is almost exclusively based on data from hospital records. The individual hospital profiles, on the other hand, consist primarily of (1) relevant observations and comments by respondents who were personally interviewed, and (2) comments by those of our respondents who filled out questionnaires, but who chose to expand or elaborate on various aspects of the structure and functioning of their respective institutions, i.e., comments that were apparently salient from the respondent's own point of view. Accordingly, although the profiles do not yield a complete picture of the community general hospital without the benefit of the more quantitative and more reliable findings which are to follow, they provide a good overall picture of how each hospital looks to many of its people.

Ten Hospitals in Profile

As already indicated, those people in each hospital who were personally interviewed, in addition to filling out a questionnaire, constitute the main source of the profile data. Included in this group are the members of the executive committee of the board of trustees, key members of the medical staff, and the hospital administrator—a total of between 14 and 24 persons from each hospital. As part of our open-ended interviews with them, these individuals were specifically asked to comment in as much detail as they wished about such things as: recent significant changes in the hospital; community characteristics that may tend to create problems for the hospital; internal problems or issues faced by the organization; any major differences in orientation concerning relationships between medical staff and trustees; things or areas in which the hospital may be considered particularly strong or particularly weak; and similar other items. Moreover, they were urged to volunteer any additional information that would give us a picture of their organization and their feelings about it.

Similarly, all respondents who filled out questionnaires were invited to amplify any of their answers and to comment freely on any subject, whether or not covered in their questionnaire, that seemed important to them. Many doctors, nurses, and department heads in each hospital used the margins and back space of their questionnaire to make such comments. A good deal of the profile materials derive from these write-in data. Finally, each hospital was requested to provide us with copies of its constitution and bylaws, as well as any other written documents, including medical staff rules and regulations, that might help us gain an understanding of its overall organization. These documents furnished the remaining part of the profile materials, but they contributed only a minor portion of the information used.

A number of different topics are covered in the profile of each hospital: the size and setting of the institution; its economic status and community reputation and support; the structure of its board of trustees and its medical staff; the character of doctor-trustee-administrator relationships; relations among the members of the medical staff; quality of medical and nursing care; communication and coordination; administration and supervision; and, generally, the major problems, weaknesses, and strengths of the institution, as seen by many of its members. Several of these subjects constitute the focus of intensive analysis in later chapters, e.g., the topics of patient care, organizational coordination, and superior-subordinate relationships. A few of the subjects in the profiles (e.g., hospital-community relations and the hospital and its setting), however, being outside the scope of the present inquiry, will not be treated further in this volume.

The nonquantitative character of most of the data in this chapter is eminently suited to the purpose at hand. For the reader who is not familiar with community general hospitals, the profile materials quickly provide a certain amount of basic information and familiarity with these organizations; for the reader who has had a good deal of experience in this field, they provide a sense of the importance of different problems faced by each hospital, and comparative perspective for viewing a number of issues across hospitals. The several profiles, however, will probably raise more questions than they can answer for the sophisticated reader. To him, each hospital's picture will still seem blurred—and it is, because a profile alone cannot be expected to tell the whole story.

For some of the topics involved there will be no clear-cut definition of the situation: some respondents may see things one way, and others may see things somewhat differently, or even in contrasting terms, depending on the issues involved and the relative importance of each to different respondents. Such ambiguity, where it occurs, however, is frequently indicative of unsolved problems or unresolved issues, and this is an important organizational phenomenon deserving consideration in its own right. For many other topics, on the other hand, there will be a good deal of agreement among the comments of different respondents, and this is just as significant and interesting. In either case, it should be remembered that the emerging picture of a particular hospital in this chapter is the result of the opinions, attitudes, perceptions, and occasionally probably stereotypes entertained by trustees, doctors, nurses, and others in each organization.

In summary, while the various qualitative materials woven together in each of the ten hospital profiles provide a great many insights into the problems and operations of the community general hospital, they cannot be used to test any hypotheses or to establish relationships between different variables. The latter is a task for the quantitative data in subsequent chapters. The main purpose of the profiles is to present as complete a picture as possible of how a number of individual respondents view their own hospital, rather than to attempt a thorough case study of each hospital or try to provide the basis for scientific comparisons across hospitals. Such comparisons had best await our presentation of additional data. Finally, while the unique features of each hospital are inevitably stressed in its profile, various characteristics that are common to all or several hospitals are not disregarded. In fact, the last section of this chapter is mostly devoted to such common themes, and the same is true of our brief sketch of the average hospital in the study.

A SKETCH OF THE "TYPICAL" HOSPITAL IN THE STUDY

Before presenting the profiles of individual hospitals, the question may be raised as to what the "typical" hospital in the study looks like. Strictly speaking, there is no such thing as an "average" or typical hospital among the ten participating institutions. As shown in the last chapter, and as confirmed in subsequent chapters, the hospitals vary a good deal from one another in many respects, despite the fact that they were all selected for study on the

Sketch of "Typical" Hospital in the Study

basis of certain common organizational characteristics (see Chapter 2). Yet, in many other respects, the hospitals are not too different from one another. Disregarding here particular interhospital differences and similarities, it is possible to construct an imaginary typical hospital, by averaging data from the ten hospitals, in a manner analogous to that employed to analyze the characteristics of the various people around the patient in the last chapter. In a sense, the background and occupational patterns which were found there to characterize the different hospital groups are also "average" or typical patterns.

A sketch of the "average" hospital in the study serves a number of useful purposes. In the first place, it provides an overview of some of the organizational background characteristics that a community general hospital of the kind here studied is likely to exhibit. Second, the characteristics of the people around the patient were earlier described on the basis of averaged data from all the hospitals in the research combined, although these people belong to different separate institutions. It would, therefore, be interesting to make it possible, for those who wish, to view the typical characteristics of the various personnel groups within the context of a typical hospital, or to associate the average characteristics of our respondents with some of the background features of the "average hospital" in which they work. Third, and more important, the brief description of our average hospital, based on real and concrete data from real hospitals, provides a modal frame of reference in terms of which one may study the individual hospital profiles in the next section, as well as the findings in later chapters, more meaningfully. In short, it serves as an introduction to the profiles, and to subsequent chapters, while summarizing some of the more salient characteristics of the participating hospitals. Let us, therefore, see what the average participating hospital was like during the fall of 1957, when the data were collected.

First, the average hospital in the study had 196 beds (more precisely, the ten hospitals together had 1962 beds, which when averaged results in 196 beds per hospital).[1] Approximately, two-thirds of these beds were for surgical and medical patients, at a ratio of about six surgical for every four medical. The remaining beds, excepting a few special beds, were almost equally apportioned between the obstetrics-gynecology service and the pediatrics service. The hospital also had 31 bassinets—equal to the number of beds in obstetrics. In addition, the typical hospital had three major and two minor operating rooms, two delivery rooms, three predelivery (labor) rooms containing about five beds, and one postoperative recovery room having seven or eight beds.

[1] The size of five of the participating institutions, however, falls between 175 and 235 beds, so that the several individual hospitals do not deviate greatly from the "average" hospital here described, in terms of size and size-related characteristics. It may also be recalled, at this point, that none of the participating hospitals has fewer than 100 or more than 350 beds.

Of the 196 beds in the average hospital, 19 percent were in private rooms, 42 percent were in semiprivate rooms, and 39 percent were in wards. The average daily occupancy of these various beds was 78 percent, which means that, on an ordinary day, this hospital had a census of 153 patients, excluding newborn. For calendar year 1957, the average participating hospital had a total of 7800 patient admissions, or between 39 and 40 admissions per bed, plus about 1300 births. The average length of patient stay in the hospital, excluding newborn, was 6.8 days, or a little less than a full week. The average gross death rate for all inpatients, excluding newborn, was 2.28 individuals per 100 patients. The infant mortality rate, excluding still births, was 1.65 infants per 100 live births.

As of the fall of 1957, with 196 beds and a daily census of 153 patients, the average participating hospital had a total of 380 full-time (or its equivalent) paid personnel, excluding students, interns, and residents (if any).[2] Thus, it had on its payroll almost two full-time paid employees for each of its beds, or about two and one-half employees per occupied bed or per patient. The average annual earnings of these employees amounted to about $2950 in 1957, although in the last quarter of that year this annual rate had risen to a little over $3000 per full-time paid employee per year. As of the fall of 1959, this figure had become $3207 (see Chapter 3 for more details on salaries). Of the 380 employees, about half were members of the nursing staff of the hospital. Personnel from the various other nonmedical jobs and departments of the institution made up the other half.

However, the above employees were not all of the people serving the patient in that hospital. In addition to its paid employees, the hospital had a core medical staff consisting of about 75 attending ("active" and "associate") doctors. And, apart from its regularly practicing physicians, it also had a good number of "courtesy" medical staff members, i.e., doctors entitled to bring a few but not all of their patients to that hospital, plus several "consulting" and "honorary" medical staff members. None of the doctors, of course, is paid by the hospital. The average hospital, moreover, had a board of trustees consisting of approximately 17 persons, all of whom offer their services to the institution without pay. The administrator of the hospital was in charge of all nonmedical personnel, services, and facilities, being directly responsible to the board of trustees for all nonmedical aspects of hospital operation. The medical staff as a whole, and through its officers, committees, and service or department heads, was in charge of all medical aspects of hospital functioning, within the framework of the hospital's constitution and bylaws. In summary, all told, for every patient or occupied bed, there were at least three persons working in or for the hospital during calendar year 1957.

[2] In the fall of 1959—the period for which most recent data are available—the average hospital in the study had 197 beds and a total of 385 full-time paid employees; i.e., it had remained practically unchanged. These figures are based on data from the 1960 "Guide Issue" of *Hospitals* (3).

Sketch of "Typical" Hospital in the Study 161

As described in the previous chapter, the large majority of the medical and nursing staff of the hospital were distributed among its four major services —surgery, medicine, obstetrics and gynecology, and pediatrics. Several medical specialties, such as anesthesiology, pathology, ophthalmology, otolaryngology, and radiology were also available, accounting for medical staff members not belonging to the four major services directly. In addition to the medical and nursing departments, of course, the hospital had an admissions department, a dietary department with dining facilities, a front office or business office, a housekeeping department, a laundry, a maintenance department, a quasi-department of personnel, and a switchboard-communications service.

The average participating hospital had the following specific medical and paramedical facilities or services: basal metabolism apparatus; blood bank; central sterile supply room; clinical-pathology laboratory; electrocardiograph; emergency room; medical library; medical records department; outpatient service; pharmacy; physical therapy service; premature nursery; radiology department, with both diagnostic and therapeutic x-ray; and several other facilities for specialized patient treatment and care. However, only two or three of the ten hospitals in the study had one of the following: a cancer program, a dental department, a nursing school, an occupational therapy department, or a social service department. The majority of the institutions had a women's auxiliary service, however, and all but one were Blue Cross participants.

During calendar year 1957, the typical hospital here described averaged a total income of about $240 per patient admission, but approximately 4 percent of its patients were classified as nonpaying. Corresponding total expenses amounted to approximately $226 per patient admission. Viewed slightly differently, the average hospital in the study had an annual income of about $9240 per bed, and annual expenses of about $8750 per bed. Its total 1957 income amounted to $1,814,500, and its total expenses to $1,719,000, leaving a "surplus" of about $95,000. At the same time, however, this hospital was likely to have an outstanding debt of about $75,000 (considering both short- and long-term debts), thus literally "breaking even" from the standpoint of income and expenditures. The largest single item in hospital expenses was the payroll, accounting for 65 percent of all hospital expenses that year. For the period between September 1958 and September 1959, the total expenses of the average hospital in the study amounted to $1,843,000, and its payroll expenses to $1,235,000 (i.e., 67 percent of total expenses), according to data from the 1960 "Guide Issue" of *Hospitals* (3).

Finally, by specification of our research design, the average hospital shared the following features with all of the hospitals in the study: it was a voluntary, nonprofit institution; it was a short-stay general hospital; it was a nondenominational, community-operated, i.e., not church-related or operated, hospital; it was governed by a lay board of trustees, and administered by a lay, male individual; it was a medium-sized hospital (had 196 beds); it was located in a Michigan city having a population greater than 10,000; and it was accredited by the Joint Commission on Accreditation of Hospitals. Such accreditation implies that the hospital meets certain specified requirements, and certain minimum standards of patient care that are acceptable to the Commission and to the medical profession in the United States.[3]

Before concluding the present section, we may also point out that normative information of the kind here presented, with which one could compare our 196-bed "average" hospital, is not available on a nation-wide or state-wide basis. There is, however, one source of similar data which, in a number of respects, approximates such normative information. We are referring to the "prototype study" of the 200-bed, nonprofit, general hospital in the United States, by Louis Block (2). This prototype study was published in *Modern Hospital*, in January 1954. The above sketch of the "average" hospital participating in the present research is, of course, based on data collected more than three years later. Yet, if one compares most of the data about our 196-bed average hospital with corresponding nation-wide data presented in Dr. Block's prototype study of the 200-bed hospital, one is struck with the many similarities rather than the relatively few differences which emerge from such a comparison. Considering the fact that Dr. Block's hospitals comprise a much more diverse universe than ours, these similarities constitute a pleasant and important surprise. Since, on the whole, our average (Michigan) hospital does not deviate markedly from the average 200-bed hospital in the United States, in terms of such basic characteristics as those discussed above, there is good reason to expect that many of the findings from our study of ten hospitals will be also applicable to a great many similar hospitals throughout the nation. The significance of the ability to generalize the findings of any research, of course, can hardly be exaggerated. In the absence of relevant studies covering a national sample of hospitals, Dr. Block's data are indeed very welcome and very encouraging, since they at least provide one factual basis for the probable generality of the results of the present research beyond the Michigan scene.

INDIVIDUAL HOSPITAL PROFILES [4]

In this section, the profiles of the individual hospitals which participated in our study will be presented. A comparative summary of the profile materials will then follow, in the next section, to emphasize some of the main differences and similarities among the ten hospitals which emerge from these materials. For

---

[3] For a recent description of this accreditation program see a discussion by the Director of the Commission, Dr. Kenneth Babcock (1).
[4] We are indebted to Dr. Franklin W. Neff, Ed.D., a member of our research staff, for excerpting the profile data from respondent interviews and questionnaires, and from various hospital documents, and for writing the initial draft of each profile.

Individual Hospital Profiles

convenience, and to allow cross references, the ten hospitals are here numbered 0 through 9, bearing the same numbers which they were assigned for the first time in Chapter 2.

Hospital #0

Located in a large city, this is one of the largest hospitals in the study in terms of number of beds, patients admitted, and size of professional and nonprofessional staffs. According to many of our respondents, the hospital is situated in a deteriorating part of the city. The immediate environment is seen as unattractive to patients, visitors, and hospital personnel. The building is described as old and costly to repair. The centrality of its site, however, is seen as advantageous, and an extensive program of area redevelopment, now in progress, is expected to increase its desirability. Some respondents also feel that the hospital is often seen as a "Negro hospital" because of recent increases in the number of its Negro patients. There is a feeling that the institution needs to improve its public image and community support, something which it is trying to do. "Our lack of public support is a weak feature," a respondent observes. Another has this to say: "This hospital's reputation is improving rapidly. It still suffers from the stigma of a poor neighborhood, standards identified with [the former name and status of the hospital], and its lack of eye appeal." Recently, the hospital underwent extensive remodeling and increased its facilities for patient care.

Like all other hospitals in the study, this institution is under the general control of a board of trustees. This board consists of 19 members. It is different from other hospital boards in the study in that ten of its members have to be doctors. Lay members are elected for life and medical members for three-year terms by the "hospital corporation." The latter consists of doctors of medicine or dentistry who have contributed a certain amount of money to the hospital. While the boards of voluntary, community general hospitals are largely, if not exclusively, made up of laymen, several members of the medical staff view the composition of this board favorably and describe it as effective. "The hospital is under the 'ownership' and guidance of physicians—a very unusual feature, which I believe is desirable," a doctor comments.

The board of trustees elects its officers—a president, a vice-president, a secretary, and a treasurer—at their first meeting following the annual meeting of the members of the hospital corporation. (A doctor, formerly president of the board, thinks it preferable to have a lay person as president, which is currently the case.) According to the bylaws of the hospital the board itself meets monthly. In addition, it appoints three or more of its members to an executive committee. The executive committee of the board of trustees can exercise most of the powers of the board. In general, the board is responsible for the hospital, its policies and finances. As in the case of the other hospitals in the study, however, the day-to-day operations of the organization are carried out under the overall direction of the hospital administrator and his administrative department heads. The administrator, appointed by and responsible to the board of trustees, is the principal manager and representative of the institution, being in charge of all nonmedical aspects of hospital functioning.

The medical staff conducts its administrative affairs through its own executive committee. This committee consists of two or three doctors from each major medical division of the hospital, such as surgery and medicine. Its members are elected annually by the attending medical staff (voting members). The executive committee then elects the staff's officers—a chief, a vice-chief, and a secretary-treasurer—from its members. The chief of staff, in turn, appoints a number of standing medical committees including a credentials and professional standards committee, a medical records committee, an education and house staff committee, and a medical audit committee. Typical of hospitals in this study, medical staff membership and privileges are recommended by the credentials committee, voted upon by the medical executive committee, and finally approved by the board of trustees of the hospital.

A number of the persons interviewed indicate that one of the strengths of this hospital is an interested board of trustees. And, although some doctors see the board oriented more toward financial aspects of hospital operation than the medical staff, some feel that "there is no difference [in the orientation of these two groups] because doctors on the staff are elected to the board of trustees." Still others perceive a general difference in approach between these two groups: "The trustees have a more general approach; the doctor is more specific to his own area. The board looks at it from a community point of view." In general, however, respondent comments suggest no conflict between doctors and trustees.

Within the medical staff, many report good relationships; ". . . the staff is close, warm, and friendly." Some doctors, however, choose to comment on the problematic nature of the relationship between doctors who are specialists and doctors who are general practitioners. "I think the most important problem we have here is the relationship between general practitioners and specialists," says one. "You know there is a tendency now to squeeze out general practitioners. Consequently, here he [the general practitioner] feels he does not want to get consultations or to participate in any education program because of the possibility of losing his patients to the specialists." This specialist-general practitioner issue is by no means peculiar to this hospital. Our study elicited many controversial comments regarding both sides of this issue, in this as well as in other participating hospitals.

The medical staff is described by some as cooperative and talented. "We have a good nucleus of teachers and specialists," one physician states. Others, however, are critical in their comments: "House doctors do not seem to take a genuine interest in patients." "A large quantity of internal medicine is done by relatively unqualified men." "Many of the doctors have no interest in research. Some of us don't stimulate them either. We would like to improve patient care, but I guess that is a universal problem."

Additional comments by doctors have to do with the organization of the medical staff. A recent revision in staff bylaws is reported to have strengthened staff relationships and eliminated some schisms. Yet, some adverse comment on the part of some staff members is also expressed. "If you look over the members of top level committees," says one, "they have been there for years—a political football rather than attempting to do the most good for the hospital." Another complains, "There are a lot of us on the staff who have very little to say because it is the corporation members who are the only ones who can hold office."

Individual Hospital Profiles 165

On the other hand, several respondents express pride in the hospital having "a strong feeling for patient's care as a sick person," and "the human relations approach to patients." Highly specialized care for such diseases as cancer and muscular dystrophy is also frequently cited as one of the strengths of the hospital. Another strength, according to many comments, is its ties with a medical school. In this connection, a doctor observes, "it's [the hospital] turning on more power for the patients. If we can't solve their problems, and the consultants [professors from the medical school] can't either, then the case is almost hopeless."

Many favorable comments are made about the administrator—"we appear to have a vigorous and interested administrator," "an open-minded, fair, highly-thought-of administrator." A department head favorably comments on the daily meetings between department heads and the administrator, and another speaks of the hospital's "progressive, democratic administration." One respondent, however, disapproves of the "administrator's professed indifference to personal problems of employees at all levels." Certain other aspects of hospital supervision and administration are criticized by some respondents: "personnel policies are changed by department heads without consulting the personnel beforehand"; "time is lost by personnel in too-frequent and nonproductive meetings"; "there is a lack of understanding by personnel of goals or plans of administrator."

Criticisms are also leveled at nursing personnel. One doctor sees the weakness of the nursing service as "particularly due to the hiring of many incompetent nurses and understaffing." Another respondent complains of "too many coffee breaks and too much loafing," "but resistance to work seems to be universal," he adds. Along the same lines, a doctor offers this opinion: "At present, there is a general attitude of employees similar to that in industry—that is, much of the old pride in participating in an important service to the community has been replaced by the attitude that working in a hospital is the same as any other job." A colleague of his, however, still reports that in hospitals there is "a certain dedication that is not necessary in industry," and a department head comments on "the eagerness of employees to learn and want to do right." Similarly, a supervisory nurse observes, "hospitals, public or private, have a sacred responsibility to humanity."

Additional comments suggest various general problems faced by this hospital. For example, doctors often mention that the segregation of Negro patients within the hospital is a source of irritation, particularly to Negro doctors. Some doctors believe that low wages and the location of the hospital make recruitment of personnel, especially nurses, technicians, and medical interns, quite difficult. In addition, there is a feeling on the part of certain respondents that the hospital's teaching programs for doctors and nurses are not as adequate as they should be. A shortage of beds is also reported, one doctor saying that the hospital's bed capacity is at the lower limits necessary for specialized departments and services. In connection with such specialized work, another doctor perceives additional difficulties: "Our large volume of cancer and cerebral vascular patients . . . spells financial difficulty as it makes for low [patient] turnover. . . . All of our community hospitals are trying to carry on this specialized work which is costly, and the cost has to be spread to the patients. I have been preaching that we need different types of hospitals [for highly specialized care]. . . . That would cut the cost of hospitalization a great deal." Perhaps not unrelated to such problems as this could be also the fact that the present hospital is one of the only two hospitals in this study actually operating on a budget.

Hospital #1

This hospital, one among the larger in this study, is situated in an industrial community. The lack of diversification in the economy of this city is reported to make for employment fluctuations, which have an unfavorable impact on the hospital. People who work in the hospital take pride in its services, reporting that it provides care for many indigents and handles a large amount of emergency work. "Its attitude toward helping people . . . regardless of race, color, religious faith, or financial status" is seen as one of its strengths. In spite of these attributes, some respondents believe that public interest and knowledge about the hospital need to be increased. "The community doesn't understand our aims and most people are not interested in finding out what those aims are," says one. However, financial support is not lacking according to another person: "We found [that the hospital] was well supported by the community. We got capital funds to help."

A board of trustees exercises general control over the affairs of the institution. Board members are traditionally elected by the board of trustees of a local church to serve for three-year terms. (There is no evidence, however, that this introduces any denominational considerations with respect to the composition of the board or with respect to the nondenominational character of the hospital itself.) The officers of the board, who comprise the executive committee, are elected annually from and by the board. As is true for the other hospitals in this study, the executive committee acts with most of the powers of the full board between board meetings. One of these powers is that of appointing the medical staff. However, a provision of the medical staff bylaws (which have been rewritten recently) makes it clear that staff membership is controlled by doctors: "In no case shall the board of trustees take action on an application, refuse to renew an appointment or cancel an appointment previously made without conference with the medical staff or the executive committee [of the medical staff]." Essentially, this arrangement obtains in all hospitals in the study.

The medical executive committee is charged with providing liaison with the board of trustees, and the chief and vice-chief of staff attend board meetings. The effectiveness of this link is not agreed upon. One doctor says, "We have a very cooperative board of trustees. . . . It brings its problems to the general medical staff and asks their opinion. You know, they're so cooperative I don't know if they look at things differently than we do or not." Yet, another reports, "There is not as good understanding between the board of trustees and medical staff as there might be. That was borne out at the meeting last night. Some of the doctors spoke and gave their views. But some trustees gave the impression they were not listening—just waiting for them to finish." Problems between the medical staff and the board are described by a doctor this way: "When the thinking members of the medical staff are apprised of the problems besetting the board through direct communication, the problems disappear. . . . The greatest trouble and source of annoyance is a lack of understanding by the medical staff of the problems of operating a hospital. . . . There has never been any attempt by the board to encroach or dictate medical policies. On a

Individual Hospital Profiles

few occasions physicians have tried to operate the hospital." According to another doctor, "the board places too much reliance on the word of the administrator," and another thinks "the weakest link is between the board of trustees and the staff. . . . The board doesn't know what the medical staff is thinking."

However, several doctors also make favorable comments about the trustees, one saying, "they appreciate the problems from a medical standpoint as well as they do from their standpoint as a lay person." Another respondent says that the hospital "always has had a strong board of trustees—representative leaders who have devoted a huge amount of time and service." The medical staff is also described as being of high quality by some respondents. One doctor, however, feels that the medical staff "is just the same as anywhere else." The hospital is reported to have been the first in the area to bring in a radiologist and a pathologist, and respondents state that only a few specialties are not represented. In this connection, some point to a need for the hospital to improve its psychiatric and pediatric services.

Several doctors comment on the cooperation among members of the medical staff: "We have a very cooperative medical staff. They seem to participate on committees surprisingly well." "From a staff viewpoint . . . there has been a gradual change in the point of view of the doctors—less individualistic, more teamwork. More tendency to ask for consultation." ". . . though we have more specialists than general practitioners, even so the chief of staff is a general practitioner, and heads of departments are also. I'd further say that, as a result, there is little factionalism." One problem, however, is reflected in the following comment by a doctor: "Radiology should be an ancillary department; but as it is, they're telling us what we can do. It pays to have a good department . . . but they're out of proportion to the rest." Some difficulties in getting doctors to complete charts are also reported, and this may account for a doctor's remark that "tension is with the records committee." "Lack of use of means of censure of poor medical practice," reported by another doctor, suggests an additional problem.

Patient care is generally described as good by various respondents, one stating that the hospital has "excellent surgery . . . good diagnostic work." Similarly, a doctor believes that "medical care is excellent by most but rather poor by a few." The relationship between nursing personnel and patients is commended by some, one seeing "a pleasant, happy personnel who work for the patients." Others, however, are less favorable in their descriptions. "A 'personal desire and interest' touch on the part of all personnel to make the patient feel at home and comfortable" is lacking, one says. Another demands, *"Bring back the good bedside nursing system along with the newest trend!"* Doctors also frequently praise hospital facilities, though some object that too much money was put into a recent expansion of x-ray facilities. A need for more space and even better facilities, mentioned in most of the hospitals studied, is also reported in this hospital.

Nursing supervision receives several criticisms. "The nursing administration is not worth a damn," states a doctor. One of his colleagues says, "They don't know who does what. Don't know who bathes patients, they go off and leave 'em one leg washed and forget to come back. . . . Nobody with a sense of responsibility." A nurse says, "I feel we need a 'supervisory person' in between the head nurse and the assistant director . . . it seems to me that it is too hard for one person regardless of who she is to handle two jobs." Another adds, "it is impossible to do the supervision I would like to and have the patient contact I would like to have." Still another nurse feels that the director of nursing "spends too much time with recruiting and students, and not enough on the floor."

Some persons comment on the ease of getting complaints to top administration; others say that many complaints come to the hospital but that nothing is done about them. Some speak of the willingness of the administration to obtain competent men and women; others say inefficient personnel are retained. Descriptions of the administrator also reflect real differences of opinion among respondents; "We have an excellent superintendent," ". . . a good administrator." Another person, however, sees the hospital as wanting "an honest to goodness man with control of his temper, and a 'doer' for an administrator."

As in most of the hospitals included in this study, there is a shortage of nurses and a feeling on the part of some respondents that nurses, as well as others, are not "as dedicated as they used to be." A doctor expresses the opinion that unionization and government backing of sit-down strikes affected employees so that wages and hours are now the important thing, pride and accomplishment seemingly are gone. Adverse comments are made about service personnel standing around talking rather than working. One person reports, "The problem is staffing with competent people. Five different girls refused one job . . . afraid of responsibility." Not all comments are unfavorable, however. A technician states that a strength of the hospital is its intelligent and efficient employees who have to deal with the public.

A variety of other concerns are suggested by additional comments. One doctor sees a "lack of good feeling and rapport among *all* the staff—too much antagonism among groups . . . staff and administrator seem to be at great odds." The emergency service does not function as some doctors wish it would. One says, "We have quite an element of Negro and poor white trash who come for free service to our emergency service. We also use this service for emergency use for strangers, people with no money or who are unconscious or who have no doctor. It is abused. People come who are not an emergency in order to get free service." Another doctor comments, "a serious case may be brought in while the lone nurse is at supper or busy . . . and may not get attention for half an hour or so." Another problem according to a doctor is that there is "no county or city hospital here, so that a lot of indigent and accident cases are brought to this hospital and this creates certain financial problems." A board member adds, "The fact that we have a large Negro population creates certain problems. Emergency treatments are so often administered and are not paid for. County welfare funds are inadequate to meet all the indigent patient charges." Finally, the reported policies of a local osteopathic hospital are also seen as sources of irritation. According to one doctor, "It creates a problem because we don't get cooperation from the osteopaths. They will send patients here in the middle of the night, and we have to take them. They are very selective in their patients and won't take anyone who can't pay."

Hospital #2

This hospital, one of the smaller in this study, is located in a relatively small urban area. In some respects, the community is roughly divided into two parts,

Individual Hospital Profiles

one being more heavily populated by low socioeconomic groups. It is in this section that the hospital is located. There is another hospital in the other section, and, although one person feels that rivalry or competition between the two no longer exists, a doctor comments on it as follows: "There is great rivalry between the two hospitals, and between the two men who head the boards of trustees. The proposal came up that the two be merged. Almost everyone was in favor of it except the board presidents. They each wanted a living memorial for himself."

Community attitudes toward the hospital, reportedly, are improving, but are not as favorable as desired. A doctor says, "The main problem has been to live down the poor relationship with the public," and another sees a weakness in "a long-standing reputation handed down from years back that the institution was mercenary." Some respondents also remark that migrant workers and Negro patients pose a problem of expenses, since they get much free care in this hospital. Other data indicate, however, that the trustees characterize the general financial condition of the hospital as adequate. (It is perhaps relevant to add here that this is one of the only two hospitals in the study which are operating on a budget.) Additional problems of operation are connected with Negro patients by various respondents. A doctor observes, for example, that a "particularly strong policy of segregation . . . causes much rearranging of beds and general unnecessary furor." Another comments: "We have not integrated patients here regardless of what the front office says. . . . I doubt that we ever will." A supervisory nurse, however, says that "there seems to be less racial discrimination than usual, both to patients and personnel."

Doctors often describe board members as being unduly concerned about finances, but a department head says, "the hospital has a progressive and interested board of trustees, willing to spend any amount to get good care for the ill in the community." Descriptions of the way the board works suggest that its president has very great influence. "For years it has been a one-man show," comments one respondent. A doctor adds, "He [the president] wouldn't even have to wait for a board meeting. The board doesn't do a thing while he is in Florida." A trustee sees the board as "a task force tackling individual problems; no regular meetings." "Actually," comments another, "I'm not close enough out there until something goes wrong. Then we learn of it and act accordingly. The president of the board devotes almost all of his time to it; when there is need for action, we all work together."

Many comment on differences between doctors and trustees. A doctor describes one difference this way: "I think the board of trustees looks at it to a large extent with a dollar sign in front of their eyes." Similarly, another comments as follows: "It is basically impossible for a businessman to think as a doctor does. He can't conceive of any institution continuing to operate while losing money. . . . The businessman is not apt to do anything that will hurt himself or his industry; whereas the doctor is willing to put his reputation, his career, and the hospital in jeopardy if he believes it to be in the best interest of his patient."

Informal channels are often used to reach organizational decisions. According to one doctor, "problems are settled at the country club or when you run into board members at lunch." Apparently, this system is not satisfactory to many doctors: "Actually we know nothing about the board—how they operate, and we never see them." "I don't know anything about the board of trustees. I don't think any of us do—no contact!" And although a board member states, "Well, we have a particularly fine liaison through the director of the hospital with the medical staff," a doctor differs: "The superintendent acts as a buffer between staff and board. The present superintendent is more 'pro-board' than usual. . . . The chief function of the board in this hospital—aided by the superintendent—is to say 'no' to staff requests and keep the hospital solvent. The latter they do very well indeed."

Another avenue which is supposed to link the board and the medical staff is described by a doctor: "At present our bylaws call for the chief of staff to be present at their board meetings, but we have never been invited. At present there is no representation of the medical staff point of view to the board." In the same connection, another says, "Pressures are exerted by the doctors but don't result in any good. We don't meet with the board and aren't welcome at their meetings. Their attitude is, 'it is none of your damn business.'" On the other hand, one doctor feels this way: "It is our fault that we do not have one or two staff men at every board meeting. Opposition to this from the administrator and from the board—which is truly present—could be easily overridden. As I see the setup there, the president of the board, whom I admire, has been dictatorial in hospital affairs for years. . . . I am not criticizing Mr. _____, I'm criticizing ourselves for letting him lead us around by the nose. He would enjoy us winning a bout and laugh with us about it."

A problem of importance to the medical staff and others concerns the medical intern program. This program has been jointly sponsored by the hospital and a university, but soon the hospital will have to assume full responsibility for the program—if it is to continue. "This problem of acquiring interns is one which is of great concern to us," a doctor remarks. Another says, however, "I don't know that that is a real problem . . . because the hospital functioned for many years without interns, and I imagine it will again." Another issue within the medical staff revolves around difficulties between specialists and general practitioners. According to one doctor, there is a "dire need for G.P.'s. . . . There is a preponderance of surgeons and other specialists. Since they represent a majority, they protect their portion by restricting the practice of G.P.'s." Another, referring to privileges of general practitioners, says "this is tending to be encroached upon, but the G.P.'s are a hardy lot and will hold their own."

In spite of these issues, a doctor describes the staff as "a unified medical staff which works well together," and many respondents see it as competent. Several refer to the number of specialists on the staff, one saying that this is unusually large for a community of this size. A doctor reports, "There is no resistance to medical progress. The staff is interested in promoting good medical care and good relations in the hospital as a unit in the community." A nurse, however, observes that "the medical staff seems disinterested in improving the hospital."

Patient care is frequently commended, respondents making such statements as: "Wonderful patient care" and "almost every type of case is handled and handled as well surgically, medically and diagnostically as anywhere else." Nursing care is also commended by some. A department head says, "I do feel that the quality of nursing care given has always been maintained at a high level." A doctor, however, complains that some night nurses sit watching television while the children in the wards need attention, such as having diapers changed. Hospital facilities are both praised and criticized. One doctor says "the facilities are excellent." Others, however, speak of crowded conditions, inefficient layout of the plant, and needed housing for the school of nursing and for nurses and interns.

Here, as in other hospitals in this study, the shortage of registered nurses is mentioned many times. Respondents also point out the need for other personnel, particularly more skilled people and more able supervisors. A trustee explains that there are "constantly personnel problems due to a lack of qualified people for supervisory positions." And a department head says that there is some inefficient use of personnel. One reason for some of these problems may be suggested by this statement from a nurse: "I think they need a more sincere personnel policy."

In the opinion of a department head, the thing most needed in this hospital is a "big improvement in cooperation between departments." Others add: "Lack of organizational meetings—or any type of planned meeting with all department heads participating." "Good lines of communication are not always established." Some respondents speak of confusion in the front office, one stating, "They annoy too many patients with their method of collecting." Another problem, according to a doctor, is "improving the morale." Others say that "there has been little effort to curb petty annoyances and grievances among personnel." Several persons, however, speak of a "friendly atmosphere." The administrator is sometimes praised but frequently criticized. "We have," a doctor comments, "a very fine hospital administrator who is quite capable and who does not interfere." Another doctor feels differently: "His task as he sees it, I think, is to stall politely and sympathetically until the present crisis, whatever it is, is solved by the passage of time, forever keeping uppermost in mind that the board frowns on expense."

A number of other areas of hospital operation are also commented upon. The emergency service, described by some as one of the strong points of the hospital, is the center of some difficulties. A department head says, "We need a change of policy in the operation of the emergency room. It is now so cluttered with 'office visits' to see specific doctors, that it is at times difficult to take care of real emergencies." The educational activities of the hospital are frequently commended. "The intern program has made a substantial contribution to the community," a board member states. A technician expresses a similar opinion: "We have an excellent school system in medical technology, x-ray, nursing, and medical internships." One person, on the other hand, thinks the school of nursing is weak. Crowded conditions, referred to earlier, also create some difficulties for hospital personnel, and several mention a need for more facilities. A technician, referring to changes in policies, procedures, and equipment, states, "as far as I can see they haven't improved the hospital much for the last five years."

Hospital #3

"Stable," "conservative," and "pretty wealthy" is the way some respondents describe the community in which this hospital is located. Both the community and the hospital are among the smaller ones in the study. Concerning hospital-community relations, a doctor says, "I think the community is proud of the hospital." And, according to a trustee, "it is a very generous community when it comes to giving." Another comments, "We take the patients in and ask questions later—requiring no financial statement as some hospitals are criticized for. Not that we'd take anybody, but we know most of these people." He also feels, however, that the hospital has a problem "of explaining to the public why the cost of hospital service is so high."

Membership in the association of this hospital, from which trustees are chosen, is obtained through donation of money or property. The membership of the board of trustees and its executive committee are apparently quite stable, a trustee saying, "I feel for the good of the hospital and community there should be some rotation as well as some continuity. . . . We never have new members unless someone dies." The president of the board is seen as having considerable influence. A recent revision of hospital bylaws is reported to have increased the responsibility of some committees and reduced the control of the president. However, a doctor comments, "[The board president] is really head. This hospital is his baby. He has business connections and influence to go on."

According to one doctor, no change in the organization of the medical staff can be made "unless you have a quorum, and it's voted on." Another comments, "The medical staff works much more as a 'committee of the whole,' so that its officers are not very important." On the other hand, one doctor says, "About a half dozen doctors really direct policy around here, and I am one of them because I am interested." "Cooperation among the staff is superior," according to another, and a nonmedical person reports, "no petty cliques, no friction, a good feeling which is unique." However, as is true for other hospitals in the study, some respondents are concerned with difficulties between specialists and general practitioners. One doctor reports the existence of "rivalry between surgical staff and G.P.'s." Another says, "The hospital is currently undergoing a change in the bylaws, segregating and drawing lines between the work of G.P.'s, specialists, etc. The general practitioners are way outnumbered. The G.P.'s are losing the type of work they want . . . and getting the least desirable part of medical practice —house calls, etc." A third doctor, however, mentions one recent change "in regard to liberalizing practice, particularly participation in surgery—increasing surgery privileges." The present issue is of interest to some trustees also, one saying "the medical personnel has taken a rather narrow technical position, whereas the board has insisted that the general practitioners should be permitted to do whatever work they are competent to do."

Relations between the board and the medical staff are, reportedly, satisfactory. One doctor states, "The board of trustees, in my experience, does not interfere in any way with the practice of medicine in this hospital." And, although respondents frequently point out the trustees' greater concern with costs, many comment that there is little friction between the two groups. A doctor reports that the board of trustees, "since I've been here, has been very cooperative." And another adds, "I'd say the board leans over backward to do what doctors want." The administrator is seen as a link between the board and the medical staff, and one doctor says he "is well suited to arbitrate between business and professional men."

The medical staff is often praised, respondents saying such things as, "an excellent medical staff." A doctor states, "I truly think that the standards of professional care here are high," and another observes, "we have an unusually competent professional staff." According to a nurse, however, "It is difficult to give an unqualified evaluation . . . since our surgeons and physicians vary from poor and mediocre to about as good as you can find anywhere." According to a trustee, "The nursing care is as good as you can get," and several doctors also compliment the nurses and their work. A doctor, however, thinks that "the quality of nursing is not as high. No Florence Nightingales today. They watch the clock." Many other respondents describe the interest and warmth of hospital personnel toward patients. A trustee states, "Patients go away feeling we have a very personal feeling for them. We tried to organize at this hospital to create an atmosphere . . . to help make them feel that way." Another says, "99 percent of our patients are satisfied and complimentary."

The emergency service seems to be a focus of some criticism. "There are complaints from the community that our emergency isn't well covered," a respondent remarks. One nurse makes a rather lengthly comment related to this facility: "I feel that the doctor exploits the hospital as a convenience, giving very little in return. . . . He frequently relies on the nurse's observations and gives orders by phone when he should come to see his patient. The nurse does many jobs for him that he would have had to do himself a few years ago. The hospital's equipment is available to him free of charge. He uses the emergency room like a second office, and for all this he gives begrudgingly a couple of days a month on emergency call." Other facilities are favorably mentioned, although some anticipate that growing community needs will make expansion necesssary before long. Several respondents also contend that the hospital should have a training program for various groups such as residents, interns, and nurses, and some think it should have psychiatric and rehabilitation facilities.

A number of favorable comments are made about the administration of the hospital. A doctor remarks, for example, "I think the hospital . . . is administered in a very efficient way." And according to one nurse, "the departments seem to cooperate together." Another nurse, however, thinks the hospital needs "meetings for department heads to discuss interdepartmental problems," and another says "employees are not consulted in these matters." Certain hospital policies are criticized. For example, a department head reports a "lack of definite personnel policies," and a nurse suggests that "there should be standard salaries set up and they should be used." Several persons feel salaries are low, and in the words of one nurse, "if the wage scale in this hospital were raised, there would be a better 'all-around' feeling." Another problem, which this hospital shares with others in the study, is that of obtaining and keeping professional nurses in the face of competition from individual doctors, industry, and other sources, according to some respondents.

Morale is frequently reported to be high, and several people comment on good relations between groups. According to a nurse, for example, "There is hardly ever any friction between departments. . . . Workers at this hospital are always trying to help and assist each other." One person, however, mentions "Very poor 'human relations' on the part of the administrator." And a nurse says, "I think nurses are too much regarded as a commodity by the administrator and the board, and they are not given credit due them for their technical skill and their skill in human relations." Most respondents, however, make comments similar to this one by a doctor: "I feel general camaraderie of employees and doctors is exceptionally high compared to other hospitals I've been in."

Hospital #4

This hospital, a medium-sized one in the study, serves an area of several counties. Various respondents describe the hospital as strong in "rapport with community members," and in having "the respect of the community." One trustee thinks, however, that the area of "keeping the public informed so that they know facts instead of fiction" is neglected. Another respondent is of the opinion that the hospital will have to expand in order to handle a new program of county care to which it has agreed. This will involve cooperation between the hospital and the county, and a doctor feels that the hospital has done only a "fair job getting along with the county board of supervisors." Others mention various problems that accompany this program.

"This hospital and staff are considered the outstanding ones [in a large section of the state]," according to one doctor. Other respondents support this view with such comments as: "high level of skill and knowledge of the medical staff"; very high professional standards"; and "the hospital has a reputation as a medical center serving an increasingly greater trading area." Several trustees hold similar views about the medical staff, one saying, "our staff would be classed number one . . ." Many doctors express similar opinions. For example, one says, "we have a super-excellent medical staff with a great majority of the specialties represented." And, another adds this: "We are represented by a wide variety of well-qualified specialists. This is important to me because it raises the quality of our service through—not competition, but—keeping us on our toes."

Concerning nursing care, a doctor reports a "well-organized and well-trained nursing staff," and a nurse says "the nursing care is excellent—the number of R.N.'s on the staff is relatively high, and the practicals are well trained." Several persons praise the attention given patients. A doctor, for example, comments on the "careful consideration of the patient," and another mentions letters from patients that express appreciation for personal attention. Another doctor, who commends the nursing staff, also feels, however, that "the nursing personnel are not very sympathetic to the patient with emotional problems." And, another says, "we have nurse aides—young girls off the streets. . . . I have no respect for them." According to a supervisory nurse, however, "the aide group is intelligent and capable."

One of the strengths of the hospital, according to a doctor, is "encouraging the citizenry in naming outstanding individuals to the board of governors [trustees]." In this connection, another respondent feels, however, that the three-year term of office for trustees "is inadequate to indoctrinate a new trustee to a place as large as this." And, although the bylaws permit re-election, a trustee has this to say: "Well, I think most of us would like to stay, but it is a case of two things: One, people on the board have a lot of other civic responsibilities. The other, it's a good idea to let other people come in as long as they are capable people."

The medical staff, comments a doctor, "works in a very harmonious way to provide excellent care for the patient." Another respondent observes, however, that the chief of staff "is a very strong-willed man, full of self-conviction about

Individual Hospital Profiles

all things . . . but we can control it through these two men [two other doctors]. He's a good doctor, but very determined about getting what he wants, and [the other two doctors] serve as a balancing wheel." It is also interesting to note, in this connection, that the members of the executive committee of the medical staff, unlike in most other hospitals, are elected for three-year terms. The specialist-general practitioner issue, though not frequently mentioned in this hospital, is not entirely absent. "I'm the oldest practicing member on the staff; I'm the rebel; I've been the one to keep the specialists from taking away the privileges of the general practitioner," says one doctor. Another sees a need for "further definition of medical staff privileges."

In connection with the area of relationships between medical staff and board of trustees, one doctor says, "Well, we have seen eye-to-eye a good many years. When we ask the governing board for something and they study it, we usually get it. Very excellent relationship." Another states that "there have been very harmonious feelings between the staff and the board here." On the other hand, a doctor feels "board members make a point of ignoring the medical staff in many matters where their advice would be invaluable." The chief of staff attends board meetings, according to one respondent, and another says the administrator provides additional liaison between board and staff. However, one doctor thinks that "proper liaison between staff and governing board is very definitely one of . . . the big things we need." Another suggests that "it would be good to have two doctors on the board as one might be biased whereas two would more nearly represent the opinions of the staff."

The relationship between administrator and medical staff is commended by one doctor. Another says, "He [the administrator] has the ear of the board. I feel he is a very good man, well trained and just." Similarly, according to a trustee, "We lean heavily on the administrator. . . . He usually makes suggestions and is well informed, knows pretty well who would fit, or work out on the various committees. He makes a thorough study of all these things and is of great help to all of us on the board." Other trustees make similar comments: "Management outstanding." The administrator is "a wonder—a top-notch guy." Some nursing personnel, however, are critical in their comments about administration. "Not adequate communication between administration and nursing department," says one nurse. Another comments as follows: "I feel that there is maladjustment between the administrator, the director of nursing, and the associate director of nursing. The director of nursing does not have the proper authority in problems which should fit within her realm, and she, in turn, wears herself out by not giving proper authority to the department supervisors."

A department head thinks the hospital is weak because of lack of "scheduled conferences with members of the medical staff and department heads to *plan* and *execute* goals." Another says "our department is never consulted." And, although a technician says, "everyone in all departments work well together for the betterment of our patients," a doctor sees a problem in getting "proper cooperation between the departments in the hospital including the medical staff." Certain personnel-related aspects of hospital operation also seem to be of concern to various respondents. According to one nurse, for example, "there is a need for written policies and procedures"; and another says there are "no proper personnel policies." Similarly, a trustee sees a problem in personnel relations: "They just expect people to work because they have jobs. That's true of all business—mechanically O.K., but skips the human element." Concerning staffing, a respondent sees a need for "supervisory and head nurse material," and another adds, "there are other areas where we wish we had more supervisors—the dietary department, physical therapy, laboratory. . . ."

The various physical facilities of the hospital are generally seen as adequate, but several respondents point to a need for more space for certain departments (e.g., laboratory, x-ray, and surgery). Various respondents also agree with a trustee who feels that "our most pressing need is an outpatient department." Other things of concern to respondents include the training program for interns, which is praised by several, and the need for training programs for nurses and other personnel. The laboratory is criticized by several doctors, and a technician has this to say: "I feel personally, as I know the doctors do also, that the work that is going out of the laboratory is getting poorer in quality as time goes on. We need a *Registered* Technician as a superior." Similarly, the dietary department is criticized by a number of persons. Finally, in connection with the new county care program, some comment on the problem of potential relations with osteopathic doctors. In the words of a medical staff member, "Our most important problem is coordination with a proposed medical facility . . . particularly relative to the utilization of our professional services by osteopaths who in the future may be allowed to use that facility."

Hospital #5

This is another medium-sized hospital. It is located in a community which is described by a doctor as "probably one of the better-educated communities in respect to the needs of the hospital and preventive medicine." The dominance of one industry in the city reportedly affects the hospital in various ways. For example, with respect to fund raising, a doctor thinks that "the public has it in the back of their minds that [this industry] will come through if support is needed." He also adds, however, that "when we went to the community three or four years ago, the community came through." Competition with the above mentioned industry for skilled personnel is also reported by some respondents. Perhaps related to this is also a doctor's comment that "unions are trying to creep in and organize some of our help; I don't know whether that's good or bad." Regarding relations with the community, other respondents speak of a "very cooperative community," and of "public interest and support through the volunteer group." One doctor comments, nevertheless, that the hospital has some problems in "getting our message across to the public."

The board of trustees consists of about a dozen members, being relatively small as compared to other hospitals. According to a doctor, it is "an excellent board," and another respondent says that it is "unusually interested and competent." Some persons ascribe much influence to the president of the board, and to a trustee who is a top official of the major industry in the city. Of the latter, a trustee says, "if we get off, he can influence us—by a couple of words he can straighten us out." Concerning relations with the medical staff, a doctor says "we've had good relations with the board . . . they have pretty well left the staff to run their own problems," and trustees generally agree on this. Another doctor reports "very good liaison" between the board of trustees and the medical staff. In this connection, a doctor also feels that the division of labor between the two groups is so nearly complete that they do not look at the same problems. And, the following comment by a trustee seems to support this contention: "I think the board is ever conscious of costs and public reaction . . . while doctors think in terms of their work and their own work alone."

The absence of a chief of staff in this hospital constitutes an interesting organizational pattern. The medical executive committee members are elected, one each year, for three-year terms. The third-year man is automatically chairman of the executive committee and is described as "nominally chief of staff." Commenting on the absence of a chief of staff, a doctor feels that this "deters from good functioning . . . . I'd want an elected chief of staff to have authority over medical practice in the hospital." Another doctor, however, says "we have none—thank God." Not unrelated to this issue may also be another comment by a doctor that "probably we are lacking in staff control of individual members."

Relations among medical staff members are often described as good, one doctor saying that, in contrast to hospitals in neighboring communities, there are no cliques in the staff. However, the issue between specialists and general practitioners receives some comments. For example, one doctor says that the staff has had "to reconsider and re-evaluate our criteria for individual staff member accreditation. . . . We can no longer assume that a G.P. is qualified to do a D. and C. [dilatation and curettage], a T. and A. [tonsillectomy and adenoidectomy], or a circumcision." Another doctor makes the following comment: "The men who have actual voting control of staff functions haven't completely grown up to a teaching or big city hospital staff. . . . Those people who are accustomed to covering the waterfront can't believe there are other capable people."

Various other respondents comment on the medical staff and on patient care. A doctor, for example, says "We've got a comparatively high caliber medical staff. We've got a few 'ringers'. . . ." Similarly, another speaks of "adequate, well-trained medical specialists," adding also that "most general practice men are of good quality." A nonmedical respondent expresses a similar view: "We have a quite well-rounded staff . . . interested in the practice of good medicine . . . there are only two or three specialties not represented." One doctor, however, has this to say about medical care: "The most important problem is which way we're going . . . whether we're going to improve the quality of service or . . . give up. Work here falls into two classifications—those qualified to do it and those not. Some are doing work that they're not qualified to do."

Several respondents speak of the attention given to patients. An aide says, "we try to make patients feel like individuals, which is sometimes lost in more understaffed or larger hospitals," and a doctor refers to "a warm atmosphere for patients" as a hospital strength. Concerning nursing, several respondents from the nursing department agree that aides and practical nurses may be doing things that they are not qualified to do, and a few feel that aides are not as good, or as well trained, as they should be. One person comments as follows: "I think P.N.'s are expected to do things that perhaps R.N.'s should do. However, training through experience and observation makes some practicals as competent as some

R.N.'s. Some practicals . . . do the same work as R.N.'s because they are asked to." Other respondents speak of a shortage of registered nurses, one nurse saying, "I feel the hospital needs more professional help; and aides and P.N.'s should be given less responsibility."

Concerning administration and supervision, respondent comments indicate both strengths and weaknesses. A trustee feels that "the hospital, on the whole, is very well administered," and a doctor says, "we've got an excellent administrator and nursing supervisor." Also, one doctor reports, "the hospital has frequent meetings with personnel and discussion groups and management committees in order to get the viewpoint of the personnel." Another doctor, however, feels that "a bit more autonomy in the office of the administrator would make for more prompt decision." Similarly, according to another, there is a "lack of designated authority on the floor, or inability to assume it. . . . Passing the buck. . . . Nobody has the right or the willingness to crack the whip on the floor." Another respondent feels that the hospital cannot attract top-flight administrative personnel, and a technician states that "most obvious in this institution is the lack of a coordinator with a working knowledge of all departments."

The emergency service and the laboratory receive some criticism, and one respondent feels that the laboratory personnel "is not as integrated into the overall hospital team as we would have liked." In the area of communication, a nurse who has been in the hospital for a relatively short time comments, "I have never been informed as to hospital rules and regulations." Several other nurses report that they have not participated in group meetings. A number of other problems are also mentioned by various respondents. "We have the problem of attracting intern staff or house staff," states a doctor, adding that the hospital has a "good house staff education program." Others say that expansion of facilities is needed, partly to keep up with a rapid community growth. As to the available facilities, one doctor says, "We have physical equipment and facilities beyond those you might expect in a hospital of similar size."

Hospital #6

This is one of the larger hospitals in the study, located in one of the larger cities in the state. The city is reported to have one main industry. And, a doctor thinks "the fact that the city is dominated by one industry and one union creates a problem. . . . You got one group that can put real pressure on. You don't dare mention the industry around here without crossing yourself." Another adds, "as go [the industry's products], so goes the hospital." According to many respondents, the increasing number of Negro patients coming to this hospital is also a source of some problems. For example, a doctor reports that "the three Negro doctors in the community bring most of their patients to this hospital, and this results in considerable financial loss to the hospital." In this connection, a trustee argues that since the industry brought in most of these people it should share in their hospitalization costs. Perhaps not unrelated to this financial issue might also be the factor of considerable unemployment, reported by some persons.

Several respondents speak of competition between this hospital and another in the city. A trustee says, however, that "we have good relations with the other hospitals." Regarding general relations with the community, several persons view the position of the hospital as favorable and improving. According to a department head, citizens in the community do not have an adequate knowledge of the hospital, but this is improving, he feels. Finally, one doctor characterizes the community as a "very stable, conservative community," adding that this sometimes "makes progress slow."

The members of the board of trustees, some of whom are women, may not be adequately informed about the hospital, according to some respondents. As an answer to a question about hospital problems, one trustee says, "I'm not qualified to answer these things." Another respondent characterizes the trustees as "people who don't—and maybe shouldn't—know what's going on at the hospital except regarding money." According to another, "none of them is too well informed, but they do a good job, considering their lack of information." This person also adds that "a lot of board members are busy otherwise and try to duck committee work." However, a doctor reports that the hospital is strong in "the interest and active participation of its lay board." In this connection, others feel that the president of the board, who is at the top level in the dominant industry, is forceful and active—a driver. "He is the determining factor in policies of this hospital and the future of it," a doctor comments. The board, according to conflicting reports, meets four to six times a year, and its executive committee meets monthly for one hour.

The proper role of trustees, as seen by one of them, is as follows: "What we are working for, as far as the board is concerned, is to have an administrator with enough progress-mindedness so that the president of the board is honorary and does not have to be concerned with detail." And, according to a doctor, responsibility is divided between board and medical staff in this manner: "Theirs is to provide the wherewithal; ours to provide medical care." Another doctor, commenting on differences in viewpoint between the two groups, has this to say: "I think generally the medical attitude initially and usually is whether it will benefit the patient and the lay board's is whether it will benefit the hospital." Another of his colleagues feels that "the present board and medical staff see things the same—a large part of this is due to a liaison committee." A trustee concurs: "We have a liaison committee . . . and we all agree that it has been a most satisfactory arrangement." Several members of the medical staff report that strained relations with the board and administration prevailed until the present administrator came, about a year prior to the study. Under the new administrator, things have improved greatly, according to many respondents.

Several persons comment on relations among members of the medical staff. A doctor says that "the good coordination of the doctors is unusual" for hospitals such as this. Another thinks that "the spirit of cooperation and friendliness and lack of cliquishness is unusual" within the staff. The specialist-general practitioner issue, apparently, is not salient in this hospital. Finally, commenting on the organizational functioning of the staff, a doctor observes that "the heads of medical departments are the ones who formulate policy . . . any change in organization has to be all done by backdoor politics with members of the senior staff—particularly the executive committee."

There is considerable pride among respondents in the quality and scope of the medical care provided at this hospital. A trustee, for example, says the hospital is "outstanding particularly in medical staff, the best you can find in this section of the state." Similarly, a doctor comments, "we have a very strong staff, a high number of board men." And, a nurse reports "outstanding medical specialists." It is also interesting to note that one member of the medical staff speaks of the existence of an informal, "secret" credentials committee for several hospitals in that area, adding this: "We have been working on overall standards of patient care for a long while, and this hospital has been the leader in it."

Regarding nursing care, one nurse sees the hospital as strong in its nursing staff. Several supervisory nurses also commend the nursing staff and its work. Problems in this area also exist, however. One doctor puts it this way: "The hospital has a problem because of inadequate quantity and, to some extent, quality of nursing care. Although the practical nurses were necessary, it did lower the standard of all nursing care." Another person reports inadequate supervision of certain nursing personnel, and an aide says "we have only one R.N. on our wing." Shortage of nursing personnel is also mentioned by others. Regarding another type of problem, a supervisory nurse feels that "there is not enough cooperation between shifts or departments." Other respondents also comment on some tension, or problems, between shifts.

Various aspects of administration are discussed by several persons. There is much praise for the administrator, who is variously seen as "excellent," "approachable," and "capable." A trustee says, "He [the administrator] has inaugurated new philosophies and new programs. He has generally developed more enthusiasm among the personnel." One problem concerning administrative personnel is mentioned by a respondent who says, "The former administrator tried to do the work that three men are doing now; he wouldn't delegate, wouldn't share decisions. As a result, people can't think for themselves." The same person also reports some "inequitable treatment of personnel because our policies are not sufficiently clear and written out." Communication practices are similarly criticized by some. A nurse comments as follows: "Some suggestions have been made and even though they were considered good, nothing was ever done. We didn't even hear why." Another respondent claims that "the suggestion box is never opened."

Several favorable comments are made about the hospital's intern, resident, and nursing education programs, although a few individuals also have certain reservations about them. The building is not adequate for present needs, according to many of the respondents. Some also speak of a need to establish an outpatient clinic. Others indicate that x-ray is inadequate. In general, although various renovations and improvements were recently made, many comments suggest that the hospital needs more beds, more space, and more equipment.

Hospital #7

Situated in a relatively large city, this hospital is of medium size in comparison to others in the study. Control of the institution changed hands about two years prior to the study. A group of citizens, forming a corporation, assumed responsibility. Many important changes are reported to have followed, and many respondents speak favorably, even enthusiastically, of them. One trustee, for example, reports that the hospital is now out of "politics," and another says it has made a "wonderful advancement." Along with changes reported in employee morale,

Individual Hospital Profiles

physical facilities, patient records, etc., comments are made about changes in relations with the community. One person says, "the remnants of bad public opinion is our only problem in this respect, and it is rapidly changing to good." Similarly, a doctor reports as a problem "the attitude of the people, relative to financial support of the hospital," but he adds that the hospital "has been able to create a marked degree of loyalty in the community recently." According to another doctor, "the citizens have responded as the hospital has improved in quality of care."

Much credit for the changes is given to the new administration. A doctor says, "As far as Mr. ——— is concerned, I feel he is a very able administrator and doing a good job." And, another comments, "This administrator is tremendous." The board of trustees also receives praise, one doctor calling it "a top-notch lay board." Similarly, a trustee sees the board as "tremendously interested in the operation and growth of the hospital." Some evidence of this interest is provided in reports that the executive committee of the board meets every week. The medical staff is also reported by some respondents to be actively concerned with the functioning of the hospital. According to one doctor, "the members of the medical staff are very interested and energetic in trying to keep the hospital running smoothly."

Relations between trustees and medical staff are almost universally described as good. One person comments on "a very fine understanding between them as to what their respective roles should be." And, a doctor says "the medical staff and the board work well together—what one needs, the other sees to it that it is worked out to the advantage of both." Another feels that the hospital is "particularly strong in its combined teamwork between the trustees, administrator, medical staff, and all other employees." A report that "the medical staff has an advisory board that meets with the trustees" suggests one factor which may facilitate such teamwork.

The organization of the medical staff is criticized by several respondents. A trustee feels that "their organization is such that they can't take rapid action." And a doctor explains that "medical departments are not autonomous—all actions taken must be approved by the executive staff and general medical staff; no *progress* can be made." As in many other hospitals in the study, some difficulties are reported between general practitioners and specialists. For example, one doctor says "general practitioners have too much power," while another comments, "our specialists attempt to exclude the general practitioners from things that they are competent to do." A third doctor observes that "staff requirements [privileges] are too easy to obtain." Along the same lines, a doctor feels that the control of the hospital "is dominated by a clique of older M.D.'s," and another feels that "doctors do not discipline themselves as well as they should." Related to these problems may also be the following comment by another doctor: "We only have four staff meetings a year, and it's difficult for the men to act democratically. They don't get a grasp of the problems."

Following such criticisms as the above, mixed reports about the work of the medical staff and the quality of patient care may not be unexpected. On the positive side, for example, a trustee says, "I feel we have excellent men on the medical staff." And, a doctor reports, "The surgery is especially strong, and pediatrics is very well developed and gives excellent service. . . . Our medical department also is manned by top-flight men who do an excellent job." On the other hand, one doctor says, "I think the quality of some of the medical staff care should be improved; records, diagnosis, and treatment in some instances are poor." Another comments as follows: "The medical staff, historically, has been a relatively poor one—a fee-splitting, selfish, and mediocre bunch, who have practiced rather poor medicine and cared less." On balance, the care picture is not particularly favorable, according to respondent comments.

Regarding nursing care, relatively few direct comments are made. One doctor says the hospital is weak in its ability "to give acutely ill patients all the care they need because of inadequately trained people doing the job. P.N.'s and aides do too much of this work now because of the scarcity of R.N.'s." Several other doctors and nurses similarly point to the shortage of registered nurses as affecting patient care adversely. Nursing organization and supervision are also criticized by some respondents. Discussing hospital weaknesses, one doctor points to "nursing organization—not enough established procedures to systematize the care of patients." Another reports "ineffective nursing administrative personnel—several in these positions who do not know administrative problems and offer little help to floor nurses."

In the area of hospital administration, while the administrator is generally praised, certain changes are also recommended by various respondents. One department head, for example, thinks that there should be department head meetings at least once a month. Another suggests better cooperation with maintenance. Communication also may not be entirely satisfactory. An aide puts it this way: "We are only aides, so we are not asked about ways to make improvement. If personnel cared about what we thought, we could make quite a number of suggestions for improvement in many things." Another aide comments, "I don't think the organization even knows of any unknown skills and abilities one may have."

Morale among hospital personnel is frequently reported as good, one nurse saying, "We have high morale in this hospital which leaves little room for improvement." Other favorable comments are made about the attitude of hospital people toward the patients. One doctor reports "strong friendliness to patients," and another commends the "personal service" to them. In this connection, however, a nurse says, "I enjoyed the nurse-patient relationship, but now with the acute shortage of R.N.'s there is little time for this." Concerning hospital facilities, some persons report that improvements have taken place, but many view the need for expansion and further improvements as pressing. A doctor comments on the inefficiency of the present architectural layout, while a trustee sees a need for "the addition of new rooms . . . two additional operating rooms, additional OB facilities, additional pediatric space, and additional dining-room facilities." Finally, as in other hospitals in this study, the emergency service is also mentioned as presenting some difficulties. According to a medical staff member, the problem is "getting doctors to cooperate in the care of patients brought into emergency."

Hospital #8

One of the smaller hospitals in the study, this institution is located in a fairly large city. Its relationships with the community, described as having been poor in the past, are reported to be good. Commenting on this area, one person says

Individual Hospital Profiles

that "this was a terrific weakness of this hospital a few years ago; don't think quite so much now—lots of acceptance by the community." A trustee similarly reports "strong community support—especially by industry—they raised a million dollars, nearly, in the last drive." Public attitudes toward the hospital may be also affected by its relation with a philanthropic organization. Speaking of this organization, a doctor comments as follows: "It tries not to be paternalistic, but it is, and this affects the community . . . adversely . . . tends to destroy initiative a little bit." Another doctor says that, if the foundation "put thumbs down," it would not be possible to make changes in the physical plant of the hospital.

Another factor in the community which raises some problems, according to some respondents, is the presence and work of osteopaths. In this connection, a doctor has this to say: "They have their own hospital. . . . Many of our patients want to go there, not realizing the difference in medical care and professional care. The osteopaths run a hospital with no standards at all—according to our standards." Some difficulties and competition with another hospital in the community are also reported, a trustee saying, "you can't get cooperation from the standpoint of community effort, so that you can't judge the whole picture of what the community need is."

Members of the board of trustees are generally seen as capable and interested, but not particularly well informed on hospital-related problems. For example, one respondent says, "I think we have a progressive board . . . interested in anything that makes a better hospital," and a doctor characterizes the board as "patient-conscientious." At the same time, one trustee says, "I don't know enough of the details. I feel I can help steer overall, and take the administrator's word on how we operate." Another comments as follows: "We had a labor problem a few years ago, and the board didn't even know about it. That shows why I can't answer some of these questions. We just don't know a lot of things." Other trustees say, "The board is quite free of politics and cliques"; and, "No 'Mr. Big'; we work as a team. A problem is settled on its merits. No one would take the first place."

Both doctors and trustees report favorable relations between the board and the medical staff, saying such things as, "close cooperation," "good relations," "work well together," and "good feeling." Many report that the two groups tend to see problems in much the same fashion. Some points of difference are also mentioned, however. Regarding costs, for example, a trustee gives this account: "The staff has the feeling that hospital rates are too high. The board feels medical men charge too high. We think that they're coming off a hell of a lot better than we are." Then, according to a doctor, the board lacks understanding of the "scientific approach to community health problems," and it does not "always understand why it is necessary to obtain certain facilities." Another issue, according to a trustee, concerns the question of disciplinary action: "Doctors don't like to do that, but they do a lot of belly-aching about it. It is hard for a board to keep a hospital committee on standards doing their job, particularly when it is an unpleasant job [such as disciplining a staff member]." On the whole, however, comments on board-staff relations are similar to this one by a trustee: ". . . strong cooperation between the two."

Several doctors report good relations among members of the medical staff also, one saying that there is "complete intermingling of the staff with no conflicts in professional services." On the other hand, another doctor sees a need for greater cooperation between departments "by having departmental reciprocation insofar as patients are concerned—i.e., referrals." Similarly, one doctor states that the hospital needs a "more conscientious medical organization—rounds, consultations, conferences." Another holds the following view on medical organization: "An attempt has been made by the staff, at least on paper, to conform to certain idiotic requirements established by the Joint Commission [on Accreditation of Hospitals]—certain standards for conduct of the staff which are really inapplicable to a smaller institution [such as this]." Other doctors, however, feel that this attempt at reorganization has been a real one: "Real attempt by the medical divisions to scientifically strengthen each department"; and "In the last few years we have completely reorganized our faculty and instituted disciplinary measures." Finally, some members of the medical staff see "a weak and vacillating attitude toward the occasional examples of medical neglect," and believe that there should be "perhaps a little greater control over the medical and surgical work done by some staff members."

The medical staff is of high quality, according to several doctors. "We have an excellent medical staff," one says, and another reports that "the number of board men and college men is exceptionally high." Some specify that certain areas of medical care are particularly outstanding, obstetrics being repeatedly mentioned in this connection. Others praise patient care, in general. For example, a nurse says, "I feel our patient care is a strong area," and another reports "progress—in regard to new methods of patient care." Not all comments are highly favorable, however. One doctor characterizes medical care as a "little better than average," for instance. And, another sees the hospital as "weak in nursing personnel," although he adds that recently there has been "better nursing care." On the whole, however, respondent comments about patient care are favorable.

Patients also evaluate the hospital favorably, according to several persons. "I have questioned patients," one says, and "years ago they were adverse, now they are favorable in their comments." Many others report a high level of concern for the patient, a doctor saying patients "like the community spirit and friendliness." Another doctor comments, "We built up such a doggone good hospital now that everyone wants to get in. The demand for beds is tremendous." Previously mentioned comments about community support for the hospital perhaps add to the validity of these expressions.

The following comment by a doctor probably provides the best summary of the patient care picture in this hospital: "In about the last four years there has been good cooperation of the administration, the board of trustees, and the medical staff. We have ironed out practically everything—except the problem of help. . . . It started with the lack of accreditation, which was partly our fault, partly the fault of the inspector [from the Joint Commission on Accreditation of Hospitals] who was determined to find things wrong. But actually it was a good thing for the hospital. Records improved. It woke lots of people up. Standards improved. It's almost unbelievable." The earlier mentioned reorganization of the medical staff apparently has had an impact.

The hospital administrator is often praised by respondents. He is described as "very good," "outstanding," and "a great organizer." A doctor comments, "The man at the head [administrator] is what makes this hospital tick. He takes his duty as being here to improve the hospital all the time." And, more generally, a trustee says that "the hospital is running well and smoothly." Other respondents, however, also point to certain problem areas of hospital administration. A department head, for example, sees a "lack of other departments understanding our function—thereby not working together with us." Another feels that "sometimes the effect of decisions on our department is not considered." And, a supervisory nurse thinks that there ought to be "more interdepartmental meetings, including anyone who might be interested."

Among the more important recent events mentioned by respondents is a substantial expansion of the building, described by one as "a hundred percent addition," and the appointment of a new director of nursing, who according to a doctor has "better control" of the situation. Plans are also reported to be under way for the creation of a special care program for acute cases, and some respondents feel that this will raise the quality of care. Concerning hospital needs, some persons feel that the establishment of an intern program would improve patient care, and recent efforts to this effect are reported. Others speak of a need for an outpatient department, but one doctor says this is something that "none of us want." According to one respondent, this hospital is not as well endowed as some other hospitals and this results in monetary problems. But according to others, the financial status of the hospital is good. Finally, although the physical plant of the hospital is seen by one person as "relatively new and modern," several respondents speak of a shortage of beds, and of the need for certain specialized facilities such as isotope laboratory equipment.

Hospital #9

Located in a middle-sized Michigan city, this is a hospital of medium size compared to others in the study. The community it serves is characterized by a trustee as "a cohesive one, one which sees eye-to-eye and pulls together." According to another trustee, the community has been static in population and economic growth. A doctor adds that there has been unemployment here, which "creates the problem of unpaid care, as well as lack of funds for giving to hospital fund-raising campaigns." Regarding fund raising, however, one trustee reports that a community organization helped raise funds for this hospital and another in the city, and that this was a remarkable job "as at no time has the city been a booming community." Relations between the two hospitals are also discussed by several persons, a trustee saying that there is very good cooperation between them. Competition is also reported by others, however, and a doctor sees "friction between the two hospitals—the personnel." Concerning broad community understanding of the hospital, a trustee says "Well, there's always the lack of understanding of the average citizen."

The board of trustees is favorably seen by some respondents. One person calls it "an excellent board," with no "bickering" among its members, and a doctor says it is "a superlative board." A trustee adds that the board members are successful and highly regarded businessmen. The president of the board is described by another respondent as "a heck of a nice fellow . . . easy to get along with . . . but he doesn't dig deep enough." Some board members apparently feel that the hospital is reasonably free of difficulties. For example, one comments as follows: "Day-to-day problems we don't get in with much. These are the responsibility of the administrator. Most of our problems are recently behind us." And, one of his colleagues agrees: "We have been working for the past two years and we have solved our problems. I do feel, we do not have any problems of major importance."

The bylaws of the institution provide for a liaison group between board and medical staff, composed of both doctors and trustees, as well as for the chief of the medical staff to be a voting member of the board—a feature unusual to hospitals in this study. Concerning staff-board relations, however, respondent reactions vary. Some trustees say such things as, "we haven't had many differences," and "we see pretty much the same in the majority of cases." A doctor also says that he sees no real problems in this area. Other respondents, however, are less favorable. A trustee has this to say: "The major conflict area would be that we on the board think of the hospital as the doctor's workshop, but the doctors think the public owes it to them. . . . They want so much in terms of physical equipment—demand it and think it's their right to have it." A doctor makes a similar comment: "Doctors are interested only in their own problems—not sympathetic to the board."

Other comments on relations between doctors and trustees are critical of the board and of the administrator. For example, one doctor calls the board "unyielding," while another says the administrator is "deaf to staff recommendations." A third doctor adds this: "The board accepts the director [administrator] over the staff. I feel he is biased and does not truly represent our viewpoints to the board of trustees." Another of his colleagues agrees: "The board of trustees views the problems essentially as the administrator and a few nonrepresentative doctors wish them to view the problems." Finally, the following comment by one doctor suggests that some of the above difficulties between board and staff may be due to a lack of balance in the organization roles of the two groups: "I think probably the big problem is that you have, on one side, the board of trustees, who feel they are solely responsible, and, on the other side, a staff of doctors who feel *they* are solely responsible, for the functioning of the hospital."

Many respondents also comment on medical staff organization and on relations among staff members. A doctor says that the medical staff has adopted a new constitution, "the operation of which has made the staff members more responsible to the community regarding the quality of medical care." Another doctor adds that this revision of medical staff bylaws has led to improved care, one type of operation having been reduced by about one-third as a result of consultations newly required. Several organizational weaknesses are also mentioned, however. Respondents feel, for example, that certain key medical committees are not sufficiently active. Others feel that a better adjustment between specialists and general practitioners is necessary. Additional comments are made about relations within the staff and relations with the hospital. According to one doctor, "the greatest need we have is improvement of personal relations between doctors for the good of the staff, the patients, and the hospital." And, according to another, there are "a lot of cliques" within the staff. Other doctors similarly comment that some members of the staff have "no loyalty to the hospital," or that "one half of the staff is always running down this hospital."

With respect to the quality of the medical staff and medical care, most respondent comments are favorable. For example, a trustee states that "we've always said that the city is blessed with some darned good doctors," and another adds,

Individual Hospital Profiles

"we have acquired a large number of young excellent doctors." Similarly, a doctor thinks that this hospital "is unique for one of this size in the quality of medicine overall," and another considers the staff outstanding in the area of training. Another doctor feels that the hospital staff is outstanding in orthopedics, and above average in internal medicine, surgery, radiology, and pathology. Some weaknesses are also indicated, however. One doctor states that there is a "lack of complete control of quality of medical care, which in some instances is grossly inadequate." Another is critical of x-ray, and two technicians describe x-ray interpretation as poor.

Many respondents feel that nursing care is outstanding or very good. A trustee says, for example, that the nursing staff is "tops." "Good nursing service" is one of the strengths of this hospital, observes a doctor. Another calls nursing care "outstanding," adding that "the nurses are far and above those I've come in contact with in large institutions." One doctor reports hearing some complaints about nursing care, but he says that personally he is satisfied. Other respondents comment more generally on the "fine attitude of the staff," a trustee saying that this makes "patients feel their [doctors', nurses', etc.] main concern is for them [the patients]." Others, similarly, mention such things as friendliness, attention, and consideration on the part of the staff: "We do hear our people [patients] receive very considerate care from the staff. They get care and courtesy not only from the nurses but kitchen help, aides, etc."

Comments about administration and the administrator vary. Several respondents praise the administrator, while others are critical of him. A doctor, commenting on important changes in the past, says that they were brought about by "one man more than any other—the administrator." Other doctors characterize him as "remarkably strong," and as doing "a good job." A trustee adds that the administrator "wants to know of any bad experiences anyone has so he can correct any improper procedures or talk it over with offending employees." On the other hand, a doctor thinks that the administrator "has no concept of personnel management," and another feels that relations between administrator and nurses need improvement. Another respondent says that the administrator does not back up his department heads.

Various other aspects of general administration and organization are also commented upon by several respondents. Some persons see a need for such things as "department head conferences," "definite policies and procedures . . . in writing," "more decentralized administration," "establishment of overall organizational goals," and "better communication practices." In this connection, a supervisory nurse remarks that "one soon learns not to make suggestions, since they are not received with even courtesy," and a department head expresses "frustration with the lack of organization." One doctor, similarly, complains about lack of concern "by the administration for improvement primarily in patient care." Finally, a number of additional aspects concerning the hospital also receive some comments. Facilities are seen by some to be "better than in many hospitals much larger than this," and the hospital is said to have been transformed and improved in the past ten years. A "new short training course for nurses" is reported to have "eased nursing shortages." And, according to a trustee, the hospital is "in good financial shape."

A COMPARATIVE OVERVIEW OF THE TEN HOSPITALS

The preceding short descriptions show both differences and similarities among the hospitals studied. They show the atypical as well as the typical, indicating what a particular hospital shares with others and what is unique to that hospital in terms of its operations and problems. The most immediately striking impression one gets from the several profiles, however, is that they clearly point to a good deal of variance across the hospitals with respect to most of the areas covered. Even though this is a relatively homogeneous group of organizations, all of the hospitals having been selected for study because they had certain important criteria in common—location in cities larger than 10,000 population, number of beds, type of service offered, length of patient stay, type of institutional control, type of administration, and institutional accreditation—the profile materials show considerable heterogeneity among these hospitals on a number of dimensions.

A portion of this heterogeneity, or variance, across hospitals is undoubtedly spurious, however, due to at least two main reasons: first, in the profiles we have deliberately emphasized the unique aspects of each organization, in order to introduce the reader to as many different patterns and facets of hospital structure and functioning as possible; and, second, the data on the basis of which the profiles were constructed are incomplete, in the manner that we have previously indicated. Accordingly, the reader should not lose sight of the various similarities and common themes characteristic of these community general hospitals. The common criteria used for the selection of these ten hospitals out of a greatly heterogeneous population of hospitals, and the similarities emerging from the profiles just presented are at least as important, and probably more important, as the differences to which the profiles point.

In this section, by way of a summary and using the ten profiles as a basis, we will attempt to pull the various pieces together by comparing and contrasting the hospitals on each of the following topics: local setting and relations with the community; boards of trustees; medical staffs; relations between doctors and trustees; medical and nursing care; administration and related aspects; and some additional subjects. We will consider these topics in order, beginning with the physical setting of the various institutions.

Local Setting and Relations with the Community

While all ten hospitals are in the lower peninsula of Michigan and in cities of over 10,000 population, only three (0, 1, 6) [5] are in very highly indus-

---

[5] In these summary paragraphs, we will refer to the various hospitals by their profile numbers, enclosing these numbers in parentheses. Thus, in the present case, (0, 1, 6) indicates that Hospital #0, Hospital #1, and Hospital #6 are the three hospitals in the most industrialized cities.

Comparative Overview of the Ten Hospitals

trialized communities. Another two (7, 9) are in communities which are relatively less industrialized. The remaining five hospitals are in communities which have their economic bases partly in industry and manufacturing and partly in agriculture. Two of the hospitals (5, 6) are in communities which are virtually single-industry towns.

The immediate physical setting for four of the ten hospitals (1, 2, 6, 9) is in an area of single family dwellings typically found in midwestern communities. Another hospital (0) is located in a large city within an area of urban transition. The other five hospitals are situated in large wooded plots of land, in parklike settings, being relatively isolated from housing or commercial structures. In terms of physical plant, three of the hospitals (3, 4, 5) have relatively new plants; all others have had one or more major additions. However, only one of the ten hospitals (0) has what may be considered an old plant, which according to our respondents is costly to repair and creates serious problems. In terms of space conditions, more than half of the hospitals (0, 1, 2, 6, 7, 8) have considerable space difficulties. In fact, in only two hospitals (3, 9) space was not mentioned as a relatively major inadequacy. Incidentally, some of the hospitals are currently under expansion, and others are planning to expand their plants in the near future.

Half of the hospitals (3, 4, 5, 8, 9) are serving relatively wealthier communities than the other half. In one of the former hospitals (9), it is emphasized that the community has been relatively stable and economically static, while in another (5) it is emphasized that the community contains a large proportion of highly educated people. The financial status of hospitals in the more industrialized areas (0, 1, 6) is said to be closely tied to fluctuations in business conditions. Four of the hospitals (0, 1, 2, 6) are concerned with the extent to which their facilities are being increasingly used by Negro patients or patients from low socioeconomic groups, this concern being primarily expressed with respect to financial aspects and difficulties in internal operations. In this connection, a strong policy of segregation of Negro patients is reported in one of these hospitals (2), while in another (1) some respondents express pride in that their hospital serves the community regardless of race, faith, or financial status; even in this latter case, some express concern about an inadequacy of funds related to indigent and Negro patients. It is noteworthy, however, that in all ten hospitals members of the boards of trustees, administrators, and other respondents, on the whole, feel that the general financial condition of their institution is good. Furthermore, only two of the ten hospitals (0, 2) are reported to be actually operating on a budget.

Relations between the hospital and the community are seen as particularly good in two hospitals (3, 4) and rather poor in a third (2); markedly improved in three others (0, 7, 8), after having been dangerously unsatisfactory; and needing improvement in all other hospitals. In nearly every one of the ten hospitals, moreover, respondents feel that public knowledge and community understanding of the hospital and its problems leave much to be desired. The problem here was nicely capsuled by a trustee in a hospital (where relations with the community were reported to be quite good) who told the interviewer, "Well, there is always the lack of understanding of the average citizen." Interestingly enough, however, most hospitals report good support on the part of their community, even though the community has relatively little understanding of the operations and needs of the hospital. Perhaps a little more emphasis on public relations on the part of these hospitals would stimulate more community interest and understanding to the benefit of all concerned.

Hospitals, like other organizations, have a number of publics, and this may create special community-hospital problems. Two of the hospitals (*5, 6*) in this study, for example, face communities dominated by one industry and one union. The public image of another (*8*) is affected by its unique relationship to a local foundation. In another hospital (*4*), while relations with the community at large are described as excellent, relations with the county board of supervisors are not seen as satisfactory. In two hospitals (*1, 8*) there is considerable concern about future relations and problems with osteopathic hospitals in the community. Some concern is also expressed in two hospitals (*2, 8*) about competition with other hospitals in the community. In this connection, we should note that all except one of the ten hospitals in the study are in cities which have at least one more hospital, and in most cases they have more; even in the case where the exception occurs, however, the hospital is located at a point which is no farther than 15 miles from several similar hospitals. Relations between hospitals in the same community are generally described as good.

Boards of Trustees

The members of the various boards of trustees serve on a voluntary basis, without pay. In most cases, as would be expected, the majority of them are laymen who hold major positions in business and industry. The number of trustees varies across hospitals, ranging from 19 in one hospital (*0*) to 12 in another (*5*). But nearly all of the boards consist of nonmedical people, with two exceptions: 10 of the 19 members in one hospital (*0*), according to the constitution, must be doctors; and the chief of the medical staff in another hospital (*9*) is a voting member of the board. Eligibility for board membership is generally determined by such factors as contribution of money or property to the hospital, recognition of past achievements in the community, status and influence in the community, business experience, former board membership, and similar other considerations. Actual board membership, however, is determined through election either by the hospital corporation—a parent organization consisting of interested people representing various segments of the community—or by the existing board of trustees which is self-perpetuating. In most hospitals, the term of office for trustees is three years, but re-election is both permissible and likely.

The primary function of the boards of trustees is one of exercising general control over the affairs of the institution, especially over fiscal matters and long-range policies on such things as hospital expansion and plant improvements, nonmedical personnel, and public relations. The day-to-day operations of the organization, excepting medical matters, are entrusted to the hospital administrator and his staff; and, all aspects of medical practice and organization are mainly under the control of the medical staff itself. The boards may meet as frequently as monthly, which is the case for one of the ten hospitals *(0)*; four to six times a year as is the case for most of the hospitals; or on no regular basis, which is the case for another of these hospitals *(2)*. However, their executive committees meet more frequently, in one hospital *(7)* as often as weekly, and are empowered to make decisions for the full board between board meetings.

In general, the various boards are seen to operate on the principle of traditional democratic procedures. In one hospital *(8)*, for example, the trustees themselves are particularly pleased with the balance they have achieved as a team of equals, without having a "Mr. Big" amongst them. Similar, though less explicit reactions on the part of various respondents, in this connection, prevail in several hospitals. In some hospitals *(2, 3, 6)*, however, the board presidents are seen as rather powerful and dominating individuals who determine policies and programs for the hospital. In all hospitals, the board presidents spend a good deal of time working with the administrator and others for their particular institution. Finally, in most cases, the boards are seen as doing an effective job for the organization, although their members' knowledge of hospital matters is frequently questioned by many respondents. In fact, some of the trustees who were interviewed in this study themselves expressed embarrassment for not being able to answer various questions about the hospital for lack of familiarity with the problems or issues involved.

Medical Staffs

The medical staffs in the various hospitals are in almost complete charge of medical policies and medical practice. They have their own organization within the overall hospital organization; have their own constitution, rules, and regulations; and are, in the main, self-disciplining bodies. They do have, however, to abide with certain fundamental hospital policies, such as maintaining adequate patient records up to date, having their membership recommendations formally reviewed by the board of trustees and, generally, operating in a manner that would not jeopardize the accreditation of the hospital. In addition, of course, medical staff members, like all others working at the hospital, depend on other people in the process of carrying out their professional functions.

From an organizational standpoint, hospital medical staffs operate through various professional and administrative committees. For example, they have a records committee, an education committee, a tissue committee, and other committees in charge of various aspects of medical practice. Similarly, on the administrative side, they have a credentials committee in charge of staff membership, and an executive committee which represents the staff at large. Members of the executive committee are either elected by the entire staff or are appointed by the chief of staff, who is elected by the staff. Such elections and appointments usually occur annually. There are some exceptions to this pattern, however, for in the case of two hospitals (*4, 5*), members of the executive committee serve for three-year terms. Medical staff executive committees are often seen as having little authority with respect to making important decisions for the entire staff, and in some hospitals (*3, 7*) they are seen as unable to move fast enough when needed. Similarly, chiefs of staff are often seen as holding an honorific position rather than a position wielding significant authority. But in the case of the only hospital in the study (*5*) which has no chief of staff, some doctors feel that because of this there is not enough control over medical practice.

Relationships within the medical staff are seen as particularly warm, friendly, and harmonious in three of the ten hospitals (*0, 4, 8*). In another three hospitals (*3, 5, 6*), they are seen as satisfactory, with no "cliques" or "friction." In the remaining hospitals, relationships among doctors are commented upon somewhat less favorably. However, in most hospitals relationships between those physicians who are specialists and those who engage in general practice are seen as entailing some problems. The issue usually revolves around the question of what and how many staff privileges should general practitioners be allowed to have, i.e., the question of setting limits to professional practice. The specialist-general practitioner issue is brought into particularly sharp focus in three of the ten hospitals (*2, 3, 5*). On the basis of our hospital profiles, it appears that the general practitioners are fighting a rear-guard action against encroachment of their privileges by the specialists.

Relations Between Doctors and Trustees

Relations between doctors and trustees in our group of hospitals are generally very good. In only two hospitals (*1, 2*) is there much evidence of problems in this area. In both of these cases, there are formal organizational devices designed to ensure satisfactory liaison between the two key groups, but they are not being used. In one of the two hospitals (*2*), the chief of staff is supposed to be invited to board meetings, for example, but he is not; and on past occasions when doctors attended board meetings, they felt that they were unwelcome. The hospital administrator, who is supposed to serve as liaison between board and staff, does not do a good job either according to the doctors, although according to the trustees he does. And, the president of the board is a dominating person according to several reports. In any event,

Comparative Overview of the Ten Hospitals

mutual contacts and consultations between the two groups appear to be very constricted. It is also worth noting, finally, that a member of the medical staff in this hospital points out that both sides will have to assume joint responsibility for improving the situation, and that the doctors ought to fight for their rights.

In the other hospital (*1*) where relationships between doctors and trustees are also strained, the medical executive committee has the responsibility for providing liaison with the board. The chief of staff and the vice-chief attend board meetings, but there is a feeling that the communication process is not functioning properly. Liaison members are not really listened to carefully until a major problem demands that "the thinking members of the medical staff" talk directly with board members. Similarly, the role of the administrator in providing liaison between staff and board is often viewed with a critical eye by various respondents.

All hospitals rely heavily on the administrator to serve in a liaison capacity between the medical staff and the board of trustees. And, some of the administrators (*3, 6, 7*) are perceived as performing this coordinative function especially well. Liaison between the two groups in the various hospitals is also provided in a number of other ways. These range from having a special joint conference committee consisting of doctors and trustees (*6, 7*), through relying on meetings between the executive committees of the two groups, to having key members of the medical staff attend board meetings as nonvoting members (*1, 4*) or even as voting members (*0, 9*). These formal devices are, of course, frequently supplemented by informal ones, such as meetings between members of the two groups at luncheon, at the country club, or even in the hospital corridor.

In most of the hospitals each group's sphere of competence is recognized and respected by the other. There is little evidence of overt power conflicts or of attempts by one group to usurp the other's authority or to establish itself as the dominant element. There is, however, some evidence of variation in the pattern of relationships between the two groups. While the division of labor between doctors and trustees is so complete in one hospital (*5*) that some members of each group wonder if there is not too much specialization in this respect, in another (*3*) the board is watching with interest the way in which the medical staff works out its internal problem of the relationship between specialists and general practitioners.

Medical and Nursing Care

The profiles show a surprising willingness in most hospitals, especially on the part of doctors, to make frank and critical evaluations of patient care in their hospital. A good number of individual doctors in each case are willing to discuss openly with researchers the problems they and the hospital face in upgrading medical and nursing performance—a very reassuring attitude indeed. As a consequence, even in this highly subjective material of the various hospital profiles, a good deal is said to suggest the quality of medical and nursing care patients receive.

The general impression one gets from the profiles is that, on the whole, the quality of patient care in this group of hospitals is quite good. However, differences across hospitals with respect to both medical and nursing care are also indicated. In two hospitals (*3, 4*) there is a good deal of agreement among respondents, both doctors and others, that medical and nursing care meet very high standards of preformance; doctors are seen as very skillful and competent, working together to provide excellent care to patients, and nurses are seen as doing an equally outstanding job. In some cases, either the quality of medical care or the quality of nursing care, but not both, is evaluated very favorably. For example, in one hospital (*6*) the quality and scope of medical care are seen as outstanding, while nursing care is only seen as good or average. Still in other hospitals (*0, 1, 5, 7*) the quality of medicine practiced is partly evaluated as very good and partly as needing improvements. The perennial problem of trying to improve medical practice, through proper controls, is mentioned by doctors in several hospitals (*6, 7, 8*).

The shortage of professional nurses is seen as a major barrier to providing adequate patient care in this group of hospitals. The need for nurses and other professional personnel is stressed by respondents in all hospitals except two (*4, 9*). In some hospitals, it is also felt by some doctors that there is not enough good bedside nursing (*1*), or that some nurses watch television instead of patients (*2*), or that nursing personnel are unwilling to assume as much responsibility as they should (*1, 5*). Conditions such as these are often attributed to inadequate direction, inadequate supervision, or inadequate administrative procedures (*1, 2, 7*). Finally, in some of the hospitals criticisms and questions are raised about the work done by such medical facilities as the laboratory (*4, 5*) and x-ray (*6, 9*) departments.

However incomplete these qualitative evaluations may be, they are both suggestive of the quality of medical and nursing practice in the various hospitals and indicative of problems and issues that lie behind the more systematically obtained quantitative data in this area. Our measures of medical and nursing care, based on quantitative data, will be presented in the next chapter, and the reader may wish to compare the standing of the various hospitals in terms of both the present qualitative evaluations and the corresponding quantitative measures.

Administration and Related Aspects

In most of the hospitals, both doctors and trustees see the administrators as performing their role of managing the hospital very effectively. In half of the hospitals (*4, 5, 6, 7, 8*) respondents commend the administrator in rather glowing terms—"tremendous," "vigorous," "top-notch," "a wonder," etc.

There are, however, some differences of opinion about the performance of the administrator in other hospitals (*1, 2, 9*). In two of the hospitals (*6, 7*), the administrators had recently been given the task of rebuilding an organization that was very poorly functioning under preceding administrators, and respondents feel that in both cases the present administrator is doing an excellent job.

On the whole, the various administrators appear to be performing their role very well. As might be expected, however, most of them are better in certain areas than in others. For example, in one hospital (*3*) respondents feel that the administrator is stronger in administrative skills than in the area of human relations. In two hospitals (*1, 2*) the administrators are weak with respect to providing adequate liaison and coordination between medical staff and trustees. And, in another two hospitals (*4, 9*) they are criticized with respect to administrator-nursing staff relationships. Furthermore, the profiles suggest that even some of the most competent administrators are doing a better job in their work with doctors and with trustees than in their work with their own subordinate staffs. Perhaps, they inevitably put more emphasis and effort to maintaining good relations at the top of the organization with the consequence that other levels are correspondingly neglected.

It is also significant that in all ten hospitals, regardless of how the administrator is personally evaluated, one finds many references to the need for better coordination, better integration and cooperation, and better communication practices among organizational groups and across organizational levels. Similar other references point to the need for written procedures and better personnel policies in some hospitals (*3, 4, 9*) as a means for increasing mutual understanding among organizational members and improving work relationships.

Some Additional Items

The profiles indicate that several hospitals (*4, 6, 8*), finding their present facilities taxed by persons who do not actually require hospitalization, yet recognizing their responsibility to the community, would like to establish outpatient departments. Certain other hospitals (*1, 2, 3, 7*) have problems with their emergency service. According to various comments, in two of these (*2, 3*), the emergency room is being misused by some doctors having patient visits there instead of at their own office; and in another case (*1*) the emergency service is being abused by low-income persons coming to obtain free medical assistance. In another hospital (*7*), related comments suggest a good deal of difficulty in getting the cooperation of doctors to cover the emergency service. In fact, problems related to the outpatient service, the emergency service, and the specialist-general practitioner issue are among the most frequently commented topics in the profiles.

As might be expected, additional materials in the several profiles show that a number of respondents in every hospital express a good deal of satisfaction and pride about the service the hospital is rendering to its patients and its community. In different hospitals, certain specialized aspects of hospital service such as orthopedics, work with cancer diseases, pediatrics, obstetrics and gynecology, and specialized surgery are highly praised by respondents. Hospital facilities, supplies, and equipment, excepting particular instances already indicated, are generally seen as adequate in this group of hospitals. Space and bed problems, on the other hand, seem to be common to nearly all of the hospitals in the study. Finally, the general financial condition of each institution, as earlier stated, is generally seen as adequate and satisfactory.

SUMMARY

In this chapter we have attempted to introduce the reader to each hospital in the study as a distinct organization with its own outlook, weaknesses, and strengths, and to all ten hospitals as a group of similar social systems which face a number of needs and problems in common. We have tried to accomplish this by (1) presenting a sketch of the "typical" participating hospital, (2) constructing a short profile for each institution studied, and (3) summarizing some of the contents of the individual hospital profiles to indicate the main differences and similarities which characterize the ten hospitals. The main objective was to provide an answer to the question of what these community general hospitals look like—what kind of organizations they are and how they operate—as seen through the comments and verbatim remarks of the respondents, who freely and generously furnished us with most of the materials incorporated in the profiles.

Because these materials are neither complete (only a proportion of the respondents from each hospital having provided the information in each case) nor entirely objective (they contain many facts, but also some respondent biases), they cannot give a thorough picture of hospital organization. A clearer and more complete picture will begin to emerge with the presentation of the more systematic, quantitative findings in the next chapters. The qualitative data presented here, however, along with the data about the people around the patient in Chapter 3, provide a great deal of information about the structure and functioning of the community general hospital. They cover a wide range of topics, issues, and problems which, in all probability, are shared not only by the few hospitals in this study but also by many other voluntary hospitals in the nation. (For a commentary on some of the issues and problems discussed here, as well as several additional ones, see Chapter 11.) Furthermore, they make it possible for the reader to compare and contrast simultaneously ten independent organizations, all of which are attempting to accomplish the same objective—that of providing adequate patient care effectively. Above all, these qualitative data provide the outsider with many insights, as well as a certain amount of basic understanding about hospital operation, and serve to confirm or deny many of the beliefs the insider may be entertaining about institutions such as these and those who work there.

REFERENCES

1. Babcock, K. B. "Accreditation," *Hospitals,* 34:43, (April) 1960.
2. Block, L. "Prototype Study: 200 Bed Hospital," *Mod. Hosp.,* 82:76–80, (Jan.) 1954.
3. *Hospitals.* Guide Issue. *Hospitals,* 34:Part Two, (Aug.) 1960.

5 ASSESSMENT OF PATIENT CARE

The individual hospital profiles in the preceding chapter tell us some things about the organization and social structure of each institution, but they do not give us an adequate indication of its effectiveness or of the kind of care it provides. Patient care, which constitutes the main objective of the community general hospital and one of our major research concerns, cannot be assessed from the limited information of these profiles. Additional data are necessary. The main purpose of this chapter is to develop, from appropriate data, measures which can be employed to evaluate and compare the quality of patient care rendered by the different participating hospitals.

Once a satisfactory assessment of patient care is attained, different aspects of hospital structure and functioning can be related systematically to the quality of care, and factors associated with better or poorer care can then be determined. This latter task we are reserving for later chapters. In the present chapter we shall be concerned only with the measurement of patient care.

The problems encountered in attempting to evaluate the quality of care which, on the aggregate, patients receive in a hospital are obviously very complex and very difficult. Even a casual reflection quickly reveals that no uniform standards are available for this purpose; nor is there consensus in this field about the sources and kinds of data that are necessary, sufficient, and feasible at the same time. The lack of suitable standardized criteria for evaluating hospital care, or the absence of valid and reliable measures, makes it necessary for the researcher to develop such measures, using whatever relevant resources that may be available. Furthermore, when no single satisfactory measure exists, it virtually becomes indispensable that several rather than one measure be developed and used, if at all possible. This is the task undertaken in the present chapter.

Our specific objective here, however, is not to develop criteria in terms of which one can appraise the quality of hospital patient care in an absolute sense, but rather to develop measures with which one can successfully distinguish the better-care hospitals from those where care is of relatively lower quality. For this purpose, it is sufficient that the measures be such as to permit us to rank-order the ten hospitals from "best" to "poorest," although in absolute terms the "poorest-care" hospital may still be one where patient care is satisfactory from a medical standpoint. In fact, it should be recalled and emphasized that all ten participating hospitals are institutions which are accredited by the Joint Commission on Accreditation of Hospitals, such accreditation implying that the hospitals at least meet minimum standards of care, i.e., meet essential requirements and prerequisites that are acceptable to the medical profession. Our aim, then, is to obtain measures capable of differentiating between better- and poorer-care hospitals and not necessarily between "good" and "bad" hospitals.

Theoretically, the problem of assessing patient care in hospitals is similar to that of evaluating other complex phenomena. For example, it is not unlike the problems encountered in appraising the effectiveness of an industrial firm, the personality of an individual, or organizational coordination (which we shall take up in the next chapter). What makes the present problem especially difficult is the relative paucity of prior research and the fact that the components of organizational input-output are much more diverse, much less tangible, less well understood, and considerably more elusive in the case of a hospital as compared to an industrial organization, for example. Both the producers and their products are substantially more variegated in the hospital situation. Patient care requires the concerted effort of many individuals in various positions with many different skills, talents, abilities, and backgrounds; and the patients are live human beings rather than passive physical objects of lesser value or complexity. Apart from these difficulties and unlike many other organizations, moreover, hospitals do not ordinarily maintain uniform, or even comparable, data regarding their output, i.e., data capable of yielding suitable measures of patient care.

Regardless of the problems involved, however, it is the task of research to provide useful answers to meaningful questions about complex phenomena, including the phenomenon of patient care in hospitals. And the researcher, at least potentially, has at his disposal various scientific tools and resources which, in principle, enable him to solve his problems more or less successfully. In this respect, the measurement of patient care presents no exception other than constituting a relatively new research venture. Knowledge of results from previous relevant studies, experience with tackling similar problems in other settings, familiarity with the issues involved, advice from experts, and information from those directly involved in hospital operations are all useful aids and, potentially, all can contribute to the development of the needed measures of hospital patient care.

Before discussing the specific measures of patient care developed in this study, it would also be useful to indicate briefly the nature of previously suggested approaches to the problem of assessment. What are the main issues?

How much agreement is there among those who have had some experience or have done relevant work in this area? What are the alternatives and their relative merits? These and similar other questions require an answer, and such an answer can serve as a basis for obtaining suitable measures. Let us therefore search for some answers.

PREVIOUSLY SUGGESTED APPROACHES

The literature on hospitals and patient care provides a good indication both of the specific difficulties and the specific possibilities and alternatives regarding the evaluation of hospital care. On the whole, it shows a good deal of agreement about some of the more general aspects of the problem of assessment, but less unanimity about concrete steps to be taken toward its solution. As we will see, however, it is not so much that people in this field are not agreed upon what should be done ideally, or in the long run, in order to obtain satisfactory measures which makes things difficult at present, as is the gap which exists between what is theoretically desirable and what is practically feasible. The main problem stems from the fact that no comparable data about the quality of patient care are readily available in hospitals, if at all available. Let us examine the literature a little more closely.

At the outset, one should point out that there is general consensus in the hospital field regarding some of the major components of a "good," or good-care, hospital. A summary of such components, given in *Lancet* (22), includes a team of good doctors, enough qualified nurses, a competent administrator, adequate diagnostic facilities, and sufficient social-welfare services. Davis (6) similarly suggests five basic elements in hospital patient care: the professionals responsible for patient care, the organization of medical practice in the hospital, the physical plant and equipment available, finances, and the patients requiring care. The literature is also replete with such statements as "The hospital is only as good as its medical staff" (18), "Committees make the staff a team" (31), "Department heads make the hospital" (5), and the like. On a general level, within the limits of present-day medical and organizational knowledge, and apart from financial and technological aspects, the quality of hospital patient care is seen to depend upon at least five major factors: (1) the training and skills of the various medical and nonmedical members of the organization; (2) the nature of medical and nursing practice; (3) the nature of administration and supervision, and the organization of the medical staff; (4) the nature of coordination, communication, and interpersonal relationships among hospital members and between them and the patients; and (5) the structure and character of the total hospital organizational system. In turn, of course, each of these factors depends upon a host of more specific variables, many of which will be spelled out in our own analyses in this and subsequent chapters.

Previously Suggested Approaches

Further, most writers, with or without medical training, tend to view the effective hospital as one which, above anything else, provides its patients with adequate care and treatment. Of course this is not surprising in view of the fact that patient care constitutes the main product of a hospital. On the other hand, this is an important consideration because it suggests that, for the hospital, organizational effectiveness and patient care are essentially equivalent which, in turn, implies that we cannot know how effective a hospital is unless we know something about the kind of patient care it provides. Accordingly, measures of patient care would not only be important from a medical standpoint, but also from an organizational and administrative standpoint.

Along the same lines, most writers also tend to agree with Hawley (13) that the quality of patient care is the "ultimate yardstick" for evaluating a hospital, as well as with Dichter (8) that it is "the *quality* rather than the *amount* of the care that the patient is wary of." The patient, who is the center and origin of all hospital functions, apparently is assured of some minimal amount of care upon entering a hospital. Beyond this, however, it is quality rather than quantity that is crucial. High quality care would almost certainly imply sufficient quantity, while the converse is not true. Consequently, the literature suggests that it is the qualitative factor that should be prominently reflected in one's measures of patient care and hospital effectiveness.

At best, these considerations can only indicate the general approach one must follow in order to obtain acceptable measures of patient care. When it comes to using specific measures, however, one finds neither standard criteria nor hard and fast rules of procedure. Nevertheless, a number of guiding principles from previous research do exist. These provide important clues about what measures may or may not be feasible and appropriate, thus helping to guard against serious pitfalls. Let us, therefore, consider some of the more important and more prevalent alternatives that have been suggested in the past, with emphasis on their relevance to our specific problem of obtaining measures which can differentiate between better- and poorer-care hospitals.

Four major approaches to assessing patient care in hospitals have been frequently proposed in recent years. For purposes of discussion, these approaches may be identified as follows: (1) the accreditation approach; (2) the statistical approach; (3) the "satisfied customer test" approach; and (4) the clinical approach. Of course, these approaches are not mutually exclusive. However, they may best be discussed separately here.

First, an obvious way to evaluate hospitals and, by extension, the care they provide is to look at their accreditation status. Accredited hospitals meet certain standards and requirements of patient care, while nonaccredited hospitals do not. The accreditation requirements have been established by the medical profession, particularly the American College of Surgeons, and the Joint Commission on Accreditation of Hospitals. This commission is the authority which awards, withholds, or withdraws accreditation, based on its own review of the situation prevailing in a given hospital. And although the review is in a sense a voluntary affair, initiated at first on the request of the hospital, it is now an institutionalized and widely accepted procedure among hospitals. In various respects, hospitals benefit from accreditation and are usually proud of being accredited. Accreditation status thus offers one criterion, crude as it may be, for judging hospital patient care. For our purposes, however, the accreditation approach is entirely inadequate. Irrespective of its merits or deficiencies, as discussed by Babcock (1), King (20), Kossack (21), Myers and Babcock (31), Rourke (36), and others (27), this approach cannot solve our problem because all of the hospitals in the study were chosen from among accredited institutions. We are interested in the extent to which the various hospitals go beyond meeting only essential requirements of patient care; they all meet minimum standards well enough to be accredited. We must therefore look elsewhere for the necessary measures of hospital care.

A second, frequently proposed, approach to evaluating patient care is to analyze statistically data from patient records and from the medical "self-audit" which is normally carried out by the staff of individual hospitals.[1] The patient record contains a wealth of information about the condition of the patient, the nature of his illness, diagnosis, drugs, therapy, progress, and discharge. Theoretically, therefore, appropriate analysis of patient records data should be very useful. The same may be said of the medical self-audit. The medical staff in the hospital, in addition to maintaining patient records, ordinarily audits part of its work in an effort to "educate" itself and to maintain and improve professional standards and patient care. The specific audit procedures and the cases being audited may vary widely from hospital to hospital, but all accredited hospitals are required by the Joint Commission on Accreditation to engage in some audit activity—and many hospitals, such as those participating in the audit program of the Commission on Professional and Hospital Activities, do a great deal more auditing than the requirements they may have to fulfill for accreditation purposes.

The current trend in hospitals is toward more and more rigorous audit, and considerable attention has in recent years been given to the nature, problems, and advantages of medical auditing in relation to improving patient care and other pertinent issues. For some interesting discussions of various aspects of the medical self-audit, the reader may wish to consult such pub-

---

[1] The medical self-audit in hospitals should not be confused with the more systematic medical audit program which, since 1956, is being carried out by the Commission on Professional and Hospital Activities in cooperation with various hospitals which have joined its program (3), or with the Commission's "Professional Activity Study" (4). The Commission's program is uniform and standardized. At the time of the present study, only two of our ten participating hospitals had joined the programs of the Commission.

Previously Suggested Approaches

lications as those by Hawley (12), Hill (14), Johnson (16, 17), MacEachern (25), McGibony (26), Sewall and Berger (37), Smith (41), or other relevant references. Here, of course, we are interested in the medical audit and in the patient record only from the standpoint of their usefulness to obtaining satisfactory measures of hospital patient care, particularly medical care.

Unfortunately, the statistical approach based on patient record and medical self-audit data, like the accreditation approach, is also inadequate for our purposes. Looking into the future, statistical analysis of patient record and medical audit data appears to hold considerable promise with respect to assessing patient care, but for the time being it is not suitable to the task at hand for several important reasons. For one thing, the different hospitals do not maintain sufficiently comparable records to provide necessary data that are amenable to scientific analysis. Across hospitals, patient records do not contain uniform data, and within hospitals there is a fairly wide variation among doctors in their handling of patient records. Furthermore, while some hospitals keep up-to-date records, others lag to a greater or lesser extent. In short, patient records are neither uniform, nor sufficiently comparable, nor equally complete from one hospital to another, or even within hospitals (notwithstanding the fact that accredited institutions must meet certain minimum requirements concerning their patient records). And although the patient record, as Bachrach (2) observes, has great potential usefulness if properly planned and executed, at present it cannot provide the assessment data we need.

Some of the most crucial information concerning the quality of patient care can be obtained only from the results of medical audit, as it does not appear on the patient record. Even the audit data (if available, and if at all recorded, for in some hospitals the audit committee deliberately prefers not to keep minutes containing audit information), however, are not amenable to effective statistical analysis. In fact, audit data, if anything, present even greater difficulties than patient records data, from the point of view of standardization and statistical treatment. The proportion of cases audited varies considerably among hospitals, sometimes being very small, and usually being unrepresentative of the total volume of patient cases. Similarly, there are wide variations in the nature and type of cases subjected to medical audit in the time periods for which audit data may be available, in the thoroughness of the audit procedures followed, in the composition of the medical committees performing the audit, in the extent to which the results of the audit are recorded, in the particular usage and consequences of the audit, e.g., whether the results are seen and used primarily for educational versus disciplinary or punitive purposes, and in many other important respects.

Because of these and other difficulties and deficiencies pertaining to data from patient records and the medical self-audit, and apart from equally serious problems of practicality and required effort, the second suggested approach to assessing patient care was also ruled out in this study. As

Hawley (12), Lembcke (24), Myers (30), and Sheps (38, 39), among others, have previously concluded, comparable and sufficient data of the type here discussed simply are not available in the different hospitals to permit one to derive "objective" measures of care from patient record and medical audit materials. Of course, this in no way detracts from the value of patient records, or from the value of the self-audit and its role in improving patient care in hospitals. Nor does it detract from the potential usefulness of audit data in connection with the problem of assessment. On the contrary, it is very likely that the medical audit in individual hospitals, and the similar but more systematic audit which, along with the related "Professional Activity Study," is currently carried out by the Commission on Professional and Hospital Activities in cooperation with a number of hospitals (3, 4, 29, 30, 32, 40), will eventually yield data that can be effectively utilized for the purpose of deriving measures of hospital patient care—hopefully in the near future.

Sometimes, the so-called "satisfied customer test" is also suggested as another approach to the problem of patient care assessment. This approach is based on two rather questionable assumptions, (1) that patients can judge the care they receive, and (2) that if the patients are satisfied with their care, then care is good. Obviously, such inferences cannot be made, especially in the absence of supportive empirical evidence. The patient is hardly in a good position to evaluate the quality of his care, either during or after hospitalization. First, as Goldwater (11) observes, the patient has limited medical (and nursing) knowledge; accordingly, although suggesting the satisfied customer test, he attaches to it this important qualification. Second, the studies of Reader, Pratt, and Mudd (35) show that the medical care expectations of patients and the way in which patients define their problems and "optimal care" are influenced by patient-physician interaction. Third, along the same lines, Phenix (34) and others correctly point out that the goals and expectations of the patient with reference to his care are often at variance with those of his doctor, depending on such things as the seriousness and nature of the patient's illness, his personal liking for his doctor, whether or not his goal is one of complete cure or mere restoration of essential functions, etc. Fourth, in short-stay hospitals, patient turnover is very rapid (the average length of stay for adult patients in the ten hospitals participating in this study was 6.79 days during 1957) and, being a transient member of the hospital system, the patient cannot be expected to familiarize himself adequately either with the many facets of the care process or with the many complexities of the hospital situation, within a brief period of time.

All the above factors would, of course, affect and "bias" the patient's judgment regarding the quality of his hospital care. Even more significant is perhaps the fact that, during hospitalization, the patient is both physically and psychologically disturbed and unstable; he does not function normally or as a relatively free and independent agent. As Dichter (7) points out, the

Previously Suggested Approaches

adult patient upon entering the hospital "feels like a child and, for a short time, regresses to the emotional level of the child," because he finds himself "all at once in a strange environment," he is "helpless and afraid," and "all his physical needs are taken care of and all decisions are made for him" by others. Moench (28) makes essentially the same point. Lederer (23), in his stimulating article "How the Sick View Their World," aptly shows that illness is a complex psychological phenomenon which involves a great many fears and anxieties on the part of the patient. Under these conditions, we could hardly expect the patients to provide us with an acceptable evaluation of patient care. We might also add that interviewing or questioning patients about their care while in the hospital itself poses great many difficulties. Some patients cannot be subjected to interviewing because they are critically ill; others can be interviewed only at a certain time during their hospital stay; nonadult patients, being incapable of mature judgment, cannot even be requested to provide information; other patients may object because of their condition or other reasons, etc.

Most of the medical and psychological forces operating during hospitalization will, of course, no longer exist after the patient has been discharged, but some of their effects may still carry over and color the judgment which the patient might make about his hospital care after recovery and discharge. Furthermore, a changed outlook due to the patient's return to normalcy, as well as errors of memory and recall, may well affect patient judgment after hospitalization. And the limitations of medical and nursing knowledge will certainly still be an obstacle to valid judgment. From another standpoint, the problem of obtaining a representative sample of discharged patients and then successfully tracing them to collect data is also a difficult one, apart from the additional problem that discharged patients do not represent all of the patients who were initially admitted to the hospital. In the light of these considerations, the satisfied customer test approach to assessing the quality of patient care was also ruled out in the present study, although some data on patient reaction toward the hospital were obtained from our medical and nursing staff respondents.

In summary, for the reasons indicated in each case, the accreditation approach based on minimum standards, the approach involving statistical analysis of data from patient records and the medical self-audit, and the satisfied customer approach based on patient judgment cannot at present provide adequate data for evaluating and comparing the quality of patient care rendered at various hospitals. The fourth major approach suggested in hospital-medical literature is the "clinical judgment" approach.[2] Briefly, this

---

[2] In addition to the four approaches considered here, other less frequently proposed techniques for measuring patient care are occasionally proposed. For example, Furstenberg and his colleagues (9) attempted to evaluate patient care in the Baltimore City
[*Footnote continued.*]

approach rests on the reasonable assumption that qualified judges, such as hospital staff physicians, can appraise patient care on the basis of their medical knowledge, clinical experience, and firsthand familiarity with the care situation at their hospital. In practice, the hospital medical staff inevitably engages in informal assessment of patient care as part of its job while, somewhat more formally, through its committees, it carries out various assessment activities, e.g., activities involving the medical audit, the policing of patient records, the conduct of clinicopathological conferences, and the like. Consequently, the hospital medical staff possesses a good deal of information about patient care and related issues.

This last approach to measuring the quality of hospital patient care, generally, seems to be the least inadequate and most feasible, partly because it does not entail most of the theoretical and practical difficulties which plague the preceding approaches. It is not surprising, therefore, that the clinical judgment approach is favored by many people in the hospital-medical field who have done rather intensive analyses of the problem of patient care assessment. Sheps (38), for example, having reviewed several possible measurement techniques—including examination of postoperative death and infection rates, examination of prerequisites, such as minimal levels of facilities, and examination of "performance elements," such as autopsy rates and Caesarian rates—which can be subsumed under the first two approaches discussed above—concludes that "qualitative clinical judgment" may be more valid since these other techniques provide only "indirect and partial" indicators of the quality of patient care. She then goes on to suggest that, in order to attain objectivity, evaluation data must be obtained from several independent judges in each case. Myers (30), in his discussion of deficiencies associated with various hospital statistics and of the work of the Commission on Professional and Hospital Activities, similarly states that the Commission hopes to complement its medical audit program with "the factor of medical judgment."

As already mentioned, hospital staff physicians would presumably be the primary judges in conjunction with the clinical approach, since they are both technically qualified and familiar with the particular conditions prevailing in their respective hospitals. In this connection, after his own review of the problem of patient care assessment, Hawley (12) explicitly feels that "the evaluation of the quality of patient care can be done only by physicians and is best accomplished by physicians of the medical staff of individual hospitals." And although this proposition may be argued to some extent—it is likely,

---

Medical Care Program on the basis of drug prescriptions, employing such criteria as the acceptability of prescriptions according to defined standards and the duration of drug therapy. An operations research approach to evaluating patient care is also being developed by Howland and others at the Ohio State University (15). See also the recent report of the Committee on Measurement of the Quality of Medical Care of the Department of Medicine and Surgery, Veterans Administration (42).

for example, that registered nurses on the staff of individual hospitals may also be capable of judging patient care, especially the nursing care component of hospital care, and our own data will show that the registered nursing staff are in substantial agreement with the medical staff in how they evaluate patient care in the participating hospitals—it both supports and reinforces the position taken by Sheps (38) and others in favor of a clinical evaluation approach.

Theoretically, it may be safely concluded that data from qualified judges should at least provide one acceptable measure of patient care. In any event, the absence of uniform standards, or more "objective" criteria, for assessing the quality of patient care in hospitals (and, by extension, hospital effectiveness) makes some form of the clinical judgment approach virtually essential and indispensable at the present time. Furthermore, as we will see in the next section of this chapter, this approach may be improved through proper handling and modification, so that "qualitative" data can be combined and transformed to yield various "quantitative" measures in terms of which one can successfully differentiate between better- and poorer-care hospitals.

THE MEASURES OF PATIENT CARE

The particular approach followed in the present study to measure patient care makes use both of clinical judgment data and data from other sources. First, the bulk of necessary data were obtained, in the form of responses to scaled questionnaire items, from medical and nursing staff respondents from each participating hospital. Second, these data were variously supplemented with: (1) certain data about patient care from other than medical and nursing staff respondents—from laboratory and x-ray technicians, the administrator and his department heads, and members of the executive committee of the hospital's board of trustees; (2) data from hospital records concerning such things as mortality rates, length of patient stay, the composition of the medical and nursing staffs, etc.; and (3) certain auxiliary data about patient reaction toward the hospital, about the public reputation of the hospital, and about accreditation. Third, the above data were supplemented with a rating of the hospitals obtained not from respondents within the hospitals but from a group of outside physicians each of whom had personal knowledge of half or more of the hospitals in the research. These outside "experts" were requested to rate the quality of medical care provided by each hospital with which they were familiar, if they felt capable of performing such a rating.

The exact nature of the ratings and of the information collected from respondents within each hospital will be discussed in detail in following sections. In order that we may better understand the measures that were derived from these data, however, we shall preface our discussion with a brief restatement of the assessment task that we have set for ourselves, and a summary of important characteristics on the basis of which the ten participating hospitals were included in the study.

Our primary aim in this chapter, it will be recalled, was to develop measures of hospital patient care with which to compare the ten hospitals with one another, and to differentiate between the relatively better-care and the relatively poorer-care hospitals. In addition, as earlier indicated, it was deemed desirable, if not indeed essential, to employ not one but several measures of patient care.[3] In this connection, our experience from reviewing the literature and from our own exploratory work in two hospitals, which preceded the collection of data from the ten hospitals in the study, made it clear that data were needed to provide at least the following four measures: (1) an *overall* measure of the quality of total care given to patients in the hospital; (2) a measure of the quality of *medical* care given to patients; (3) a measure of the quality of *nursing* care given to patients; and (4) a measure of the quality of total care given to patients in the hospital *in comparison* to the total care given to patients in similar other hospitals, i.e., a comparative measure of overall care. Accordingly, the different kinds of data outlined in the preceding paragraph were designed to yield these four measures, making it possible to compare and contrast the various hospitals in terms of the principal aspect of care reflected in each measure.

Before presenting the specific measures, along with additional data which supplement and validate them, however, it is also useful to remind ourselves of the major institutional characteristics of the hospitals which will be compared on the basis of these measures. Briefly, the ten participating hospitals, as pointed out in an earlier chapter, share the following characteristics: (1) they all are hospitals of medium size—between 100 and 350 beds; (2) they all are short-stay general hospitals; (3) they all are community, voluntary, nonprofit organizations; (4) they all are nondenominational institutions; (5) they are all administered by male, lay administrators and governed by a board of trustees; (6) they are all located in Michigan cities of a population larger than 10,000 and (7) they are all accredited by the Joint Commission on Accreditation of Hospitals. On all of these important criteria the hospitals in the study are very similar, and with this similarity in mind one will be better equipped to interpret the meaning of interhospital differences in patient care that may be established by our measures.

We shall now present and examine the particular measures of patient care that were developed in this study. The four main measures will be presented in this order: the nursing care measure, the medical care measure, the (non-

---

[3] As employed in this study, the concept of "patient care" refers both to "cure" and to all other aspects of the care process. A conceptual distinction between patient "care" and "cure" may be meaningful and desirable when dealing with long-term hospitals or with mental hospitals, but when dealing with short-stay hospitals such a distinction is both of doubtful theoretical value and nearly impossible methodologically.

comparative) measure of overall patient care, and the comparative measure of overall care. In each case, the measure will be described first, followed by a discussion of its internal consistency and validation.

THE NURSING CARE MEASURE

To ascertain the quality of nursing care given to patients in the various participating hospitals, respondents from each institution were asked this multiple-choice question:

(On the basis of your experience and information) How good, would you say, is the nursing care given to patients in this hospital? (Check one.)
_____(1) Nursing care in this hospital is outstanding
_____(2) Excellent
_____(3) Very good
_____(4) Good
_____(5) Fair
_____(6) Rather poor
_____(7) Nursing care in this hospital is poor

The response alternatives offered by the question form a seven-point scale, which makes it possible to combine the answers of any group of respondents and then to compute the arithmetic mean, or average, of all answers. In the present question, as well as in other questions about patient care, seven rather than fewer response alternatives were used for three main reasons: (1) to permit as much discrimination among as many different degrees of quality of care as might be reasonably expected for hospitals of the kind studied; (2) to allow the respondents relatively great freedom of choice in their answers; and (3) because the results of the pretest of our research instruments had demonstrated that the majority of respondents mostly tend to check alternatives toward the favorable end of the scale, thus making it necessary to design a scale permitting rather fine distinctions, especially on the favorable side.

Our measure of the quality of nursing care is based on the answers given to the above question by the following groups of respondents from each hospital: medical staff respondents; registered nursing staff respondents; laboratory and x-ray technicians; and by the hospital administrator, the nonmedical department heads, and the members of the executive committee of the board of trustees of the hospital. The specific number of respondents represented in each group (separately for every hospital in the study), the manner in which respondents were chosen to participate in the research, and their background characteristics have already been described in Chapters 2 and 3.

Of a grand total of 902 individuals comprising the above respondent groups

882, or almost 98 percent, actually answered the question about nursing care.[4] This response rate exceeded our best expectations, suggesting that, since all potential respondents were given the opportunity and were free not to answer the question if they so chose, these individuals felt both capable and comfortable to evaluate the nursing care which patients receive in their particular hospital.

The data from the question on nursing care are summarized in Table 20. This table shows the percentage of group members who evaluated the quality of nursing care in their hospital as "outstanding" or "excellent," i.e., the percentage who selected the first two of the seven response alternatives listed after the question. Figures are shown separately for each respondent group and each hospital involved, as well as for the ten hospitals combined. In the tabulation, however, because of their small number, the administrator, the department heads, and the trustees from each hospital have been collapsed into a single group to yield more stable percentage figures. The data also happen to show that these latter groups of respondents are very similar in their answers, all tending to evaluate nursing care very favorably.

Before examining the data in Table 20, it should be noted that the complement of each percentage shown, i.e., its difference from 100 percent, represents in every case the percentage of respondents who evaluated nursing care as other than "outstanding" or "excellent," i.e., those who selected one of the other response alternatives available. However, none of the respondents chose the least favorable alternative "nursing care in this hospital is poor," and only 1 percent of all respondents chose the next to the least favorable alternative which indicates that nursing care is "rather poor." As a consequence, the complements of the percentages shown virtually represent only the "very good," "good," and "fair" alternatives. Of course, the figures actually appearing in the table refer only to the percentage of respondents who assessed nursing care as "outstanding" or "excellent."

What are some of the major conclusions that one can draw from the data in Table 20? First, it is obvious that, regardless of which respondent group is considered, the ten hospitals differ from one another in terms of the proportion of respondents who evaluate nursing care as "excellent" or "outstanding." Looking at the first row of percentages, for example, we find that 59 percent of medical staff respondents in Hospital #9 say nursing care is outstanding or excellent, while only 9 percent of the medical respondents in Hospital #5 give the same evaluation. Similarly, the comparable figures for Hospitals #3 and #2 are 50 percent and 19 percent, respectively. Again, if we look at the evaluation of nursing care by the technicians group, we find that

[4] The overall response rate was 97 percent for medical staff respondents, 98 percent for registered nursing staff respondents, 98 percent for laboratory and x-ray technicians, and 97 percent for the remaining respondents combined. The total number of respondents representing each hospital ranges between 75 and 113.

The Nursing Care Measure 211

while not a single one of the 14 technicians in Hospital #6 evaluates nursing care as outstanding or excellent, 57 percent of technicians in Hospital #3 do. Similar differences among the hospitals are found when we examine the percentage figures for the registered nursing staff group and for the administrative group of respondents. In short, as anticipated, irrespective of whose respondent group's evaluation we examine, we find that in some of the hospitals nursing care is considerably better than in others, according to the data; i.e., the quality of nursing care varies a good deal from hospital to hospital (despite the many important similarities of these hospitals which we have indicated earlier in this section).

TABLE 20. Percentage of Members from Each Respondent Group in Each Hospital Who Evaluated Nursing Care as "Outstanding" or "Excellent"

Respondent Group		#0	1	2	3	4	5	6	7	8	9	Group Total (All Hospitals)
						(percent)						
Medical staff respondents			32	20	19	50	45	9	38	29	46	59	35
	(N =		34	25	21	26	20	22	21	28	26	22	245)
Registered nursing staff respondents *			27	24	15	38	42	29	22	38	31	47	30
	(N =		44	34	41	32	45	31	50	24	39	32	372)
Laboratory and x-ray technicians			33	33	13	57	20	40	0	40	44	38	31
	(N =		21	18	8	7	10	10	14	10	16	8	122)
Administrator, executive trustees, and nonmedical department heads †			64	46	58	62	64	69	33	69	63	88	62
	(N =		14	13	12	13	14	13	18	13	16	17	143)
All four groups combined			34	28	22	47	44	32	24	40	42	58	37
	(N =	113	90	82	78	89	76	103	75	97	79	882)

* Includes all registered nurses in supervisory positions, from head nurse on up through the director of nursing, and a representative sample of nonsupervisory registered nurses in each case.
† Does not include the director of nursing who is also a nonmedical department head, but who has been included in the registered nursing staff group in each case.

It is also clear from the same data that the various respondent groups show certain differences in their evaluation of nursing care. In general, for all hospitals combined, the registered nurses group gives the most critical, or least favorable, evaluation among the four respondent groups, while the lay-administrative group is the least critical. Only 30 percent of all nurse respondents evaluate nursing care as outstanding or excellent; by contrast,

62 percent, or twice as many, of the administrative respondents evaluate nursing care so highly (and the tendency of administrative respondents to give a more favorable evaluation holds consistently true for our other measures of patient care, as well as for most items about which data were collected). The corresponding percentages for medical respondents and for technicians are very close to the percentage figure for nurses—35 percent of medical respondents and 31 percent of the technicians assess nursing care as outstanding or excellent. Similar differences among the respondent groups can be observed also when we consider the data for individual hospitals rather than all hospitals together.[5] In general, however, it should be noted that respondent group differences exist mainly between the lay-administrative group on the one hand and the medical, nursing, and technician groups on the other; the latter three groups evaluate the quality of nursing care quite similarly.

What is perhaps more important to know in relation to the above results is the fact that the obtained differences among respondent groups have little effect on the relative standing of the hospitals on nursing care. If we examine the data in Table 20 more carefully, we find that certain hospitals place consistently high, and others consistently low, on nursing care, across respondent groups. Hospital #9, for example, in terms of the percentage figures shown, always places among the five better nursing care hospitals, while Hospitals #1 and #2 always place among the five poorer nursing care hospitals according to the evaluation of nursing care by each and all of the respondent groups involved. Similarly, Hospitals #3, #7, and #8 place among the five better nursing care hospitals according to the evaluations given by three of the four respondent groups, and exactly the reverse holds true for Hospitals #0 and #6. The data, then, show a good deal of consistency when the evaluations of the different respondent groups are compared, in addition to discriminating well among the ten hospitals with respect to nursing care quality. Consequently, it would be feasible to rank-order the hospitals on nursing care, using the percentage data in Table 20 as a basis.

Although it would be possible to rank-order the ten hospitals on nursing care quality in terms of the percentages given in Table 20, and then use that rank-order as the measure of nursing care, such a measure would still be inadequate on two important counts. First, these percentages do not take full advantage of all the different answers given by the respondents simply because the percentages are based on one particular kind of grouping of the data; they represent the proportion of respondents who evaluated nursing care as "excellent" or "outstanding" without differentiating either between these two alternatives or among any of the other response alternatives that were checked by respondents. In other words, the percentages do not reflect

---

[5] These results in part confirm an earlier finding by O'Malley and Kossack (33) that occupational groups differ in their ratings of certain hospital areas.

The Nursing Care Measure

such distinctions as between "very good" and "good" or "fair" nursing care, even though the respondents actually made these discriminations in answering our question about nursing care.

The second difficulty with using a rank-order based on percentages stems from the composition of the respondent groups involved. Whereas the technicians group consists of all the technicians from every hospital, and the lay-administrative group includes all of the department heads, all of the members of the executive committee of trustees plus the administrator from every hospital, the other two respondent groups do not include all of the doctors or all of the registered nurses. The medical staff group consists of two subgroups: all doctors who hold staff offices or major committee and administrative positions in the hospital, plus a representative *sample* of the remaining active members of the staff. The registered nursing staff group also consists of two subgroups: all registered nursing personnel in supervisory positions, from head nurse on up through the director of nursing, plus a representative *sample* of the remaining registered nurses on the staff. When samples of this kind are involved, the data must be weighted according to the sampling rate with which respondents were selected into the sample, if they are to be combined with the data obtained from the other respondent groups, and herein lies the difficulty.

To handle the problems posed by using percentages to represent the quality of nursing care, we made use of means, i.e., arithmetic averages, instead of percentages. The procedure followed to derive the nursing care measure is relatively simple. First, separately for every hospital, using the answers of the members of each group of respondents, and based on the scale values to which particular answers correspond (the scale values for different answers are shown by the numbers preceding the various response alternatives listed under the question about nursing care), the arithmetic mean of responses was computed to represent the entire group's evaluation of nursing care. In other words, the answers of all respondents belonging to a given group were properly combined and averaged, separately for each hospital in the study. This procedure was applied without modification in the case of the technicians group and in the case of the lay-administrative group of respondents.

In the case of the medical group and of the nursing group or respondents, which consist of two subgroups each, the answers of the respondents were averaged after being weighted according to their respective sampling rate (the sampling rates for the different respondent groups and subgroups from each hospital have been presented in Chapter 2). Finally, to derive a single measure representing the quality of nursing care in each hospital, the obtained means for the four respondent groups involved themselves were properly combined and averaged, separately for every hospital. This last step yielded a single overall mean for each participating institution, reflecting the evaluation of nursing care by all of the different respondents. These overall means constitute our main quantitative measure of the quality of nursing care given to patients in the various hospitals and are presented in Table 21, below.

Table 21 shows the relative standing of the ten hospitals based on the measure of nursing care just described. It shows how the different hospitals score, both according to the evaluation of nursing care by all respondents combined, i.e., the overall mean obtained for each hospital, and according to the evaluations of the different respondent groups considered separately, i.e., the individual means obtained for each hospital based on the separate evaluations of the respondent groups involved. In addition to the mean-scores received by each hospital, Table 21 also shows the ten hospitals rank-ordered from 1 to 10 (i.e., from high to low quality of care, or from the hospital ranking most favorably in relation to the rest, in terms of its mean-score on nursing care, to the hospital ranking least favorably) according to their respective mean-scores in each case. In all instances shown, smaller means, and corresponding smaller ranks, represent more favorable evaluations of nursing

TABLE 21. The Quality of Nursing Care in Each Hospital as Evaluated by Certain Groups of Respondents, and the Relative Standing of the Ten Hospitals on Nursing Care *

First Row: Respondent group's mean response about nursing care
Second Row: Rank-order of hospitals according to mean response

Respondent Group	#0	1	2	3	4	5	6	7	8	9
Medical staff respondents	3.33	3.80	3.58	2.54	2.63	3.37	2.96	3.14	2.54	2.40
	7	10	9	2.5	4	8	5	6	2.5	1
Registered nursing staff	3.36	3.12	3.55	2.56	2.69	2.83	2.78	2.71	3.06	2.74
	9	8	10	1	2	6	5	3	7	4
Laboratory and x-ray technicians	3.48	3.39	3.38	2.43	3.30	2.90	3.57	2.90	2.69	2.88
	9	8	7	1	6	4.5	10	4.5	2	3
Administrator, nonmedical department heads, and executive trustees	2.20	2.51	2.38	2.14	2.33	2.29	2.84	2.21	2.47	1.78
	3	9	7	2	6	5	10	4	8	1
All preceding respondent groups combined †	3.18	3.32	3.26	2.44	2.64	2.91	2.90	2.76	2.73	2.44
	8	10	9	1.5	3	7	6	5	4	1.5

* Smaller means, and corresponding smaller ranks, represent more favorable evaluations of care in this and subsequent tables.

† This is subsequently used as the main measure of the quality of nursing care in the various hospitals.

The Nursing Care Measure

care or higher quality of nursing care, with larger means and ranks representing poorer quality.

What exactly do the findings in Table 21 indicate? On the whole, they are congruent with the percentage results presented in Table 20, but they provide both a clearer and more accurate picture of the quality of nursing care in the various hospitals. Two major impressions will strike the reader in examining Table 21. The first concerns the rather considerable differences in nursing care which characterize the various hospitals, as shown by the mean-scores which represent the evaluation of nursing care by the different groups of respondents. The second impression concerns the rather high consistency which prevails among the evaluations of nursing care by the different respondent groups, as shown by comparing the several ranks of each hospital.

First, with regard to interhospital differences, looking at the assessment of nursing care by the medical staff, we see that the mean-scores for the ten hospitals range from 2.40 for Hospital #9, the hospital whose nursing care is evaluated most favorably, to 3.80 for Hospital #1, the least favorably scoring hospital. According to the medical staff's evaluation, the former hospital is the best nursing care hospital, while the latter is the poorest nursing care hospital. The difference between 2.40 and 3.80 is of course considerable. The former score roughly represents almost "excellent" nursing care, while the latter represents just "good" nursing care; an intermediate score of 3.00 would represent "very good" nursing care. Further examination of the medical staff's evaluation shows that Hospitals #3 and #8 are tied for second best place with a score of 2.54, and Hospital #2 places second poorest among the ten institutions. The remaining hospitals occupy intermediate standings. Finally, similar, though less pronounced, differences in nursing care among the ten hospitals can be also observed when we examine the evaluations of nursing care by the remaining groups of respondents—nurses, technicians, and administrative personnel. Thus, the data on nursing care quality discriminate quite well among the participating hospitals.

Equally important is the fact that the individual hospitals place quite consistently in relation to each other on the evaluations they received from the different groups of respondents. Table 21 shows, for example, that Hospitals #1 and #2 place consistently low among all hospitals. More specifically, Hospital #1 ranks 10, 8, 8, and 9, respectively, according to the assessment of nursing care by doctors, nurses, technicians, and administrative personnel. The corresponding ranks for Hospital #2 are 9, 10, 7, and 7. By contrast, Hospitals #3 and #9 always rank very favorably; the former ranks 2.5, 1, 1, and 2, and the latter ranks 1, 4, 3, and 1, according to the evaluations of the same respondent groups. When the data from the four respondent groups are combined to yield the single overall measure of nursing care shown in the last row of means in Table 21, we again find that Hospitals

#3 and #9 are the top two hospitals on nursing care, both ranking 1.5, while Hospitals #1 and #2 are the bottom two hospitals, respectively ranking 10 and 9 among the ten institutions. The remaining hospitals, of course, occupy intermediate positions and, as might be expected, do not rank as consistently across respondent groups as the four hospitals which occupy the extreme positions.

As already indicated, the final measure of the quality of nursing care used in this study incorporates the evaluations of all four of the respondent groups involved. This measure, rather than a measure based on the assessment of nursing care by a single respondent group, was finally adopted because of the following principal reasons:

1. It was considered desirable that the judgment of all respondent groups be represented in the final measure for, regarding nursing care in hospitals, the judgment of these groups undoubtedly carries very great weight. Although the medical staff and the registered nursing staff may be better qualified by training and experience to evaluate nursing care, the technicians group is in frequent interaction with both doctors and nurses and familiar with various nursing activities, while the administrative group consists of the people who hold the key lay positions in the entire hospital organization and who have a good deal of knowledge of the nursing situation.

2. Combining the respondent groups is appropriate in view of the consistency of their evaluations, which were discussed above and which will be further commented upon below.

3. Combining the respondent groups yields more stable means and, therefore, a more reliable measure, because in this manner the quality of nursing care in each hospital is assessed by a larger number of respondents.

4. We had no compelling theoretical or empirical grounds on the basis of which any one of the four respondent groups, particularly doctors or nurses, could be singled out as the group whose assessment of nursing care is the most valid and the most significant. Thus, it was decided that the final measure should reflect the assessment of nursing care by all of the respondent groups involved.

Returning once more to the question about the consistency of the data, partly discussed above, a more precise picture emerges from the correlations presented in Table 22. Table 22 shows (1) the degree of relationship among the specific evaluations of nursing care by doctors, nurses, technicians, and the administrative group, and (2) the relationship between each of these four evaluations and the final measure of nursing care, i.e., the assessment of nursing care by all respondent groups combined. The separate evaluations of the four respondent groups are positively intercorrelated, the specific correlations ranging from a low of .41, which measures the relationship between the evaluation of nursing care by the nurses group and its evaluation by the administrative group, to a high of .65, which measures the relationship between the evaluations by doctors and by nurses. On the average, of the different evaluations of nursing care, the one by the administrative group of respondents agrees least well with the others. But, across the ten hospitals, there is significant agreement between the quality of nursing care as assessed by doctors, on the one hand, and by nurses and technicians, on the other.

Even more important, insofar as the measurement of nursing care is concerned, is the existence of high positive relationships between the final nursing care measure and the separate assessment of nursing care by doctors, nurses, and technicians, as shown by the last column of correlations in Table 22. As assessed by the final measure, the quality of nursing care in the various hospitals correlates .95 with the quality of nursing care as evaluated by doctors alone, .83 with the quality of nursing care as evaluated by the registered nursing staff alone, .72 with the quality of nursing care as evaluated by x-ray and laboratory technicians alone, and .54 with the quality of nursing care as evaluated by the administrative group alone. Therefore, the separate data on nursing care from doctors, nurses, and technicians agree very well with the final measure of nursing care here developed. On the aggregate, these results suggest that the obtained final measure of the quality of nursing care prevailing in the various hospitals is stable and reliable.

TABLE 22. Rank-order Intercorrelations Among the Evaluations of the Quality of Nursing Care by Various Groups of Respondents *

Evaluation by:	1	2	3	4	5
1. Medical staff respondents	—	.65	.62	.43	.95
2. Registered nursing staff		—	.51	.41	.83
3. Lab and x-ray technicians			—	.52	.72
4. Administrator, nonmedical department heads, and executive trustees				—	.54
5. All preceding respondent groups combined					—

* All correlations are based on an N of 10 hospitals. Coefficients larger than .56 are significant at the .05 level, and those .75 or larger are significant at the .01 level.

Two supplementary pieces of evidence supporting the stability of the final measure of nursing care should also be mentioned at this point. The first concerns a comparison between the weighted and the unweighted basic data from which the measure of nursing care was constructed. In this connection, it will be recalled that the final measure of nursing care was computed after the data had been weighted according to the sampling rates with which respondents had been selected. Now, had the data been left unweighted—and this would be statistically inappropriate because of the sampling involved for certain respondent groups—the final measure of nursing care which would have been obtained is found to correlate .92 with the measure which was actually derived from the weighted data and which is the correct measure. The second, and more important, piece of supplementary evidence relates to the general question of controls. Specifically, the question arises as to whether within a given respondent group, e.g., nurses, there is divided opinion about nursing care, or whether a subgroup of nurses tends to evaluate nursing care more highly than another subgroup because of such things as differences in shift of work, age, length of service in the hospital, and the like. Empirical evidence demonstrates that this is not the case.

Considering first all nonsupervisory registered nurse respondents from the ten hospitals, we find the following: (1) no significant difference between younger (under 30) and older R.N.'s in their evaluation of nursing care; (2) no difference in the evaluations of nursing care by full-time and part-time R.N.'s; (3) no difference between R.N.'s on the same job in the same hospital for one year or less and those with longer service; (4) no difference between R.N.'s in different shifts, considering the three shifts two at a time, e.g., no difference in the evaluation of nursing care by R.N.'s on the day shift and R.N.'s on the afternoon shift; (5) no significant difference between R.N.'s working in one service area and those working in another, i.e., no difference across the major services—these include medicine, surgery, obstetrics and gynecology, and all other services combined—taken two at a time, although there is a slight tendency for R.N.'s in surgery to evaluate nursing care somewhat more favorably than R.N.'s in medicine; and (6) no difference in the evaluation of nursing care between the nonsupervisory registered nurse respondents, to which the above statements apply, and the supervisory registered nurse respondents in the study.[6]

Considering next the medical staff respondents from all hospitals combined, the results show: (1) no significant difference between how "general practitioners" and how the rest of the medical staff evaluate nursing care; (2) no difference in the evaluation of nursing care by doctors holding staff offices or major committee and administrative responsibilities and by the rest of the doctors; and (3) no differences across major services taken two at a time, e.g., no difference between doctors in surgery and doctors in obstetrics and gynecology—the major services being surgery, medicine, obstetrics and gynecology, and all other services together.

However, we find that younger doctors (under 40) and doctors associated with the hospital for less than five years (the two groups overlap very greatly,

[6] The statement that there is no difference means that no statistically significant difference at the .05 level exists between the mean-scores on nursing care which are obtained from the two subgroups of respondents in each case. As a specific illustration, we may point out that the mean on nursing care for the 178 supervisory nurse respondents in the study is actually 2.90, and the corresponding mean for the 194 nonsupervisory nurse respondents is exactly 3.00. The difference between these two means is not significant, in the present case amounting to practically no difference at all.

The Nursing Care Measure

age and length of association correlating .80) tend to be somewhat more critical in their evaluation of nursing care than older doctors and doctors associated with the hospital for five or more years. It turns out, however, that this tendency on the part of older doctors and doctors with longer service to evaluate the quality of nursing care more favorably than their other colleagues has no biasing effect whatsoever upon the obtained final measure of nursing care. Had this tendency affected the measure, we would expect those hospitals which have proportionately more doctors in the older age bracket, or in the longer service category, to score more favorably on nursing care. Actually, if anything, the data show a reverse tendency, although not a statistically significant one. Specifically, we find that (1) the proportion of doctors in the various hospitals who are 40 years old or older correlates —.23 with the obtained measure of nursing care, i.e., with the relative standing of the different hospitals on nursing care quality as assessed by our final measure, and (2) the proportion of doctors who have been associated with the hospital for at least five years correlates —.07 with the nursing care measure.

The preceding findings demonstrate further the consistency of the data from which the nursing care measure was derived while, at the same time, they indicate that the differences in nursing care which were found to characterize the various hospitals according to our measure are apparently "genuine" differences rather than differences which could be attributed to such factors as those examined above. To put it differently, the interhospital differences established by our measure of nursing care are not due to any of the major characteristics which differentiate the respondents who provided the data, i.e., the characteristics discussed above. The same findings also serve to provide support for the face validity of the nursing care measure. We now turn to a more direct examination of the question of validity—how valid is the obtained measure of nursing care, or to what extent can we be sure that it measures what it purports to measure.

Validation of the Nursing Care Measure

In addition to the consistencies of the data from which the measure of nursing care was constructed, as discussed above, and in addition to the relationships of this measure with the other measures of patient care which will be presented later in this chapter, certain other data were collected in this study for the purpose of ascertaining the validity of the nursing care measure. These data fall into three categories: (1) Spontaneous, volunteered comments about nursing care and the nursing staff from physicians and other respondents who were personally interviewed in addition to filling out a questionnaire, and answers by different respondents to two open questions, one about what they considered as "the most important strengths," the other about what they considered as "the most important weaknesses" of their hospital. Most of these qualitative data have been summarized in Chapter 4, where we presented a brief profile for each of the ten participating hospitals. (2) Data concerning the composition of the nursing staff of each hospital, or the proportions of staff members who are registered nurses, practical nurses, and aides. (3) Auxiliary questionnaire data obtained from certain respondents in each hospital and having to do with "the kind of job the nursing staff does for the hospital" and with "how well the nursing department is doing in relation to what it should be accomplishing." To ascertain the validity of our measure of nursing care, we must find out what relationships, if any, there are between these data and the nursing care measure.

First, we shall consider the data falling in the first of the above categories. In Table 21, we have seen how the ten hospitals rank in relation to one another according to the final measure of nursing care developed in this study. When the rank-order of the hospitals on this measure is compared with the volunteered comments of different respondents about nursing care, we find that those hospitals which place high in terms of our quantitative measure also receive many favorable comments about nursing care in their respective profiles shown in Chapter 4. Conversely, those hospitals which place low according to the nursing care measure also receive many negative, or unfavorable, comments about nursing care in their profiles. For example, Hospital #9, which ranks 1.5 (tied in first place) on the nursing care measure, in its profile materials in Chapter 4 receives such comments as: nursing care is "outstanding," the nursing staff is "tops," "good nursing service," "the nurses are far and above those I've come in contact with in large institutions," and the like. Similarly, Hospital #3, which also ranks 1.5 on nursing care, is generally commended by respondents for its quality of nursing care, as shown in its profile, and the same is true for Hospital #4, which ranks third among the ten hospitals according to the nursing care measure.

By contrast, the individual hospital profiles show a reverse picture in the case of hospitals ranking low according to the nursing care measure. In the case of Hospital #1, for instance, which ranks tenth among the hospitals, we find a good deal of spontaneous criticism about nursing in general, and nursing supervision in particular: "A 'personal desire and interest' touch on the part of all personnel to make the patient feel at home and comfortable is lacking"; "The nursing administration is not worth a damn"; "They don't know who does what, don't know who bathes the patients, they go off and leave 'em one leg washed and forget to come back. . . . Nobody with a sense of responsibility." Hospitals #0 and #2, respectively ranking eighth and ninth on nursing care, similarly receive several unfavorable comments about their nursing in their respective profiles. In short, the relevant qualitative data from the various hospitals agree remarkably well with the standing of the hospitals on nursing care, as assessed by our quantitative measure.

Additional qualitative data point to the same conclusion. Specifically, the doctors, the trustees, and the administrator from each hospital were asked to

The Nursing Care Measure

indicate on a list of nine different items the *"three* items with which you are *most concerned* at present." The nine items, in order of their listing, were: "improvements in nursing care"; "improvements or expansion of the hospital building or equipment"; "improvements in wages, hours, working conditions, or employee benefits for hospital personnel"; "changes in the organization of the board of trustees"; "changes in the organization of the medical staff"; "improvements in the quality or in the completion rate of medical records"; "changes in the qualifications, rights, or responsibilities expected for members of the medical staff"; "improvements in the economy and efficiency of operation in offices or departments"; and "improvements in training programs."

The data from this question show that in the case of Hospital #1, which ranks tenth, or poorest, among the participating hospitals on our measure of nursing care, the administrator selected "improvements in nursing care" as one of the three items of greatest concern to him. Similarly, the trustees selected the same item more frequently than any of the other eight items, except for the item on economy of operations. And, the two subgroups of doctors (the special medical staff, and the general medical staff) both selected "improvements in nursing care" most frequently of all items on the list, as one of the three items of greatest concern to them. In the case of Hospital #2, which ranks second poorest among the ten hospitals on the nursing care measure, we find essentially the same results. The only exception is that "improvements in nursing care" was the third most frequently selected item by the trustees, who chose expansion and training programs somewhat more frequently (but, training programs are closely related to nursing care). Moreover, in none of the remaining hospitals do we find the same pattern of results, i.e., "improvements in nursing care" was not of as great concern in these other hospitals as it was in Hospital #1 and in Hospital #2, apparently because nursing care was more satisfactory in the other institutions. (Incidentally, for all hospitals combined, both the administrators and the trustees selected expansion, economy of operation, and employee benefits as the three items of greatest concern to them; the doctors selected improvements in nursing care, expansion, and improvements in training programs.)

The preceding results establish a good deal of confidence in the validity of the quantitative measure of nursing care which was developed in this study. A similar conclusion can be drawn, moreover, when the nursing care measure is compared against the composition of the nursing staff in the various hospitals. The quality of nursing care in a given hospital should in part depend upon the skill and qualifications of its nursing staff. Accordingly, hospitals whose nursing staff consists predominantly of registered nurses should presumably have better nursing care than hospitals whose nursing staff consists predominantly of aides. Based on this assumption, we related our measure of nursing care to the composition of the nursing staff in the various hospitals. The obtained findings are as anticipated.

First, we find that the higher the proportion of nursing staff members who are registered nurses, the higher the quality of nursing care as assessed by our final measure of nursing care. The correlation between these two variables is .71, which, based on an N of 10 hospitals, is statistically significant at better than the .05 level. Second, and by contrast, the higher the proportion of nursing staff members who are aides, the lower the quality of nursing care; here the correlation is —.73, which is also significant. And third, the higher the proportion of nursing staff members who are practical nurses, the higher the quality of nursing care (although not as high as for the proportion of staff members who are registered nurses); here the correlation is .61 which, although smaller than the other two correlations, is again statistically significant at the .05 level. (Apparently, whatever little training practical nurses have received—usually one year of special training—which distinguishes them from aides contributes positively and significantly to the quality of nursing care, in view of these findings.) In other words, those hospitals which are "loaded" with aides, as against registered or practical nurses, are also shown to rank low on nursing quality as assessed by our measure, in comparison to hospitals which have proportionately fewer aides.[7] These results again serve to enhance confidence in the validity of our measure of nursing care.

An analysis of certain auxiliary data that should also provide some indication of the kind of nursing care rendered at the various hospitals yields results which reinforce the preceding findings concerning the validation of the nursing care measure. These data were obtained using the following two questions: (1) "How well is the nursing department doing in relation to what it should be accomplishing?", and (2) "On the whole, what kind of a job would you say each of the following does for this hospital? . . . The Nursing Staff? . . ." The first question was designed to yield an evaluation of the performance of the nursing department based on the expectations of the nursing staff of the particular hospitals. The question provided the respondents with five response alternatives, ranging from "the nursing department is doing extremely well in relation to what it should be accomplishing" to "it is not doing well at all considering what it should be accomplishing," and forming a five-point scale. It was answered by the registered nursing staff respondents, supervisory as well as nonsupervisory. The second question also had five response alternatives, ranging from "(the nursing staff does) an excellent

[7] The proportion of nursing staff members belonging to each category is based on full-time staff, but when part-time nurses are included in the analysis the results remain substantially the same. Across hospitals, excluding the few orderlies involved, the proportion of full-time nursing staff who are registered nurses (both supervisory and non-supervisory, but excluding directors of nursing) varies from a high of 47 percent to a low of 23 percent, the average being 35 percent. The corresponding figures for aides vary from a high of 66 percent to a low of 21 percent, the average being 41 percent. And, those for practical nurses vary from 43 to 7 percent, the average being 24 percent.

job" to "a rather poor job," and it was answered by the medical staff respondents.

To the extent to which the quality of nursing care in the various hospitals depends upon the performance of the nursing department, and chances are that it does to a large degree, to that extent we should expect a positive and significant correlation between the measure of the quality of nursing care and nursing department performance, the latter as evaluated in response to the first of the above two questions. And, similarly, the extent to which the quality of nursing care depends upon the overall performance of the nursing staff—and excepting very unusual circumstances it should to a large degree—to that extent the data from the second of the above questions should also relate significantly to our measure of nursing care. What do the actual findings show?

We find that the quality of nursing care in the various hospitals, as assessed by the measure developed in this study, correlates .73 with how well the nursing department of each hospital is doing in relation to what it should be accomplishing, as viewed by our registered nurse respondents. This correlation, based on an N of 10 hospitals is statistically significant at better than the .05 level, thus furnishing additional support for the validity of the nurs.ng care measure. Similarly, we find that the quality of nursing care, as measured in this study, correlates .92 with how good a job the nursing staff as a whole does for the hospital, as viewed by our medical staff respondents. This relationship is of course also significant, it too providing added support for the validity of the nursing care measure.

In summary, the evidence presented in the preceding pages leads to the conclusion that the quantitative measure of the quality of nursing care which was developed and used in the present study is both valid and reliable, successfully differentiating among the various participating hospitals. Since the measure of nursing care was discussed first among the four measures of patient care presented in this chapter, and since the data from which the other measures of care were derived are similar to those on which the nursing care measure is based, the latter was examined in somewhat greater detail than some of the other measures. Let us now turn to a discussion of the remaining measures of patient care, beginning with a description of our measure of the quality of medical care.

THE MEDICAL CARE MEASURE

Our measure of the quality of medical care is based on the answers of medical staff respondents from each hospital to the following question:

On the basis of your experience and information, how good, would you say, is the *medical care (including surgical work)* given to patients in this hospital? (Check one.)

_____(1) Medical care in this hospital is outstanding

_____(2) Excellent

_____(3) Very good
_____(4) Good
_____(5) Fair
_____(6) Rather poor
_____(7) Medical care in this hospital is poor

This question is exactly parallel to that asked about nursing care, and the earlier discussion about the latter with respect to question form, response alternatives, and computation of means is equally applicable to the present question.

Although the final measure of medical care here derived is based solely on data from medical respondents, supplementary data for validation purposes were also collected from nonmedical respondents, using the same question. All respondents were of course free not to answer the question, if they so elected, whether because of lack of sufficient knowledge or for any other reasons. As in the case of the question about nursing care, however, only a few respondents did not answer the medical care question. Of a total of 252 medical respondents from the ten hospitals in the study, 243 (or an average of 24 doctors per hospital) answered the question, yielding a response rate of 96 percent. Of the medical respondents who answered, 14.8 percent evaluated medical care as "outstanding," 39.5 percent evaluated it as "excellent," 33.7 as "very good," 11.5 percent as "good," and the remaining .5 of 1 percent (i.e., just one respondent) evaluated it as "rather poor."

Thus, an average of about 54 percent of all doctor respondents from all ten hospitals evaluated the quality of medical care in their hospitals as "outstanding" or "excellent," the remaining giving a less favorable evaluation.[8] Needless to say, the individual hospitals differ considerably from one another in terms of the percentage of their physician respondents who evaluate medical care as outstanding or excellent. These percentage figures range, across hospitals, from a high of 84 percent to a low of 36 percent—the average being 54 percent, as indicated above. Based on these percentage data, the two most highly evaluated hospitals are Hospital #4 and Hospital #6 and the two least highly evaluated are Hospital #1 and Hospital #2. The percentages of physician respondents assessing medical care in these four hospitals as outstanding or excellent, respectively, are 84, 82, 36, and 38 percent.

For the reasons discussed in connection with the nursing care measure, however, the above percentages provide neither the best nor the most ap-

[8] Corresponding data from the other respondent groups show that: (1) 99 percent of the 378 registered nursing staff respondents from the ten hospitals answered the question about medical care, and of those who answered 44 percent evaluated medical care as outstanding or excellent; (2) 97 percent of the 125 technician respondents answered the same question, and of those who answered 52 percent evaluated medical care as outstanding or excellent; and (3) 97 percent of the administrative group of respondents answered the question, and of those answering 75 percent evaluated medical care as outstanding or excellent. Once more, the administrative group is the one which differs most from the other respondent groups, always tending to give a more favorable evaluation than the others. The nurses group is again the most critical.

propriate measure of the quality of medical care characteristic of the various hospitals. Means rather than percentages are required to take advantage of the full potential of the data. Accordingly, the final measure of medical care obtained from the data is based on hospital means that were computed using the answers medical staff respondents from each hospital gave to the above question.

Before computing the hospital means which constitute the final measure of the quality of medical care, two operations were performed on the data: (1) As in the case of the nursing care measure, because the medical group of respondents consists of two subgroups, one of which includes a representative sample rather than all of the active staff members who hold no office or administrative responsibility, the data were properly weighted according to the sampling rates with which staff members from each hospital had been included into the study as respondents. (The sampling rates and sizes of the two medical staff subgroups for every hospital have been presented in Chapter 2.) This procedure was methodologically necessary. (2) In addition to weighting the data in this manner, and unlike the case of the nursing care measure, we assigned somewhat more weight to the answers of certain key medical respondents from each hospital, on theoretical rather than methodological grounds. The specific procedure through which this was done will be specified below, following an explanation of the theoretical rationale underlying it.

The medical respondents from each hospital whose answers to the question about the quality of medical care received extra weight are: the chief, or president, of the medical staff; the chairman of the executive committee of the medical staff, if not the same as the chief of staff; the chief pathologist, or director, of the clinical laboratory; the chief radiologist, or head of the x-ray department; the chairman of the medical records committee; the chairman of the tissue committee; and the chairman of the audit committee, for institutions having such a committee (not all hospitals have an audit committee, this normally being a combined medical records and tissue committee but sometimes being an additional standing committee). For a brief description of these and other committees, the reader may wish to refer to an article by Myers and Babcock (31).

For all ten hospitals combined, a total of 44 doctors holding the above key positions, or an average of 4.4 physicians from each hospital, are involved in the present procedure. Even though the positions indicated would imply a larger number than this, the total number of individuals involved reduces to 44 because: (1) an individual doctor often holds more than one of these key positions in a particular hospital, e.g., being chief of staff and chief radiologist simultaneously; (2) not all of the positions exist as separate positions in every hospital involved, e.g., the chief of staff is usually also chairman of the executive committee; and (3) few of the hospitals have an audit committee in addition to their medical records and tissue committees.

The main reason for giving more weight to the responses of the above key physicians rests on the assumption of "greater expertness." It is assumed that because of their special roles in the hospital these doctors have both a broader, i.e., a more hospital-wide, and a deeper, i.e., a more detailed or more accurate, knowledge of the medical situation in their hospital than other staff members. Therefore, their evaluation of the quality of medical care is likely to be "superior" on the average than the evaluation of medical care by an equal number of other staff members. Moreover, within a particular hospital, medical organization and medical practice and progress are undoubtedly affected very significantly by what these few key members of the staff think, feel, do, or say. Our early exploratory work in two hospitals, prior to collecting data from the ten participating hospitals, made it clear that both doctors and the top administration felt that the members of the staff who occupy the above key positions would be best qualified to evaluate the quality of medical care in their respective hospitals. Subsequent discussions with other doctors from participating hospitals, as well as doctors not on the staff of participating institutions, confirmed our earlier experience on this matter.

The underlying reason for this generalized consensus that staff members in the above special roles would be best qualified to evaluate medical care is that the positions held by these members are precisely the ones which are most centrally and most inclusively concerned with the quality of medical care. These positions, more than any others, are charged with such "policing" functions as the maintenance and improvement of professional standards, the maintenance and control of staff discipline, the maintenance and improvement of medical records, the clinical evaluation of surgical and medical work in the hospital, the implementation of many of the important patient care requirements specified by the Joint Commission on Accreditation, and the like. In addition, the men who fill the positions in question are practicing doctors in the hospital, they are likely to be respected and trusted by other staff members, and they are most frequently in contact with the administration, board of trustees, and others in the organization. In brief, their respective key positions themselves serve to give them an advantage over their colleagues from the standpoint of personal knowledge and other information both about medical care and about the hospital in general.

The chairmen of the tissue and audit committees, for example, have as much, or more, information about medical care as anybody else in the hospital because it is the function of these committees to evaluate a portion of the surgical and, to some extent, medical work done by the staff. The chief pathologist, among other things, examines the tissues removed in surgery and is in a good position to know the extent of "unnecessary" or inappropriate surgery (e.g., unjustified removal of healthy tissues) in his hospital. Similarly, the chief radiologist is frequently in a good position to compare diagnoses made by the staff with what actual x-rays show. The extent to which keeping thor-

The Medical Care Measure

ough and up-to-date patient records is an indication of medical performance, as many people in the field assert, the chairman of the records committee ought to know a great deal about medical care in the hospital.

In summary, the few key medical respondents from each hospital whose evaluation of medical care was given added weight hold the most crucial set of jobs from the standpoint of medical practice, professional medical organization, and medical care in the hospital. In a sense, the adoption of this device of extra weight is a practical substitute (compensates to an extent) for the unavailability of uniform data from medical records and the medical self-audit which we have discussed at the beginning of this chapter.

Having explained the theoretical bases for assigning greater weight to the answers given by certain key medical respondents to our question about medical care, we may now examine more precisely how this weighting procedure enters the derivation of the medical care measure. Briefly, the specific steps leading to the construction of the final measure of medical care were as follows:

1. For each individual hospital, we first computed the mean of the answers given by *all* medical respondents to the question concerning medical care quality. (Means were also computed for all medical respondents *excluding* the special key staff members whose answers received extra weight.) In the process, the data were properly weighted according to the sampling rates involved. The means obtained from this first step are presented in the first row of figures in Table 23, followed by a rank-ordering of the ten hospitals based on the magnitude of their respective mean-scores.

2. Then, separately for each hospital, we computed the mean of the answers given to the medical care question by the few key doctors whose responses were given more weight (i.e., chief of staff, chief pathologist, chief radiologist, and the chairmen of the medical audit, tissue, and records committees). It may be noted, at this point, that these doctors had been included in the study automatically, comprising part of the medical subgroup whose members hold staff offices or major committee and administrative assignments in each hospital. (Accordingly, their responses to the medical care question have also been incorporated in the means obtained from the preceding step.) The hospital means derived from this second step, and representing the evaluation of medical care by the special key doctors alone, are presented in the third row of Table 23.

3. The final measure of the quality of medical care was next obtained by summing for each hospital (a) the mean of the answers of all medical respondents—including the special key staff, as described in step (1) above, and (b) the mean of the answers of the special key doctors considered separately, as described in step (2) above, and then dividing the product by two. In effect, this procedure results in giving some extra weight to the assessment of medical care by the few key expert doctors described above. The individual hospital

scores derived from this third step, and representing the final measure of medical care, are presented at the bottom of Table 23.

TABLE 23. The Quality of Medical Care in Each Hospital as Evaluated by Medical Staff Respondents, and the Relative Standing of the Ten Hospitals on Medical Care *

First Row: Respondent group's mean response about medical care
Second Row: Rank-order of hospitals according to mean response

Respondent Group	#0	1	2	3	Hospital 4	5	6	7	8	9
All medical staff respondents	2.55	2.88	2.80	2.42	1.59	2.64	1.91	2.91	2.36	2.53
	6	9	8	4	1	7	2	10	3	5
All medical staff respondents except special key staff	2.51	2.83	2.88	2.43	1.62	2.60	1.84	2.88	2.35	2.49
	6	8	9.5	4	1	7	2	9.5	3	5
Special key staff respondents only †	2.67	2.75	2.33	2.33	1.33	2.40	1.80	2.80	2.40	2.40
	8	9	3.5	3.5	1	6	2	10	6	6
Final medical care measure: average mean for all medical staff respondents *and* special key staff ‡	2.61	2.81	2.56	2.37	1.46	2.52	1.85	2.85	2.38	2.46
	8	9	7	3	1	6	2	10	4	5

* Smaller means, and corresponding smaller ranks, represent more favorable evaluations of medical care in all cases.
† This group consists of the chief of staff, chief pathologist, chief radiologist, and the chairmen of the tissue, medical audit, and records committees of each hospital. However, since one individual often holds more than one of these positions, the group averages 4.4 respondents per hospital. The small size of this group results in somewhat less stable means than is the case for the other respondent groups, and this accounts for the several ties in the rank-order of the hospitals which is based on the mean response of this group.
‡ This measure, which in effect gives some extra weight to the data from the special key staff group, is subsequently used as the main measure of the quality of medical care in the various hospitals. The measure is derived by summing for each hospital the mean for all medical staff respondents and the mean for the special key staff respondents and then dividing the product by two.

The Internal Consistency of the Medical Care Measure

We have indicated that two weighting operations were performed on the data before obtaining the final measure of medical care, one because of methodological considerations, the other because of theoretical considerations. To appraise the consistency of the obtained measure, among other things, we would like to know how each of these operations affected the final measure. In this connection, the evidence shows that the weighting effects were actually

The Medical Care Measure

very small. First, weighting the data according to the sampling rates involved had little effect on the hospital means which were obtained. The means based on the evaluation of medical care by all medical respondents (first row of figures in Table 23), which were computed after the data had been weighted by the sampling rates, correlate .95 with the hospital means that would have been obtained from the same data, had the data been left unweighted (which would have been methodologically incorrect). Since the means based on weighted data correlate so highly with the corresponding means from the unweighted data, it is clear that the first of the two weighting operations had a negligible effect upon the final measure of medical care.

The second weighting operation, which resulted in giving added weight to the data from the special key doctors, also produced a relatively small effect insofar as the final measure of medical care is concerned. In the first place, we find that the hospital means based on data from all medical staff respondents (first set of means in Table 23), which constitute one of the two components of the final measure of medical care (last set of means in Table 23), correlate .78 with the means which are based on the data from the special key staff members (third set of means in Table 23) and which constitute the second of the two components of the final measure. In short, the two sets of means which serve as components of the final measure of medical care are highly (though far from perfectly) intercorrelated. This relationship is a significant one, moreover, even though the "all medical respondents" group also includes the "special key staff members," for we also find that the hospital means based on data from "all medical respondents *except* the special key members" (second set of means in Table 23) correlate .68 with the means based on data from the special key staff respondents alone. This latter correlation is statistically significant at better than the .05 level.

Secondly, using the different sets of means shown in Table 23 as a basis, we find that the final measure of medical care correlates .95 with the evaluation of medical care by all medical respondents, .91 with the evaluation of the same by all medical respondents *except* the special key members, and .89 with the evaluation of medical care by the special key members alone. Considered together, these intercorrelations show that the extra weight given to the data from the few key doctors has had a rather small effect upon the obtained final measure of medical care. It is very interesting to note, in fact, that the final measure of medical care turns out to correlate even a little more highly (.95) with the evaluation of medical care by all medical respondents than with its evaluation by the special key staff members alone (.89), although the data from the latter were deliberately assigned extra weight.

The above results suggest that the internal consistency of the data from which the measure of medical care was derived is quite high. There is a good deal of consensus regarding the assessment of the quality of medical care in the various hospitals by the several subgroups of medical respondents. In this connection, an examination of Table 23 provides an even clearer demonstration of how consistently medical care in the various hospitals was evaluated by the different subgroups of doctors, or how consistently the ten hospitals place on medical care in relation to one another. For example, Hospital #4 always ranks first among the ten hospitals, according to the assessment of medical care by the final measure and according to its separate evaluation by all medical respondents, by all medical respondents except the special key staff members, and by the key staff members alone. Similarly, Hospital #6 always ranks second best among the ten hospitals. At the other extreme, Hospital #7 always places last among the ten institutions, and Hospital #1 always places next to last. As a matter of fact, there is only one discrepancy of any magnitude among all the rank-orders shown in Table 23: according to the final measure of medical care Hospital #2 ranks 7, also ranking 8 according to the evaluation by all medical respondents and 9.5 according to the evaluation by all medical respondents except the special key members; but according to the evaluation by the special staff members it ranks 3.5 among the ten hospitals. Excepting this single discrepancy, the consistency with which the ten hospitals rank on medical care in relation to each other is very high, indicating that our final measure of medical care is stable and reliable.

As anticipated, the results presented in Table 23 also show considerable variation in the quality of medical care from one hospital to another, i.e., the measure shows appreciable interhospital differences in medical care quality. According to the final measure of medical care, for example, Hospital #4 received a mean-score of 1.46, which roughly signifies almost "outstanding" medical care in terms of the scale value to which it corresponds. By contrast, the poorest medical care hospital, Hospital #7, received a score of 2.85, which signifies only "very good" medical care (a score of 2.00 would signfy "excellent" medical care). Similarly, the hospital placing second best in medical care, Hospital #6, received a score of 1.85, signifying "excellent" medical care, while the hospital placing second poorest among the ten institutions, Hospital #1, received a score of 2.81, signifying "very good" medical care. For a group of only ten hospitals which, as repeatedly stated, are very similar in a number of important characteristics, the obtained range on medical care quality is unquestionably high. Thus, in addition to the internal consistency of the data, we find that the final measure of medical care here developed discriminates very well among the participating hospitals—and it is this discriminatory power of the measure which enables one to rank-order, and to compare and contrast, the various hospitals successfully.

With reference to the issue of consistency, it should finally be pointed out that the differences in quality of medical care among the various hospitals, as established by the measure here developed, cannot be attributed to the personal characteristics of the respondents whose answers were used to derive the measure. Instead, they are apparently "genuine" differences (a conclusion further supported by the validating evidence which will be presented in the following subsection). More specifically, when subgroups, or categories, of respondents having different characteristics are compared with respect to the manner in which they evaluated medical care, the following findings emerge:

1. Comparing the answers of medical respondents who hold staff offices, administrative positions, and committee chairmanships (a total of 117 individuals from the ten hospitals) with the answers given by the remaining medical respondents participating in the study (a total of 126 individuals), we find no significant difference in the evaluation of medical care by the two subgroups. The data from the former subgroup yield a mean evaluation score of 2.29 and the data for the latter yield a score of 2.50, the difference between the two means being statistically nonsignificant. In short, one subgroup does not evaluate medical care more favorably than the other.

2. Similarly, considering the respondents' major field of interest, we find no differences in the way in which "general practitioners" from the ten hospitals combined evaluate the quality of medical care, as against the way in which "surgeons" and medical respondents in "all other fields" evaluate the same. The data show a mean evaluation score of 2.55 for the general practitioner respondents, one of 2.57 for the surgeon respondents, and one of 2.58 for the remaining medical respondents. The three scores could hardly have been more similar than they are.

3. We, likewise, find no differences in the evaluations of the quality of medical care by medical respondents who, at the time of the study, indicated that they were working in different service divisions. For all hospitals combined, the mean evaluation score of medical care by respondents working in "medicine" is 2.48, for those in "surgery" it is 2.64, for those in "obstetrics and gynecology" it is 2.78, and for those in "all other divisions" (e.g., pediatrics, etc.) it is 2.45. Taken two at a time, these means do not yield any significant differences. Respondents working in medicine, for instance, do not evaluate the quality of medical care any more favorably or unfavorably than respondents working in obstetrics and gynecology, and so on.

4. In fact, of all the controls which we examined, we find that only the age of the respondents and the length of their association with the hospital (these two variables correlate highly and positively [.80], i.e., they overlap so that older doctors are generally the ones who have been associated with the hospital longer) yield a difference. Specifically, the younger doctors (under 40) and doctors who have been associated with the hospital for less than five years tend to be somewhat more critical, or to give a less favorable evaluation of the quality of medical care, than do older doctors (40 or over) and doctors who have been associated with the hospital for at least five years. The difference is greater with respect to age than with respect to length of institutional association; and, in terms of mean evaluation scores, the data from the older sub-

group of respondents yield a score of 2.37, while the data from the younger subgroup yield a score of 2.83.

Careful study of the data shows, however, that the relative standing of the various hospitals, as assessed by the final measure of medical care, is not even affected by the above differences connected with respondent age and length of institutional association. First, we find no significant relationship between the proportion of older doctors (40 or over) on the staff and the quality of medical care in participating hospitals. And, if the age of respondents had affected our measure of medical care, such a relationship should be obtained since older respondents, as individuals, tend to evaluate medical care more favorably than their younger colleagues. Second, we find no statistically significant relationship between the proportion of doctors who have been associated with the hospital for five or more years and the quality of medical care in the ten hospitals. Hospitals having a higher proportion of older doctors, or doctors associated with the hospitals for at least five years, do not rank more favorably on medical care quality than hospitals having a smaller proportion of doctors in these categories. In view of these findings, it is obvious that the tendency of younger doctors, and doctors associated with the hospital for a relatively short time, to be somewhat more critical in their evaluation of medical care than their other colleagues has not affected our final measure of medical care; it has not affected the relative standing of the ten hospitals on medical care quality. (A parallel conclusion was also reached earlier in connection with the nursing care measure.)

In summary, then, the preceding analysis reveals that the differences in quality of medical care among hospitals, which were established by the medical care measure here developed, cannot be attributed to such respondent characteristics, or "controls," as major field of interest or specialty, hospital division where working, position on the staff, length of institutional affiliation, and age. On the whole, the findings presented thus far clearly show high internal consistency for the data from which the final measure of medical care was derived, suggesting that the measure is stable and reliable, in addition to discriminating well among the various hospitals. We now turn to a discussion of the validity of the measure. To what extent can we be sure that the obtained measure is actually measuring the quality of medical care in participating hospitals?

Validation of the Medical Care Measure

Data for the validation of the present measure were obtained from five sources:

1. Spontaneous comments about medical care and the medical staff that were either volunteered by interviewed medical and nonmedical respondents from each hospital or were written by respondents on their questionnaires to

The Medical Care Measure

elaborate some of their answers. These data have been summarized in the individual hospital profiles in Chapter 4.

2. A special rating of the quality of hospital medical care, performed by a group of outside doctors, who were not on the staff of any of the participating hospitals but who were familiar with the medical situation in most of these hospitals.

3. Certain information from hospital medical records, as specified below.

4. Questionnaire data regarding the extent to which each hospital excels in meeting accreditation requirements, and the use of test materials for diagnostic purposes on the part of the medical staff.

5. An evaluation of the quality of medical care by nonmedical respondents from each hospital, who answered the same question about medical care as the medical respondents did, but whose answers were not included in the measure of medical care developed in this study.

To validate our measure of medical care, we compared it against each of these five sets of data, following the above order. The results of this comparative analysis will now be presented, beginning with a comparison of our measure with the free comments of respondents about medical care and medical practice.

According to the final measure of medical care shown in Table 23 above, Hospital #4 ranks first, i.e., places best, among the ten hospitals in the study, and Hospital #6 ranks second. At the other extreme, Hospital #7 ranks tenth, i.e., places poorest in medical care among the ten hospitals, and Hospital #1 ranks ninth. What do the profile materials in Chapter 4 show about medical care in these hospitals? In general, these spontaneous, qualitative materials confirm what the quantitative measure of medical care indicates. In the case of Hospital #4, which is the best medical care hospital according to our measure, we find such respondent comments in its profile as: "We have a super-excellent medical staff . . ."; "The hospital has a reputation as a medical center . . ."; and "Our [medical] staff would be classed number one . . ." Similarly, in the profile of Hospital #6, which is the second best hospital according to the medical care measure, we find such remarks as: "[The hospital is] outstanding, particularly in medical staff, the best you can find in this section of the state . . ."; "We [doctors from a number of hospitals] have been working on overall standards of patient care for a long while, and this hospital has been the leader in it . . . ; and "[This hospital has] outstanding medical specialists."

As a contrast, in the profile of Hospital #7, which places last on medical care, we find a few favorable comments and a great many negative remarks, especially concerning different aspects of medical organization: "Staff requirements [professional privileges] are easy to obtain . . ."; "[The hospital] is dominated by a clique of older M.D.'s . . ."; "General practitioners have too much power . . ."; and the like. In the case of Hospital #1, which ranks second poorest according to the medical care measure, we similarly find mixed comments, with the balance on the unfavorable side. The absence of completely negative comments regarding medical care in the hospitals placing on the poor side is of course due to the fact that, although comparatively these are "poor" medical care hospitals, in an absolute sense, they still provide reasonably satisfactory medical care (all being accredited institutions). On the whole, the volunteered comments of many respondents from each hospital, as shown in the individual hospital profiles, corroborate very well the standing of the various hospitals on medical care, as shown by our quantitative measure.

An even more crucial test of the validity of the measure in question can probably be made in terms of the evaluation of medical care by the outside group of doctors. In the early phases of the study and prior to the collection of data from the participating hospitals, in view of the difficulties involved in securing valid and reliable measures of patient care from hospital medical records, we examined the possibility of locating outside doctors who had knowledge of the medical situation in the participating institutions, in order to obtain from them a rating of the quality of medical care provided in these hospitals. After considerable exploration and contacts, it became apparent that certain outside doctors were in fact in a position to perform the desired rating, in the view of informants from the fields of medicine, hospital administration, and public health. Furthermore, it became evident that the dozen or so of our informants agreed very well amongst themselves in their independent suggestion of specific doctors as potential raters, i.e., a certain few doctors were nominated by several informants. Some of the informants themselves felt qualified to rate the participating hospitals; all of them suggested several potential raters. In the end, out of a suggested total of ten outside physicians, eight felt qualified to perform the requested rating and agreed to do so, after we personally contacted each of them and explained to him the purposes of the research and the nature of the rating.

The outside doctors who rated the quality of medical care prevailing in the various hospitals, of course, did the rating independently of one another, and were assured of both personal anonymity and confidential treatment of the information they gave us. Accordingly, we are not free to identify them. In terms of their general characteristics, however, each of them, at the time of the rating, was in some manner associated with one of these organizations: the Joint Commission on Accreditation of Hospitals, the University of Michigan Hospital and Medical Center, the Michigan State Department of Health, the Michigan Crippled Children Commission, and one other institution. It should be emphasized, in this connection, however, that every rater performed the rating as an individual person and *not* as a representative of any of these organizations. The point that we wish to make by listing these organizations is not to imply any involvement or approval on their part, but only to indicate that each individual rater had personal knowledge and a good deal of information about medical care in most of the participating hospitals.

Irrespective of his knowledge, each rater was still urged to rate only those of the hospitals about which he felt sure and not to hesitate to omit any number of them. At the same time, it was decided in advance that we would consider as capable raters only those doctors who would at least rate half of the ten hospitals (of course, this was unknown to the raters), in order that we might be reasonably sure that each rater had a comparative perspective of the medical situation in the group of hospitals studied. As it turned out, however, none of the eight doctors rated fewer than six of the ten hospitals and, consequently, no rater was eliminated.

The several raters performed their rating of medical care independently of one another, and following certain standard instructions. These instructions appeared on a single-page form which was especially designed for recording the ratings. In part, this form read as follows:

University of Michigan
Institute for Social Research

Hospital Study

On the basis of your experience and information, please rate the few hospitals listed below as *"A"* (*most favorable rating*), *"B,"* or *"C"* on (their quality of overall medical care to patients). You may use *plus* or *minus* signs after the letter you choose, if you wish to make a finer distinction. Leave out any hospital which you do not feel you can [judge]. Your individual rating will be used for research purposes only, along with similar ratings from other experts, and shall remain strictly anonymous and confidential. . . . Please keep in mind the period from January 1, 1957 to date as a time-basis for your rating.

The various hospitals were listed alphabetically on the same form, under these instructions, being identified only by their official name and city of location. And a column, titled "quality of overall medical care to patients," was provided for recording the rating given to each hospital. It was not feasible to obtain the ratings from all eight doctors at the same time, but all ratings were completed by the summer of 1957 (actual data collection from the ten hospitals did not begin till later in the fall of the same year), and all referred to the period beginning January 1, 1957.

Five of the ten hospitals were rated by all eight doctors, another two were rated by seven doctors, and the remaining three were respectively rated by six, five, and four doctors. Of the eight doctors, three rated all ten hospitals, one rated nine hospitals, three rated eight hospitals, and the remaining doctor rated six of the ten hospitals. On the average, each hospital was rated by seven out of a total of eight individuals. The several ratings were finally combined and averaged, separately for each hospital, and each hospital was given an average score depending on the ratings it received. More specifically, "A+" and "A" ratings were assigned a score of 1, ratings of "A—", "B+", and "B" were assigned a score of 2, and ratings of "B—" or lower were assigned a score of 3, in computing the average rating scores for the various hospitals. Only scores of 1, 2, and 3 were assigned to maintain simplicity and because we felt finer discrimination might reduce the overall reliability of the ratings. This procedure, it was decided, would yield sufficiently different average scores to permit a rank-ordering of the ten hospitals in relation to one another, and this actually proved to be the case.

Following the above scoring procedure, we computed the average rating score for each hospital. The individual ratings received by each hospital were assigned the appropriate numerical scores indicated above and, then, these scores were summed and divided by the total number of individuals rating the hospital to obtain the average rating score. Theoretically, the obtained scores could range from 1.0 (if a hospital were rated as "A" or "A+" by all those who rated it) to 3.0. The actual obtained range was from 1.37, signifying the best scoring hospital, and roughly corresponding to an average rating of "A" with respect to the quality of its medical care, to 2.50, signifying the poorest scoring hospital and roughly corresponding to a "C+" or "B—" average rating. Taking into consideration the relatively small number of raters involved, the obtained range is exceptionally good.

Having obtained the average rating score for each hospital, we then rank-ordered the ten hospitals in relation to one another, according to the magnitude of their respective scores. The best rated hospital was ranked 1, the next best was ranked 2, and so on, with the poorest rated hospital being given a rank of 10. In effect, this rank-order represents an outside measure of the quality of medical care rendered by the various hospitals.[9] How does the standing of the various hospitals according to the results of the outside doctor rating compare with their standing according to our final measure of medical care, which was discussed in the preceding section and was derived from the evaluations of medical respondents inside the hospitals? The correlation between the two is .61, which is statistically significant at better than the .05 level. In other words, the independent evaluation of medical care by outside doctors agrees with the final measure of medical care developed in this study, the former serving to validate the latter.[10]

[9] The split-half, odd-even reliability of the present outside rating measure is .67; i.e., the evaluation of half of the eight raters correlates .67 with the evaluation of the other half of the raters who furnished the data. Based on an N of 10 hospitals, this correlation is statistically significant at better than the .05 level, although in an absolute sense the reliability is not very high, due in large part to the small number of raters involved.

[10] In this connection, it is also worth mentioning that Hospital #4, which placed best on medical care among the ten hospitals according to our final measure of medical care shown in Table 23 above, also placed first according to the rating of outside doctors; and Hospital #6, which placed second best according to our measure, again was rated second best in medical care by the outside doctors. By contrast, Hospital #7, the poorest

Supplementary Validating Evidence

Thus far, the medical care measure was validated in terms of the volunteered comments of various respondents from each hospital and in terms of the rating of medical care by the outside group of doctors. Further validating evidence was obtained by relating our measure of medical care to certain fairly uniform data from hospital medical records. Two kinds of data were used: (1) data about the composition of the medical staff in each hospital, and (2) data concerning patient death rates. Although these data are not as detailed and as adequate as we would like them to be, they are still useful and interesting in that they provide some auxiliary evidence which is consistent with the validating evidence already presented.

With respect to the composition of the medical staff, there exists among medical and hospital circles a rather widely held assumption that, other things being equal, in hospitals whose medical staff includes a relatively high proportion of specialist "board certified" members, medical care will be of higher quality. Since board certification implies greater competence and more experience and skill for the certified doctor over his noncertified colleagues in the same field, on the face of it, this assumption seems reasonable. The question then arises as to what relationship, if any, is there between our measure of medical care and the proportion of medical staff members in the various hospitals who are "board men." A positive correlation between the two would provide additional validating evidence for the medical care measure. Accordingly, we computed the proportion of active medical staff members who are certified (not merely eligible for certification) by established medical specialty boards, and then related the distribution of the ten hospitals on this measure to their distribution on our measure of medical care.[11]

The results show that, for the ten hospitals in the study, the rank-order correlation between the proportion of medical staff members who are "board men" and the quality of medical care, as assessed by our measure, is .49.[12]

---

medical care hospital according to our measure, was also evaluated as poorest, i.e., placed tenth among the hospitals, by the outside doctors. Similar, though not as pronounced, consistencies between the two measurements characterize the remaining hospitals.

[11] Across hospitals, the percentage of active staff members who are "board men" varies from a high of 53 percent (in Hospital #6, which ranks second among the ten hospitals on medical care quality)·to a low of 27 percent (in Hospital #7, which also happens to rank poorest according to the medical care measure), the average for the ten hospitals being 38 percent.

[12] In this connection, it is also interesting to note that the correlation between the proportion of board men in the medical staff and the quality of medical care, as rated by the outside group of doctors, is .31, which is not statistically significant. This is an important finding because it shows that the outside doctors did not rate medical care on the basis of the proportion of board men in the various hospitals. Apparently, they used other criteria. Consequently, the outside rating and the proportion of board men constitute independent validating variables.

This relationship, although not statistically significant at the .05 level—which would require a correlation of .56, is both in the anticipated direction and large enough to be suggestive. Hospitals with proportionately more board men on their staff, if anything, tend to have better medical care than other hospitals.

Data from hospital medical records concerning patient death rates were also examined in relation to the medical care measure, in a manner similar to that employed in connection with the proportion of board men. Specifically, the medical care measure was compared against (1) the average gross death rate for inpatients, excluding newborn, and (2) the infant mortality rate prevailing in the various participating hospitals.[13] The results may be summarized as follows:

1. The average gross death rate of patients, excluding newborn, expressed as the percentage of patients who died in each hospital, during 1957, correlates —.10 with our measure of medical care. The correlation is in the right direction, but obviously not statistically significant. Death rates for specific and uniform categories of illness and diagnosis, and for specific patient groupings, would ideally be the rates against which to relate the quality of medical care (because of variations among hospitals in these respects), but unfortunately such refined rates were not available in the different hospitals.

2. The infant mortality rate, excluding still births (obviously a "purer" rate than the above), expressed as the percentage of newborn who died in the hospital, during 1957, correlates —.47 with the medical care measure. This correlation does not reach statistical significance at the .05 level, but it is suggestive of a tendency for the better medical care hospitals to have somewhat smaller infant mortality rates, as might be anticipated. In fact, if we consider the five hospitals shown to be the top five institutions according to our measure of the quality of medical care, i.e., the five most favorably ranking hospitals, we find that four of them also rank among the five institutions which have the smallest infant mortality rates. And, conversely, of the five poorer medical care hospitals, four have higher than median infant mortality rates.

It is, therefore, reasonable to interpret the above relationship between infant mortality rate and medical care as supportive of the validity of the medical care measure. Moreover, it is also worth pointing out in this connection that other findings from the study show a significant negative correlation of —.66 between infant mortality rate and the quality of nursing care in the participating hospitals. That is, the poorer the quality of nursing care in the hospital, the higher the infant mortality rate is likely to be. It is perhaps also relevant to add here

---

[13] As defined below, across the ten hospitals in the study, these rates were found to range as follows: (1) the gross death rate during 1957, excluding newborn, ranged from 1.19 to 3.99 per hundred patients, the average for the ten hospitals being 2.28; and (2) the infant mortality rate during 1957, excluding still births, ranged from 1.06 to 2.06 per hundred live births, the average for the ten hospitals being 1.65.

that the quality of medical care correlates positively and significantly with the quality of nursing care in the various hospitals, as will be shown in a later section of this chapter. The finding that the infant mortality rate correlates more strongly with the nursing care measure than it does with the medical care measure ($-.66$ compared to $-.47$) must be attributed to the fact that it is the nurses, and not the doctors, who keep constant vigilance over the newborn in the hospital. The newborn is unable to make his health needs known verbally or clearly, and much depends upon the alertness and performance of the nursing staff who surround him, and who are supposed to watch him and make sure that he is given proper care and, if necessary, prompt medical attention.

The findings pertaining to the gross death rate and the infant mortality rate, as of themselves, certainly do not establish the validity of our measure of medical care quality. Nevertheless, they are both illuminating and consistent with the validating evidence which we have already presented. The main problem with the above and similar other rates [14] still is that which we discussed at the beginning of this chapter: as yet, the different hospitals do not maintain uniform records of sufficiently detailed and accurate data that could be used with confidence to measure the quality of hospital patient care adequately. Moreover, to make matters more difficult, even if better and more specific rates were available from hospital medical records, rates such as these reflect not only the quality of medical care but also the quality of nursing care and of overall patient care as well, and our objective was to use measures which distinguish among these different aspects of patient care.

Questionnaire data concerning the accreditation status of participating hospitals constitute still another source of validating evidence for the medical care measure developed in this study. These data were obtained from all medical staff respondents, who were asked this question:

> In your opinion, to what extent does this hospital meet more than minimum accreditation requirements? (Check one.)
>
> _____(1) This hospital just meets the minimum accreditation requirements

[14] For example, maternal mortality rates and postoperative death rates are also of potential relevance here. However, we found that most of the hospitals in the study had zero, or nearly zero, maternal mortality rates in 1957 and, consequently, it was not possible to differentiate among them on this variable. In the case of postoperative death rates, we obtained information from the various hospitals, but the accuracy and uniformity of this information is questionable. Accordingly, no specific findings will be presented regarding the relationship between the medical care measure and postoperative death rate, other than a mention of the fact that our pertinent analysis did show a negative relationship between the two, as would be expected. In connection with these rates, we might also note that the average length of patient stay in the various hospitals, during 1957, is not significantly related either to the medical care measure or to the nursing care measure; the correlations are negative in both cases, but they are too small ($-.10$ and $-.32$) even to suggest that the longer the stay, the poorer the care.

_____(2) It does a little better than merely meeting the minimum accreditation requirements
_____(3) It does noticeably better than merely meeting the minimum accreditation requirements
_____(4) It does much better than merely meeting the minimum accreditatation requirements
_____(5) This hospital is definitely way ahead of the minimum accreditation requirements

Of a total of 252 doctor respondents from the ten hospitals, 243 actually answered this question. Across hospitals, the means computed from the obtained data range from 3.94, the most favorable score (attained by Hospital #6, which ranks second among the ten hospitals according to our measure of medical care), to 2.75, the least favorable score (attained by Hospital #7, which ranks in last place according to our measure of medical care).

Based on these data, our analysis shows that the extent to which the various hospitals go beyond merely meeting accreditation requirements correlates .55 with our measure of medical care quality, this relationship being practically significant at the .05 level (significance at this level requires a correlation of .56). Therefore, this auxiliary evidence also serves to enhance confidence in the validity of the medical care measure. We also find that the rating of medical care by the outside doctors (which is positively and significantly related to our measure of medical care) likewise correlates positively and significantly (.59) with the above measure of how well the various hospitals meet accreditation requirements. Viewed together, these results indicate that accreditation requirements were probably included among the criteria used by the outside doctors to rate the quality of medical care rendered in each hospital.

Some additional auxiliary evidence regarding the validity of the medical care measure is provided by data from the following question:

> What is your opinion about the number and quantity of laboratory and x-ray tests and other items of this type that the medical staff uses for diagnostic purposes? (Check one.)
> _____(1) In general, the staff makes excessive use of this type of materials for diagnostic purposes
> _____(2) In general, the staff uses perhaps a little more than what it should
> _____(3) In general, the staff uses the right number and quantity of these materials
> _____(4) In general, the staff uses perhaps a little less than what it should
> _____(5) In general, the staff does not use enough of this type of materials for diagnostic purposes

This question was asked of the general medical staff group in each hospital. The data show that, for all hospitals combined, 7 percent of the respondents felt that the staff uses "perhaps a little less than what it should," 8 percent felt that the staff makes "excessive use" of the materials in question, 39 percent

The Medical Care Measure

felt that the staff uses "perhaps a little more than what it should," and 46 percent felt that the staff uses the "right" amount. Across individual hospitals, the percentage of respondents who felt that the medical staff uses the "right" amount of test materials for diagnostic purposes ranges from a high of 73 percent (in Hospital #4, which ranks first among the ten hospitals on the medical care measure) to a low of 27 percent (in Hospital #5, which ranks sixth).

When these data are related to the medical care measure, we find that the extent to which the medical staff uses the "right" amount of test materials for diagnostic purposes correlates .71 with the quality of medical care. And, similarly, the extent to which the staff uses either the "right" amount or "perhaps a little more than what it should" correlates .74 with the medical care measure. Both of these correlations are statistically significant at the .05 level. Assuming that the quality of medical care in hospitals depends in part upon good diagnosis, and assuming that good diagnosis depends in part on a proper use of test materials by the medical staff ("proper use" referring to use that is neither insufficient, as when the staff uses less materials than it should, nor wasteful, as when the staff makes excessive use of test materials), proper use of test materials would be expected to relate positively to the quality of medical care. The obtained correlations show that such a relationship exists, thus providing some validating evidence for our measure of medical care.

The final piece of evidence in support of the validity of the medical care measure derives from an evaluation of the quality of medical care by respondents from each hospital. As earlier noted, although our final measure of medical care was constructed exclusively using the answers of doctors, we did ask registered nursing staff, technician, and administrative respondents to give us their own evaluations of the quality of medical care in their respective hospitals, using a question identical to that asked of medical respondents (the question has been presented earlier in this section). Based on the answers of these nonmedical respondent groups, mean-scores were computed, separately for each hospital, to obtain a supplementary appraisal of medical care in the various hospitals. This appraisal was then related to our principal measure of medical care to determine the relationship between the two.

The relevant findings may be summarized as follows:

1. The quality of medical care in the various hospitals, as appraised by all nonmedical respondents from each hospital (supervisory and nonsupervisory registered nurses, x-ray and laboratory technicians, and the lay-administrative group of respondents), correlates .70 with the final measure of medical care developed in this study, which is based solely on the evaluation of medical care by medical respondents (see Table 23 above). This relationship, based on an N of 10 hospitals, is statistically significant at better than the .05 level, thus providing additional validating evidence for the measure under examination.

2. Similarly, the quality of medical care in the various hospitals, as evaluated by registered nursing staff respondents alone, correlates .61 with our final measure of medical care, this relationship too being significant at better than the .05 level.

In short, nonmedical respondents, as a group, agree significantly with medical respondents in their assessment of the quality of medical care characteristic of their respective hospitals. And, parenthetically, this finding casts some doubt on the often made assertion in the literature that doctors alone can evaluate the quality of hospital medical care. This is only of secondary importance to our main concern here, however, which is the validation of the medical care measure. From the standpoint of validation, the finding that nonmedical respondents agree with medical respondents about the quality of medical care is the important one.

In summary, the results of the various analyses reported in the preceding pages lead to the conclusion that the final measure of the quality of medical care which was developed in this study is both reliable and valid, thus permitting one to rank-order and to compare and contrast the various participating hospitals on this variable with confidence. As in the case of the nursing care measure, described earlier in this chapter, the research evidence which we have presented assures us that our effort to measure the quality of medical care, by properly combining the judgments of medical staff respondents from each participating hospital, has been successful. We thus have two reasonably satisfactory measures of hospital patient care up to this point—a measure of the quality of nursing care, and a parallel measure of the quality of medical care that patients receive in the various hospitals. But we are still lacking a measure of the quality of total care given to patients. And even though the quality of overall patient care would be largely determined by the quality of medical care and nursing care, a separate measure of overall care is highly desirable, both because other variables may enter the determination of total care and because we would want to be able to compare the various hospitals on total care. Such a measure was, therefore, also developed and will be presented next.

THE MEASURE OF OVERALL PATIENT CARE

The quality of total patient care in the various hospitals was measured using data from the medical staff, registered nursing staff, technicians, and the administrative group of respondents. Members of these groups from each hospital were requested to rate the quality of overall patient care in their hospital by answering the following question:

> On the basis of your experience and information, how would you rate the quality of *overall care* that the patients generally receive from this hospital? (Check one.)

The Measure of Overall Patient Care

_____(1) Overall patient care in this hospital is outstanding
_____(2) Excellent
_____(3) Very good
_____(4) Good
_____(5) Fair
_____(6) Rather poor
_____(7) Overall patient care in this hospital is poor

This question is very similar to the earlier questions about nursing care and medical care. We shall, therefore, dispense with methodological details here, noting only that the treatment of the data from this question followed a procedure identical with that employed in deriving the nursing care measure.

For all hospitals combined, of a total of 902 respondents, 880 answered the question about overall care, the average response rate being almost 98 percent and ranging from 96 percent in the case of medical staff respondents to 99 percent in the case of registered nursing staff respondents. With reference to the respondent groups involved, the data show that 60 percent of medical respondents from all hospitals evaluated overall patient care as "outstanding" or "excellent," compared to 36 percent of nurse respondents, 42 percent of technician respondents, and 79 percent of lay-administrative respondents. As in the cases of nursing and medical care, the administrative group evaluated overall care most favorably, while the registered nursing staff group was again the most critical.

Considering all respondents from all ten hospitals, we find that 51 percent of them rate overall care as "outstanding" or "excellent," 30 percent rate it as "very good," 16 percent rate it as "good," and the remaining 3 percent rate it as "fair" or "rather poor." These figures, of course, vary a good deal for individual hospitals, as might be expected. For example, considering the percentage of all respondents who evaluate overall care as outstanding or excellent in the various hospitals, we find a range from a low of 30 percent in the case of Hospital #2, which previously ranked ninth on nursing care and seventh on medical care, to a high of 72 percent in the case of Hospital #3, which previously tied for first place on nursing care and ranked third among the ten hospitals on medical care. In other words, well over twice as many respondents in the latter hospital evaluate overall care as outstanding or excellent in comparison to respondents in the former hospital.

The final measure of overall care is not based on percentages such as the above. It takes into account the total distribution of responses to the question about overall care. More specifically, the measure was derived by computing the arithmetic mean of the responses of the members of each of the four respondent groups, for each hospital separately, and then combining properly these four means into an overall hospital mean or a single mean-score. Therefore, like the nursing care measure, the measure of overall care incorporates the evaluations of all four respondent groups. Table 24 shows the standing of

244   ASSESSMENT OF PATIENT CARE

the ten hospitals on the quality of overall patient care, according to our measure. The first line of figures in Table 24 shows the mean-score on overall care received by each hospital; the second line shows the ten hospitals rank-ordered in relation to one another according to the magnitude of their mean-score; and the third line shows the total number of individual respondents from each hospital who rated the quality of overall patient care.

TABLE 24. The Quality of Overall Patient Care in Each Hospital as Evaluated by Four Respondent Groups Combined, and the Relative Standing of the Ten Hospitals on Overall Care *

	Hospital									
	#0	1	2	3	4	5	6	7	8	9
Hospital mean-score on quality of overall patient care †	2.78	2.94	2.83	1.99	2.24	2.42	2.63	2.56	2.32	2.37
Hospital's rank, according to its mean-score	8	10	9	1	2	5	7	6	3	4
Total number of individual respondents from each hospital	112	92	82	76	89	75	103	75	98	78

* Smaller mean-scores, and corresponding smaller ranks, represent more favorable evaluations of overall care. The mean-scores are based on data from medical staff respondents, registered nursing staff respondents, x-ray and laboratory technicians, and the administrative respondents participating in the research. For each hospital, the data have been weighted according to the sampling rates with which respondents have been selected into the study.

† This is subsequently used as the main measure of the quality of overall patient care in the various hospitals.

The decision to combine the answers of the different groups of respondents in deriving the measure of overall care was based essentially on the same reasons which were discussed in connection with the nursing care measure. One reason is that all four respondent groups were considered relevant. Another reason is that with respect to the relative standing of the various hospitals on overall care—which constitutes our main concern here—the evaluations of the different respondent groups are fairly consistent with one another. Not shown in Table 24, the relative standing of the ten hospitals on overall care, as evaluated by a given respondent group, correlates positively (though not always significantly) with the standing of the hospitals on overall care as evaluated by the other respondent groups. We find, for example, that the evaluation of overall care by medical staff respondents correlates .71 with the evaluation by registered nursing staff respondents, .50 with the evaluation by technicians, and .51 with the evaluation by the administrative group of respondents. Another, and more important, reason is the fact that the obtained final measure of the quality of overall patient care, shown in Table 24, correlates positively and signifi-

The Measure of Overall Patient Care

cantly with the separate respondent group evaluations which it incorporates.

The quality of overall patient care, as evaluated by the four respondent groups combined, correlates .95, .84, .62, and .57, respectively, with its separate evaluation by medical staff respondents, by registered nursing staff respondents, by technician respondents, and by administrative respondents. Based on an N of 10 hospitals, all of these correlations are statistically significant at better than the .05 level, indicating that the obtained final measure significantly reflects the several separate evaluations of overall care. It is also important to note that the same correlations show that the medical staff's evaluation of overall care agrees most closely (correlates .95) with the final measure of overall care, and the nursing staff's evaluation agrees with it next most closely (correlates with it .84). Consequently, we are assured that the evaluations of overall care by the most revelant, and probably most competent, of the four respondent groups involved are the ones which are best represented in the final measure of overall patient care.

As anticipated, Table 24 shows that the various hospitals differ in the quality of the overall care they provide their patients. Moreover, the obtained interhospital differences on overall care, as in the cases of medical and nursing care previously discussed, cannot be attributed to response differences due to the particular characteristics of the respondents. Considering the largest two of our respondent groups—medical staff and registered nursing staff, for example —we find that such control factors as shift of work, hospital division where working, full-time as against part-time work, and medical specialty do not affect differentially the respondents' evaluations of overall care.

First, examining the data from our nurse respondents, we find no significant difference between the mean evaluations of overall care by: (1) full-time versus part-time nurses, (2) younger versus older nurses, (3) nurses in different shifts, and (4) nurses working in different hospital divisions—medicine versus surgery versus obstetrics and gynecology versus all other. Second, examining the data from medical respondents, we likewise find no significant differences between the mean evaluations of overall care by the following subgroups: (1) doctors holding administrative positions versus other doctors; (2) general practitioners versus surgeons versus all other doctors; and (3) doctors working in medicine versus those working in surgery versus those working in obstetrics and gynecology versus those working in all other areas. The only significant difference which we have found is that younger doctors tend to be more critical in their evaluations than older doctors (for all hospitals combined, the mean evaluation score of overall care for the former is 2.90 versus 2.32 for the latter). Even this difference, however, for the reasons which we presented when discussing the same finding with respect to our measure of medical care, has no perceptible effect upon the final measure of overall care —i.e., insofar as the relative standing of the ten hospitals on overall care, shown in Table 24, is concerned.

Validation of the Overall Care Measure

In large part, the quality of overall patient care is undoubtedly determined by the quality of medical care and the quality of nursing care given to patients in the various institutions. Therefore, one would expect positive and significant relationships between the measure of overall care, on the one hand, and the measures of medical and nursing care, on the other. Such relationships actually exist.[15] Similarly, if one were to compare the standing of the ten hospitals on overall care, as shown in Table 24 above, with the various qualitative comments of respondents about patient care, as shown in the individual hospital profiles in Chapter 4, he would find that, on the whole, the volunteered remarks of respondents from each hospital are quite consistent with the ranking of the various hospitals on the overall care measure. The evidence from these two sources, however, is not sufficient to establish adequately the validity of the measure of overall care. Other relevant results must also be examined.

The reader will recall that one of the criteria of patient care often suggested in the literature is the "satisfied customer test," i.e., what patients think of their hospital care. And although this criterion would be entirely inadequate for measuring patient care, because of the reasons presented early in this chapter, an indication of patient reaction toward the hospital could be used for validating purposes. Provision was therefore made by the study to obtain some information about patient reaction. But, since patients were not included in the study as respondents, this information was collected from hospital personnel, who were asked this question:

On the basis of your experience and information, how do the patients feel about this hospital? (Check one.)

_____(1) All patients without exception speak very well of this hospital
_____(2) Nearly all of the patients speak very well of this hospital
_____(3) The large majority of the patients speak very well of this hospital
_____(4) A little over half of the patients speak very well of this hospital
_____(5) About half of the patients speak very well of this hospital
_____(6) Less than half of the patients speak very well of this hospital
_____(7) Only a few of the patients speak very well of this hospital

Those who answered this question in each hospital were the medical staff respondents, the registered nursing staff respondents, the technicians, and the

---

[15] Table 27 (p. 258) shows that the overall care measure here examined correlates .67 with the medical care measure and .91 with the nursing care measure, both correlations being statistically significant at better than the .05 level. Moreover, if we relate the overall care measure to the average standing of the various hospitals on both nursing care (shown earlier in Table 21) and medical care (shown earlier in Table 23)—the "average standing" being obtained by summing and averaging each hospital's ranks on medical care and on nursing care—the resulting correlation between overall care and the average standing of the hospitals on medical-nursing care is .92. This relationship shows that the quality of overall patient care is, to a great extent, a function of the quality of nursing care and the quality of medical care that patients receive in the hospital.

administrative group of respondents, the first two groups obviously being the most relevant because of their more frequent and more intensive contact with the patients. Of a total of 902 individual respondents, only 23 failed to answer the question, with the administrative group of respondents showing the highest nonresponse rate—7 percent. Based on the answers of our respondents from each group and each institution, in the usual manner, the data were converted into means using the seven-point scale corresponding to the response alternatives offered by the question. These means indicate the approximate proportion of patients who speak very well of the hospital and, by inference, about the care they received there, according to the respondents. The obtained means, considering the data from all respondent groups combined, range across hospitals from 2.17, the most favorable score (received by Hospital $\neq$3 which, among the ten hospitals, respectively ranks 1.5, 3, and 1 on our measures of nursing, medical, and overall care), to 2.96, the least favorable score (received by Hospital $\neq$2 which respectively ranks 9, 7, and 9 on nursing, medical, and overall care).

Correlational analysis of the data shows that "customer satisfaction" is higher in those hospitals which rank better on the measure of overall patient care shown in Table 24. Those hospitals which rank more favorably on overall patient care also tend to be the ones where a higher proportion of the patients speak very well of the hospital, according to our respondents. More specifically, we find that the quality of overall patient care correlates .82 with the relative proportion of patients who speak favorably of the hospital, as assessed by all respondents from each hospital, .81 with the same variable, as assessed by medical staff respondents only, and .78 with the same variable, as assessed by nurse respondents only. (Parenthetically, it may also be added that patient reaction as assessed by medical respondents correlates .89 with patient reaction as assessed by nurse respondents.) These relationships, based on an N of 10 hospitals, are all significant at better than the .01 level. Consequently, it may be concluded that the validity of the measure of overall patient care receives good support from these supplementary data about patient reaction toward the hospital.

Additional validating evidence derives from data concerning the reputation each hospital enjoys in its community. Frequently, hospital people maintain that the effectiveness of a community general hospital and, by extension, the quality of its overall service, or total patient care, may in part be gauged by the kind of reputation the institution has in its community, since the hospital's primary aim is to serve the community. By implication, the assumption is made that, if a hospital has a good reputation, it must generally meet the expectations of its community, which roughly means that the hospital provides adequate patient care to those members of the community who seek its services. In turn, of course, this assumption is based upon a second one, namely, that the community has a fairly good image of the hospital, or some minimum knowledge about it, which presumably is reflected in the kind of reputation the hospital comes to enjoy. With these assumptions in mind, and disregarding for the moment the particular problems which they pose, if anything, one is led to expect a positive relationship between the hospital's quality of overall patient care and the hospital's public reputation. As in the case concerning patient reaction toward the hospital, therefore, the study made provision to obtain some measure of the community reputation of each hospital, and then to relate this measure to our measure of the quality of overall patient care for validation purposes.

To obtain the required measure of hospital reputation, once more we had to rely on data supplied by hospital personnel, since no community members other than the people working in the hospital were included in the study. The medical staff, registered nursing staff, technician, and administrative respondents from each institution provided the data by answering the following question:

What kind of reputation does this hospital have in the community? (Check one.)

_____(1) This hospital has an excellent reputation in the community
_____(2) A very good reputation
_____(3) A good reputation
_____(4) A fair reputation
_____(5) This hospital has a rather poor reputation in the community
_____(6) I can't judge

The overall nonresponse rate to this question, including "I can't judge" answers, was merely 4 percent, with only 35 of the 902 respondents involved feeling unqualified to evaluate the public reputation of their respective hospitals.

The answers of respondents from each hospital were properly combined and converted into means to yield a measure of the reputation of their hospital. Across hospitals, using data from all four respondent groups combined, the obtained means on hospital reputation range from 1.49, the most favorable score, to 2.41, the least favorable score.[16] The former score signifies a reputation midway between "excellent" and "very good," while the latter signifies a reputation midway between "very good" and "good." It is also of interest to point out that the hospital scoring most favorably on community reputation

[16] For the present variable, as well as most other variables in this study, the range, or variability, of hospital scores is smaller when the score is based on data from the different respondent groups combined than when based on data from a single respondent group. Concerning the present case, for example, based exclusively on data from the technicians group, hospital reputation scores range between 1.56 and 3.12. And although a wider range may be more desirable than a narrower one, a narrower range resulting from combining the data from several respondent groups to obtain a single score, other things being equal, is more preferable because measures based on data from more respondents are more reliable and more stable measures. Furthermore, since the present study focuses upon the hospital as a total organization, frequently it is also theoretically preferable to combine data from different respondent groups—a procedure resulting in scores of a relatively narrower range.

(Hospital #3) is the same one which scored best on patient reaction toward the hospital, while the hospital scoring least favorably on reputation (Hospital #2) is the same one which scored poorest on patient reaction. More generally, hospital reputation, as assessed by all respondents combined, actually correlates .73 with patient reaction, as assessed by the same respondents. This relationship implies that, as might be expected, the reputation which a hospital comes to enjoy in its community is probably dependent, to a considerable degree, upon how well the patients, before and after discharge, speak of the hospital.

When the public reputation of the various hospitals, as measured by the above data, is related to the quality of overall patient care, we find:

1. Hospital reputation, as evaluated by the four respondent groups in each hospital, correlates .61 with the quality of overall patient care, i.e., better-reputation hospitals also tend to rank better on our measure of overall care shown in Table 24.

2. As evaluated by medical staff respondents only, hospital reputation correlates .68 with the quality of overall patient care.

3. As evaluated by registered nursing staff respondents only, hospital reputation correlates .58 with the quality of overall care. (Hospital reputation as assessed by doctors itself correlates .81 with hospital reputation as assessed by nurses.)

4. As evaluated by technician respondents only, hospital reputation correlates .15 with the quality of overall care.

5. And, as assessed by administrative respondents, hospital reputation correlates .53 with the quality of overall patient care.

Based on an N of 10 hospitals in each case, the first three of the above correlations are statistically significant at better than the .05 level, the fourth is not significant, and the last approaches significance at the .05 level. Considered together, the results suggest a positive overall relationship between the kind of reputation each hospital enjoys in its community—reputation as appraised by hospital personnel—and the quality of overall patient care each hospital provides. Consequently, there is some merit to the hypothesis that better-care hospitals also tend to be better-reputation hospitals. What is more important to our purposes here, however, is that the findings just discussed reinforce the evidence which we have already presented in support of the validity of the measure of the quality of overall patient care developed in this study.

THE COMPARATIVE MEASURE OF OVERALL PATIENT CARE

Thus far, we have presented three of the four measures of hospital patient care that were developed in this study—a measure of the quality of nursing care, a measure of the quality of medical care, and a measure of the quality of overall patient care. The fourth, and last, measure also concerns the quality of total patient care, but it differs in one important respect from the overall care measure that was described in the preceding section. Specifically, it differs in that it is a *comparative* measure, i.e., a measure of the quality of overall patient care a hospital provides *in comparison to* the quality of overall care similar other hospitals provide. In this case, instead of having the respondents rate the quality of overall patient care in their hospital in terms of a scale ranging from "outstanding" to "poor," and without any reference to other hospitals, we had them rate it in terms of how it compares with the quality of overall care rendered by similar other institutions. Throughout the book, this last measure of patient care is referred to as the measure of the quality of comparative overall care, or as the comparative measure of overall patient care.

Frequently, a comparative measure such as the present measure is superior to a noncomparative one, because it furnishes the respondents who provide the data with a particular frame of reference in terms of which they can appraise a given situation. In the present case, being interested in measuring the quality of hospital patient care, the relevant referent is patient care in other hospitals which are similar to those in the study. Another and more crucial reason for using a comparative measure stems from previous research findings. Several studies of organizational behavior have shown that the members of a group, or organization, can generally compare the performance, and other characteristics, of their group with the performance of similar other groups successfully. In many organizations—in some of which excellent criteria of performance were available—it was found that group performance, as evaluated by the members of the organization, correlated very highly with performance as assessed on the basis of such "hard" criteria as productivity figures arrived at through time-study techniques and obtained from company records. In other words, on the average, the members of the more effective productive groups correctly rated their group's performance high, while the members of the less effective groups correctly rated their group's performance low, when asked to evaluate the performance of their group in comparison to the performance of similar other groups.

Kahn and Katz (19) report, for example, that (1) in a study of a large insurance company employees in high-producing groups actually evaluated their group more favorably in comparison to other groups with respect to getting the job done, pride in the group, and similar other variables, and (2) in a study of a manufacturing company, employees in better-producing groups evaluated the performance of their group more highly in response to the question "When it comes to putting out work, how does your group compare to others?" Kahn and Katz also point out that "There was no difference between high and low producers in the characteristics they ascribed to their groups in the areas of skill, know-how, education, and the like." Similarly, in a comparative study of organizational effectiveness in a multiunit company engaged in the delivery of retail merchandise, where particularly good measures of performance were available, Georgopoulos and Tannenbaum (10) found that "those directly involved with the operations of the organization can make [correct] judgments about the performance of their respective units [groups]."

Of course, successful comparative evaluations of organizational performance such as those cited here presuppose that the members of a given group have some familiarity with the situation prevailing in similar other groups with which they compare their own, as well as that such groups actually exist to provide the referent for comparative judgment. In the present study, fortunately, both of these conditions are satisfied as we will show below, when discussing the validity of the comparative measure of overall patient care. One is also impressed by the fact that hospitals and their product are in many ways different from those organizations in which the above studies were conducted and that, consequently, some caution is necessary in expecting hospital members, like the members of these other organizations, to appraise successfully the quality of hospital performance—or, more precisely, the quality of overall patient care—as compared to that in similar other hospitals. Yet, the evidence in point derives from sufficiently complex and sufficiently different organizational settings to argue in favor of such an expectation.

Still another important reason for utilizing a comparative measure of overall patient care is the recommendation of researchers in the hospital field who, having struggled with the whole problem of hospital patient care assessment, concluded that comparative measures are essential at this stage of our knowledge. Sheps (39) in her discussion of approaches to measuring hospital care quality, for example, has explicitly stated that, in the absence of an objective standard, comparative judging and evaluation are needed. Similarly, Kossack (21) has pointed out that, to measure the quality of a hospital with respect to patient care or other dimensions, we need to show how the whole hospital rates in comparison with other hospitals of its size and type. In short, a comparative measure of the quality of total patient care has much merit on its own right, apart from its usefulness as an additional measure to the three measures of patient care which we have already presented in this chapter. Accordingly, appropriate data were collected from each participating hospital in order to enable us to construct a comparative measure of overall patient care—the fourth and last measure of patient care developed in this study of community general hospitals. We now turn to a more detailed description of this measure.

Data for the measurement of the quality of comparative overall care were collected by means of this question:

How would you rate the quality of *overall patient care* in this hospital as compared to similar other community general hospitals? (Check one.)

_____(1) Overall patient care in this hospital is outstanding compared to most other hospitals of this kind

_____(2) Much better

_____(3) Generally better
_____(4) About the same
_____(5) Somewhat poorer
_____(6) Generally poorer
_____(7) Overall patient care in this hospital is much poorer than in most other hospitals of this kind

The question was asked of the same respondents as the previous questions about patient care, but the final measure of comparative care is based exclusively on data from the medical respondents representing each hospital. For all hospitals combined, the average response rate to the present question was 96 percent for medical respondents, and 95.5 percent for both medical and non-medical respondents. Concerning the distribution of responses, the data show that, for all hospitals together, 47 percent of all respondents indicated that overall patient care in their hospital was "outstanding" or "much better" in comparison to other similar hospitals; another 29 percent indicated that it was "generally better," 22 percent said that it was "about the same," and 2 percent felt that it was poorer compared to other hospitals. The corresponding figures for medical staff respondents are 48, 33, 16, and 3 percent, respectively, being fairly similar to the average figures for all respondents combined. Of the four respondent groups involved, the administrative group again gave the most favorable evaluation of comparative overall care, while the technicians group gave the most critical evaluation. The registered nursing staff group was somewhat less critical than the technicians, but somewhat more critical than the medical group.

The data show considerable interhospital differences in the quality of comparative overall care, suggesting that the measure discriminates well among the various hospitals. For example, while 19 percent of medical respondents in Hospital #1 rate the quality of overall patient care in their hospital as "outstanding" or "much better" compared to overall care in similar other hospitals, fully 70 percent of medical respondents in Hospital #4 do so, the average for all hospitals being 48 percent. Similarly, 35 percent of medical respondents in Hospital #2 versus 68 percent in Hospital #3 rate the quality of overall care in their hospital as outstanding or much better compared to overall care in other hospitals of the same kind. Similar differences among the ten hospitals, moreover, can be also observed when means rather than percentages are used to present the data. The data from the question about comparative overall care, converted into means, are summarized in Table 25. Mean-scores representing the quality of comparative patient care, as evaluated by each respondent group and by the four respondent groups combined, are shown separately for every hospital. In addition, the rank-orders in Table 25 indicate the relative standing of the ten hospitals on comparative overall care.

The first row of means in Table 25, based exclusively on data from medical staff respondents—between 20 and 33 doctors per hospital, with an average of 24 doctors—constitutes the final measure of the quality of comparative overall care. According to this measure, Hospital #4 with a score of 1.81 ranks first, or best, among the ten hospitals, while Hospital #1 with a score of 3.61 ranks tenth, or poorest. Roughly, the former score indicates that, compared to similar other hospitals, overall patient care in Hospital #4 is "much better," while according to the latter score overall care in Hospital #1 is "about the same" as in other hospitals (an intermediate score of 3.00 would indicate that care is "generally better" than in other hospitals).

TABLE 25. Comparative Evaluation of the Quality of Overall Patient Care by Certain Respondent Groups in Each Hospital, and the Relative Standing of the Ten Hospitals on Comparative Overall Care *

First Row: Respondent group's mean response about comparative overall care
Second Row: Rank-order of hospitals according to mean response

Respondent Group	Hospital #0	1	2	3	4	5	6	7	8	9
Medical staff †	2.88	3.61	3.00	2.18	1.81	2.40	2.61	2.65	2.37	2.50
	8	10	9	2	1	4	6	7	3	5
Registered nursing staff	3.23	3.13	3.35	1.93	2.15	2.43	2.57	2.64	2.38	2.60
	9	8	10	1	2	4	5	7	3	6
Laboratory and x-ray technicians	2.80	2.83	3.43	1.86	2.40	2.62	3.62	2.44	2.19	2.88
	6	7	9	1	3	5	10	4	2	8
Administrator, nonmedical department heads, and trustees	2.29	2.38	2.23	1.93	2.15	2.33	2.44	2.21	2.19	2.47
	6	8	5	1	2	7	9	4	3	10
All preceding respondent groups combined	2.92	3:17	2.99	2.01	2.06	2.38	2.65	2.49	2.31	2.55
	8	10	9	1	2	4	7	5	3	6

* Smaller mean-scores, and corresponding smaller ranks, represent more favorable evaluations of comparative overall care.
† This is subsequently used as the main comparative measure of the quality of overall patient care in the various hospitals.

Further examination of the results in Table 25 reveals that the relative standing of the ten hospitals on comparative overall care, based on data from the medical group of respondents, remains remarkably consistent when we consider it in relation to the evaluations of comparative care by the other three groups of respondents. Hospital #4, for example, ranks 1, 2, 3, 2, and 2 among the ten hospitals, according to the evaluations of comparative care by medical respondents, by registered nursing staff respondents, by technicians, by administrative respondents, and by all four respondent groups combined. Correspondingly, Hospital #3 ranks 2, 1, 1, 1, and 1. At the other extreme,

Hospital #1 not once places better than seventh among the ten institutions, and Hospital #2 ranks ninth or tenth in all cases except one (according to the evaluation by administrative respondents, it ranks fifth). The separate evaluations of the quality of comparative overall care are thus in substantial agreement with one another.

The stability of the comparative measure of overall patient care is perhaps better demonstrated by the results in Table 26. This table presents the specific intercorrelations among the evaluations of comparative overall care by the different respondent groups. In general, based on an N of 10 hospitals and ranging between .49 and .95, these correlations are positive and significant, as expected. Among other things, these findings show that the quality of comparative care in the various hospitals as assessed by the final measure, i.e., as evaluated by medical respondents, correlates .94, .67, .53, and .95, respectively, with the quality of comparative care as assessed by nurse respondents, by technician respondents, by administrative respondents, and by all respondents combined. Those hospitals which are rated highly on comparative care by the medical staff are also evaluated highly by the other respondents. Accordingly, our comparative measure of the quality of overall patient care, like the previous three measures of patient care, may be considered as stable.

TABLE 26. Rank-order Intercorrelations Among the Evaluations of the Quality of Comparative Overall Patient Care by Various Groups of Respondents *

Evaluation by:	1	2	3	4	5
1. Medical staff respondents	—	.94	.67	.53	.95
2. Registered nursing staff		—	.68	.49	.92
3. Lab and x-ray technicians			—	.83	.82
4. Administrator, nonmedical department heads, and trustees				—	.67
5. All preceding respondent groups combined					—

* All correlations are based on an N of 10 hospitals. Coefficients larger than .56 are significant at the .05 level, and those .75 or larger are significant at the .01 level.

Other findings, in addition to illuminating further the internal consistency of the comparative measure of overall care, show that the interhospital differences which are established by this measure (see Table 25) cannot be accounted for in terms of the particular characteristics of the respondents who provided the data. Specifically, considering all medical staff respondents from the ten hospitals, we find:

1. No statistically significant difference between how the younger doctors (under 40) and the older doctors evaluate the quality of comparative hospital care; the mean evaluation score based on data from the former subgroup is 2.94 and for the latter subgroup of respondents it is 2.69.

2. No significant differences in how favorably general practitioners, as against surgeons, as against all other doctors, evaluate the quality of comparative care; the mean evaluation scores for the three subgroups are 2.68, 2.65, and 2.94, respectively.

3. No significant differences in the evaluation of comparative care by doctors working in medicine, doctors in surgery, doctors in obstetrics and gynecology, and doctors in all other services, when the four subgroups are examined two at a time, except that doctors in obstetrics and gynecology tend to give a somewhat more critical evaluation than their colleagues in medicine.

4. Doctors associated with their hospital for five or more years, however, assess the quality of comparative hospital care significantly more favorably than doctors associated with their hospital for a shorter time; the data from the former subgroup yield a mean evaluation score of 2.66 compared to a score of 3.10 for the latter subgroup.

The conclusion to be drawn from these results is that the evaluation of the quality of comparative overall care was not affected perceptibly by the personal characteristics of the physicians who provided the data. Even the single significant difference between doctors associated with the hospital for five or more years and the remaining doctors does not affect the relative standing of the various hospitals on comparative care, as assessed by our measure. In this connection, additional analysis shows that there is no relationship whatever between the comparative measure of overall care (i.e., the relative standing of the ten hospitals on comparative overall care shown in Table 25) and the proportion of doctors in the various hospitals who have been associated with the hospital for at least five years. The rank-order correlation between these two variables is −.13, which is not significantly different from zero and which, if anything, is in the opposite direction than one would be led to expect on the basis that respondents associated with their hospital for five or more years evaluate comparative care more favorably than the remaining respondents.

The conclusion that the interhospital differences established by the comparative measure of overall patient care cannot be attributed to the personal characteristics of the medical respondents who provided the data for the measure is also supported indirectly by findings involving the characteristics of nurse respondents. The latter's evaluation of comparative care was not incorporated in the final measure. It will be recalled, however, that the quality of comparative care, as evaluated by nurse respondents, was found to correlate very highly (.94) with the quality of comparative care as evaluated by medical respondents. It would be instructive, therefore, to know whether or not nurses with different characteristics evaluate the quality of comparative care differently. The answer, as in the case of medical respondents, is negative. We find no significant difference in how favorably different subgroups of nurse respondents evaluate the quality of comparative overall care. Specifically, we find no significant difference between: full-time and part-time nurses; younger (under

30) and older nurses; nurses on the same job in the same hospital for less than a year and nurses of longer standing; nurses in one shift and nurses in another, the three shifts taken two at a time; or between nurses in one major service and those in another, the four services—medicine, surgery, obstetrics and gynecology, and all others areas—considered two at a time.

Validation of the Comparative Measure of Overall Care

The measures of the quality of nursing care, medical care, and (noncomparative) overall care were validated independently of one another, i.e., each was compared against a different set of available relevant data. The comparative measure of overall care will be here validated by relating it to the other three measures of patient care, which have already been validated, and by means of certain ancillary information.

When the comparative care measure is related to the other three measures of hospital patient care, we find that it correlates positively and highly with each of them. It correlates .96 with the noncomparative measure of overall care, .78 with the measure of medical care, and .82 with the measure of nursing care. Each of these relationships, based on an N of 10 hospitals, is statistically significant at better than the .01 level. Hospitals scoring favorably on the comparative measure also score favorably on each of the other three measures. It is also of interest to note that the quality of comparative overall care correlates more closely with the quality of noncomparative overall care than with the quality of medical care or the quality of nursing care. The two measures of overall care correlate .96. This relationship is in fact so high as to suggest that, for practical purposes, the comparative and the noncomparative measures of overall care could be used interchangeably. Theoretically, however, the two measures have different bases, if not different meanings, and for this reason they will both be used as separate measures in all subsequent analyses.

In view of the above results, it may be said that if the previous three measures of patient care are valid—and the relevant evidence shows that they are—the comparative measure of overall care is also valid. The validity of the comparative measure also depends, however, upon whether or not the respondents who evaluated the quality of overall care comparatively were actually in a position to perform such an evaluation. In this connection, it will be recalled, the respondents had been asked to rate the quality of overall care in their hospital *as compared to* the quality of overall care in similar other hospitals. But this assumes (1) that the respondents were familiar with the care situation in "similar other hospitals," and (2) that "similar other hospitals" operated nearby, so that regional differences between the respondent's hospital and the other hospitals with which he compared his own did not obscure the rating.

Apparently, both of these two assumptions are tenable according to available data. First, in response to the question "Are you on the staff of any other hospitals at present?" 83 percent of all medical respondents from the ten participating hospitals said "yes." In other words, the great majority of the medical respondents who rated the quality of overall care comparatively were, at the time of the rating, on the staff of at least one additional hospital, thus having a concrete referent on the basis of which to make the required comparison. In fact, at the time of the rating, at least 80 percent of the medical respondents from eight of the ten hospitals were also on the staff of another hospital (which presumably was located nearby). Moreover, in addition to their "current" experience with the care situation in these other hospitals, the respondents involved undoubtedly have had previous familiarity with similar general hospitals, either as students and trainees or as practicing physicians. It is safe to assume, therefore, that the medical respondents indeed had a frame of reference in terms of which to perform the comparative rating of overall patient care requested of them (and the comparative measure of overall care is exclusively based on the ratings of these respondents).

The second of the above assumptions—that "similar other hospitals" operated in the same area at the time of the comparative rating—is also substantially sound. All except one of the ten participating hospitals are located in cities having at least one additional short-stay general hospital. Furthermore, the single hospital which constitutes the exception itself is located at a point within 15 miles of which there are several other general hospitals. (Parenthetically, as might be anticipated, this is also the hospital with the lowest proportion of medical respondents reporting that they are on the staff of additional hospitals.) And although most of the other hospitals located in the same cities as the participating hospitals are not similar in every major respect to the hospitals in the study (see the criteria used for including hospitals in the research), they still are short-stay general hospitals. The assumption under examination is therefore upheld by the available evidence.

In summary, based on all of the evidence discussed in the preceding pages, we conclude that our comparative measure of the quality of overall patient care, like the other three measures of patient care developed in this study, is both a reliable and a valid measure. We now turn to a brief examination of the interrelationships among the four measures.

RELATIONSHIPS AMONG THE FOUR MEASURES OF PATIENT CARE

Table 27 presents the intercorrelations among the four measures of hospital patient care described in the preceding sections. All the intercorrelations are positive and statistically significant, as might be expected. Hospitals scoring high, or favorably, on any one measure are also likely to score high on each of the remaining measures, e.g., the better medical care hospitals also tend to be the ones which have better nursing care and better overall care. The degree of relationship between any two of the four measures, however, varies considerably, depending on the particular measures viewed. The highest relationship obtains between the two measures of the quality of overall care, these being correlated .96. The smallest relationship obtains between the medical care and the nursing care measures, these being correlated .60. Accordingly, these relationships show hospitals which score high on (noncomparative) overall care are much more likely to score high on comparative overall care than hospitals which score high on medical care are likely to score high on nursing care. The obvious reason for this condition is that the difference between medical and nursing care is greater than the difference between overall patient care and comparative overall patient care; both of the latter refer to the quality of total patient care, while each of the former represents one component of total care.

TABLE 27. Rank-order Intercorrelations Among Four Measures of Patient Care *

Patient Care Measures:	1	2	3	4
1. Measure of the quality of nursing care	—	.60	.91	.82
2. Measure of the quality of medical care		—	.67	.78
3. Measure of the quality of overall care			—	.96
4. Comparative measure of the quality of overall care				—

* All four measures have been described in this chapter. The correlations are based on an N of 10 hospitals in each case. Coefficients larger than .56 are significant at the .05 level, and those .75 or larger are significant at the .01 level.

When we compare the standing of the ten hospitals on the two measures of overall patient care, shown earlier in Table 24 and Table 25, we find that the top two hospitals on overall care are also the top two hospitals on comparative overall care, while the bottom two hospitals on the former measure are also the bottom two on the latter. The same is true when we consider the top three hospitals and the bottom three hospitals, or when we consider the top five hospitals and the remaining five hospitals. But when we compare the standing of the various hospitals on the nursing care measure, shown in Table 21, with their standing on the medical care measure, shown in Table 23, a variety of patterns emerges. For example, while Hospital #9 ties in first place with Hospital #3 on the quality of nursing care, it ranks fifth among the ten hospitals on the quality of medical care. Conversely, while Hospital #6 places second on the quality of medical care, it ranks sixth on nursing care among the ten institutions. Hospital #7, ranking fifth on nursing care but tenth on medical care, shows a reverse pattern. In general, these institutions tend to rank relatively high on either nursing care or medical care but not on both. Hospitals ranking high, or low, on both measures also exist. Hospital #3 ties in first place on nursing care and ranks third on medical care; Hospital #8 ranks fourth on both medical and nursing care; and Hospital #4 ranks third on nursing care and first on medical care. At the other extreme, Hospital #1 ranks tenth on nursing care and ninth on medical care; Hospital #2 ranks ninth on nursing care and seventh on medical care; and Hospital #0 ranks eighth on both medical and nursing care.

The above results show that hospitals having good medical care do not necessarily also have good nursing care, or vice versa, although on the average there is a significant tendency for the better medical care hospitals to be among the better nursing care hospitals, and vice versa—the correlation between medical care and nursing care being .60 for the hospitals in this study. In the light of this conclusion, those interested in assessing the quality of hospital patient care would do well to obtain separate measures of the quality of medical care and of the quality of nursing care.

The specific relationships among the four measures of patient care shown in Table 27 also suggest another important observation concerning the nature of the measures. On first inspection, since the two measures of overall patient care correlate .96, it might appear that these two measures could well be used interchangeably and that, therefore, either one of the two measures would suffice for assessing the quality of total patient care in hospitals. More careful study of the intercorrelations, however, suggests that the two measures of overall care do not behave alike in relation to nursing and medical care, i.e., do not produce the same relational patterns with the medical and nursing care measures. While the comparative measure of overall care correlates to about the same degree with medical care (.78) and with nursing care (.82), this is not true of the noncomparative measure of overall care. The latter correlates .91 with nursing care but only .67 with medical care—the first correlation accounting for about 80 percent of the variance and the second accounting for only 45 percent of the variance involved.[17]

These results provide one important reason for retaining both of the measures of overall care in subsequent analyses. Another reason for not treating these two measures as interchangeable is the fact that while the comparative measure was derived exclusively from an evaluation of overall care by medical respondents, the noncomparative measure is based on data from all four of the respondent groups involved in this part of the study. Still another important reason stems from theoretical considerations. Theoretically, rating the quality of overall patient care in a hospital, without reference to other similar hos-

[17] Further analysis along these lines might be directed toward ascertaining the specific effects and consequences of the quality of medical care, and of the quality of nursing care, for the quality of total patient care in the hospitals, whether total care is measured comparatively or noncomparatively. Such analysis would require, among other things, partial and multiple correlations between medical and nursing care, on the one hand, and total care on the other. Unfortunately, however, with only ten hospitals in the study, the application of partial and multiple correlation techniques would be methodologically unsound, being incapable of yielding accurate and conclusive results. The analysis here suggested, nevertheless, would be both an important and fruitful one to pursue in future studies which may include a larger number of hospitals than the present one.

pitals, is quite different from rating it by comparison to the care rendered by other institutions. And although in the present study the two ratings happened to correlate very highly, one can still conceive of cases where this correlation could be low. For instance, one can readily think of a hospital where, in absolute terms, the quality of overall care is moderately good but not excellent or outstanding. Now, were such a hospital to be located amidst a number of poor-care hospitals, it could be easily rated as providing excellent overall care by comparison. The reverse pattern is also conceivable; a moderately good-care hospital amidst excellent-care hospitals could well be rated comparatively as a rather poor-care institution. In view of the above considerations, in subsequent analyses, we shall treat all four of our patient care measures separately, including the two measures of overall care, even though the four measures cannot be considered as being independent of one another. Being all concerned with the quality of patient care in hospitals, as anticipated, the four measures are interrelated in the manner shown by the correlations in Table 27. And, parenthetically, the fact that the different measures intercorrelate significantly provides added confidence in the measures.

SUMMARY

Our task in this part of the study was to develop appropriate measures of patient care capable of distinguishing between better- and poorer-care hospitals. The main objective of this chapter was to present the several measures which we were able to develop. Following a discussion of the problems and issues of assessing the quality of patient care in hospitals, and a review of previously suggested approaches for measuring patient care, four measures were described in detail: (1) a measure of the quality of nursing care patients receive in the various hospitals based on the evaluation of nursing care by doctors, registered nurses, laboratory and x-ray technicians, and certain administrative respondents from each hospital; (2) a measure of the quality of medical care patients receive based on the evaluation of medical care by doctors from each hospital; (3) a measure of the quality of overall patient care based on the evaluation of overall care by the same respondents who evaluated nursing care; and (4) a comparative measure of the quality of overall patient care, i.e., the overall care in each hospital rated by comparison to the overall care in similar other hospitals, based on data from medical respondents.

With reference to each measure, the data used to derive the measure were first discussed, along with the rationale underlying the procedure of constructing the measure from the original data. Then, the measure was examined from the standpoint of its stability, or the consistency and reliability of the data on which it is based. Finally, certain findings from an analysis of supplementary data were reported in connection with each measure. This analysis was

Summary

mainly designed to test the validity of the measure, i.e., to ascertain whether or not the obtained measure in fact measures what it purports to measure.

Each measure of patient care was validated using a different set of data for this purpose. The nursing care measure was validated by comparing it against (1) data from hospital records regarding the composition of the nursing staff in the various hospitals, (2) questionnaire data on how good a job the nursing staff does for the hospital, and on how well the nursing department is doing in relation to what it should be accomplishing, and (3) volunteered comments by different respondents from each participating hospital about nursing care and the nursing staff. The medical care measure was validated by comparing it against (1) a special rating of the quality of medical care in the various hospitals performed by a group of outside doctors who were familiar with most or all of the hospitals in the study, (2) certain data from hospital medical records concerning the composition of the medical staff and patient death rates, (3) questionnaire data about the extent to which each hospital surpasses minimum accreditation requirements, (4) an evaluation of the quality of medical care by certain nonmedical respondents from each hospital, and (5) spontaneous, qualitative comments on the part of various respondents from each institution regarding medical care and the medical staff.

The overall care (noncomparative) measure was similarly validated by comparing it against (1) data on how well the patients speak of the hospital, according to medical and nonmedical respondents from each institution, (2) data about the reputation each hospital enjoys in its community, in the view of medical and nonmedical respondents, and (3) free, qualitative comments by various respondents about patient care in each hospital. Finally, the comparative measure of the quality of overall patient care was validated by comparing it with each of the other three measures of patient care developed in this study, and against certain data demonstrating that the medical respondents who rated overall patient care comparatively had a realistic frame of reference in terms of which to perform such a rating.

The last section of the chapter, following the presentation of the different measures, was devoted to a discussion of interrelationships among the measures. The four measures were found to be positively and significantly related with one another, as they normally should. However, as anticipated, the size of the particular intercorrelations was found to vary from a low of .60 to a high of .96, depending on the specific measures being considered. The smallest correlation was obtained between the nursing care measure and the medical care measure, while the highest was obtained between the comparative and the noncomparative measures of total patient care. These differential relationships are, of course, easily explained if one takes into account the fact that the former two measures represent aspects of hospital patient care that are more different than the aspects of patient care reflected in the latter two measures.

In summary, several important conclusions emerging from our discussions in the present chapter may be pointed out. First, the four measures of patient care which were developed in this study are sufficiently different from one another—excepting the single case when the two measures of overall care are compared with each other—to indicate a need for treating them separately in subsequent analyses and future studies. Second, each of the four measures discriminates well among the "better" and "poorer" patient care hospitals, according to the data. Third, in light of the multiple evidence presented in this chapter, the reliability and validity of each measure appear to be sufficiently high and adequate to warrant confidence in its use. Fourth, the nature of the obtained measures makes it possible to compare, contrast, and rank-order the ten hospitals in the study successfully with respect to the quality of nursing, medical, and overall care which they provide their patients. Finally, because of these characteristics of the measures, it becomes possible to relate, in later chapters, the quality of patient care to other important aspects of hospital structure and functioning. Before engaging in this task, however, we shall take up the subject of internal coordination which, like patient care, constitutes a major objective in this research.

REFERENCES

1. Babcock, K. B. "Accreditation," *Hospitals,* **34**:43, (April) 1960.
2. Bachrach, C. A. "The Patient Record as a Source of Useful Statistics," *Hospitals,* **29**:67–71, (Oct.) 1955.
3. Commission on Professional and Hospital Activities. Report 13: The Medical Audit Program. Commission on Professional and Hospital Activities, Ann Arbor, Mich., 1960.
4. ———— The Professional Activity Study. Commission on Professional and Hospital Activities, Ann Arbor, Mich., 1960.
5. Danhorst, H. E. Department Heads Make the Hospital. *Mod. Hosp.,* **84**:81–82, (Jan.) 1955.
6. Davis, M. M. *Medical Care for Tomorrow.* New York: Harper, 1955.
7. Dichter, E. "A Psychological Study of the Hospital-Patient Relationship: How 'Secure' Is Your Hospital?" *Mod. Hosp.,* **83**:61–63, (Nov.) 1954.
8. ———— "A Psychological Study of the Hospital-Patient Relationship: What the Patient *Really Wants* from the Hospital." *Mod. Hosp.,* **83**:51–54 and 136, (Sept.) 1954.
9. Furstenberg, F. F., Taback, M., Goldberg, H., and Davis, J. W. "Prescribing an Index to Quality of Medical Care: A Study of the Baltimore City Medical Care Program," *Am. J. Pub. Health,* **43**:1299–309, (Oct.) 1953.
10. Georgopoulos, B. S., and Tannenbaum, A. S. "A Study of Organizational Effectiveness," *Amer. Sociol. Rev.,* **22**:534–40, 1957.
11. Goldwater, S. S. *On Hospitals.* New York: Macmillan, 1947.
12. Hawley, P. R. "Evaluation of the Quality of Patient Care," *Am. J. Pub. Health,* **45**:1533–537, (Dec.) 1955.
13. ———— "Hospital Standards Are for Patients," *Mod. Hosp.,* **80**:51–53, (Jan.) 1953.
14. Hill, F. T. "Maintenance of Professional Standards," *Mod. Hosp.,* **67**:86–88, (July) 1946.

References

15. Howland, D., et al. "The Development of Methodology for the Evaluation of Patient Care." Mimeographed progress notes, Parts I-III, Operations Research Group, Ohio State University, 1958.
16. Johnson, L. W. "Make the Most of the Medical Audit," *Mod. Hosp.*, 84:96-104, (April) 1955.
17. ——— "Questions Concerning the Medical Audit," *Mod. Hosp.*, 84:106-12, (March) 1955.
18. Jones, E. W. "The Hospital is Only as Good as its Medical Staff," *Mod. Hosp.*, 70:54-55, (Jan.) 1948.
19. Kahn, R. L., and Katz, D. "Leadership Practices in Relation to Productivity and Morale." In Cartwright, D., and Zander, A. (eds.). *Group Dynamics: Research and Theory*. Evanston, Ill.: Row, Peterson, 612-28, 1953.
20. King, F. "So You Meet Minimum Standards, but What About the Maximum?" *Mod. Hosp.*, 66:50-51, (April) 1946.
21. Kossack, C. F. "To Measure the Quality of a Hospital," *Mod. Hosp.*, 81:71-79, (July) 1953.
22. *Lancet*. "What Makes a Good Hospital?" *Lancet*, 1:633-34, (April) 1950.
23. Lederer, H. D. "How the Sick View Their World," *J. Soc. Issues*, 8:4-15, 1952.
24. Lembcke, P. A. "Lack of Data Complicates Hospital Care Comparison," *Pub. Health Rep.*, 70:198-99, (Feb.) 1955.
25. MacEachern, M. T. "Examining the Present Status of the Medical Audit," *Hospitals*, 26:49-51 and 71-73, (Dec.) 1952.
26. McGibony, J. R. *Principles of Hospital Administration*. New York: Putnam, 1952.
27. *Modern Hospital*. "A.M.A. Committee to Review Accreditation," *Mod. Hosp.*, 85:49-52, (July) 1955.
28. Moench, L. G. "Reaction of the Medical Patient to Hospitalization," *Rocky Mountain M. J.* 52:519-25, (Jan.) 1955.
29. Mooi, H. R. "Doctors Do Take Records Seriously," *Mod. Hosp.*, 83:59-61, (July) 1954.
30. Myers, R. S. "Hospital Statistics Don't Tell the Truth," *Mod. Hosp.*, 83:53-54, (July) 1954.
31. Myers, R. S. and Babcock, K. B. "Committees Make the Staff a Team," *Mod. Hosp.*, 83:64, (Nov.) 1954.
32. Myers, R. S., and Slee, V. N. "Medical Statistics Tell the Story at a Glance," *Mod. Hosp.*, 93:72-75, (Sept.) 1959.
33. O'Malley, M., and Kossack, C. F. "A Statistical Study of Factors Influencing the Quality of Patient Care in Hospitals," *Am. J. Pub. Health*, 40:1428-436, (Nov.) 1950.
34. Phenix, F. L. "Coordination of Services," *Physical Therapy Review*, 35:229-34, (May) 1955.
35. Reader, G. G., Pratt, L., and Mudd, M. C. "What Patients Expect from Their Doctors," *Mod. Hosp.*, 89:88-94, (July) 1957.
36. Rourke, A. J. J. "Must Minimum Standards Be So Minimum?" *Mod. Hosp.*, 85:81-82 and 146-48, (Aug.) 1955.
37. Sewall, L. G., and Berger, D. G. "A Medical Audit Plan for Psychiatric Hospitals," *Mental Hospitals*, 10:7-9, 1959.
38. Sheps, M. C. "Approaches to Measuring Hospital Care Quality," *Pub. Health Rep.*, 70:198, (Feb.) 1955.
39. ——— "Approaches to the Quality of Patient Care." *Pub. Health Rep.*, 70:877-86, (Sept.) 1955.
40. Slee, V. N. "Statistics Influence Medical Practice," *Mod. Hosp.*, 83:55-58, (July) 1954.

41. Smith, A. W. "The Medical Audit Gives the Answer," *Mod. Hosp.*, **80**:88–91 and 144, (March) 1953.

42. Veterans Administration, Department of Medicine and Surgery. Report of the Committee on Measurement of the Quality of Medical Care. Department of Medicine and Surgery, Veterans Administration, Washington, D.C., 1959.

6 ORGANIZATIONAL COORDINATION[1]

One of the paramount and most difficult problems faced by all complex organizations is the problem of internal coordination—how best to fit things together, gearing resources and facilities to attain the objectives of the organization in the most effective manner. In this study, like patient care, coordination occupies a prominent place, constituting one of our major research objectives. But what does the problem of coordination involve, and why is it so important?

The need for achieving and maintaining adequate coordination is by no means peculiar to social systems alone. Most complex systems, whether social or mechanical, are confronted with coordination requirements. In fact, any structure which consists of multiple parts that have some relation to one another has to come to terms with the question of articulating these parts into a coherent whole. From an organizational standpoint, for example, a new car is neither a decorative object nor a pile of undifferentiated metal. It is a rather intricate instrument, consisting of numerous parts that are arranged, according to certain ordering principles, in precise positions, each part being designed to perform a given function at a certain time and in relation to the functions performed by other parts, so that in the end the system as a whole can accomplish a certain objective—in this case, controlled self-motion. This arrangement, or articulation of parts according to certain temporal and spatial principles, is a matter of coordination. In the case of a new car the problem of coordination has been solved mechanically, at least for the time being. It will arise again with use, or if any of the parts in the system get out of gear. Then adjustments, or repairs, may be needed in order to improve or reestablish coordination.

Next, take a look at your watch and think for a moment of what is going

[1] We are indebted to Dr. Paul E. Mott, Ph.D., for his contribution to the part of the study dealing with coordination. Although he joined our staff, as Assistant Study Director, after the data had been collected, he became centrally involved in the analytical phases of the research, and he wrote preliminary drafts for several sections of Chapter 6 and Chapter 7.

on inside it. If you are willing to risk it, better yet, open the back cover and glance inside. What you will see is many gears, parts, and gadgets that are arranged in certain ways to work in relation to each other's functions; little wheels and big wheels interlocking, fixed at certain points, and a wound-up spring providing the needed pressure to be transmitted through the wheels, so as to produce and maintain a certain movement which enables you to read hours, minutes, and seconds on the face of the mechanism. The various parts of the watch are "coordinated," and as long as they remain adequately coordinated you will be able to tell the time. If one or more parts happen to be disturbed or removed, the whole thing goes awry—if it does not indeed break down completely—and you no longer have the correct time.

In a gross way, you have just studied the coordination of a mechanical system, but this is only of peripheral importance to you as well as to us. Leaving mechanical systems aside, therefore, let us move to the consideration of human ones. First, let us view a single human being. Any nurse will be able to give you a fair account of what would happen if insulin were withheld from a diabetic patient, if ice chips were applied on the forehead of a patient with high fever, or if a shot of Adrenalin were administered to another. She will be less likely, however, to elaborate for you the various underlying connections among the functions of affected body organs in each case, although it is certain that, if you ask her, she will make it clear for you that the deficiency of one specialized organ somehow affects other organs and the balance of the organism is thrown off—the formerly healthy person gets sick.

The point is that the complex organization, called human body, to function properly, must maintain a certain chemothermal equilibrium. To achieve adequate balance, its various organs must each function according to the needs, or requirements, of the others and of the total system. If a deficiency or disturbance occurs in some organ it must be corrected, or compensated for by other organs, so that the equilibrium of the organism may be re-established to a satisfactory degree.[2] The human body as a system provides an excellent illustration of the problem of coordination. Specific physical parts of the body are articulated with one another, physiological and chemical processes are geared to each other, and both affect the psychomotor functions and well-being of the total organism. Like automobiles, watches, and human beings, complex social organizations, such as the hospital, all have their share in the problem of coordination.

Let us next consider a fairly simple social system. If you have ever seen a football game, you saw two opposing teams, together with some officials, in action. Each team was an organization—a social system. And, forgetting

---

[2] Whether equilibrium is re-established through general homeostasis, through specific compensatory activity, or through medico-surgical intervention and treatment is another matter, which for the moment is irrelevant. What is relevant and important is the idea of coordination itself.

Organizational Coordination

for the moment the other team, the officials, and the audience, that system was organized to play a particular game. The term "organized," among other things, immediately implies and suggests coordination phenomena, both in the physical sense (motor coordination of players) and the organizational sense (role and task coordination among players). In the football field, and for a given team, in addition to the precise bodily movements of the players, a number of specialized skills and assignments had to be articulated with one another into a coherent pattern so that cooperative effort could be maximized and unnecessary duplications, errors, and interference could be minimized. Each player, not unlike the parts in our automobile or watch, had to work in terms of what others had to do, or were doing. Furthermore, and more importantly, he had to understand each play and think in terms of the needs and problems of his teammates, while participating in its execution. Positions in the team, player skills, and task assignments had all to be coordinated in time and space.

The Problem of This Chapter and of Chapter 7

As we move from relatively simple mechanical or "closed" systems, through transient social systems such as a football team in action, into more complex social systems such as a hospital, coordination phenomena become more complex and more important to society. Indeed, the very concept of coordination becomes more difficult to grasp and more difficult to study. This is especially true of those social organizations which, while they demand the varied skills of many specialists and the accomplishment of many particular tasks by different people working interdependently, are not amenable to extensive routinization and mechanization. For some organizations, e.g., power plants and oil refineries, automation itself is a major mechanism (if not the main one) of internal coordination.[3] For most large-scale organizations, however, coordination is dependent upon human activity mechanisms and, more or less, continuous efforts and adjustments on the part of the members of the organization. In social systems there is not such a thing as a perfect state of coordination. The factors giving rise to the need for coordination, the principal means of coordination, and the coordination problems requiring solution are to be found in the efforts and interactions of people—in the social and psychological forces which characterize the organizational situation. The hospital as an organization is no exception in this respect.

More than an assembly line or a football team in action, the hospital represents a case of remarkable differentiation and specialization of skills and activities, and of divided authority and responsibility among its members.

---

[3] Automation is here used in the same sense in which Diebold (5) and Mann and Hoffman (12) employ the concept, i.e., it is used to refer to the continuous electronic or mechanical monitoring and feedback of information to maintain the functioning of a production system within specified limits.

Indeed, one would have great difficulty, even in present-day society, finding any other organization whose internal differentiation and structural heterogeneity could match that of a large hospital, excluding the interesting case of complex government systems. (A large university might approximate a hospital in this respect, but it seldom faces the imperative of dealing with acute emergency conditions.) Between patient admission and discharge, workflow processes in the hospital are carried out by a staggering variety of people—people ranging in education, skill, training, and status from the most highly professionalized physician to the most unskilled dishwasher, from the trained graduate nurse to the untrained aide, from the specialized laboratory technician to the maintenance man who is a jack of all trades, and from the hospital administrator who is in charge of hundreds of nonmedical personnel of varying backgrounds to the messenger who is only in charge of himself. In fact, in his study of one hospital, Wessen (21) reports that there were 23 different occupations represented in a *single* ward.

But the many roles and activities represented in a hospital are neither unrelated nor independent of one another. They are, on the contrary, mutually complementary or supplementary, all focusing and converging on the common objective of providing adequate treatment and care to the patient. Every person working in the hospital, irrespective of his authority, professional role, and organizational position, and regardless of skill and training, depends on some other person or persons in the process of performing his particular role or tasks. For example, the doctor depends on the nurse, and vice versa, they both depend on the dietitian or the laboratory technician, and the patient depends on all of them. Because of this internal differentiation of roles and activities which characterizes the action structure of the hospital, and because of the interdependence of its parts, the need for coordination and integration is both inevitable and essential. The various elements in the system, as Parsons and his associates observe, "must be coordinated either negatively, in the sense of the avoidance of disruptive interference with one another, or positively, in the sense of contributing to the realization of certain shared collective goals through collaborated activity" (15, p. 197). Furthermore, because internal differentiation is so extensive and so highly developed in hospitals, the question of coordination is a crucial one to the effective functioning of organizational units and of the total system. For the same reason, the hospital provides an excellent site for the study of coordination phenomena in all their complexity.

The main problem of this chapter and of the next one is to study organizational coordination in hospitals as a phenomenon in its own right before examining, in later chapters, the importance of coordination for other aspects of hospital functioning, especially patient care and organizational performance. The main objective of the two chapters is to measure coordination and identify factors which make for more adequate coordination in the hospital, as a total system, and in one of its key units, the nursing department. Using coordination as a dependent variable, our task is fourfold: (1) to clarify the nature of the concept and specify its main aspects; (2) to measure organizational coordination in hospitals; (3) to specify conditions and variables which are expected to be associated with adequate or good coordination; and (4) to test a number of corresponding hypotheses about coordination in the next chapter. And, although it is the community general hospital which provides the site and context for this study, theoretically, our approach is not confined to hospital organization alone. It could be easily applied to most social systems, particularly other large-scale organizations, including industrial ones.

The contents of the present chapter have been organized into three main sections. In the first section, below, we will be concerned with some further theoretical considerations about coordination in an attempt to elaborate some of the most important aspects of this concept. In the second section, we will describe and examine our measures of coordination. In the third section, we will specify several sets of variables that are expected to affect coordination, i.e., certain categories of independent or conditioning variables. The measures of these independent variables and the findings which establish relationships between them and organizational coordination in the hospital will be presented and discussed in the next chapter.

THEORETICAL CONSIDERATIONS: THE CONCEPT OF ORGANIZATIONAL COORDINATION

One of the main impacts of the Industrial Revolution on society was the destruction of the old home and guild industries, where each worker embodied all skills essential to the manufacture of some product. The newly emerged complex machine technology was much too severe a competitor for the small home manufacturer. It produced more goods more rapidly, more efficiently, and of uniform and perhaps superior quality compared with that of the home versions of the same products. However, it also demanded a span of skills beyond the comprehension of any one individual worker. The worker, formerly sufficiently skilled to complete the entire product, now sought to master only a segment of the productive process. Thus, the expanding machine technology was giving rise to an age of specialization and the development of modern large-scale organizations.[4] In the process, specialists in pursuing their goals came to depend on other specialists, both across organizations and within the same organization. This meant that, for an organization to attain its objective, a conscious effort to articulate the varied activities of its many specialists had to be made. The problem of coordination, relatively insignificant in earlier times, now assumed great importance.

[4] For a specific illustration of this evolution of specialization, and a discussion of accompanying consequences, see Warner and Low's study of the shoe industry (19).

An analogous chain of events was at work in the hospital field. When Lister and his colleagues, for example, introduced aseptic techniques in hospital practice, a new set of functions was created. Similarly, the role of nurse evolved in response to newly created requirements. Whereas nurses at an earlier period were often recruited from such strange places as prisons, they now had to be recruited from schools giving special training in the techniques of the emerging profession. Along with the development of new functions and specialists, medical techniques and equipment rapidly expanded in scope and range to an extent beyond the ability of any single mind to master. Consequently, the division of labor increased many times over. Furthermore, the expense and knowledge required for the use of new and extensive techniques and equipment prevented physicians from being able to operate effectively as independent practitioners. The centralization and easy availability of such techniques and equipment in hospitals, however, made it possible for doctors to avail themselves both of superior equipment and of the talents of many medical specialists and, thus, to provide their patients with more adequate care. But, with this extensive variety of specialists in medicine, nursing, and other areas (some of whom did not even work directly for the organization, as in the case of the large majority of doctors), the hospital faced the problem of coordinating these numerous and highly diversified roles and activities on behalf of the patient. Moreover, problems of coordination assumed special significance here because the organizational product was neither shoes nor cars but the health and well-being of people—a product so highly and so unquestionably valued by society.

Coordination Defined

Historically, these are some of the most important factors which gave rise to complex coordination phenomena in large organizations, among which the modern hospital is only one important organizational species. Considered together, these factors suggest that coordination presupposes three essential elements: (1) division of labor among organizational members; (2) specialization of organizational roles and functions; and (3) interdependence among members, roles, and functions arising from division of labor and specialization. In commensal relationships, where all of the members of the organization perform the same, similar, or parallel functions, the problem of articulating their activities is almost by definition nonexistent. It is the condition of functional interdependence among organizational parts and operations—the fact that organizational activities are contingent on one another rather than independent—that gives rise to the need for coordination processes. Coordination processes are those organizational processes through which functionally interdependent parts and activities in the system are articulated with one another so as to ensure the system will operate effectively. The adequacy of coordination, or producing sufficient articulation which enables the hos-

The Concept of Organizational Coordination

pital to achieve its objectives, constitutes an important object of research in the present study.

Organizational coordination is often confused with organizational effectiveness, and a great deal of care is required to avoid such a pitfall. Adequate coordination is necessary to effective organizational functioning, but it is not a sufficient condition by itself. Other important factors such as quality of skill, technology, and adequacy of organizational resources and facilities, human as well as material ones, must too be taken into account to ensure organizational effectiveness. Organizational effectiveness says something about how well an organization is doing in achieving its objectives, while coordination says something about the articulation of diverse organizational parts and functions. Coordination, in Goldwater's words, "suggests a more perfect adaptation of means to ends" (9, p. 14), while effectiveness suggests successful attainment of ends. Since, in a later chapter, we will also want to study the relationship between coordination and quality of patient care in hospitals, the concepts of coordination and effectiveness should be kept theoretically distinct.[5]

Sometimes coordination is also confused with decision making and administrative expertness. However, as Simon points out, these are two different concepts: "Coordination should be clearly distinguished from *expertise*. Expertise involves the adoption of a *good* decision. Coordination (on the other hand) is aimed at the adoption by all the members of the group of the *same* decision, or more precisely of mutually consistent decisions in combination attaining the established goal" (17, p. 139).

The term "goal" itself—or organizational objective as we are using the concept—also requires some clarification in relation to coordination. It is sometimes implied in the literature that coordination can be studied only with reference to specific goals, and an organization may have several such goals. According to this position, it could be argued that what may be adequate coordination with respect to a given goal may be detrimental with respect to a second goal. This argument, however, assumes that organizations have mutually contradictory goals. And while it is not impossible that this may be the case with respect to various secondary objectives of an organization, it could hardly apply to the overall goals, or main objectives, of the system. If the system-wide objectives of an organization were contradictory with one another, that organization would not last very long. A proposition to the contrary would be very difficult to maintain. First, it is unlikely that an organization can come into being, and then survive, while pursuing system-wide objectives which are incompatible or contradictory. Second, while short-run incompatibilities among the system-wide objectives of an organization may conceivably arise, long-term incompatibilities of this kind are very unlikely, if at all possible, without jeopardizing the integrity of the organization. Al-

---

[5] For a detailed discussion of the concept of organizational effectiveness, see Georgopoulos and Tannenbaum, "A Study of Organizational Effectiveness" (8).

most by definition, an organization is identifiable as a distinct system partly because it has certain major objectives which are different from those of other types of organizations. With respect to coordination, it is these major objectives that deserve special attention.

The major objectives of an organization are not only important in their own right, i.e., as desirable ends, but they also constitute the essence of the controlling principle in the organizational system. As Feibleman and Friend point out, "it is not simply the fact of linkages but rather the principle according to which all linkages fall together into one controlling order, which makes an organization" (7, p. 21). And, it is the major objectives of the organization which define this "principle." The main purpose of a rifle, as an organizational system for example, is to discharge a bullet at high velocity toward a target. The principle of organization of the various parts of the rifle serves to implement this main function, and it represents something different from the parts themselves or their respective "goals," i.e., their specific tasks. It becomes patently important for the study of coordination not to confuse overriding organizational objectives that are systemwide with the subgoals of particular organizational parts. The latter may, at times, be at variance with the overall goals or with one another, but even then this would provide the very *raison d'être* for organizational coordination.

The concept of organizational coordination should, therefore, be geared to the overall objectives of organizations—to the "wholeness" of the system. As Barnard puts it, "what is required is a sense of things as a whole, the persistent subordination of parts to the total, the discrimination from the broadest standpoint of the strategic factors from among all types of factors . . ." (1, p. 256). What is required is that the main objective, or the system-wide objectives, of the organization be taken into consideration. In most large-scale organizations, Georgopoulos and Tannenbaum (8) observe, the main objectives of the system include such things as: high output, whether quantitatively or qualitatively, or both; adjustment to endogenous and exogenous changes; and the preservation of human and material resources and facilities. In hospitals, the first and the last goal, the primary and ultimate objective of the system is to provide adequate patient care and treatment to those persons who enter the system as patients, eventually releasing them to their community with their health restored. It is this system-wide objective that provides the organizing principle and controlling order for the community general hospital. All other goals, such as research, education, employment, etc., are subservient to the paramount goal of patient care. Hospital people at all levels and in all roles are both very conscious and very outspoken on this point.

One final caution is in order before defining the concept of organizational coordination. Coordination should not be equated with cooperation. The latter may affect the former, and the former may facilitate the latter, but they are two different concepts. Cooperation means working together for the accomplishment of some goal, while coordination means that the efforts and work activities of group members are regulated, articulated, and related to one another in certain ways, in terms of time and space and according to certain principles. And, while people who cooperate with one another within an organization may have or share a common goal, the goal they share need not necessarily be one sponsored by the organization as a whole system, as Simon (17) has indicated. In the case that it is not an organizational objective members are pursuing, moreover, their "cooperative" activity may actually be detrimental both to coordination and to organizational functioning. In summary, therefore, coordination must be conceptually differentiated from such other phenomena as organizational effectiveness, administrative expertness, and cooperation.

Coordination presupposes division of labor among organizational members, specialization of organizational roles and functions, and a certain amount of interdependence among them. It involves those organizational processes through which functionally interdependent parts and activities in the system are interrelated and articulated with one another so as to ensure the system as a whole will move in a desired direction.[6] Articulation is achieved by means of combining, ordering, and arranging the differentiated elements of the organization into proper time sequences and space positions, and into definitive functional relationships with one another and with the total organizational system. These processes take place according to the means-ends dimensions of the organization, and are aimed toward the prevention and correction of overlappings, duplications, errors, conflicts, and waste on the part of organizational members, and toward the channeling of concerted member efforts in the direction of the overall objectives of the system.

Coordination may, therefore, be viewed as representing the internal adjustment state and processes of articulation in a system; and adequacy of coordination may be viewed as representing the degree to which the various parts and activities of an organization are adjusted in relation to one another and in relation to the whole system. In line with this position, we propose the following definition for the concept of organizational coordination: *Coordination represents the extent to which the various interdependent parts of an organization function each according to the needs and requirements of the other parts and of the total system.* Of course, the preceding detailed discussion of the concept provides a more accurate and more thorough definition; the brief definition here can only give us a shorthand version of the phenomenon which it represents.

[6] In a discussion of the significance of coordination for collective planning and organizational behavior, Mary Parker Follett made a similar observation nearly 30 years ago. After contrasting coordination with *laissez faire,* she spoke of it both as a continuing process of organizational self-adjustment, and as "the reciprocal relating of all the factors in a situation" (14, p. 297–314).

Bases and Means of Coordination

All factors which give rise to the need for coordination constitute the bases of coordination. There are many such factors in organizations. Most of them, however, can be subsumed under the three general factors which we have already indicated: division of labor, specialization, and interdependence. The division of labor, accompanied as it is by specialization of functions, creates the initial basis of coordination. It is the condition of functional interdependence, however, that constitutes the basic need for coordination in organizations. Each specialty in a system, as Hawley (11) points out, contains its own unique set of functions and rhythms. But, if each set of functions were carried out without concern for other functions in the system, it would have no meaning. It is only when the various sets of specialized functions are linked together, according to some organizing principle, or for the purpose of contributing to the realization of the objectives of the system, that they gain meaning and utility. This linking together illustrates the concept of functional interdependence.

Functional interdependence means that the various roles, skills, and activities in an organization must come into play at the appropriate time and place, and in a certain order, if the organization is to achieve its objectives. The various sets of functions of specialized parts in the system must complement or supplement each other, in a manner that maximizes the convergence of diverse efforts on a given target and minimizes interference or disruptions in the process. Think, for example, of what it takes in order to process an emergency case in the hospital from the point of admission to the point of discharge or, better yet, consider all that is involved in performing an operation on a patient, and you immediately realize both the fact of interdependence and the sequence of events such interdependence entails—a sequence which demands timing and ordering of workflow, with certain things taking priority over others and all things being articulated into a coherent pattern.[7]

In mass-producing organizations, such as an automobile assembly line, much of the timing, spacing, and articulation of activities is accomplished by the use of machines, i.e., through mechanical coordination. Organizations with lower levels of routinization and mechanization such as a hospital, however, require the expenditure of considerable and continuous human effort to achieve and maintain adequate coordination. In these organizations, moreover, it is difficult to evaluate how well the system is functioning, and this is even more difficult if coordination is not well developed. The motivation

---

[7] In their description of the operating room, Burling, Lentz, and Wilson (2, pp. 260–72) give a graphic account of the interdependence and teamwork involved in the performance of operations. Elsewhere, Turner speaks of teamwork as "the bedrock of the hospital structure" (18), and Phenix (16) makes a good case for the need of coordinating various services in the hospital.

Bases and Means of Coordination

to evaluate the effectiveness of the system and of its parts—almost a universal phenomenon arising from a desire to maximize the economic posture or improve the standing of one's organization—constitutes a rather subtle basis of coordination. In many cases, the only way to evaluate the performance of various parts of the system is to relate and compare them with one another and evaluate the relative contribution of each. This process implies coordination.

Another basis for coordination arises out of the inevitability that certain parts in the system come to be more influential than others. As Hawley (11) suggests, differential influence among organizational parts or groups is characteristic of most organizations, which stems from the fact that certain parts in the system have greater control over the allocation of resources and facilities. But, when such a hierarchy of parts is developed on the basis of the type and amount of resources each part controls, an accompanying tendency by the less dominant parts to align themselves with the more dominant parts also develops. This tendency, coupled with the motivation of the dominant parts to structure the system so as to maximize their own objectives, results in a need for organizational coordination in order to avoid throwing the system out of equilibrium. This need for checks and balances entails coordinative activity.

If these are the major bases of coordination, what are the means for achieving coordination? The range of methods and mechanisms by which coordination may be attained in large-scale organizations is almost infinite. The process of coordination may be formal or informal and, in either case, it may be intentional or unintentional. Organizations often create administrative and liaison positions and committees, whose main purpose is coordination. In fact, the authors know of one industrial organization which has gone much further in this direction, by establishing the position of "coordinator of management methods." Similarly, some hospitals have a so-called "Joint Conference Committee," consisting of trustees, doctors, and the administrator, whose main functions include coordination. In other cases, various functional roles in the organization are assigned a good deal of coordinative responsibility as, for example, the role of the registered nurse in the hospital. Sometimes, as suggested above, parts of the system will also line themselves up with a more dominant part without any intentional effort at coordination.

The constitution, bylaws, and other written documents of an organization also serve as instruments of coordination. The patient chart in the hospital, for example, constitutes a mechanism of coordination of efforts among medical, nursing, and administrative staffs. Formal and informal meetings, conferences, and exchanges among organizational members whose activities are in some way related illustrate additional means of coordination. The system of superior-subordinate relationships in organizations constitutes, among other things, a mechanism for coordinating activities. Finally, one of the less obvious but more important means of coordination is to be found in the attitudes and values of organizational members. The development of common norms, shared expectations, and mutual understanding among different people in the system is probably the best guarantee that adequate coordination can be achieved and maintained. Alongside the administrative plans and directives, alongside the written rules and regulations, and alongside all other aspects of the formal organizational structure are these extensive and often all too important informal aspects.

The motivations, expectations, and attitudes of organizational members constitute powerful social-psychological forces which, if neglected, could make the problem of coordination very formidable. If properly channeled, on the other hand, so as to supplement and support the formal plans and means of coordination, the task of coordination will be correspondingly easier. There are several reasons for this assertion. First, no formal plan can be expected to provide complete and detailed prescriptions for all organizational activities in all their complexity and ramifications. Second, even if this were possible, such a plan would be difficult to communicate to organizational members. Third, even if successful communication were assured, members would find it difficult to comprehend the plan thoroughly and follow its prescriptions. Fourth, the preceding requirements rest on the assumption that members accept the basic objectives of the organization and are willing to follow the coordination plans and programs presented to them. Finally, even if such acceptance and willingness were present, coordination still could not be guaranteed. What would be required, in addition, is that members develop and maintain shared frames of reference and mutual expectations which will enable them to relate their own performances to those of other members.

Planning, communication, and sharedness or complementarity of expectations among members, all constitute important means for coordination. Under each, a number of more specific items can be easily subsumed. In a hospital, for example, planning includes a variety of activities, ranging from the structuring of member roles and functions (e.g., the role of the nurse in relation to the role of the doctor with respect to the patient or with respect to one another, or the role of the administrator in relation to the role of trustees and the role of doctors), through the articulation of work among different shifts, to the establishment of routines and schedules for the everyday activities of different departments. Communication, in addition to written rules and regulations or other documents governing the work relationships and performances of organizational members, includes telephone conversations and intercommunication devices, formal and informal meetings, the "grapevine," and a host of other things all of which can serve as coordination mechanisms. Social-psychological mechanisms include such things as the extent of mutual or reciprocal understanding between doctors and nurses, or between doctors and trustees, the ease with which members can communicate with one another about their work relationships or about common problems, the readiness of people in interrelated jobs to assist each other when needed, the willingness of people to accept and follow rules and regulations, and similar other factors. Potentially, all of these can serve as means of coordination.

Types of Coordination

Regardless of the coordination means employed or emphasized in a given organization, coordinative behavior may vary according to its particular scope, or according to the objectives to which it is directed and the motivations underlying it. For example, coordinative activity may be initiated in response to an existing problem; it may be initiated to prevent certain problems from arising at all; or it may be initiated without any reference to a particular problem in order, for instance, to implement a new plan. Accordingly, it is possible and convenient to group coordinative activities into various types. In the present study, we have distinguished four major types: *corrective, preventive, regulatory,* and *promotive* coordination.

If the particular objective of a set of coordinative activities is to rectify an error or to correct a dysfunction in the system after it has occurred, the type of coordination involved is corrective. If, for example, the chief of the medical staff discovered that the x-ray department was having difficulty in sending its reports to the surgery division on time and he developed a schedule which, if implemented, would expedite the routing of the reports, he would be engaging in corrective coordination. On the other hand, if he had anticipated that unless such a schedule were developed the above problem would have arisen, and he had developed the schedule in question to forestall or avoid the problem, he would have been engaged in preventive coordination. While corrective coordination takes place after a problem has occurred, preventive coordination takes place in anticipation of a problem of malfunction.

Another type of coordination does not involve cognizance of any particular malfunctions or problems, whether in retrospect or anticipation. Rather it is aimed at the maintenance of the status quo of the system, i.e., it is aimed at the preservation of existing structural and functional arrangements in the organization. Essentially a conservative activity, this type of coordination may be called regulatory. Still a different type of coordination is involved in the case where a positive attempt is made to improve the articulation of the parts of the system, or to improve the existing organizational arrangements, without regard for a specific problem. Such coordination activity does not stem from an awareness of particular problems in the system, or from a depth of understanding of organizational imperatives, but rather from the simple assumption that the system is imperfectly coordinated, at any given time, and that there is always some room for improvement. The type of coordination represented by such a positive attempt may be called promotive coordination.

An organization may be more likely to engage in some of these four types of coordination than others, and this may have corresponding implications for the system. Regardless of which is the prevalent type in a particular organization, however, most organizations at one time or another engage in all four types. Furthermore, a given set of coordinative activities may involve two types of coordination at the same time, e.g., it may involve both preventive and promotive coordination. The four types discussed here, therefore, are intended to serve as convenient devices for organizing data rather than to suggest that all coordination phenomena in an organization are purely corrective, preventive, regulatory, or promotive. As analytical devices, these may be very important tools, for what makes for good coordination of a given type may not necessarily make for good coordination of another type. Adequate promotive coordination, for example, may require certain things not required by adequate corrective coordination, and vice versa.

We have just differentiated coordinative activities into four types, according to their particular scope in each case. Other kinds of differentiation are also possible. We will mention one of these here because it has already received some attention in the literature. According to this way of looking at coordination phenomena, all coordinative activities in an organization may be divided into two broad categories: those which involve programming, and those which do not. In this study, we will refer to the former as *programed coordination,* and to the latter as *general coordination.* The concept of programed coordination, as used here, corresponds closely to what March and Simon (13) have called "coordination by plan," while the concept of general coordination is similar to what they have called "coordination by feedback."

Programed coordination concentrates primarily on a special set of the means of coordination which we have discussed earlier, namely those means listed under planning. Furthermore, in contrast to general coordination, programed coordination does not emphasize the importance of social-psychological forces such as motivation, reciprocal understanding, and complementary expectations among organizational members. Rather, it proceeds mainly according to pre-established schedules and involves an approach which relies on the specification of functions to be associated with the various roles in the organization. On the basis of this specification, activities are "programed," i.e., they are timed and regulated, and role linkages in the system are established and articulated to fit the program involved. General coordination, on the other hand, makes allowance for adjustments which are required to meet organizational needs that arise in the day-to-day operations of the system—needs that cannot be satisfied through advance formal planning. Most activity in most organizations is neither sufficiently routinized nor sufficiently predictable to permit exclusive, or even predominant, reliance on programed coordination. Thus, organizations engage in both programed and general coordination. Finally, since programed coordination could be initiated with respect to any of the objectives that correspond to the four types of coordination described above (i.e., corrective, preventive, regulatory, and promotive), we shall refer to it as a major category of coordination activity rather than as a type of coordination. And, the same applies for general, or nonprogramed, coordination.

MEASUREMENT OF COORDINATION IN HOSPITALS

Coordination was conceptualized as the degree of articulation among interdependent organizational parts, and was viewed as representing the processes of adjustment associated with such articulation. More specifically, coordination was defined as the extent to which the various interdependent parts of an organization function each according to the needs and requirements of the other parts and of the total system. A distinction was furthermore made between programed and general coordinative activity, and four types of coordination—preventive, corrective, regulatory, and promotive—were described.

The measures of coordination we employed in this study have been geared to different types of coordination and were designed to represent both categories of coordinative activity, i.e., programed and general or nonprogramed. The main purpose of the measures is to provide us with an indication of the adequacy of overall coordination in the various hospitals, distinguishing between better-coordinated and less well-coordinated institutions. Therefore, all measures use the hospital as the unit of analysis, i.e., they were constructed to refer to the hospital as a total system rather than to individual units within the hospital. One section of the next chapter, however, will be specifically devoted to coordination in a key hospital unit—the nursing department. There, instead of the total hospital, the nursing department will serve as the unit of analysis.

The Measures of Coordination

The task of devising measures for a concept such as coordination is at best a complex one, partly because of lack of sufficient prior research in this area and partly because the concept is not easy to operationalize. There is no magic single way available that could be used objectively to provide a standard, valid, and reliable measure. Therefore, as in the case of patient care in the preceding chapter, we had to develop a series of measures in order to assess coordination. The measures were constructed on the basis of information obtained from the following groups of respondents in each hospital: nonmedical department heads, and the hospital administrator; supervisory and nonsupervisory registered nurses; medical staff members having administrative responsibilities, and members without such responsibilities; and x-ray and laboratory technicians. Because of their position in the organization, members of these groups are familiar with different aspects of hospital operation that involve coordination phenomena. In addition, the registered nurses and those with administrative positions carry out many coordination functions as part of their organizational role. The background characteristics of those groups have been discussed in Chapter 3.

To obtain the necessary data, members of the above groups were asked a series of questions about coordination. Seven questions were used, each representing a particular coordination variable. These questions were not all asked consecutively in the separate questionnaire forms which were filled out by the various respondent groups; they were interspersed among other questionnaire items. In the different questionnaire forms, however, every question about coordination was identically worded. Furthermore, exactly the same questions were asked of the same respondent group in each of the ten hospitals. In short, all of the procedures employed to collect the data were in every respect uniform for every hospital, and the same respondent group across hospitals followed the same steps in the process of answering the questions. The seven questions used are as follows:

1. How well do the different jobs and work activities around the patient fit together, or how well are all things geared in the direction of giving good patient care? (Check one.)
    _____(1) Perfectly
    _____(2) Very well
    _____(3) Fairly well
    _____(4) Not so well
    _____(5) Not at all well

2. To what extent do the people from the various interrelated departments make an effort to avoid creating problems or interference with each other's duties and responsibilities? (Check one.)
    _____(1) To a very great extent
    _____(2) To a great extent
    _____(3) To a fair extent
    _____(4) To a small extent
    _____(5) To a very small extent

3. To what extent do people from different departments who have to work together do their job properly and efficiently without getting in each other's way? (Check one.)
   (Same five response alternatives as for preceding question.)

4. In general, how do the patients feel about how smoothly the various personnel around them work together? (Check one.)
    _____(1) The patients feel that the personnel work together completely smoothly
    _____(2) The patients feel that the personnel work together very smoothly
    _____(3) The patients feel that the personnel work together fairly smoothly

_____(4) The patients feel that the personnel do not work together smoothly
_____(5) The patients feel that the personnel do not work together smoothly at all

5. To what extent are all related things and activities well timed in the everyday routine of the hospital? (Check one.)
_____(1) All related things and activities in the everyday routine are perfectly timed
_____(2) They are very well timed
_____(3) They are fairly well timed
_____(4) They are not so well timed
_____(5) They are rather poorly timed

6. How well planned are the work assignments of the people from the different departments who work together? (Check one.)
_____(1) Extremely well planned
_____(2) Very well planned
_____(3) Fairly well planned
_____(4) Not so well planned
_____(5) Not well planned at all

7. In general, how well established are the routines of the different departments that have to work with one another? (Check one.)
_____(1) Their routines are extremely well established
_____(2) Very well established
_____(3) Fairly well established
_____(4) Not too well established
_____(5) Their routines are not well established

The last three questions on the list are concerned with the evaluation of certain concrete aspects of hospital functioning which involve a good deal of organizational planning and programing—the timing of interdependent activities, the planning of work assignments of people whose work is related, and the establishment of routines of cooperating departments. Therefore, they represent variables of programed coordination. The first four questions, on the other hand, represent different aspects of what we have called general coordination. In terms of types of coordination, the first and fourth questions imply positive efforts at coordination and represent the promotive type. The second and third questions deal with the avoidance of problems or disruptions and represent the preventive type. The remaining questions mainly represent the regulatory type of coordination, since they deal primarily with existing arrangements in the system (although they could also represent promotive coordination, if they reflected general positive attempts at coordination without reference to specific problems).

None of the seven questions represents the corrective type of coordination, which is probably one of the most frequently used but least effective types from the standpoint of achieving and maintaining adequate overall coordination in organizations. In most organizations, including hospitals, administrators, managers, and supervisors are both tempted and likely to operate on the assumption that the system is well coordinated, until specific problems concerning the articulation of activities arise, in which case they will engage in corrective coordination to re-establish equilibrium. This is an assumption which easily leads to a patch-work kind of coordination rather than to more rational, more positive, and more thorough and encompassing coordination plans. Regardless of its efficacy, it will be recalled, corrective coordination always takes place with reference to specific problems and after the problem has occurred. Because of this and because of its relatively high prevalence, moreover, this type of coordination is easier to grasp but more difficult to operationalize than the other three types. Different hospitals, for example, are more likely than not to face different specific problems requiring corrective coordination at a given time. This makes the development of standard methods to study corrective coordination uniformly and comparatively across hospitals an extremely complex task. In the face of these methodological problems, and without sufficient prior research in this area, measures of corrective coordination were not obtained in the present study.

In each hospital, all seven questions were asked of nonmedical administrative department heads, nonsupervisory registered nurses, and laboratory and x-ray technicians. In addition, all except the fourth and seventh were asked of supervisory nursing personnel and of the hospital administrator; and all except the third and sixth were asked of medical staff members. In all cases, each question required the respondent to answer by selecting one of the five response alternatives listed under the question; of course, a respondent was also free not to answer any of the questions, but instances of nonresponse averaged less than 5 percent for each question in the hospitals studied. The response alternatives offered by each question form a five-point scale, with assigned scale values ranging from 1 to 5. This feature makes possible the use of certain standard procedures for handling the data elicited by the questions.

The specific procedures used to derive measures of coordination are very similar to the procedures used to derive patient care measures in the preceding chapter. For each variable or question about coordination, and separately for each hospital in the study, the following steps were taken:

1. Using the answers of the members of each group of respondents involved, and based on the scale values corresponding to these answers, the arithmetic mean, or group average, was computed to represent the entire group's evaluation of coordination.

2. The particular means obtained for each of the several respondent groups answering the same question were then combined and averaged to yield an overall mean-score for each hospital, separately for each question about co-

Measurement of Coordination in Hospitals

ordination. (To obtain these overall means for each hospital, the separate group means were first weighted by their respective sampling ratio interval, which had been used originally to select members from each group as respondents, and then the resulting products were summed up and divided by the sum total of the sampling ratio intervals involved. The specific sampling ratios used to select the respondents participating in this study have also been described and discussed in Chapter 2, along with the number of respondents selected from each group.)

3. Following the completion of the preceding two steps, seven overall means, one for each specific coordination variable, were obtained for each of the ten hospitals. These constitute seven separate measures of coordination. The ten hospitals were then rank-ordered according to the magnitude of their respective score in each case to show their standing on these separate measures. The hospital with the lowest mean (or most favorable scale score) was given first place and assigned the number 1, followed by the hospital with the next lowest mean, etc., until the hospital with the highest mean (or least favorable score) was given last place and assigned the number 10 to complete the rank-order. The seven rank-orders thus obtained are shown in Table 28 below. They will be discussed after the presentation of four additional measures. These are overall, composite measures of coordination which were constructed using the above seven rank-orders and the corresponding hospital mean-scores as a basis.

Measure #1 of overall coordination takes into account data from all seven coordination variables, and was computed as follows: (1) With respect to each question about coordination, the ten hospitals were rank-ordered in relation to one another according to the magnitude of their respective overall mean in each case, as discussed above. (2) Having rank-ordered the ten hospitals with respect to each of the seven coordination variables involved, we next summed up each hospital's seven ranks and divided the resulting product by seven to obtain each hospital's mean-rank, or average rank on the entire series of variables. These hospital mean-ranks constitute one measure, measure #1 of overall coordination in this study. The ten hospitals were subsequently rank-ordered again, according to the magnitude of their respective mean-rank to show their relative standing on this measure of coordination (see Table 28 and Table 30).

Measure #2 of overall coordination also takes into account the data from all seven coordination variables, but it was computed somewhat differently. Instead of using the seven ranks of each hospital, the seven overall means corresponding to these ranks were used as components. These means, already described above, were summed up and divided by seven to yield a grand mean-score of coordination for each hospital. This constitutes the second overall measure of coordination. Again, the hospitals were rank-ordered according to the magnitude of their respective grand mean-score to show their relative standing on this measure (see Table 30 below). The remaining two measures were obtained in a similar manner. *Measure #3* was computed like measure #2, except that it makes use only of four component means instead of all seven for each hospital. The means involved are those pertaining to the first four questions about coordination listed earlier in this section; these four questions represent different aspects of general coordination and, for this reason, they were here treated together to provide an overall measure of general coordination. Finally, the last three questions on the list, representing different aspects of programed coordination, were used in a similar manner to provide an overall measure of programed coordination, *Measure #4* in this series. The ten hospitals were also rank-ordered in the usual manner to show their standing on each of the last two overall measures of coordination (see Table 30).

In summary, in addition to the seven measures of coordination obtained from the seven questions used in the present study, four overall measures of hospital coordination were developed and will be used in subsequent analyses. Measure #1 represents the overall mean rank-order of each hospital on all seven coordination variables studied. Measure #2 represents the grand mean-score of each hospital on the same seven component variables. Measure #3 represents the grand mean-score of each hospital on the first four coordination variables, as listed earlier and as shown in Table 28 below, being an overall measure of general coordination. And the last measure, measure #4, represents the grand mean-score of each hospital on the last three coordination variables shown in Table 28, being an overall measure of programed coordination.

Consistency of Measures and Their Interrelations

Table 28 presents the rank-orders of the ten hospitals on the seven coordination variables, which correspond to the questions listed earlier, as well as the mean rank-order of the hospitals on all these variables combined, which represents overall measure #1 of coordination. The table shows rather graphically the stability of the different ranks (i.e., coordination measures) of each hospital. Considering Hospital #3, for example, we find that it consistently ranks first or second among the ten hospitals, i.e., it ranks very favorably. Rank 1 is the most favorable and rank 10 is the least favorable in all cases, since low ranks correspond to more favorable coordination scores. For only one of the measures does Hospital #3 rank below second place—the extent to which work assignments are seen as well planned. A similar situation obtains in the case of Hospital #8. These two hospitals, respectively, place first and second in terms of their mean-rank, or the overall measure #1 of coordination. In the case of Hospital #1 and Hospital #2, the picture is reversed. These two hospitals consistently rank eighth, ninth, or tenth on the several coordination items, both ranking 9.5 in terms of overall measure #1. The remaining hospitals, as might be expected, show less consistent ranks across the different items measured. Complete consistency of this kind would not be possible, however, if the variables involved actually represent different aspects of coordination, as intended.

TABLE 28. Hospitals Rank-ordered According to Their Score on Each of Seven Coordination Variables *

Coordination Variable	#0	Hospital 1	2	3	4	5	6	7	8	9
How well different jobs and activities fit together	8	10	9	1	5	2.5	7	6	2.5	4
Extent members make an effort to avoid creating problems or interference	2	8	9	1	10	4	5	6	3	7
Extent members do their jobs properly without getting in each other's way	3	9	10	1.5	8	6	7	5	1.5	4
Extent patients feel personnel around them work together smoothly	7	8	10	1	3	6	9	2	4	5
How well timed activities are in the everyday routine	6	10	9	2	5	7	8	3	1	4
Extent work assignments are well planned	2	10	9	4.5	8	6.5	6.5	4.5	3	1
How well established are the routines of interdependent departments	5	10	9	1	8	7	4	6	2	3
Overall mean rank-order: † (Overall measure #1 of coordination)	5	9.5	9.5	1	8	6	7	4	2	3

* In all cases, the smaller ranks represent higher scores, i.e., more favorable scores on coordination.
† This is used subsequently as one of four overall measures of coordination.

In large part, the obtained consistency across measures is of course due to the fact that the several items measured are not unrelated. Since they were all designed to represent coordination, they should bear some relationship with one another on theoretical grounds. That this is also empirically the case is demonstrated by the specific intercorrelations among the variables involved. Based on the rank-orders shown in Table 28 above, these intercorrelations are presented in Table 29. The results are generally as expected. Consider the variable "how well different jobs and activities fit together," for example. We find that it correlates with the remaining items as follows: .51 with the extent to which organizational members make an effort to avoid interference, .69 with the extent to which members do their job without getting in each other's way, .72 with the extent to which patients feel that personnel work together smoothly, .77 with how well timed activities are, .49 with how well planned work assignments are, and .71 with how well established the routines of interdependent departments are.

Table 29 shows similar correlations when any other of the above measures is considered in relation to the rest. As expected, all 21 possible correlations among the seven measures are positive. The particular coefficients range from .30 to .89, 15 of them being statistically significant at the .05 level or better. It is also worth noting that of the six coefficients which do not reach statistical significance three are contributed by the item "extent to which patients feel. . . ." This suggests that very probably the respondents used, as they should, a frame of reference other than their own in answering this particular item. The criteria that patients themselves would employ in answering the same item would be expected to differ from the criteria actually employed by our respondents, who were nurses, doctors, and other hospital personnel rather than patients. The pattern of correlations in Table 29 is consistent with this expectation.

TABLE 29. Rank-order Intercorrelations Among Seven Coordination Variables *

Coordination Variable	1	2	3	4	5	6	7
1. How well different jobs and activities fit together	—	.51	.69	.72	.77	.49	.71
2. Extent members make an effort to avoid creating problems or interference		—	.83	.30	.48	.59	.73
3. Extent members do their jobs properly without getting in each other's way			—	.62	.85	.85	.89
4. Extent patients feel personnel around them work together smoothly				—	.85	.41	.49
5. How well timed activities are in the everyday routine					—	.73	.77
6. Extent work assignments are well planned						—	.85
7. How well established are the routines of interdependent departments							—

*. Correlations are based on an N of 10 hospitals in each case. All coefficients larger than .56 are significant at the .05 level, and those .75 or larger are significant at the .01 level. These correlations were computed using the appropriate rank-orders shown in Table 28, with the hospital serving as the unit of analysis.

The individual correlations contributed by the item of how patients feel reveal certain interesting results. In addition to producing half of the six nonsignificant correlations in Table 29, this item also contributed the two smallest correlations. Specifically, it produced a correlation of .30 with the item concerning personnel efforts to avoid interference, and one of .41 with the item concerning the planning of work assignments—two items with which patients would not be expected to be familiar. On the other hand it produced the highest correlation, one of .85, with the item concerning the timing of activities—precisely the one of all items with which patients would likely be most familiar. Such aspects of timing as giving medications, baths, and food, answering patient calls, and taking temperatures at certain times are things very familiar and important to the patients, probably constituting one of the major factors in terms of which our respondents evaluated the item involved and in terms of which patients themselves would be likely to evaluate the same item.

Other correlations in Table 29 provide support for additional kinds of consistency among the various measures of coordination. First, we find that the three items which were designed to measure programed coordination, the last three items on the table, are highly and significantly associated with one another: how well timed activities are correlates .73 with how well planned assignments are, and .77 with how well established routines are, while the latter two items correlate .85. In other words, these items exhibit a good deal of clustering. Second, we similarly find that the first and fourth items on the table, which were designed to represent promotive coordination, correlate .72; and the second and third items, designed to measure preventive coordination, correlate .83. Finally, as might be expected, we also find that: (1) the extent to which organizational members do their job without getting in each other's way correlates most highly, .89, with how well established routines are, being also highly related to activity timing and assignment planning—the items pertaining to programed coordination; and (2) the extent to which different jobs and activities fit well together is most closely related to how well timed activities are in the hospital. On the whole, consistencies such as these lend a certain amount of validity to the measures used.

From a methodological standpoint, it is also useful to know that the data show no consistent correspondence between the correlations presented in Table 29 (which were computed using the appropriate rank-orders shown in Table 28, with the hospital serving as the unit of analysis), and the parallel set of correlations obtained when instead of the hospitals the individual respondents serve as the unit of analysis. For example, if the answers of the individual respondents from all hospitals combined pertaining to variable 3 are related to their answers pertaining to variable 4 (for the specific variables mentioned here see Table 29), a correlation of .22 is obtained, which is not statistically significant. Similarly, on the individual level, variables 3 and 5 correlate only .17, which likewise is nonsignificant. By contrast, Table 29 shows that both of these pairs of variables yield significant correlations at the hospital-group level of analysis. On the other hand, whereas on the hospital level variables 2 and 4 do not correlate significantly, they correlate .36 on the individual level, this relationship being statistically significant. Still other pairs of variables, e.g., variables 1 and 5, yield significant relationships on both the hospital level and the individual level, although in the latter case the correlations are generally smaller, and considerably smaller in most instances. On the whole, these results demonstrate that the individual respondents have not answered the different questions about coordination similarly, or on the basis of a generalized "response set"; i.e., as expected, the respondents did not tend to answer all questions indiscriminately, either in a favorable-positive or in an unfavorable-negative manner. The absence of a generalized response set or of "halo effects," of course, enhances confidence in the data. (Additional evidence for the absence of halo effects is presented in a technical methodological note, at the end of this chapter.)

Up to this point, we have seen that the seven variables used to measure coordination intercorrelate positively (i.e., on the hospital level of analysis), while exhibiting certain consistency patterns. Moreover, 15 of the 21 possible correlations among them were found to be statistically significant. However, as it had been anticipated, these correlations are far from perfect, i.e., can account for only a portion of the variance involved in each case. Accordingly, the four overall measures of coordination, described earlier, are very important. Since each of them incorporates three or more of the specific measures, it is a more stable and more reliable indicator of coordination, thus representing hospital coordination better than any of the specific measures. Table 30 and Table 31, below, deal with the overall measures of coordination.

Table 30 shows how the ten hospitals rank in relation to one another on each of the four overall measures of coordination. It also shows that each hospital ranks consistently across the four measures. For example, Hospital #3 ranks first on all measures, and Hospital #8 ranks second. On the other hand, Hospital #1 and Hospital #2 rank least favorably among the ten hospitals. The consistency in ranks for the remaining hospitals is also high. These results suggest that the four measures intercorrelate very highly, and this is actually the case. The rank-order correlation between any two of the four measures is .90 or higher, which is statistically significant beyond the .01 level. The smallest

TABLE 30. Hospitals Rank-ordered According to Their Score on Each of Four Overall Measures of Coordination *

Coordination Measure †	#0	1	2	3	Hospital 4	5	6	7	8	9
Overall measure #1	5	9.5	9.5	1	8	6	7	4	2	3
Overall measure #2	6	10	9	1	7	5	8	4	2	3
Overall measure #3	6.5	9	10	1	6.5	5	8	3	2	4
Overall measure #4	5	10	9	1	8	7	6	4	2	3

* Measure #1 represents the mean-rank of each hospital on the seven coordination variables shown in Table 28; measure #2 represents the grand mean of each hospital on the same seven variables; measure #3 represents the grand mean of each hospital on the first four variables in Table 28; and measure #4 represents the grand mean of each hospital on the last three variables shown in Table 28.

† The rank-order intercorrelations among these four overall measures of coordination, based on an N of 10 hospitals, are as follows: .97 between measures #1 and #2; .95 between measures #1 and #3; .98 between measures #1 and #4; .97 between measures #2 and #3; .94 between measures #2 and #4; and .90 between measures #3 and #4. All are statistically significant beyond the .01 level.

Measurement of Coordination in Hospitals

correlation, one of .90, obtains between overall measure #3, which represents general coordination, and overall measure #4, which represents programed coordination. Since, unlike any other pair of overall measures, these two measures are based on different components, it is not surprising that they correlate somewhat less highly—though, in absolute terms, a correlation of .90 is very high.

Further examination of the four overall measures reveals that each correlates positively and significantly with all of its components. Table 31 presents the specific correlations. First, considering overall measure #1, we find that it correlates very highly with each of its seven components, the particular correlations ranging from .71 to .96—all being statistically significant at better than the .05 level. The comparable correlations concerning the other three measures are very similar; in all cases, the overall measure is positively and significantly related to each of its particular components. These relationships are important for, if each component did not correlate significantly with the overall measure, we would be very skeptical of using the overall measure to represent organizational coordination. The findings in Table 31, in conjunction with the findings in Table 29, regarding the intercorrelations among the seven

TABLE 31. Rank-order Correlations Showing the Relationship Between Four Overall Measures of Coordination and Their Component Items *

Component Item	Measure #1	Measure #2	Measure #3	Measure #4
How well different jobs and activities fit together	.78	.88	.86	— †
Extent members make an effort to avoid creating problems or interference	.73	.64	.62	—
Extent members do their jobs properly without getting in each other's way	.96	.90	.87	—
Extent patients feel personnel around them work together smoothly	.71	.78	.87	—
How well-timed activities are in the everyday routine	.90	.93	—	.89
Extent work assignments are well planned	.83	.76	—	.84
How well established are the routines of interdependent departments	.91	.84	—	.95

* Correlations are based on an N of 10 hospitals in each case. All coefficients larger than .56 are significant at the .05 level, and those .75 or larger are significant at the .01 level. These correlations were computed using the appropriate rank-order shown in Table 29 and Table 30.

† Where dashes appear, that particular item is not a component of that particular measure.

items which were used as components of the overall measures, indicate both that these items represent a common phenomenon—coordination—and that the four overall measures can be used with confidence to represent essentially the same phenomenon.

Further Results About the Consistency of Measures

In an effort to establish additional confidence in our measures of coordination, we also correlated each of the seven specific measures and each of the four overall measures with two variables which were not used as measures of coordination in this study but which, we have reasons to believe, could have been used for this purpose. The first of these two variables represents the extent to which each hospital has achieved singleness of direction in the efforts of its members. In an earlier study, Weiss (20) described the process of organizational coordination as pertaining to how an organization achieves singleness of direction in the efforts of its members. A well-coordinated organization should, therefore, have achieved greater singleness of direction than a less well-coordinated one. If this were actually the case, our measures of coordination should be significantly related to a measure of singleness of direction in the efforts of hospital people. In view of these considerations, provision had been made for obtaining such a measure in the present study.

To obtain the required measure, the following question was used: "In your opinion, to what extent has the hospital been able to achieve singleness of direction in the efforts of its many groups, departments, and individuals?" The response alternatives offered by this question ranged from "to a very great extent" to "to a very small extent," forming a conventional five-point ordinal scale. The question was asked of the following groups of respondents in each hospital: supervisory and nonsupervisory registered nurses, laboratory and x-ray technicians, medical staff members, and nonmedical administrative department heads, including the hospital administrator. In the usual manner, means were computed using the answers of each respondent group from each hospital, and then these means were properly combined and averaged to yield an overall mean for every hospital, i.e., to yield a measure of singleness of direction for each institution. Based on the five-point scale corresponding to the response alternatives, these means ranged from 2.06 to 2.68. Then, the ten hospitals were rank-ordered according to the magnitude of their mean-score and the resulting distribution was correlated with the rank-orders of the hospitals on the seven specific measures of coordination (Table 28) and on the four overall measures of coordination (Table 30). The correlational results are presented in Table 32. As hypothesized on theoretical grounds, these results show empirically that singleness of direction is positively and significantly related to every measure of coordination developed in the present study; all eleven possible correlations are statistically significant at the .05 level or better. These results lend additional support to our measures of coordination.

Table 32 also presents the results obtained from relating the several measures of coordination to the second variable which could have been used to measure coordination but which was not included among our measures. This variable is represented by a question which was designed to elicit a "direct" measure of coordination, by providing the respondents with what amounted to a definition of the concept of coordination and asking them to evaluate coordination on the basis of that definition. The question used was as follows: "In this hospital, how well organized or tied together are the efforts of its many groups and individuals toward providing 'the best possible patient care'?" The response alternatives ranged from "extremely well" to "not at all well," forming a five-point scale. The question was asked of all supervisory registered nurses, including the director of nursing, in each hospital. Based on the responses of

TABLE 32. Relation of Coordination Measures to Singleness of Direction and Articulation of Organizational Efforts *

Coordination measures	Extent to which the hospital has achieved singleness of direction in the efforts of its members †	How well articulated the efforts of hospital members are for providing the best possible care †
Overall measure #1	.67	.72
Overall measure #2	.64	.75
Overall measure #3	.59	.81
Overall measure #4	.63	.62
How well different jobs and activities fit together	.56	.59
Extent members make an effort to avoid creating problems or interference	.78	.45
Extent members do their jobs properly without getting in each other's way	.86	.67
Extent patients feel personnel around them work together smoothly	.61	.65
How well timed activities are in the everyday routine	.75	.70
Extent work assignments are well planned	.66	.66
How well established are the routines of interdependent departments	.57	.43

* All figures shown are rank-order correlations, based on an N of 10 hospitals in each case. Coefficients larger than .56 are significant at the .05 level, and those .75 or larger are significant at the .01 level.

† The rank-order correlation between these two variables is .64 which, based on an N of 10 hospitals, is statistically significant at the .05 level.

these nurses, and on the five-point scale corresponding to the response alternatives used, means were computed. Across hospitals, these means ranged from 1.60 to 2.68. The ten hospitals were then rank-ordered according to the magnitude of their mean-score, and the resulting distribution was correlated with the rank-orders of the hospitals on each of the various measures of coordination (shown in Table 28 and Table 30). The findings are presented in Table 32.

The correlations in Table 32 confirm our expectations. The four overall measures of coordination correlate .72, .75, .81, and .62, respectively, with how well the efforts of hospital members and groups are tied together toward providing the best possible patient care. These relationships are statistically significant at better than the .05 level. Moreover, the seven specific measures of coordination also correlate positively with the same variable, the particular coefficients ranging from .43 to .70. Five of these seven correlations are significant beyond the .05 level. In short, as in the case of the results from the question about singleness of direction, the several measures of coordination come out very well also when compared against the evaluation by supervisory registered nurses of how well articulated are the efforts of organizational members. (Incidentally, singleness of direction correlates .64 with articulation of efforts—a relationship which is statistically significant but which accounts for only 41 percent of the variance involved.)

These results take even greater significance when we consider the following relevant points: (1) The overall measures of coordination correlate better with the above measure of articulation of efforts than do the seven specific measures; this should be the case, since the item about articulation provided a definition of overall coordination rather than emphasizing any specific aspects of the concept. (2) The same item, in addition to providing such a definition, also supplied the respondents with a referent of coordination in specifying articulation of efforts "toward providing the best possible patient care"—the main organizational objective toward which coordination efforts are presumably directed in hospitals. (3) Only supervisory registered nurses were asked this item, whereas our measures of coordination are based on the combined evaluations of several respondent groups in each case, including supervisory registered nurses. Members of this last group are in an especially advantageous position to evaluate coordination because they hold coordinating positions in the hospital, and because they are familiar both with different aspects of coordination and with patient care.

These considerations, in conjunction with the other findings discussed in this section, provide a good deal of support for the reliability and validity of the measures of coordination developed in the present study. Finally, it should also be noted that the relative standing of the hospitals according to the quantitative measures of coordination, shown in Table 28 and Table 30, corresponds fairly well to whatever limited qualitative data about coordination

Factors Expected to Affect Coordination

and coordination problems were obtained from volunteered comments by hospital personnel; these comments were presented earlier in the profiles of the various hospitals, in Chapter 4. The profiles of Hospital #1 and Hospital #2, for example, show a number of comments by various respondents regarding coordination weaknesses, especially lack of adequate liaison between key hospital groups, such as doctors and trustees. In terms of the quantitative measures of coordination, these two hospitals rank least favorably among the ten hospitals in the study. By contrast, most comments relevant to coordination in the profiles of Hospital #3 and Hospital #8 are positive. In terms of the quantitative measures, these two hospitals rank most favorably on coordination.

FACTORS EXPECTED TO AFFECT ORGANIZATIONAL COORDINATION

We will now discuss certain aspects of organizational functioning, which, on theoretical grounds, should be related to the adequacy of coordination in formal organizations. Six sets of independent variables will be considered: organizational planning, sharedness or complementarity of expectations and cooperation among organizational members, intraorganizational strain, problem awareness and problem solving, communication, and certain variables representing structural aspects of organization. The operations used to measure specific variables belonging to these categories, and the particular relationships between these variables and organizational coordination, will be presented in the next chapter.

Organizational Planning

In our discussion concerning the means of achieving coordination, we touched on the role that organizational planning activities play in this connection, especially with respect to programed coordination. The range of behaviors included among such activities may run from the creation of an overall master plan for the organization to the everyday task of laying out and integrating the work of a few subordinates. But regardless of the range of planning activity in a given situation, we may expect the quality of planning to have an effect upon coordination. The excellence of planning itself, however, is largely dependent upon the skill of the planners. Accordingly, we expect a positive relationship between the skill with which planning is carried out in an organization and coordination.

The relationship of organizational planning to coordination, however, may manifest itself most clearly in the reactions of organizational members toward the plans involved, i.e., in the application and implementation aspects of planning rather than the initial quality of the plans and the skill behind them. Organizational planning involves, among other things, the regulation of the behavior of members in the system, through the promulgation of standards, rules, and policies. Such rules and standards are usually designed to implement plans which will presumably facilitate the achievement of organizational objectives. These coordinative purposes, however, can only be realized if the rules underlying them are sufficiently clear to those organizational members who are affected by them, and if members will ultimately adhere to the rules. Consequently, we expect that both the clarity of definition of rules and the willingness of members to follow them will be directly related to organizational coordination.

Sharedness of Expectations, Complementarity of Expectations, and Cooperation Among Members

The nature of member expectations is very important to organizational functioning. By expectations, we mean here the anticipations that organizational members have with respect to how other organizational members with whom they interact will act or think under given circumstances. When the mutual expectations of different members show a poor fit, adequate organizational coordination becomes difficult to attain and maintain. In the presence of poorly fitting expectation systems, as Cumming and Cumming (3) found out in their study of a mental hospital, the organization tends to become "granulated," i.e., segmented and compartmentalized rather than integrated. And, segmentation, among other things, means that the organization is likely to respond and function by parts rather than as a unified structure. If, for example, members from different roles and departments in the hospital fail to see one another's viewpoint in their work relationships, they will tend to think and act exclusively according to their own particular norms and frames of reference. As a consequence, serious deficiencies in communication and intergroup tensions will be likely to arise and to impair effective organizational planning.

Member adherence to organizational plans and rules, which is a precondition to attaining adequate coordination, is contingent upon the norms and mutual expectations of the members in the system. The extent to which members share the same or similar norms or, at least, complementary and supplementary rather than contradictory or divergent expectations, will affect both the chances that organizational plans will be effectively implemented and the chances that the interdependent activities of different members will be adequately coordinated. If both sharedness of norms and complementarity of expectations characterize the different members of an organization, the various parts of the system will be likely to function according to one another's needs and according to the needs of the entire organization—assuming, of course, that members accept the basic objectives of the system or follow norms which do not contradict such objectives.

Under certain conditions of member norms being contrary to organizational goals, complementarity of expectations among members might prove detrimental to coordination. This would be a likely outcome if the members sharing organizationally undesirable norms cooperated with one another against the plans and objectives of the total system. However, under conditions of acceptance by members of the plans and goals of their organization and conditions of complementarity of expectations, cooperation among members should facilitate coordination.[8] Under these conditions, assuming that organizational channels of communication are open and in use, members will be more likely to develop an awareness of each other's role in the system and mutual understanding of each other's problems and needs in the process of pursuing organizational goals.

In view of these considerations, we hypothesize a direct relationship between organizational coordination and: (1) the degree to which members in the system share similar or congruent viewpoints about the operations of the organization; (2) the degree of reciprocal understanding of work problems and needs among members occupying different but interdependent positions in the system; and (3) the extent of cooperation among members whose work activities are related.

Intraorganizational Strain

Shared expectations and mutual understanding on the part of different members in an organization, in addition to contributing to better coordination, minimize the likelihood of strain among members in the system. Intraorganizational strain, in the form of tensions and pressures among interdependent parts of the action structure of the system, makes it more difficult and less likely for members to adhere to the coordination imperative of meeting each other's needs while pursuing the objectives of the total organization. Tensions and pressures build up hostilities, distrust, and barriers to mutual understanding among members, with the result that coordination in the system suffers correspondingly. Under these circumstances, moreover, organizational efforts to improve the situation through corrective coordination are likely to face inertia difficult to overcome. And, although a certain amount of intraorganizational strain is undoubtedly, and perhaps inevitably, present in any social organization, relatively high levels of strain are dysfunctional from the point of view of achieving adequate coordination. We, therefore, expect a negative relationship between the degree of tension among interdependent parts in the system and organizational coordination.[9]

---

[8] An experimental study by Deutsch (4) has already provided some support for the hypothesis that cooperation will be positively related to coordination. Deutsch concluded that in a cooperative situation improved coordination of efforts can be expected.

[9] In this connection, it is also interesting to note that, in a study of an industrial organization, Georgopoulos and Tannenbaum (8) found an inverse relationship between intraorganizational strain and organizational effectiveness. Groups with high tension between supervisors and workers were characterized by low productivity, low overall performance as judged by management, and low flexibility of response to change.

The relationship between tension and coordination, however, is likely to be a circular one. High tension makes for inadequate coordination, but inadequate coordination is likely to create, increase, or perpetuate tension in the system since the articulation of member activities is, by definition, defective. In his study of restaurants, for example, Whyte (22) relates a case where tension was high between cook and waitresses because, while the former considered himself higher in status than the latter, the waitresses were literally telling him what to do when shouting customer orders to him. Another restaurant did not have this problem because the waitresses could not see or talk to the cook; instead, they wrote their orders on tickets and placed them on a board where the cook received them. In this latter case, coordination between the activities of cook and waitresses was such that it created neither disjunctures in the pattern of the organizational activity involved nor tension between the affected parties. In hospitals, personnel of varying status are similarly initiating action for one another, and related problems of tension can and do likewise develop. Careful coordination, which takes into account these problems, can be an important organizational mechanism for mitigating tensions and alleviating conflicts in the action structure.

Problem Awareness and Problem Solving

In a hospital, as well as any other organization, problems that remain unresolved or undetected may cause tensions in the system and contribute to poor coordination. Organizational planning and coordination, almost by definition, require that planners and coordinators resolve problems existing in the organization. Problem solving, however, depends on whether or not those charged with this activity are aware of the problems involved. To engage in corrective or preventive coordination, for example, one must first be aware of the particular problems or malfunctions which create the need for these types of coordination.

Adequacy of coordination will, therefore, depend both on the detection and resolution of existing problems. A certain amount of awareness is only a necessary condition, however; it will not by itself ensure good coordination. Adequate coordination will further necessitate that the problems involved be resolved satisfactorily and promptly. If the solution of a given problem means the creation of another difficulty, for example, coordination is not likely to improve. Similarly, if the problem is not solved soon enough, tensions and conflicts are likely to be accentuated and additional difficulties are likely to arise. These would render the solution of the original problem more difficult and, sometimes, even meaningless. Consequently, we expect that coordination will be better in those hospitals where persons in coordinative positions are aware of existing problems and, at the same time, these problems are handled satisfactorily and settled promptly.

Communication

Communication variables constitute another important set of factors that may condition or directly affect coordination. In our earlier discussion of the relationship between coordination and sharedness of expectations on the part of organizational members, we touched on the role which communication plays in that connection. In a later chapter, Chapter 10, moreover, the importance of different communication patterns among nursing personnel with respect to various aspects of hospital functioning, including coordination, will be examined in detail. At this point, it is sufficient to note briefly that we expect certain relationships between communication variables and organizational coordination. There are several reasons why this should be the case.

First, communication, or lack of it, can be instrumental in promoting or impeding the development of complementary expectations and mutual understanding among organizational members whose work activities are interrelated. Second, it can be instrumental in increasing or diminishing tensions and conflicts in the organization. Third, it can be instrumental in facilitating or impeding problem awareness and problem solving. In general, the exchange or transmission of adequate and relevant information among different parts of the system is a matter of communication, and factors which make for adequate communication should also facilitate coordination. The openness of the communication network in an organization, for example, affects the likelihood of detecting and resolving dysfunctions which, in turn, would affect the articulation of member efforts and activities. Accordingly, the ease with which persons holding interdependent roles in the hospital can exchange information and discuss problems when needed should influence the adequacy of organizational coordination. Other similar communication variables should produce similar effects. For example, the extent to which doctors explain the needs of their patients to nursing personnel, the extent to which patient charts are complete, and the extent to which the administrator's communication to medical staff members is adequate, should all facilitate coordination in the hospital.

Structural Features of Organization

The last set of factors which are expected to affect coordination deals with certain structural aspects of organization. Of the many possible variables in this area, we shall consider two kinds: size and size-related variables, and work force composition variables. With respect to size, it will be recalled, the present study was designed to include hospitals which are neither too large nor too small (between 100 and 350 beds). This design was partly premised on the assumption that in very large hospitals extensive specialization, differentiation, and interdependence make coordination problems more complex, while in very small hospitals differentiation is not sufficiently extensive to permit an adequate study of coordination phenomena. This assumption suggests that the larger the organization, the more difficult it would be to achieve and maintain good coordination. This hypothesis, however, should hold only if larger size also means more specialization of tasks and functions, higher interdependence of organizational skills and roles, and more parts in the system requiring articulation.

Mere size is not the important consideration insofar as coordination is concerned. An organization which has a large number of personnel doing essentially independent work or the same thing will have fewer coordination problems than an organization with a smaller number of personnel whose specialized work activities are interdependent. However, in the case of organizations with similar differentiation and specialization, an increase in size will entail more coordination problems and complications, thus affecting coordination in the system. In the present study, therefore, we expect a negative relationship between hospital size and coordination. But, since our ten hospitals all fall within a rather restricted size range, as previously indicated, this relationship is not expected to be very pronounced or as strong as it would probably be for a sample of hospitals representing a wider size range.

The second kind of variables to be examined is concerned with the composition of organizational work force. Organizations, including hospitals, can be categorized in terms of the number of positions and roles which they have to fill and in terms of which they have to allocate their personnel. More generally, they can be characterized in terms of the unique skill demands they make and can be arrayed in terms of their unique skill supply in each case. Coordination implies a certain amount of congruence between skill demand and supply and, in this sense, there should be a relationship between work force composition and coordination. If in a given hospital, for example, the supply of any of its many personnel categories is inadequate to meet corresponding organizational needs, personnel from other positions must carry out the functions involved with the result that intraorganizational strain is likely to develop and coordination is likely to suffer.

A shortage of registered nurses, for instance, means that in all probability practical nurses will have to take over some of the functions of the registered nurse role while, at the same time, available registered nurses must do more things than they would normally be called upon to do. Imbalances of this nature, not infrequent in organizations, are expected to make coordination more difficult. What is the optimum apportionment of personnel in a particular organization from the standpoint of coordination is, however, an empirical question. Therefore, while we will examine the association between coordination and such aspects of work force composition as the proportion of medical staff members who are specialists or general practitioners, and the proportion of nursing staff members who are registered nurses, practical nurses, or aides, we cannot hypothesize in advance specific relationships.

A TECHNICAL METHODOLOGICAL NOTE

Earlier, in discussing the consistency of the measures of coordination, we presented evidence demonstrating the absence of generalized "response set" on the part of the individual respondents who provided the data from which the several measures were derived. Results from an additional special analysis provide further evidence for the absence of set or halo effects while, at the same time, establishing empirically the existence of different types of coordination, and demonstrating the independence of some of the variables which have been hypothesized to affect organizational coordination. This special analysis was a factor analysis which, using certain data from doctors and nurses, was carried out separately for each of three hospitals. After a brief discussion of the procedure followed, we will summarize below the main results of this factor analysis.

Because of the cost, effort, and the complexity of the procedure involved, three of the ten hospitals were chosen by means of random numbers to represent the institutions studied. The particular hospitals turned out to be Hospital #4, Hospital #5, and Hospital #9. Then, of the various respondent groups, the general medical staff group and the nonsupervisory registered nurses group were chosen for inclusion in the analysis. Apart from the matter of economy, the reasons for selecting these two groups were: (1) both groups had been asked most of the specific questions in which we were interested here, i.e., both had provided the majority of the data which we wished to analyze; (2) the number of respondents from each hospital belonging to these two groups was sufficiently large for the desired analysis; and (3) the homogeneity of the membership of each group was relatively high, and the relevant data supplied by each group happened to be very similar (correlated) in most instances with the corresponding data supplied by the other group. These latter conditions would presumably maximize the appearance of halo effects, if the individual respondents had actually answered the different questions on the basis of a generalized (favorable or unfavorable) response set.

Next, of the more than 100 questionnaire items which had been answered by doctors and nurses in the various hospitals, we selected a total of 27 items, or variables, for factor analysis. This set of 27 items was made up of a number of subsets of fairly similar or homogeneous items. Specifically, included among the 27 items were the following subsets: the seven coordination variables shown in Table 29 of this chapter; four variables concerning sharedness and complementarity of expectations among organizational members (for the specific variables and their measurement, see the next chapter); three variables concerning certain aspects of communication; three variables concerning organizational rules and formal instrumentalities (clarity of rules, conformity with rules, and the adequacy of patient charts); and two items concerning the evaluation of the quality of nursing care and medical care in the hospital by the respondents included in the factor analysis. (Our measures of the quality of patient care, as described in the preceding chapter, are not the same as these two items.) The remaining eight items were selected to represent certain aspects of superior-subordinate relations, certain aspects of change in the hospital, and nursing department coordination (for most of these items, data were available from nurses only), which are not directly relevant to our present purposes.

The data from the general medical staff and the nonsupervisory registered nurses (an average total of 38 individuals from Hospital #4, 29 from Hospital #5, and 30 from Hospital #9—the exact number varying from one item to another) pertaining to the above 27 items were then intercorrelated and factor-analyzed, treating each of the three hospitals separately. Technically, the factor analysis was carried out using the centroid method and orthogonal varimax rotation. It was effected by means of I.B.M. electronic equipment available at The University of Michigan, using the "principal axes solution" program. The particular restrictions imposed were that: (1) the factors, or dimensions, emerging from the above specified domain of data should account for 95 percent of the variance, (2) the communalities should be stabilized at the .01 level, and (3) at least six estimates should be made. The entire procedure was, of course, to be carried out using data from each of the three hospitals separately, but with the data from doctors and nurses treated together.

The principal relevant findings of the factor analysis may now be summarized. First, the analysis of the 27 variables (items) yielded six different dimensions, or factors, in the case of Hospital #4, five in the case of Hospital #5, and six in the case of Hospital #9. To obtain so many factors out of a relatively few variables (an average of one factor for every four to five variables), especially when many of the variables involved had been deliberately designed to measure essentially the same phenomenon (e.g., three variables had been designed to measure programed coordination), would be virtually impossible if generalized response set had operated. That is, it would be practically impossible in view of the fact that several subsets of rather homogeneous variables constituted the domain represented by the 27 variables in the analysis. Moreover, judging from the communalities of the factors obtained for each hospital, we find no single evaluative factor in any hospital that could account or nearly account for the domain of the data involved. Accordingly, we have here added empirical evidence to the effect that set and halo effects, if any, are very negligible in the data examined.

Second, the nature of the extracted factors is also of interest, particularly in relation to the different types of coordination which were theoretically distinguished earlier in this chapter. In this connection, the analysis yielded the following results:

1. Of the six factors obtained in the case of Hospital #9, three are coordination factors. One of these is a preventive coordination factor. The preventive coordination item "people . . . avoid creating problems . . ." shows a loading of .981 on this factor—the highest loading of any of the 27 items in the analysis (for a full statement of this item, as well as the other coordination items, see Table 29). A second factor involves one of our programed coordination items, the item about how well planned work assignments in the hospital are. This item shows a loading of .821 on this factor, being the highest-loading item of all items in the analysis. The third coordination factor is a nursing department coordination factor (nursing department coordination is discussed in the next chapter); the highest-loading item in this instance is the item about intershift coordination in

A Technical Methodological Note

the nursing department, which shows a loading of .955 on the present factor.

2. Similarly, of the six factors obtained in the case of Hospital #4, two are coordination factors. For one of these, the item of highest loading is again the preventive coordination item "people . . . avoid creating problems . . . ," with a loading of .601. For the other factor, the item of highest loading is the programed coordination item of how well planned work assignments are, with a loading of .761. A promotive coordination item, the item on how well activities fit together, shows the second highest loading on this same factor.

3. Of the five factors obtained in the case of Hospital #5, one is a programed coordination factor. The item of highest loading on this factor is the one referring to how well established hospital routines are, having a loading of .799. (For the specific coordination items to which we have referred, see Table 29 and accompanying discussion.)

The above results establish empirically the existence of some of the types of coordination discussed earlier in this chapter. In addition, they show that distinct coordination factors were found to exist in each of the hospitals included in the analysis. As a by-product, moreover, the communalities obtained for each item in the analysis provide us with a good estimate of the lower limit of reliability of our measures of the different coordination items (and the other items in the analysis). In this connection, using the numbers given to the seven coordination measures in Table 29, page 286, in order to identify each measure, we find the following average communalities (i.e., the h^2 for each coordination variable, averaged for the three hospitals in the analysis) for each measure or item: a communality of .716 for item 1, one of .729 for item 2, one of .719 for item 3, one of .559 for item 4, one of .622 for item 5, one of .748 for item 6, and one of .640 for item 7. These communalities indicate that our various specific measures of coordination are highly reliable, confirming the results of prior relevant analyses.

To complete the present methodological discussion, we will also comment briefly on the nature of the noncoordination factors that were obtained from the above factor analysis in each hospital. The three noncoordination factors extracted in the case of Hospital #9 are: a factor which involves the items about clarity of organizational rules and the extent of member conformity to these rules (these items are among the independent variables that were earlier hypothesized to affect coordination, and are discussed in Chapter 7); a factor concerning the adequacy of communication in the hospital (this item too was hypothesized to affect coordination, and is discussed in the next chapter); and a factor concerning the promptness with which organizational members adjust to changes in the hospital, and the extent to which members accept these changes.

The four noncoordination factors extracted in the case of Hospital #4 are: a factor involving the clarity of organizational rules and the adequacy of patient charts; a factor involving variables of complementarity of expectations among interacting organizational members, particularly the extent to which doctors understand the problems and needs of the nursing staff (complementarity was also hypothesized to affect coordination, and it too is discussed in Chapter 7); a factor again involving the adequacy of communication, and an item measuring the extent to which nurses perceive their immediate superiors as having a good understanding of the employees' viewpoint; and a rather mixed, impure factor which involves some cooperation variables that were hypothesized to affect coordination, and which are also discussed in the next chapter.

Finally, the four noncoordination factors obtained in the case of Hospital #5 are: one factor concerning clarity of rules; one factor concerning complementarity of expectations between doctors and nurses; one factor concerning adequacy of communication in the nursing department, and the skill of nursing supervisors at planning and scheduling the work, as perceived by nurse respondents; and one factor involving the evaluation of the quality of nursing care and medical care by the respondents included in the factor analysis (not the measures of care discussed in Chapter 5). As evaluated by the general medical staff and the non-supervisory registered nurses, the variable of the quality of medical care in the hospital loaded .780, and of the quality of nursing care loaded .588, on this factor.

In summary, the importance of this last series of findings from the factor analysis is twofold. First, we find that certain particular factors, or dimensions, recurred in at least two of the three hospitals in the analysis. The factors involving clarity of organizational rules, complementarity of expectations among organizational members, and adequacy of communication are such recurring factors (in addition, of course, to the coordination factors discussed above). And, second, according to the above results, the variables concerning organizational rules, complementarity of expectations, and communication apparently constitute distinct sets of independent variables, as it had been anticipated.

SUMMARY

Because the specialized roles and activities of organizations are interrelated and not independent of one another, organizations constantly face the problem of coordination. While the importance of this problem as a crucial organizational phenomenon has been recognized for some time, and while serious scientific interest in this area has not been lacking in the past, surprisingly little systematic effort has been made to relate coordination to other social-psychological aspects of organizational structure and functioning. Since the early works of Fayol (6), Mary Parker Follett (14), and Gulick and Urwick (10), the tendency on the part of those concerned with problems of departmentalization, coordination, and administration has generally been to view both coordination and its determinants in narrow, mechanistic terms, paying little or no attention to the human variables of organization. As the relevant critique by March and Simon (13) shows, administrative science theories, which encompass most of what is already available about coordination, have been found wanting on many important counts. Among their major shortcomings are their inadequate motivational assumptions, their failure to consider the effects of intraorganizational conflict upon behavior, and their viewing of organizational members not as individuals who are able to feel, think, reason, and adjust but as passive instruments, like any other objects in the organizational machinery,

Summary

performing tasks more or less blindly and according to organizational specification.

In this chapter, we have been interested in the problem of organizational coordination as it relates to other important aspects of the organization, with special emphasis on the hospital situation. We have been concerned with laying out the theoretical bases in terms of which coordination, as a social-psychological phenomenon, and problems of coordination can be studied and understood. The purpose of the chapter has been threefold: (1) to discuss the importance of coordination for the organizational system and to clarify the concept; (2) to indicate the bases and mechanisms of coordination, and to measure coordination in hospitals; and (3) to specify various sets of factors which are expected to affect coordination in large-scale organizations, in general, and in the community general hospital in particular.

Coordination was viewed as representing the processes of articulation and the state of adjustment among the different elements of an organization, and was defined as the extent to which the interdependent parts of the organization function each according to the needs and requirements of the other parts and of the total system. All the coordinative activities of organizations were considered as falling into two broad categories, programed and general or nonprogramed, and different types of coordination were specified and discussed. These are promotive, preventive, corrective, and regulatory coordination. Finally, certain sets of independent variables, i.e., variables expected to affect coordination, were also specified. These are: organizational planning, communication, sharedness and complementarity of expectations among organizational members, cooperation, intraorganizational strain, problem awareness and problem solving on the part of members in key organizational roles, and certain aspects of organizational structure, such as the composition of work force.

In the past, communication, complementarity of expectations, intraorganizational strain, problem awareness and problem solving, and cooperation—precisely the variables which are central in the present study of coordination—have been almost entirely disregarded as independent variables. Similarly, previous studies have been almost exclusively concerned with programed, formal coordination, with a consequent failure to recognize that a good deal of coordinative activity in organizations is nonprogramed. The present research focuses on both programed and nonprogramed coordination, with emphasis on the latter.

In this study, several measures of coordination were developed, using data collected from the ten hospitals participating in the research. The measures were fully reported and discussed in this chapter. Similarly, for each of the above sets of independent variables, a number of specific variables were measured on the basis of data from the same hospitals. These measures will be discussed in Chapter 7. The empirical findings which establish relationships between these variables and coordination will also be presented in Chapter 7. Thus, this and the next chapter complement and supplement each other in various respects, together providing a full account of our study of coordination. It is also worth reiterating, in this connection, that while in these two chapters coordination is being treated as a dependent variable, i.e., as a phenomenon in its own right, in later chapters that deal with patient care it will be viewed and used as an independent variable.

REFERENCES

1. Barnard, C. I. *The Functions of the Executive.* Cambridge, Mass.: Harvard University Press, 1938.
2. Burling, T., Lentz, E. M., and Wilson, R. N. *The Give and Take in Hospitals.* New York: Putnam, 1956.
3. Cumming, J., and Cumming, E. "Social Equilibrium and Social Change in a Large Mental Hospital." In Greenblatt, M., Levinson, D., and Williams, R. (eds.). *The Patient and the Mental Hospital.* Glencoe, Ill.: The Free Press, 1957.
4. Deutsch, M. "An Experimental Study of the Effects of Cooperation and Competition upon Group Process," *Human Relations,* 2:199–232, 1949.
5. Diebold, J. *Automation: The Advent of the Automatic Factory.* Princeton, N.J.: Van Nostrand, 1952.
6. Fayol, H. *Industrial and General Administration.* London: Pitman, 1930.
7. Feibleman, J., and Friend, J. W. "The Structure and Function of Organization," *Philosophical Rev.,* 54:19–44, 1945.
8. Georgopoulos, B. S., and Tannenbaum, A. S. "A Study of Organizational Effectiveness," *Amer. Sociol. Rev.,* 22:534–40, 1957.
9. Goldwater, S. S. *On Hospitals.* New York: Macmillan, 1947.
10. Gulick, L. H., and Urwick, L. (eds.). *Papers on the Science of Administration.* New York: Institute of Public Administration, 1937.
11. Hawley, A. H. *Human Ecology.* New York: Ronald, 1950.
12. Mann, F. C., and Hoffman, L. R. *Automation and the Worker: A Study of Social Change in Power Plants.* New York: Holt, 1960.
13. March, J. G., and Simon, H. A. *Organizations.* New York: Wiley, 1958.
14. Metcalf, H. C., and Urwick, L. *Dynamic Administration: The Collected Papers of Mary Parker Follett.* New York: Harper, 1942.
15. Parsons, T., and Shils, E. A. (eds.). *Toward a General Theory of Action.* Cambridge, Mass.: Harvard University Press, 1952.
16. Phenix, F. L. "Coordination of Services," *The Physical Therapy Review,* 35:229–34, (May) 1955.
17. Simon, H. A. *Administrative Behavior.* New York: Macmillan, 1947.
18. Turner, J. G. "Teamwork: Bedrock of the Hospital Structure," *Hospitals,* 28:79–81, (Jan.) 1954.
19. Warner, W. L., and Low, J. "The Factory in the Community." In Whyte, W. F. (ed.). *Industry and Society.* New York: McGraw-Hill, 1946.
20. Weiss, R. S. *Processes of Organization.* Ann Arbor, Mich.: Institute for Social Research, 1956.
21. Wessen, A. F. "The Social Structure of a Modern Hospital." Doctoral Dissertation. Yale University, 1951.
22. Whyte, W. F. "The Social Structure of the Restaurant," *Am. J. Sociol.,* 54:302–08, 1949.

7 FACTORS AFFECTING COORDINATION IN HOSPITALS

The results which show the specific empirical relationships between the various factors discussed in the preceding chapter and coordination in the ten hospitals participating in the research will now be presented.

First, we shall present a series of findings about hospital coordination, using the total institution as the unit of analysis. These findings establish relationships between our measures of coordination, on the one hand, and the various sets of independent variables which we described in Chapter 6, on the other. The latter, it will be recalled, include different aspects of organizational planning, sharedness and complementarity of expectations among organizational members, cooperation, strain, problem awareness and problem solving, communication, and certain aspects of organizational structure. The measures of coordination include the four overall measures and their seven specific components, as discussed in Chapter 6, i.e., both programed and general coordination are represented, as are preventive and promotive coordination. In the second major section of this chapter we shall present certain comparable findings about coordination in the nursing department. In the third section we shall contrast the most adequately with the least adequately coordinated hospital. And in the last section we will summarize the principal findings of this part of the study, together with some of their implications.

Data for the measurement of the independent variables were collected from several groups of respondents in each hospital, using multiple-choice questions similar to those employed for the measurement of coordination. Moreover, the particular measures were derived from the data using the same procedures which were applied in the case of coordination. Separately for each variable and hospital involved, respondent group means were first computed. These means were then properly combined and averaged to yield an overall hospital mean, which constitutes the final measure used in the analysis. The ten hospitals were subsequently rank-ordered according to the magnitude of their mean-score on each variable, and the resulting distribution was correlated with the rank-order of the hospitals on coordination, to ascertain the relationship between coordination and each independent variable studied. The respondent groups which provided the necessary data will be indicated in every case.

RESULTS CONCERNING HOSPITAL COORDINATION

If organizational coordination is a function of, or depends upon, such factors as planning, strain, communication, and the other independent variables we have discussed in Chapter 6, the data should demonstrate that hospital coordination is significantly related to our measures of these variables. Let us, therefore, present and examine the empirical findings of the study to see whether, and to what extent, they support this proposition.

Organizational Planning in Relation to Coordination

In large-scale, bureaucratic organizations such as the community general hospital, the formal planning of activities is an integral part of organizational life. Much of this planning involves the establishment and maintenance of policies and operational rules and regulations that govern work and work relations in the system. It is in part through the mechanism of these products of planning that coordination can be effected. As we have indicated in Chapter 6, however, the actual implementation and efficacy of organizational rules and policies will depend on many conditions. These include the definitional clarity of existing policies and rules, the extensiveness of organizational member adherence to rules and plans, and the skill with which planning is carried out. Theoretically, it was earlier hypothesized, each of these variables should be related to coordination. The empirical data support this hypothesis.

Definitional clarity was measured using the responses of nonsupervisory registered nurses, x-ray and laboratory technicians, and nonmedical department heads from each hospital to the following question: "How clearly defined are the policies and the various rules and regulations of the hospital that affect your work?" the response alternatives ranged from "they are defined as clearly as they should be defined" to "they should be defined much more clearly." The findings in Table 33 show that, as expected, the more clearly defined policies, rules, and regulations are, the better the coordination is likely to be. The degree of clarity correlates .62 with overall measure #1 of coordination, .57 with measure #2, .59 with measure #3, and .53 with measure #4. In addition, not shown in the table, similar relationships are obtained when definitional clarity is related to the specific components of the overall measures of coordination which were discussed in the preceding chapter. The correlations are highest, however, with the two components pertaining to preventive coordination (.82 with the extent to which organizational members avoid creating interference, and .74 with the extent to which they do their work without getting in each other's way). Apparently, the definitional clarity of organizational rules is particularly important for preventive coordination.

To measure extent of conformity, or adherence to rules, this question was used: "In general, to what extent do people in the different jobs and departments follow the policies and the various rules and regulations set up by the hospital?" In each hospital, the question was asked of registered nurses, technicians, nonmedical department heads including the hospital administrator, and medical staff members having no administrative responsibilities. There were five response alternatives, ranging from "everyone without exception follows the policies and the rules . . ." to "about half or less than half of the people do." The results in Table 33 show a high positive relationship between extent of conformity and coordination. Conformity correlates .83, .78, .70, and .87, respectively, with the four overall measures of organizational coordination, each correlation being statistically significant at better than the .05 level. When conformity is related to the components of the overall measures of coordination, we find similar positive and significant relationships with five of the seven components—the three components pertaining to programed coordination, and the two components pertaining to preventive coordination. Hospitals with more extensive conformity are, therefore, likely to have better overall coordination in general and, as might be expected, better preventive and programed coordination in particular.

Table 33 also presents the results concerning the relationship between skill with which planning activities are carried out in the hospital and coordination. Planning skill was measured by asking registered nurses, technicians, and nonmedical department heads the following question: "How good is your immediate superior in planning, organizing, and scheduling the work?" Again, there were five response alternatives, ranging from "excellent" to "very poor."

TABLE 33. Relation Between Certain Aspects of Organizational Planning and Coordination *

Organizational Planning	Overall Measures of Coordination †			
	Measure #1	Measure #2	Measure #3	Measure #4
How clearly defined hospital rules, regulations, and policies are	.62	.57	.59	.53
Extent to which people from different departments follow the rules, regulations, and policies	.83	.78	.70	.87
How good immediate superior is at planning, organizing, and scheduling of work	.40	.30	.33	.36

* All figures are rank-order correlations, based on an N of 10 hospitals in each case. Coefficients larger than .56 are significant at the .05 level, and those .75 or larger are significant at the .01 level.

† These are the same measures as those appearing in Table 30, page 288.

The correlations between this variable and coordination are positive and in the right direction, but they are not statistically significant. Furthermore, when planning skill is related to the components of the overall measures of coordination, only two significant relationships are found: a correlation of .73 with the extent to which organizational members avoid creating interference, and one of .57 with the extent to which they do their job without getting in each other's way, i.e., the two preventive coordination items. These findings suggest a limited significance for the skill with which planning activities are carried out insofar as overall coordination is concerned. However, like definitional clarity of rules and regulations and conformity with rules, planning skill is positively and significantly related to preventive coordination. Accordingly, it cannot be dismissed as an unimportant variable.

The findings in Table 33 provide a clear demonstration of the importance of different aspects of organizational planning in relation to coordination. More significantly, perhaps, they emphasize the role of planning with respect to preventive coordination, being consistent with earlier theoretical expectations. The results also show that the extent of conformity with rules and regulations relates more highly to coordination in comparison to the definitional clarity of rules and the skill with which planning activities are carried out in the hospital. Extensive conformity with organizational requirements on the part of members is at least as essential to achieving adequate coordination as having clearly defined policies, rules, and regulations.

Sharedness of Expectations, Complementarity of Expectations, and Cooperation among Organizational Members in Relation to Coordination

One of the best guarantees that organizational plans will be effectively implemented and that adequate coordination can be attained lies in the nature of the expectations and attitudes of organizational members. In the first place, even if we assume a basic motivation on the part of members to fulfill formal organizational requirements, adherence to plans and rules is not an automatic affair. It depends on whether or not the different members share the same or similar attitudes about organizational operations, on the extent to which members in different but interdependent positions appreciate each other's needs, and on the extent of cooperation among members. Secondly, these normative factors are not only important to coordination through conscious rational planning, but are also important to coordination through the daily efforts of members to respond according to one another's work problems and needs in their interactions. They are important to both programed and general coordination. If the mutual expectations of members whose work is related tend to be contradictory or disparate, rather than congruent or complementary, the organization will be unable to move in a consistent direction or achieve adequate coordination.

In this study, several variables representing sharedness or complementarity of expectations and cooperation were examined in relation to organizational coordination. One measure of sharedness of expectations, emphasizing the extent of generalized consensus among organizational members, was obtained by asking nonsupervisory registered nurses and x-ray and laboratory technicians in each hospital the following question: "How much agreement is there among people in the various related jobs and departments about the everyday operations of the hospital (or to what extent do these people see eye-to-eye on things about the everyday operations of the hospital)?" The response alternatives, forming the usual five-point scale, ranged from "there is complete agreement; people see eye-to-eye very fully" to "there is no agreement; people do not see eye-to-eye at all." A related measure, which emphasizes attitudinal sharedness about work relationships among members, was obtained by this question: "To what degree do people from different departments see the other person's viewpoint in connection with their mutual working relationships?" The five response alternatives in this case ranged from "to a very great degree" to "to a very small degree." This question was asked of registered nurses, medical staff, technicians, and nonmedical department heads, including the hospital administrator.

The relevant findings in Table 34 show a strong, positive, and significant relationship between coordination and each of the two variables concerning sharedness. Those hospitals whose members tend to see eye-to-eye more fully about everyday operations have better coordination. And the same is true with respect to the degree to which members see each other's viewpoint in their work relationships. The overall measures of coordination respectively correlate .74, .74, .79, and .68 with seeing eye-to-eye about hospital operations, and .86, .82, .75, and .83 with seeing each other's viewpoint at work. It is also significant that both programed coordination (measure #4) and general coordination (measure #3) are highly related to the two measures of sharedness of expectations. Furthermore, not shown in the table, essentially the same relationships obtain when instead of the overall measures of coordination their components are used in the analysis.

Concerning complementarity of expectations among organizational members, two measures were related to coordination. These measures were derived from data elicited by the following questions: (1) "On the whole, to what extent does the nursing staff understand and appreciate the problems and needs of the medical staff?" and (2) "On the whole, to what extent does the medical staff understand and appreciate the problems and needs of the nursing staff?" These questions had identical response alternatives, ranging from "they have an excellent understanding" to "they have a rather poor understanding," and were asked only of medical staff and registered nursing staff respondent groups in each hospital. Both questions emphasize complementarity in the form of reciprocal understanding between the two largest and most central groups in the hospital.

TABLE 34. Relation of Certain Aspects of Sharedness or Complementarity of Expectations and Cooperation to Coordination *

Sharedness or Complementarity	Overall Measures of Coordination			
	Measure #1	Measure #2	Measure #3	Measure #4
Extent people from different jobs and departments see eye-to-eye on things about the everyday operations of the hospital	.74	.74	.79	.68
Degree to which members see each other's viewpoint in their work relationships	.86	.82	.75	.83
Extent medical staff understand and appreciate the problems and needs of the nursing staff	.85	.78	.70	.89
Extent nursing staff understand and appreciate the problems and needs of the medical staff	.68	.66	.57	.72
Cooperation				
Degree of willingness of people in related jobs to assist each other when needed	.69	.71	.79	.58
Extent people from different departments do their full share so as to make things easier for others	.54	.52	.53	.47
Extent members' work contacts with other departments produce satisfactory results	.52	.53	.55	.39

* All figures are rank-order correlations, based on an N of 10 hospitals in each case. Coefficients larger than .56 are significant at the .05 level, and those .75 or larger are significant at the .01 level.

The results which show the importance of complementarity of expectations for coordination are also presented in Table 34. First, we find that the better the medical staff understand the problems and needs of the nursing staff, the better the coordination in the hospital. Second, the extent to which the nursing staff understand the problems and needs of the medical staff similarly correlates with coordination positively and significantly. These relationships remain essentially unchanged, moreover, both (1) when instead of the overall measures of coordination their components are used in analysis, and (2) whether the complementarity measures incorporate the responses of both doctors and nurses or use the responses of either group only. The results in Table 34 are also interesting in that they show each of the four overall measures of coordination correlate better with the extent to which the medical staff understand the problems of the nursing staff than with the extent to which the nursing staff understand the problems of the medical staff. In this connection, other data from the study also indicate that doctors and nurses in the various hospitals agree that doctors have a poorer understanding of the problems of nurses than nurses have of the problems of doctors. The relatively poorer understanding of doctors may well be related to their relative independence from direct administrative relationships and controls. These findings should be of practical importance with reference to the tactics one should choose for improving coordination at the hospital.

To investigate the importance of complementarity in the case where organizational members are somewhat peripheral to the interaction structure, we also obtained a measure of the extent to which trustees understand the problems and needs of the medical staff, and vice versa. The study shows rather interesting results in this connection. First, the extent to which doctors understand and appreciate the problems of trustees is not related significantly to any of the overall measures of coordination. However, it correlates significantly with the degree to which the hospital has been able to achieve singleness of direction in the efforts of its various members (.66), and the degree to which members avoid creating interference with one another (.61). Second, the extent to which trustees understand the problems and needs of the medical staff is also significantly related to singleness of direction (.86). In addition, unlike the former, this latter measure correlates significantly with most of the components of the overall measures of coordination and approaches significance at the .05 level with respect to the overall measures.

It therefore seems that from the standpoint of coordination it is more important that trustees have a good understanding of the problems and needs of doctors rather than the other way around. It is more important that the problems of professional members are well understood by the administrative and nonprofessional members than the opposite. The lack of more significant relationships between doctor-trustee complementarity and coordination can be partly accounted for in terms of the fact that, unlike doctors and nurses, trustees are not involved in everyday interaction within the hospital. They are neither direct nor frequent participants in the work structure of the organization, nor have they many contacts with the medical staff. And although trustees may affect coordination indirectly, e.g., through policy making which requires appreciation of the problems and needs of the medical staff, it is not crucial for coordination that members of the medical staff also have a high degree of understanding of the problems of trustees. On the other hand, as shown above, it is of the greatest importance for coordination that doctors have a high degree of understanding and appreciation of the problems and needs of nurses with whom they interact both frequently and directly.

Thus far we have examined the significance that sharedness and complementarity of expectations among organizational members have with respect to coordination. The importance of cooperation among members was studied in a similar manner, by relating three aspects of cooperation to the various measures of coordination. The three cooperation variables were measured by data obtained from these questions: (1) "How willing are people in the different related jobs to assist each other when needed?" (2) "Do people from different departments who have to work together do their full share so that each contributes to making the other person's work a little easier?" and (3) "In general, do your various work contacts with people in other departments produce satisfactory results (i.e., do they help your mutual working relationships)?" In each hospital, the first question was asked of registered nurses, medical staff, x-ray and laboratory technicians, and nonmedical department heads including the hospital administrator; the second question was asked of the same groups, excepting medical staff; and the third question was asked of the same groups, excepting medical staff and the administrator. The response alternatives offered by each question formed the usual five-point scale on the basis of which hospital means were computed and used as measures of cooperation.

The findings regarding the relationship between cooperation and coordination in the hospitals studied are presented in Table 34. The results show that only the first of the above three aspects of cooperation is significantly related to coordination. Hospitals whose members are more willing to assist one another when needed are likely to have better coordination than other hospitals. Specifically, the degree of willingness of people in related jobs to assist each other correlates .69, .71, .79, and .58, respectively, with the four overall measures of coordination. According to these results, moreover, it correlates better with general than with programed coordination (measure #3 vs. measure #4), being apparently more important to those requirements of coordination that organizational planning cannot fulfill by itself. The other two aspects of cooperation here examined also tend to relate positively with coordination, but this tendency does not quite reach statistical significance (although several of the coefficients approach such significance at the .05 level). Doing one's full share, and having work contacts that produce satisfactory results are, therefore, less important to coordination than the willingness of organizational members in related jobs to cooperate when the need arises. However, all three of these aspects of cooperation tend to facilitate coordination in the hospital.

Intraorganizational Strain in Relation to Coordination

Among the factors which were earlier hypothesized to affect coordination is that of intraorganizational strain. In this case, a negative relationship between the degree of prevailing strain among interdependent parts in the system and organizational coordination was predicted. This hypothesis was tested, using measures of two kinds of intraorganizational strain. First, strain was measured in terms of the amount of tension or friction prevailing between interacting hospital groups considered in pairs, e.g., friction between nurses and laboratory technicians, or between housekeeping and maintenance. Second, strain was measured in terms of the degree of experienced "unreasonable" pressure for better performance on the part of nonmedical members.

Intraorganizational strain in the form of tension between groups was

Results Concerning Hospital Coordination

measured on the basis of data from the following tabular-type, multiple-item question:

> On the whole, would you say that in this hospital there is some tension or conflict (friction) between the two groups in each of the following pairs? (Check one for every pair of groups.)

Between:	A very great deal of tension (1)	A great deal of tension (2)	Some tension (3)	A little tension (4)	No tension at all (5)
Administrator *and* trustees	☐	☐	☐	☐	☐
Doctors *and* trustees	☐	☐	☐	☐	☐
Doctors *and* administrator	☐	☐	☐	☐	☐
Doctors *and* other doctors	☐	☐	☐	☐	☐
Doctors *and* nurses	☐	☐	☐	☐	☐
Doctors *and* x-ray service	☐	☐	☐	☐	☐
Doctors *and* records department	☐	☐	☐	☐	☐

This question was asked of medical staff respondents in each hospital, and of trustees and the administrator. In a slightly modified form, moreover, it was also asked of technicians, nonmedical department heads, and registered nursing staff respondents. The modification referred to here affected only the pairs of groups about which different respondents provided information; the stem of the question and the response alternatives were identical in all cases. This was necessary in order that respondents give their evaluation of prevailing tension for only those groups with which they interact or with which they are most familiar. In effect, certain respondents in each hospital, e.g., registered nurses, were asked the question about more pairs of groups than other respondents. And, similarly, tension concerning certain pairs of groups was evaluated by two or more respondent groups.

Relevant data were collected about a total of 26 pairs of groups in the hospital, as follows:

1. Medical staff respondents from each hospital supplied data concerning tension between: administrator and trustees, doctors and trustees, doctors and administrator, doctors and other doctors, doctors and nurses, doctors and x-ray service, doctors and laboratory service, doctors and records department, doctors and admissions, and between doctors and the front office or business office.

2. Supervisory and nonsupervisory registered nurses supplied data concerning tension between: nurses and doctors, nurses and the laboratory, nurses and

x-ray, nurses and admissions, nurses and dietary department, nurses and housekeeping, nurses and maintenance, nurses and patients, nurses and front office, nurses and the hospital administrator, and about tension between nurses and other nurses.

3. Technicians supplied information about tension between: nurses and x-ray, nurses and the laboratory, x-ray and front office, laboratory and front office, laboratory and x-ray, doctors and x-ray, and doctors and laboratory.

4. Nonmedical department heads supplied information for tension between: administrator and department heads, department heads and other department heads, and between maintenance and housekeeping.

5. Trustees supplied data for tension between: doctors and trustees, doctors and other doctors, administrator and trustees, and between doctors and the administrator.

6. The hospital administrator supplied information about tension concerning every pair of groups listed here.

Based on these data, two measures of tension were constructed. Using the evaluations of all respondent groups involved in each case, and with reference to each of the 26 pairs of groups listed above, hospital means were first computed in the usual manner. Each of these means indicates the degree of tension prevailing between two particular groups or departments in each hospital. However, being interested in the overall level of tension characteristic of each hospital as a total organizational system, rather than in the tension characteristic of particular subgroups within the hospital, it was necessary to obtain overall measures of tension. Two such measures were developed, one which takes into account the data from all 26 pairs of groups, and another which makes use only of tension data concerning the more central of these group pairs, as specified below.

Tension *measure #1* was obtained in the following manner: (1) with respect to each of the 26 pairs of groups, and according to the corresponding hospital means mentioned above, the ten hospitals were divided into five "high" tension and five "low" tension hospitals (i.e., using the median point of the distribution of the ten hospital means which represent the tension for a given pair of groups, we separated the hospitals into above and below median tension hospitals); (2) then, each hospital was given an overall tension score equal to the number of its "high," or above median, tension group pairs. In terms of actual scores, in the highest tension hospital 17 of the 26 pairs of groups involved had above median tension; in the lowest tension hospital, only 9 pairs had above median tension. Tension *measure #2* was obtained through an identical procedure, except that instead of using data for all 26 group pairs, only data concerning the following ten central pairs were used: doctors and administrator, doctors and trustees, doctors and other doctors, nurses and doctors, nurses and administrator, nurses and other nurses, nurses and patients, administrator and trustees, administrator and department heads, and department heads and other department heads. In terms of this second measure of overall tension, actual scores ranged from 10 to 1. That is, in the highest tension hospital all ten pairs of central groups had above median tension, while in the lowest tension hospital only one of the ten pairs had above median tension. The two measures of tension correlate .81, which indicates that tension among central groups in the hospital is very closely related to tension among organizational groups in general.

As might have been expected, the data also show that the degree of tension characteristic of a particular pair of groups, e.g., tension between doctors and nurses, varies from one hospital to another. Moreover, within the same hospital there is considerably higher tension between some groups or departments than between other groups. More importantly, some pairs of groups exhibit consistently higher tension across hospitals than other pairs. In general, both medical and nonmedical respondents indicate that more tension exists between doctors and other doctors in their respective hospitals than between any other two groups about which data are available. Considering the top groups in the hospital, we find greater average tension between doctors and other doctors *than* between doctors and nurses *than* between doctors and the administrator *than* between doctors and trustees, in that order. In all hospitals combined, for example, 81 percent of all medical respondents indicate varying degrees of tension between doctors and other doctors, while only 38 percent of them do so regarding tension between doctors and trustees; the comparable figures for trustee respondents are 90 percent and 48 percent, respectively.[1]

What is of even greater significance to our interest in coordination, however, is the fact that certain hospitals exhibit consistently higher levels of overall tension among their different groups than other hospitals. For example, according to tension measure #1, Hospital #1 and Hospital #2 show more tension than any of the remaining eight hospitals. On the other hand, Hospital #3 and Hospital #8 show less overall tension than the remaining institutions. In the case of Hospital #1, we find that 17 of the 26 pairs of groups involved show higher than median tension. By contrast, exactly the same number of group pairs, 17 of 26, in the case of Hospital #3 show lower than median tension. The results are even more dramatic according to tension measure #2, i.e., with respect to overall tension among several central groups in the hospital organization. Using this measure, we find that in the case of Hospital #1 all ten pairs of groups involved show higher than median tension, and in the case

[1] These results point to the need for research on a heretofore neglected aspect of strain in the hospital—the tensions prevailing within rather than between specific organizational groups. They also tend to contradict rather than support the widely held view that ideological differences between professional and lay personnel constitute the primary source of frictions in the hospital, or that most conflicts occur between professional and nonprofessional groups such as between doctors and trustees. This view requires re-evaluation.

of Hospital #2 nine of the ten pairs show the same. By contrast, in both Hospital #7 and Hospital #8 only one pair of groups shows higher than median tension, i.e., nine of the ten pairs show less than median tension. For supplementary qualitative data, which indicate problems of tension in the various institutions, the reader may wish to review the individual profiles of the ten hospitals. These profiles, presented in Chapter 4, contain information which is generally consistent with the findings here reported.

In addition to the two measures of intergroup tension, intraorganizational strain was also measured in the form of unreasonable pressure for better performance prevailing in each hospital. Again, two measures were developed, using data from the following question: "On the job, do you feel any pressure for better performance over and above what you think is reasonable?" Respondents answered in terms of six alternatives, ranging from "I feel a great deal of pressure over and above what is reasonable" to "I feel no pressure at all over and above what is reasonable." In each hospital, the question was asked of the following respondent groups: nonmedical department heads and the hospital administrator, supervisory registered nurses, nonsupervisory registered nurses, practical nurses, aides and orderlies, and x-ray and laboratory technicians. However, the members of each group were asked the question only about the pressure that they themselves experience.

Pressure *measure #1* was developed by computing the mean pressure characteristic of each of the six respondent groups involved, and then combining these six means into an overall hospital mean, separately for every hospital. According to this measure, Hospital #6 ranks highest among the ten hospitals in overall pressure, followed by Hospital #1 and then Hospital #2, while Hospital #8 ranks lowest, followed by Hospital #4 and then Hospital #3— showing a pattern of results very similar to the pattern obtained from the two tension measures. It may also be of interest to note that the same data show which of the respondent groups involved report more unreasonable pressure across the various hospitals. In this connection, members of groups with administrative and supervisory responsibilities are the ones who experience the greatest pressure. For all hospitals combined and in order of degree of pressure, the various groups place as follows: (1) nonmedical administrative department heads, (2) supervisory registered nurses, (3) x-ray and laboratory technicians, (4) nonsupervisory registered nurses, (5) aides and orderlies, and (6) practical nurses—the group whose members experience the least pressure.

Pressure *measure #2* was computed somewhat differently, but using the same data. Having obtained the mean pressure characteristic of a particular respondent group in each hospital, we rank-ordered the ten hospitals according to the magnitude of their means from lowest to highest pressure hospitals and assigned to them corresponding ranks from 1 to 10. This procedure was repeated for each of the six respondent groups involved, resulting in a total of six ranks for every hospital. These ranks were subsequently summed up for

Results Concerning Hospital Coordination

each institution, and the ten hospitals were given a pressure score equal to the sum of their particular ranks. This constitutes measure #2 of overall unreasonable pressure. Using this measure, Hospital #6 again places highest in overall pressure among the hospitals in the study, with a score of 45, followed by Hospital #2, with a score of 41. At the other extreme, Hospital #8 and Hospital #3 are the lowest pressure hospitals, both having a tie score of 22. Theoretically, according to the procedure used here, the highest possible score for a hospital could be 60, while the lowest possible score could be 6. The two measures of pressure correlate .87.

In summary, four measures of intraorganizational strain were developed. Two of them deal with strain in the form of intergroup tension in the hospital, while the other two deal with strain in the form of experienced unreasonable pressure for better performance by people in certain organizational roles. The former two measures correlate .81 and the latter correlate .87. Although these correlations are relatively high, they are far from perfect (the first accounts for about 65 percent of the variance involved and the second accounts for about 75 percent of the variance) and, consequently, all four measures are retained in the analyses which follow. In addition to these relationships between the measures of tension and between the measures of pressure, we find that tension measure #1 correlates .65 with pressure measure #1 and .60 with pressure measure #2, while tension measure #2 correlates .72 with pressure measure #1 and .64 with pressure measure #2. These relationships show that those hospitals which have relatively high intergroup tension are also likely to be characterized by relatively high "unreasonable" pressure, and vice versa.

With respect to each of the four measures of intraorganizational strain, the ten hospitals were rank-ordered in relation to one another, from the highest to the lowest strain hospital. The resulting distributions of the hospitals on strain were then related to the hospital distributions on the various measures of coordination. Table 35 presents the findings concerning the relation of intraorganizational strain to organizational coordination. On the whole, these findings strongly support our initial hypothesis that intraorganizational strain, whether in the form of tension or in the form of pressure, will be negatively related to coordination. The data show that hospitals with more tension, or more unreasonable pressure, have poorer coordination than hospitals with less tension or pressure.

The first four rows of correlations in Table 35 show that each of the overall measures of coordination is inversely related to each measure of intraorganizational strain, all 16 correlation coefficients being statistically significant at better than the .05 level. For example, considering overall measure #1 of coordination, we find that it correlates —.88 with tension measure #1, —.62 with tension measure #2, —.66 with pressure measure #1, and also —.66 with pressure measure #2. Similar relationships obtain when we consider the

TABLE 35. Relation Between Intraorganizational Strain and Coordination *

Coordination Measures	Tension Measure #1	Tension Measure #2	Pressure Measure #1	Pressure Measure #2
Overall measure #1	−.88	−.62	−.66	−.66
Overall measure #2	−.85	−.62	−.75	−.76
Overall measure #3	−.88	−.69	−.75	−.82
Overall measure #4	−.92	−.65	−.67	−.58
How well different jobs and activities fit together	−.70	−.50	−.69	−.82
Extent members make an effort to avoid creating problems or interference	−.51	−.32	−.19	−.41
Extent members do their jobs properly without getting in each other's way	−.78	−.59	−.63	−.65
Extent patients feel personnel around them work together smoothly	−.79	−.74	−.81	−.85
How well timed activities are in the everyday routine	−.90	−.84	−.88	−.81
Extent work assignments are well planned	−.64	−.47	−.50	−.34
How well established are the routines of interdependent departments	−.85	−.55	−.50	−.45

* All figures are rank-order correlations, based on an N of 10 hospitals in each case. Coefficients larger than −.56 are significant at the .05 level, and those −.75 or larger are significant at the .01 level.

remaining three measures of hospital coordination. The same results also demonstrate that both programed coordination (overall measure #4) and general coordination (overall measure #3) are highly and significantly related to strain in the organization. The greater the strain, the poorer the coordination is in all cases.

Of the four measures of strain, tension measure #1 produces the highest relationships with overall coordination. This measure, representing the total level of tension characteristic of 26 pairs of groups within the hospital, correlates −.88, −.85, −.88, and −.92, respectively, with the four overall measures of coordination. Tension measure #2, representing the level of tension characteristic of only ten central pairs of groups, produces the lowest correlations with overall coordination, even though all of these correlations are also statistically significant. These results indicate that: (1) it is the level of tension which more closely reflects the situation of the entire structure of the hospital, rather than certain central units of the organization only, which is of the greatest significance to coordination; and (2) since a very important component of tension measure #2 is the tension between trustees and each of certain other groups, it appears that it is the tension between groups directly involved in the action structure of the hospital that weighs most heavily with respect to coordination—trustees being a group not directly involved in the action structure. It is also possible, but unlikely, that tension measure #1 produces stronger relationships in part because it may be a somewhat more reliable measure than tension measure #2, which is based on fewer pairs of groups.

Table 35 also presents the relationships between strain and each of the seven specific components of the overall measures of coordination. Here too, the total pattern of findings clearly substantiates the proposition that intraorganizational strain is negatively associated with coordination. For example, how well different jobs and activities in the hospital fit together correlates —.70 with tension measure #1, —.50 with tension measure #2, —.69 with pressure measure #1, and —.82 with pressure measure #2. The four measures of strain yield similar relationships with the extent to which organizational members do their job without getting in each other's way, the extent to which patients feel that personnel around them work together smoothly, and with how well timed everyday activities are in the hospital. The remaining three component items of the overall measures of coordination are also negatively related to the various measures of strain, although most of the correlations here do not quite reach statistical significance.

With reference to the various types of coordination, the findings show that strain consistently tends to be more closely associated with promotive coordination; it correlates negatively both with the extent to which patients feel hospital personnel work together smoothly, and with how well different activities in the hospital fit together. It is important to note, however, that of the seven component items of coordination the one which produces the highest relationships with strain is "how well timed activities are in the everyday routine." This item correlates —.90 with tension measure #1, —.84 with tension measure #2, —.88 with pressure measure #1, and —.81 with pressure measure #2. It will be recalled that how well timed activities are is one of the three items used to represent the category of programed coordination. But, since the other two components of programed coordination (how well established routines are, and how well planned work assignments are) are among the coordination items which are least highly related to strain, we should not conclude that strain relates particularly well to programed coordination.

We should perhaps point out that, regardless of the type of coordination most closely associated with intraorganizational strain, the timing of activities *per se* seems to be a crucial variable with respect to both strain and coordination. In addition to supporting the hypothesis that strain relates negatively to coordination in general, and to the timing of activity in particular, the above findings suggest that the better the timing of activities the less the strain is likely to be. If timing actually affects the level of strain in an organization, which appears to be the case, then we are confronted with a kind of a vicious circle since good timing is an essential aspect of adequate coordination. Hospitals with high levels of strain have difficulty in attaining good coordination, while poor coordination in the form of inadequate timing of activities increases the likelihood for the development of high strain in the system. In short, deficient timing impedes overall coordination while it facilitates strain which, in turn, is detrimental both to the attainment and maintenance of good overall coordination.

Returning now to the question of the relationship between intraorganizational strain and coordination, the findings may be summarized as follows:

1. Hospitals with higher levels of intraorganizational strain have poorer coordination than hospitals with lower levels of strain.

2. The degree of strain relates negatively and significantly to both programed and general coordination.

3. Strain relates highly and consistently to the promotive type of coordination, i.e., it obstructs promotive coordination, but it relates most highly to the coordination item of how well timed activities are in the everyday routine of the hospital.

4. Of the four measures of intraorganizational strain, tension measure #1 produces the highest correlations with the overall measures of coordination and with most of the specific components of these overall measures.

5. From a functional standpoint, both kinds of strain, i.e., strain in the form of intergroup tension and strain in the form of experienced unreasonable pressure for better performance, behave similarly with respect to coordination—they both yield significant negative relationships, as expected.

The hypothesis of an inverse relationship between intraorganizational strain and coordination, therefore, receives strong support from the data.

Problem Awareness and Problem Solving in Relation to Coordination

In part, coordination represents the results of a more or less continuous process of solving problems that arise in the work relationships of organizational members. Adequate coordination is thus predicated upon the successful solution of such problems. It is not enough that problems be resolved, however. They must be handled satisfactorily, taking into account the concerns of all relevant parties, and must be settled on time so as to mitigate existing tensions and alleviate the development of new ones. Furthermore, the solution of a problem ordinarily depends upon an awareness that the problem exists, and the role of persons holding key positions in the organization may be a crucial one in this connection. Whether or not the administrator and the director of nursing, for example, are aware of the problems faced by different organizational members may have important consequences for coordination, since these two individuals have as one of their main responsibilities the coordination of the activities of numerous other people in the hospital. On the other hand, mere awareness of the presence of a difficulty is not a sufficient condition for its solution. These considerations led us to study the relationship between coordination and: (1) how satisfactorily problems of working together are handled, (2) how promptly such problems are settled, (3) how fully aware of problems are those who hold key positions in the hospital, and (4) how effective they are in solving problems.

A measure of how satisfactorily problems are handled at the hospital was obtained using the following question:

> When people from different departments have to work together in order to accomplish something in common, various problems are likely to arise. In your experience while working here, how are such problems of working together and fitting into the overall pattern handled? (Check one.)
> _____(1) These kinds of problems are handled completely satisfactorily for all concerned
> _____(2) They are handled very satisfactorily
> _____(3) They are handled fairly satisfactorily
> _____(4) They are handled rather unsatisfactorily
> _____(5) These kinds of problems are not handled satisfactorily at all

In each hospital, the question was asked of the following groups of respondents: medical staff members, nonsupervisory registered nurses, administrative department heads, and technicians. In addition, the same respondents, except medical staff members, were also asked to indicate "how quickly" the problems referred to in the above question are settled. Data from the two questions were transformed into hospital means, and these means were used as measures of how satisfactorily problems are handled and how promptly they are settled. The relationships between these variables and coordination are presented in Table 36.

The findings clearly show that the more satisfactorily problems of working together are handled in the hospital the better the coordination is. How satisfactorily problems are handled correlates .87, .83, .85, and .85, respectively, with the four overall measures of coordination. These correlations are significant at better than the .01 level. Furthermore, not shown in the table, the same variable produces positive correlations with each of the seven components of the overall measures of coordination, five of these correlations being statistically significant at the .05 level or better. The promptness with which problems are settled, which incidentally is not significantly related to how satisfactorily problems are handled, is also positively related to overall coordination. In this case, as shown in Table 36, three of the four correlations are significant at the .05 level. With reference to the components of the overall measures of coordination, promptness correlates significantly with how well established departmental routines are and with the extent to which members do their job without getting in each other's way; it also correlates positively with the remaining components but the correlations are not statistically significant. In view of these findings, we conclude that both how satisfactorily problems are handled and how promptly they are settled facilitate coordination, although the former is a much more important factor than the latter.

TABLE 36. Relation of Problem Awareness and Problem Solving to Coordination [*]

Awareness of Problems and Problem Solving	Measure #1	Measure #2	Measure #3	Measure #4
How satisfactorily problems of working together are handled in the hospital	.87	.83	.85	.85
Promptness with which problems of working together are settled	.62	.53	.58	.59
How fully aware the administrator is of problems faced by organizational members	.42	.27	.36	.44
How fully aware the director of nursing is of problems faced by members	.31	.39	.32	.33
How fully aware both the administrator and the director of nursing are of problems faced by members	.54	.49	.55	.58
How effective the administrator is in solving conflicts arising in the organization	.42	.32	.43	.47
How effective the director of nursing is in solving conflicts arising in the organization	.57	.61	.51	.54
How effective both the administrator and the director of nursing are in solving conflicts	.70	.73	.67	.72

[*] Rank-order correlations, based on an N of 10 hospitals in each case. Coefficients larger than .56 are significant at the .05 level, and those .75 or larger are significant at the .01 level.

Probably the two most crucial organizational roles in the hospital, from the standpoint of coordination, are those of the administrator and of the director of nursing. The former is in charge of all nonmedical personnel and all nonmedical aspects of hospital operation, while the latter heads the largest department in the hospital—a department, moreover, which carries out more coordinating functions than any other organizational unit in addition to having patient care responsibilties. It would, therefore, be important to know whether the relative problem awareness of the administrator and of the director of nursing, and their relative effectiveness in solving conflicts that arise in the organization, have any relationship to coordination. To this effect, a series of questions were asked of certain respondents in each hospital to provide necessary measures. Nonmedical department heads and those members of the medical staff who

Results Concerning Hospital Coordination

have administrative responsibilities or major committee functions were asked to indicate, on a five-point scale, the extent to which the administrator is aware of problems faced by others in the hospital and how effective he is in solving conflicts that arise in the organization. Similarly, supervisory registered nurses were asked the same questions about the director of nursing. Using these data, measures were constructed in the form of hospital means and related to coordination.

Table 36 shows that hospitals whose administrators are more fully aware of problems faced by organizational members tend to have somewhat better overall coordination, but this tendency is not statistically significant. The same applies in the case of the director of nursing. Therefore, better problem awareness on the part of individuals in key roles does not necessarily result in better coordination. Further analysis reveals, however, that the administrator's awareness of problems is positively and significantly related to two of the components of overall coordination, namely the components which deal with preventive coordination (problem awareness correlates .62 with the extent to which members make an effort to avoid creating interference and .58 with the extent to which they do their job properly without getting in each other's way). This finding is consistent with the nature of preventive coordination, as discussed earlier in this volume but, since no comparable significant results obtain about the awareness of the director of nursing, the data show no consistent pattern of relationships. In this connection, we should add, however, that the relative awareness of the director of nursing is not related to that of the administrator in this group of hospitals; the correlation between the two is —.30, which is not significant.

Apparently, the problem awareness of a given person occupying an important position in the organization is not a sufficient condition for adequate organizational coordination. However, the fact that no relationship exists between the awareness of the administrator and the awareness of the director of nursing in the hospitals studied suggests the possibility that those in these positions may have to be aware of different problems and that their combined problem awareness may be the important thing. That is, it may be that the problem awareness of the administrator is complemented or supplemented by that of the director of nursing. If this were true, to the extent that a relationship between problem awareness and coordination exists, we should expect the combined awareness of persons in key roles to be significantly related with overall coordination.

The relevant findings, also presented in Table 36, actually show that the combined problem awareness of the administrator and the director of nursing produces better correlations with coordination than does the awareness of either of them separately. It correlates .54, .49, .55, and .58, respectively, with the overall measures of coordination, the last correlation being statistically significant at the .05 level and the others approaching such significance.

Furthermore, combined awareness is also significantly related to three of the components of the overall measures—the two components to which the administrator's awareness had been found to relate plus the component of how well timed activities are. Taking into consideration all of the above results concerning problem awareness, we may conclude that the combined awareness of persons in key organizational positions to an extent facilitates coordination, although it does not necessarily guarantee good coordination, and that coordination is affected more by the combined awareness of such persons rather than by the awareness of a single individual in a crucial role.

An analysis similar to that concerning problem awareness was also carried out with respect to the relative effectiveness of persons in key roles in solving conflicts that arise in the organization. Again, the roles of the administrator and of the director of nursing served as the referents of the analysis. The results are presented in Table 36. First, we find that the effectiveness of the administrator in solving conflicts tends to be positively related to the four overall measures of coordination, but the correlations are not statistically significant; and the same is true when his effectiveness is related to the components of the overall measures. Second, the effectiveness of the director of nursing in solving conflicts is only somewhat better related to the overall measures of coordination as compared to the effectiveness of the administrator. In this case, two of the four correlations are statistically significant; but with reference to the components of overall coordination significant relationships are obtained only with the two preventive coordination items.

When the combined conflict-solving effectiveness of the administrator and the director of nursing is related to coordination, it produces highly significant results. It correlates .70, .73, .67, and .72, respectively, with the overall measures of coordination. Furthermore, not shown in the table, it produces comparable significant relationships with most of the components of the overall measures. These results are especially important if we also consider the fact that there is no relationship between the conflict-solving effectiveness of the administrator and that of the director of nursing in this group of hospitals; the correlation between the two is —.12. As in the case of problem awareness, only to a greater degree, it is the combined conflict-solving effectiveness of persons in key organizational roles that affects organizational coordination.

These findings have certain interesting practical implications. First, they are consistent with the current trend in many hospitals to make the director of nursing an "assistant administrator." Second, since it is the combined conflict-solving (or problem-solving) effectiveness of persons in key organizational roles that is important to coordination, one would expect those hospitals which have both an administrator and a director of nursing who rate high on this variable to be in an advantageous position over other hospitals with respect to coordination. The data show that this is the case. The three of our ten hospitals which have both an administrator and a director of nursing rated high, or above median, on conflict-solving effectiveness (Hospitals #3, #8, and #0) are also among the top five hospitals in terms of overall coordination—two of them ranking first and second on coordination. Third, one might ask the following question: aside from a hospital having both an effective administrator and an effective director of nursing, would it be better for coordination to have in these positions two individuals who are both moderately effective in solving conflicts, or would it be preferable to have a very effective individual in one of the two roles while having a relatively ineffective person in the other? And, while we are here dealing only with two organizational roles, the same issues are undoubtedly applicable also to the case where more than two key roles are involved. An answer to the question here raised would be very important to those concerned with the administration of organizations. Unfortunately, the question cannot be examined further in this study because the number of hospitals with which we are dealing is not sufficient to permit the required analysis.

Our discussion of problem awareness and problem solving on the part of persons in key roles at the hospital in relation to coordination would be incomplete without a consideration of the role of the chief of the medical staff and the role of the president of the board of trustees. Both of these individuals, like the administrator and the director of nursing, occupy very important positions. However, their roles are somewhat tangential from the standpoint of organizational coordination. The president of the board of trustees actually carries no major coordinative functions. In a sense, he is only an interested outsider insofar as the work structure of the organization is concerned. Although he plays a crucial part with respect to general hospital policies and finances, he neither has a full-time job in the hospital nor is he very familiar with the day-to-day operations of the institution. For these and related reasons, we expected no direct relationships between coordination and the extent to which the president of the board is aware of problems faced by organizational members or his effectiveness in solving conflicts that arise in the organization. Nevertheless, appropriate data were collected from medical staff respondents who have administrative functions in the hospital (and are, therefore, familiar with the president of the board) to test this hypothesis. The data substantiate our expectations. We find no relationship between problem awareness or conflict-solving effectiveness on the part of the president of the board of trustees and coordination, whether the overall measures of coordination or their components are used in the analysis.

The case of the chief of the medical staff is similar to that of the president of trustees, but for partly different reasons. In the hospitals studied, the chief of staff has no major coordinative functions outside the medical staff although he, along with other staff members, often represents the staff vis-à-vis the board of trustees. He has jurisdiction only over medical matters, and his limited authority is subject to the influence of the general medical staff and its various committees. More importantly, in most cases the office of the chief of staff is more of an honorific rather than a functional one, many chiefs being elected on bases other than administrative or professional expertness. In addition, with rare exceptions, their term of office is only one year, and re-election is unlikely in contrast to the case of the president of the board of trustees. Like the president of trustees, on the other hand, the chief of the medical staff is neither an employee nor a "full-fledged" member of the organization. In many cases, nevertheless, the person in this role may be extremely influential in the affairs of the institution and very much interested in what is going on. On the whole, however, the role of the chief of staff does not appear to be important or especially relevant to organizational coordination in comparison to the role of the administrator or of the director of nursing.

Because of these reasons, as in the case of the president of the board of trustees, we expected no relationship between the problem awareness of the chief of staff, or his conflict-solving effectiveness, and coordination. The data tend to confirm this expectation, but not completely. We find that the relative problem awareness of the chief of staff, as appraised by medical staff respondents who have no administrative responsbilities, does not relate either to the overall measures of coordination or to any of their seven components. However, his effectiveness in solving conflicts that arise in the organization, as appraised by the same respondents, produces certain rather surprising results. It correlates −.47, −.54, −.58, and −.38, respectively, with the four overall measures of coordination. One of these correlations, namely the correlation with general coordination (measure #3), being −.58, is statistically significant at the .05 level. Even though only one out of four correlations is significant, it deserves further examination because it is negative; and being negative, it implies that the higher the effectiveness of the chief of staff in solving conflicts, the poorer the coordination.

It could be that this negative correlation is the result of chance factors, especially since the other three correlations are not significant. A correlation as large as this actually could have occurred by chance 5 out of 100 times. It also happens that the effectiveness of the chief of staff in solving conflicts correlates highly and significantly (.83) with his problem awareness, but the latter was found to bear no relationship to any of our coordination measures. This enhances the possibility of a chance outcome. There is one more relevant element, however, that should be taken into consideration. The conflict-solving effectiveness of the chief of staff also correlates −.58 with two of the seven components of the overall measures of coordination, the two components representing promotive coordination (how well different jobs and activities fit together, and the extent to which patients feel that personnel work together smoothly). If these two correlations were also the result of chance, no further interpretation would be necessary; if not, another explanation should be sought.

An alternative interpretation, which may be more applicable here than the chance theory, is possible. First, being effective in solving conflicts does not also mean that the solution itself is satisfactory to all affected parties. To the exent to which the conflict solutions supplied by the chiefs of staff are unsatisfactory to that exent we may expect coordination to be adversely affected, in view of the earlier finding that how satisfactorily problems are handled is positively related to coordination. Second, it is not unlikely that those chiefs of staff who are more effective in solving conflicts are also the ones who tend to provide one-sided or biased solutions, with the net effect that promotive coordination suffers. Events within the medical staff have repercussions in other parts of the hospital, often affecting nonmedical members, and it is possible that while conflict solutions within the medical staff may protect the interests of doctors they could, at the same time, create problems for others. Third, it is also possible that chiefs of staff who are effective in solving conflicts were elected to their position precisely because their hospital was facing conflicts. Subsequently, however, some of the conflicts remained unresolved during the short term of office (one year) of most chiefs of staff. These conside.ations alone, or together with the possibility of a chance outcome, might account for the three negative correlations between the effectiveness of the chiefs of staff in solving conflicts and coordination. Our tentative conclusion is that there is little evidence for a direct relationship between these two variables in the hospitals studied, although the results are certainly not clear-cut. Further research will be necessary to explore more fully the possibilities here suggested.

In summary, the findings about problem awareness and problem solving in relation to coordination may be stated as follows:

1. There is a positive relation between how satisfactorily problems of working together are handled in the hospital and coordination.

2. The promptness with which such problems are settled also tends to be positively associated with coordination, although to a smaller degree.

3. The combined problem awareness of the administrator and the director of nursing yields several positive correlations with coordination; but the problem awareness of the president of the board of trustees or of the chief of the medical staff is unrelated to organizational coordination.

4. The combined effectiveness of the administrator and of the director of nursing in solving conflicts that arise in the organization is positively related to coordination.

5. The effectiveness of the president of the board of trustees in solving conflicts is unrelated to coordination, while the corresponding effectiveness of the chief of staff yields inconclusive results.

6. In any event, it is the combined rather than the individual problem awareness or conflict-solving effectiveness of persons in relevant key roles (administrator and director of nursing) in the hospital that is important to coordination.

Communication in Relation to Coordination

In a complex organization, problem awareness and problem solving imply the transmission and exchange of information among the parties involved. Thus, communication may affect coordination indirectly, through the facilitation of problem solving. Communication may also affect coordination directly. The synchronization of various interdependent parts and activities in the system, which is an essential aspect of coordination, would be virtually impossible without the exchange of relevant and necessary information among organizational parts. To initiate and carry out a surgical procedure in the hospital, for example, requires a good deal of communication which, in addition to the surgeon and his immediate assisting staff, may involve administrative personnel, the business office, the admissions department, the x-ray department and the laboratory, nursing personnel in different shifts, and other members of the organization, as well as the patient's family and other outsiders, such as legal agencies and authorities.

In addition to daily communication among members, many of the written documents, schedules, rules, and regulations which one finds in an organization are but devices designed to promote or ensure coordination. One of the major functions of the patient chart (record) in the hospital, for example, is coordination between medical staff and nursing staff and coordination among different personnel within the nursing staff and within the medical staff. The mechanical intercommunication system performs similar functions. In addition to serving as an important and direct means for coordination, communication may affect coordination in still another way—a way which may even be more important and more powerful. Specifically, it can affect coordination through the development of shared norms and through the development of complementary expectations and reciprocal understanding among organizational members whose activities are related. In brief, formal and informal communication may affect coordination directly as well as indirectly. For these reasons, in this study, we have examined several aspects of communication in relation to coordination.

First, it will be recalled that in our discussion of organizational planning earlier in this chapter, we found that the definitional clarity of hospital rules and regulations is positively related to coordination. One of the reasons for this relationship is that clarity makes for better communication, which in turn makes for better planning. Second, our study of communication patterns among registered nurses in the hospital, which is fully reported in Chapter 10, shows that communication is positively related to coordination within the nursing department. More specifically, the frequency with which registered nurses talk with their immediate superior, relative to talking with the person with whom they communicate most in the hospital, about such task-related topics as "ways to improve patient care" and "ways to improve nursing supervision" is positively and significantly related to nursing department coordination. These findings are reported elsewhere and will not be discussed further at this point; instead, we will turn our attention to additional results concerning relationships between communication and coordination.

In this area, theoretical considerations argued for more emphasis on the nature of communication than on absolute volume or frequency. Accordingly, instead of collecting data about the amount of time members spend communicating, or the number of meetings and conferences held among members, we mostly inquired about such things as the relative openness of communication channels and the extent to which communication is perceived as helpful, informative, or adequate. First, with respect to the openness of communication channels, we asked nonsupervisory registered nurses and x-ray and laboratory technicians in each hospital the following question: "How easy is it for you to get together and exchange information and ideas about the work with people in other departments whose jobs are related to yours?" The response alternatives ranged from "it is very easy" to "it is very difficult," forming a five-point scale. The responses of nurses and technicians were converted into hospital means to provide a measure of openness of communication channels. It is worth noting, however, that the responses of nurses correlated very highly and significantly (.78) with those of the technicians, suggesting good agreement as to the relative ease of communication in the various hospitals.

The relationship between openness of communication channels and coordination is shown by the first row of correlations in Table 37. We find that those hospitals which have relatively greater openness in communication channels tend to have better coordination. The ease with which people can meet to exchange information and ideas about work correlates .59, .55, .62, and .47, respectively, with the overall measures of coordination. Two of the first three correlations are statistically significant at the .05 level and one is almost significant. The smallest correlation, which incidentally pertains to programed coordination, is not significant, however, indicating that openness of communication channels is more important for general rather than programed coordination. This conclusion is also supported by additional results concerning the relationship of ease of communication to the various components of the overall measures of coordination. We find that ease of communication is positively and significantly related to three of the four components of general coordination, while it is similarly related to only one of the three components of programed coordination, namely the component of how well established departmental routines are in the hospital. These results show

TABLE 37. Relation Between Certain Aspects of Communication and Coordination *

Communication	Overall Measures of Coordination			
	Measure #1	Measure #2	Measure #3	Measure #4
Ease with which people in related jobs can get together to exchange information and ideas about work	.59	.55	.62	.47
Frequency with which people from related jobs get together to discuss work problems and differences	.45	.39	.39	.36
Extent to which members feel that decisions which affect their work are explained to them adequately	.68	.64	.73	.62
Extent to which medical staff members perceive the communication they receive from the hospital administrator as adequate	.54	.48	.54	.54
How adequately doctors explain the condition and needs of their patients to nursing personnel	.48	.45	.33	.53
Degree of adequacy of patient charts at nursing stations in the hospital, as evaluated by medical staff members	.23	.16	.16	.25
Degree of adequacy of patient charts at nursing stations in the hospital, as evaluated by registered nurses	.69	.78	.74	.65

* All figures are rank-order correlations, based on an N of 10 hospitals in each case. Coefficients larger than .56 are significant at the .05 level.

that the openness of communication channels in the hospital significantly affects the coordination of the institution, especially its nonprogramed coordination.

Frequency of communication is another variable which was examined in relation to coordination. Our measure of this variable is based on the following question: "How often do people from different jobs and departments get together when needed to discuss and try to do something about problems and differences arising in their work relationships with one another?" Again, the response alternatives constituted a five-point scale, ranging from "always" to "less than half of the time." In each hospital, the question was asked of registered nursing personnel, technicians, and nonmedical department heads, and hospital means were computed using the answers of these respondents. Table 37 shows that there is no significant relationship between frequency of communication, as measured by the above question, and any of the overall measures of coordination; the relevant correlations are all positive but none is statistically significant. Moreover, when frequency of communication is related to the components of the overall measures of coordination, we find that it relates significantly to only two of the seven components, the components dealing with preventive coordination (i.e., with the extent to which people make an effort to avoid creating problems, and the extent to which they do their job without getting in each other's way).

Apparently, there is very little relationship between frequency of communication and coordination. The fact that people get together to discuss their problems more frequently in some hospitals than others does not necessarily mean that their communication is more successful or that they actually do better in solving their problems. However, the fact that frequency of communication is positively related to preventive coordination suggests that frequent communication is not altogether irrelevant to coordination. Perhaps getting together to discuss problems on a frequent basis at least helps people to avoid the creation of new problems and to prevent undesirable interferences. However, unlike the ease with which people can communicate or the openness of communication channels, frequency of communication seems to be of limited importance to coordination. This is the more interesting, if we take into account the added fact that frequency of communication correlates positively and significantly (.73) with the openness of communication channels in this group of hospitals.

Another important aspect of communication, in any organization, has to do with the implementation of decisions which affect the work of the members. How adequately or inadequately decisions are communicated and explained to those concerned may have serious implications for coordination, as well as for other aspects of organizational functioning. This variable, therefore, was also measured and related to coordination. The question used in this case was: "When decisions that affect your work are made, how adequately are such decisions explained to you?" Respondents answered the question in terms of five alternatives ranging from "completely adequately" to "inadequately." In each hospital, the question was asked of registered nursing personnel, i.e., supervisory and nonsupervisory registered nurses, and of nonmedical administrative department heads—precisely those respondent groups whose members perform most of the day-to-day coordinative functions in the hospital.

Table 37 shows that the extent to which organizational members feel that decisions which affect their work are explained to them adequately is, as expected, positively and significantly related to coordination. It correlates .68, .64, .73, and .62, respectively, with the overall measures of coordination. The smallest correlation obtains with the measure of programed coordination and the largest with the measure of general coordination, but all four correlations are statistically significant at better than the .05 level. Furthermore, not shown in the table, when the adequacy with which decisions are explained to members is related to the components of the overall measures of coordination it produces similar relationships. First, it correlates positively with all of the components of the overall measures of coordination. Second, while it yields high and signficant correlations with three of the four components of general coordination, it does so with one of the three components of programed coordination, namely, with how well timed activities are. Third, it relates best to the two components of preventive coordination; it correlates .81 with the extent to which members make an effort to avoid creating problems or interference, and .77 with the extent to which members do their job properly without getting in each other's way. It is, therefore, clear that the adequacy with which decisions are explained to members affects coordination very significantly, being especially important to preventive and nonprogramed coordination.

Apart from these relationships, it is also important to add that the adequacy with which decisions are explained to members is positively and significantly related to both the openness of communication channels (.70) and the frequency with which members get together to discuss problems (.66). In view of the fact that these latter two communication variables are also significantly interrelated (.78), as noted above, it appears that some hospitals are consistently characterized by better overall communication practices than others. Those hospitals whose members feel that it is easy for them to get together for communication purposes are also likely to be the ones where frequency of communication is higher and where the adequacy with which decisions are explained to members is similarly higher. And although these three variables are not of equal importance to coordination (frequency of communication being the least important), as the findings show, it is safe to conclude that communication practices such as those examined here definitely facilitate organizational coordination.

In each hospital, medical staff respondents with no administrative responsibilities (and, therefore, members having no formally established communication ties with their hospital administrator) were asked to indicate how adequate they feel the communication which they receive from the administrator is. In this connection, Table 37 shows that the extent to which doctors perceive the communication which they receive from the administrator as adequate correlates .54, .48, .54, and .54, respectively, with the overall measures of coordination. These correlations do not quite reach statistical significance at the .05 level, but they approach such significance very closely. In other words, there is some tendency for adequacy of communication to be associated with better coordination in the various hospitals. With respect to the components of the overall measures of coordination, we find that the adequacy of the administrator's communication to doctors correlates .67 with the extent to which people do their job without getting in each other's way, .57 with how well planned work assignments are, and .65 with how well timed activities are in the hospital. Since the last two variables constitute two of the three components of programed coordination, the data show that the adequacy of the communication which doctors receive from the administrator has a positive effect on programed coordination in the hospital.

The last three rows of correlations in Table 37 deal with communication between doctors and nurses, and with the adequacy of patient records in relation to coordination. Concerning the former, all registered nursing staff and medical staff respondents from each hospital were asked to give us their judgment about how adequately doctors explain the condition and needs of their patients to nursing personnel. As Table 37 shows, this variable yields no significant relationships with any of the overall measures of coordination. Furthermore, additional analysis shows that it correlates significantly with only one of the seven components of the overall measures of coordination; it correlates .72 with how well established departmental routines are in the hospital. Apparently, the adequacy with which doctors explain the condition of their patients to nurses is not a crucial factor insofar as coordination is concerned.

It is likely that doctors are not actually expected by nurses to give an adequate explanation of the patient's condition. They may be expected to explain essential technical aspects relating to treatment and, other than that, nurses probably rely heavily on what the doctors write on the patient chart and on their own judgment. Certain findings, to be reported below, support this interpretation. The lack of significant association between adequacy of explanation and coordination can also be due to other considerations. It so happens, for example, that the judgment of medical respondents as to how adequately doctors explain things to nurses is not related to the comparable judgment of nurse respondents; the correlation between the evaluations of the two groups is practically zero (−.04). Incidentally, the data show that in five of the ten hospitals doctors evaluate their explanation to nurses more favorably than nurses do, while the opposite occurs in the other five hospitals. The lack of agreement between the two respondent groups may or may not be important. However, even when we measure how adequately doctors explain things to nurses using exclusively the responses of doctors, or exclusively the responses of nurses, we still find no significant relationships between adequacy of explanation and any of the overall measures of coordination or any of their components. This outcome tends to support our first interpretation that the communication variable here examined has no bearing on coordination.

One more communication variable was related to coordination in this study. It concerns the patient's record, which serves as an important means of communication in the hospital structure. While the patient is under care, nurses and doctors make extensive use of his chart in order both to communicate about him and to regulate his treatment. Therefore, on the assumption that the patient chart may be an important mechanism for coordination, medical staff and registered nursing staff respondents from each hospital were asked the following question: "How complete, or how adequate, are the patients' charts (records) at the nurses' stations?" The response alternatives ranged from "they are completely adequate" to "they are inadequate," constituting a five-point scale and permitting the computation of hospital means as measures of the adequacy of the patient chart.

When the adequacy of patient charts at the nursing stations, as judged by both doctors and nurses, is related to the overall measures of coordination we find only moderate positive correlations. These correlations, varying from .47 to .52, and based on an N of 10 hospitals, are not significant at the .05 level. They suggest only a tendency for the adequacy of patient charts to be associated with overall organizational coordination. Similarly, with regard to the components of the overall measures of coordination, the adequacy of patient charts produces moderate positive correlations with all seven components, but only two of these correlations are statistically significant (a correlation of .63 with the extent to which different jobs and activities fit together in the hospital, and one of .64 with the extent to which members do their job without getting in each other's way). Further examination reveals, however, that the adequacy of patient charts as evaluated by nurses produces entirely different results from the adequacy of charts as evaluated by doctors.

Additional analysis was carried out because the data showed that the adequacy of patient charts as evaluated by doctors is not related to the adequacy of charts as evaluated by nurses. The correlation between the two evaluations is —.09, i.e., practically zero. In eight of the ten hospitals incidentally, doctors evaluate the adequacy of patient charts more favorably than nurses. The lack of agreement between doctors and nurses suggests that the two groups employed different criteria, or different frames of reference, in their evaluations. It is possible, for example, that doctors evaluated the adequacy of patient charts primarily in terms of what they themselves write on them. It is also possible that doctors evaluated the charts partly on the basis of how the charts look when they complete them, after the patient has been discharged; nurses can only evaluate the charts on the basis of how they look while still at the nursing station, prior to completion. These considerations, in addition to the fact that, unlike doctors, nurses engage in considerable coordinative activity as part of their organizational role, argued for separate treatment of the evaluations given by doctors and by nurses. Table 37 incorporates the results of this analysis.

We find that the degree of adequacy of patient charts at the nursing stations, as evaluated by medical respondents, is not related to any of the overall measures of coordination. Furthermore, not shown in Table 37, it correlates significantly (.62) with only one of the seven components of the overall measures, namely with the extent to which members make an effort to avoid creating problems or interference. By contrast, very significant relationships exist between the nurses' corresponding evaluation and coordination. First, the adequacy of patient charts as evaluated by nurses correlates .69, .78, .74, and

.65, respectively, with the overall measures of coordination; these correlations are statistically significant at better than the .05 level. Second, similar correlations obtain with five of the seven components of the overall measures of coordination. Specifically, the adequacy of charts, as appraised by nurses, correlates positively and significantly with all three components of programed coordination and with the two components of promotive coordination. These correlations range from .56 to .80, the highest correlation obtaining with the promotive coordination component of how well the different jobs and activities around the patient fit together. These results indicate that the patient chart is more of an instrument for promotive and programed coordination than for preventive coordination.

At this point, the question arises why the adequacy of patient charts as seen by nurses is positively associated with coordination, while no such relationship exists between coordination and the adequacy of charts as seen by doctors. One reason is probably the fact that nurses, unlike doctors, carry out coordinative functions in the organization. The patient chart is thus more useful to nurses insofar as coordination is concerned. Another, related, reason is that the patient chart is probably a more important referent for the nurses than for the doctors. In the first place, nurses see the doctors once or twice a day for brief periods of time, and they have to depend heavily on what the doctor has written on the chart in order to carry out their responsibilities. Second, unlike doctors, nurses change from one shift to another, at times when the doctor is usually absent, having to rely on mutual reports and on the patient chart for the continuity of their work. Finally, doctors probably prefer to rely more on the oral reports of the nurses than on the patient chart when visiting their patients; the observation by some nurses that doctors often fail to study the comments recorded by nurses on the chart seems to support this point. These reasons suggest that, theoretically, the adequacy of patient charts as seen by nurses is more relevant to organizational coordination than the adequacy of patient charts as seen by medical staff members, as the data indicate.

The main results concerning relationships between communication variables and organizational coordination may now be summarized:

1. The relative openness of communication channels, or the ease with which people in the hospital can get together to discuss their problems, facilitates coordination, especially general coordination.

2. On the whole, the mere frequency or volume of communication is not significantly related to coordination, even though it is positively and significantly correlated with the openness of communication channels.

3. The adequacy with which decisions affecting their work are explained to members is positively associated with overall coordination, being especially related to preventive coordination.

4. The extent to which doctors perceive the communication which they

receive from the administrator as adequate appears to facilitate coordination, particularly programed coordination.

5. The adequacy with which doctors explain the condition and needs of their patients to nursing personnel, as perceived by both doctors and nurses or by either of them separately, is unrelated to coordination.

6. The adequacy or completeness of patient charts at the nursing stations, as evaluated by both doctors and nurses or by doctors alone, bears no significant relationship to coordination; however, as evaluated by nurses, it is positively and significantly related to coordination, especially to promotive and programed coordination.

7. Finally, previous results indicated that the definitional clarity of hospital rules and regulations is also associated with good coordination.

Hospitals characterized by the communication practices here outlined are likely to have better coordination than hospitals where communication practices are less adequate.

Certain Aspects of Hospital Structure in Relation to Coordination

The last series of independent variables studied in relation to coordination includes certain aspects of organizational size and work force composition, i.e., structural variables. As pointed out in the preceding chapter, coordination may be affected by the size of an organization, as well as by the distribution of its members in specialized roles or the nature of the composition of its work force. Other things being equal, it would seem that the larger the organization, the more difficult it would be to effect and maintain adequate coordination because coordination would require the articulation of more activities and efforts. Larger size usually means more specialization of roles, greater heterogeneity of functions, more elaborate interdependence among members, and generally a more complex organizational structure whose numerous parts and activities are contingent upon one another. Primarily because of reasons such as these, the present research was focused from the beginning on hospitals of medium size rather than on very large hospitals (or very small hospitals where problems of coordination are relatively simpler). However, by focusing on hospitals whose size falls within a relatively restricted range some of the possible effect of size on coordination has been precluded or "controlled for," i.e., we are dealing with limited variance and, consequently, whatever relationships between size variables and coordination are here established ought to be viewed as products of an exploratory attempt. On the other hand, this caution is not required with respect to the measure of work force composition that were employed because size does not necessarily affect these measures. In this particular study, moreover, no significant relationships exist between the measures of size and those of work force composition.

Results Concerning Hospital Coordination

Three different, but highly intercorrelated, measures of size were related to coordination: (1) physical size, or the number of beds each hospital had at the time of the study; (2) the average daily census of the hospital, or its average number of patients per day; and (3) the number of paid personnel in each hospital expressed in full-time equivalents, and including all members of its work force except medical staff and medical residents and interns. Based on ten hospitals, the rank-order correlation between measures (1) and (2) is .96, between (1) and (3) it is .89, and between (2) and (3) it is .88. Relationships between these measures of size and the overall measures of coordination are presented in Table 38. All the correlations are negative, varying between −.30 and −.53. As expected, these findings are indicative of a tendency for organizational size to be negatively associated with organizational coordination. However, none of them is statistically significant at the .05 level and, consequently, the evidence is not sufficient for a conclusive statement regarding the relationship of size to coordination.

Results from additional analyses reinforce the possibility of a negative relationship between organizational size and coordination but, again, they are far from conclusive. These results, in the form of correlations between each size measure and the seven components of the overall measures of coordination, are as follows: (1) Hospital size, as measured by number of beds, correlates negatively with each of the seven components. The correlations range from −.01 to −.59, but only the largest one is statistically significant at the .05 level. The significant correlation obtains between size and the promotive coordination component of how well the different jobs and activities around the patient fit together. It suggests that the larger the size of the hospital the less adequate, and probably more difficult, its promotive coordination is likely to be. (2) Hospital size, as measured by the average daily census of patients, produces similar results. It correlates negatively with all but one of the seven components of the overall measures of coordination, the correlations varying between .03 and −.58. The highest correlation is the only significant one at the .05 level, and again it involves the component of how well jobs and activities fit together. (3) Finally, size, as measured by the number of full-time paid personnel working at the hospital, likewise yields negative correlations with all seven components. These correlations range between −.07 and −.47, the highest obtaining also with the item of how well jobs and activities fit together.

Considered as a whole, the results indicate that organizational size is likely to impede coordination, especially promotive coordination. However, since only a few of the correlations are statistically significant, more research will be needed to uphold this conclusion. It would also be very desirable, in this connection, for future studies to investigate additional and more varied measures of organizational size. For example, number and size of hierarchical levels in an organization, and the number or proportion of specialized roles in the organization could be utilized as measures of size. The ten hospitals in the study, being very homogeneous with respect to hierarchical structure and role differentiation, were not suitable for the use of measures such as those proposed here. However, certain structural variables which pertain to the work force composition of the hospital were examined.

Measures of work force composition were obtained for the nursing staff and for the (active) medical staff of each hospital. In the case of the medical staff, we computed the proportion of doctors who are "board men," i.e., who have actually been certified as specialists in various fields by accrediting national boards of medical specialties. Similarly, we computed the proportion of medical staff members who are "general practitioners," i.e., who are engaged in general practice rather than in particular specialized fields of medicine or surgery. For the ten hospitals in the study, the correlation between these two measures was found to be only —.38, which is not statistically significant. We then related these measures to the various measures of coordination, on the assumption that since they represent an aspect of specialization they may be associated with organizational coordination.

Table 38 shows that there is no significant relationship between the proportion of medical staff members in the hospital who are board men, or the proportion who are general practitioners, and any of the overall measures of coordination. Furthermore, supplementary results show no significant rela-

TABLE 38. Relation Between Certain Hospital Structure Variables and Coordination *

Hospital Structure Variables	Measure #1	Measure #2	Measure #3	Measure #4
Hospital size (number of beds)	—.40	—.53	—.47	—.39
Average daily census (number of patients)	—.33	—.48	—.41	—.30
Number of paid personnel	—.37	—.49	—.43	—.38
Proportion of medical staff members who are "board men"	—.17	.04	—.08	.29
Proportion of medical staff members who are "general practitioners"	.14	.25	.31	.09
Proportion of nursing staff members who are registered nurses	.29	.29	.21	.37
Proportion of nursing staff members who are practical nurses	.67	.69	.67	.70
Proportion of nursing staff members who are aides	—.66	—.67	—.63	—.70

* All figures are rank-order correlations, based on an N of 10 hospitals in each case. Coefficients larger than ±.56 are significant at the .05 level.

tionship between any of the seven components of the overall measures of coordination and the proportion of board men in the hospital. The same holds true also for the proportion of general practitioners, with one exception: this measure correlates .59 with one of the seven components of coordination, namely the extent to which patients feel personnel work together smoothly. It therefore appears that the degree of specialization of the medical staff is not crucial, one way or another, to hospital coordination. High specialization *per se* is not inimical to good coordination, and low specialization does not necessarily facilitate coordination.

A similar analysis was carried out in the case of the nursing staff. For each hospital, using full-time personnel as a basis, we computed the proportion of nursing staff members who are registered nurses (both supervisory and nonsupervisory), the proportion who are practical nurses, and the proportion who are nurse aides. These three measures of work force composition were then related to coordination. The results are presented in Table 38. We first find that the proportion of nursing personnel who are registered nurses does not correlate significantly with any of the overall measures of coordination, or any of their components. In all instances the correlations are positive but of small size. Therefore, hospitals with a higher proportion of registered nurses among their nursing personnel have neither poorer nor appreciably better coordination than other hospitals. Since registered nurses are more specialized than practical nurses or aides, the present results essentially confirm those concerning specialization in the medical staff.

When instead of using the proportion of nursing staff members who are registered nurses, the proportion of members who are practical nurses, or aides, is used as the independent variable, an interesting pattern of relationships with coordination emerges. This is shown by the last two rows of correlations in Table 38. The higher the proportion of nursing staff members who are practical nurses the better the coordination and, conversely, the higher the proportion of aides the poorer the coordination is. In either case, the correlations with the overall measures of coordination are all significant at better than the .05 level, being positive for the proportion of practical nurses and negative for the proportion of aides. In short, while the presence of a high proportion of practical nurses within the nursing staff facilitates coordination, a high proportion of aides impedes coordination. From the standpoint of coordination, practical nurses are valuable personnel whereas aides are not. This finding questions the operating assumptions of those administrators who have felt that the more readily and less expensively obtainable aides can be used in their hospitals to compensate for shortages in practical or registered nurses. The present data, as well as subsequent findings concerning patient care, raise very serious doubts about such an assumption.

The above relationships remain essentially unchanged when instead of the overall measures of coordination their particular components are used in the analysis. Specifically, we find that: (1) the proportion of members who are practical nurses correlates positively with each of the seven components, yielding four statistically significant correlations at the .05 level or better; (2) by contrast, the proportion of aides correlates negatively with each of the seven components, also yielding four significant correlations. In the former case, the particular correlations range from .38 to .85, and in the latter from —.43 to —.83; and, in both cases, the highest correlation obtains with the programed coordination item of how well timed activities are in the everyday routine of the hospital. The two series of correlations are almost identical in magnitude while they differ in direction. This can be explained mainly as due to the existence of a very high negative correlation (—.95) between the proportion of nursing staff members who are practical nurses and the proportion who are aides in the various hospitals. The proportion of nursing personnel who are aides also correlates negatively, though to a smaller degree (—.61) with the proportion of members who are registered nurses, but no significant relationship exists between the proportion of members who are practical nurses and the proportion who are registered nurses (the correlation between these last two measures being only .39). These relationships among the proportions of nursing personnel who belong to the various classifications here examined indicate that hospitals who have more nurse's aides on their staff are likely to have both fewer practical nurses and fewer registered nurses—a condition which apparently impairs coordination, according to the findings.

That the presence of a relatively high proportion of aides in the nursing staff correlates negatively with coordination is not hard to explain in view of the characteristics of this group. Aides constitute the least educated, least trained, least professionalized, and least specialized nursing group in each hospital. At the same time, this is the largest of the nursing groups in terms of numbers, but a group which is not particularly stable according to such criteria as length of service in the hospital, turnover, and absenteeism. Because of these factors, the nurse's aides group is at best very hard to fit in the overall nursing structure, yet it is essential that the efforts and activities of the members of this group be coordinated with the efforts of practical and registered nurses and other hospital personnel. But coordinative functions are not carried out by aides; they are performed by registered and practical nurses who, as a consequence, have to carry all coordinative responsibilities rather than share them with the aides. Furthermore, this situation is particularly aggravated in hospitals which have comparatively more aides because, as we have already seen, having more aides also means having fewer practical nurses and fewer registered nurses. The net result is that in hospitals which are loaded with aides coordination suffers. The same factors may also be used to explain the finding that hospitals whose nursing staff includes a relatively high proportion of practical nurses, as against aides, tend to have better coordination. As a group, practical nurses are better trained, more professionalized, and a more stable component of the work force than aides (and even more stable than registered nurses in terms of length of service at the hospital).

The only remaining question is why the proportion of nursing personnel who are registered nurses does not produce significant positive correlations with coordination while the proportion who are practical nurses does. This is difficult to interpret, but certain relevant considerations can be enumerated. First, the higher stability of practical nurses in terms of length of service at the hospital, in conjunction with a higher annual turnover characteristic of registered nurses, places the practical nurse group in a somewhat more advantageous position with respect to coordination. Second, the constant shortage of registered nurses being experienced by hospitals in recent years probably constitutes another pertinent factor. It is possible that, because of this shortage, many of the coordinative functions which registered nurses would normally perform have been given to, left to, or taken by, practical nurses. Third, practical nurses are likely to fit better than registered nurses into the traditional dominance-submission pattern of relations among organizational members in the hospital—a pattern which, although on its way out as nursing becomes increasingly professionalized, is still in evidence in many hospitals. Finally, the finding that the proportion of registered nurses at least produces small positive correlations with all of the measures of coordination suggests that, if anything, having more registered nurses is a facilitative condition for coordination—especially since there is no significant relationship between the proportion of nursing staff members who are registered nurses and the proportion who are practical nurses.

Summary

The findings presented in this section show the extent to which organizational coordination, viewed as a dependent variable, is associated with other important aspects of hospital structure and functioning which are viewed as independent variables. The results clearly demonstrate how coordination is a function of the many different factors which were examined in detail in the preceding discussion. These factors were subsumed under the following general headings: structural features of organization; organizational planning; problem awareness and problem solving; communication practices; sharedness or complementarity of expectations and cooperation among organizational members; and intraorganizational strain. Several specific variables from each of these areas were found, as expected, to be significantly related to coordination.

Some of these variables, such as the degree of tension among interdependent groups in the hospital or the extent to which members experience unreasonable pressure in the work structure, i.e., variables representing intraorganizational strain, had been earlier hypothesized to be inversely related to coordination. The data substantiated this hypothesis; hospitals with higher levels of strain have poorer coordination than hospitals with lower levels of strain. Most of the other variables studied, such as the degree of complementarity of expectations among hospital personnel whose work is related, had been expected to be positively related to coordination, and the data also confirmed this expectation. In fact, nearly all of our initial hypotheses as to the correlates and determinants of organizational coordination received strong empirical support from the data. The major findings about overall hospital coordination will be summarized at the end of this chapter, after a discussion of coordination in the nursing department.

COORDINATION IN THE DEPARTMENT OF NURSING

The research design calls not only for the study of coordination using the entire hospital system as the unit of analysis and hypothesis testing, but also for a supplementary attempt to examine factors affecting coordination in the nursing department of each hospital. The relationships reported in the preceding section are generally expected to apply also in the case where some organizational part, such as a department, is used as the unit of analysis, provided that the department consists of people in different but interdependent roles, i.e., it can be considered as a social system. In other words, many of the variables which were found to affect overall organizational coordination should also affect intradepartmental coordination, or the coordination of specific departments within the total organization. In the present study, the nursing department was chosen to serve as a test case for this proposition. Using the nursing department rather than the hospital as the unit of analysis, permits us to investigate the generalizability of some of the findings presented in the preceding section, through replication, as well as to investigate some additional independent variables.

Measures of Nursing Department Coordination

Coordination within the nursing department occurs in three major directions. First, nursing personnel have to relate their functions with the functions of personnel in other hospital units, e.g., the medical staff, the administrative staff, the housekeeping staff, etc. This kind of coordination, however, can best be viewed as pertaining to the entire hospital rather than the nursing department. Second, coordination within the nursing department may involve the patterning of relationships among nursing personnel belonging to different classifications or performing different tasks but working on the same shift. For example, in the day shift, registered nurses have to coordinate their activities with practical nurses and aides. Similarly, nursing personnel working in the operating room have to coordinate their work with nursing personnel working on the floors, and nursing supervisors have to coordinate the work of nursing personnel in different medical divisions. Third, coordination within the nursing department may involve the continuity of work. Continuity of jobs and

Coordination in the Department of Nursing

work from one shift to another must be assured, and personnel coming to work at a given shift must succeed the preceding shift and be succeeded by the following shift in a smooth and orderly manner. Ensuring maximum continuity with minimum disruption among shifts constitutes the kind of coordination within the nursing department with which we shall be primarily concerned in this section.

Data for the measurement of nursing department coordination were obtained only from nurse respondents, by means of the following three questions: (1) "How easy is it for one shift to take over without confusion from where the previous shift left off?" (2) "When you come to work, how hard is it for you to find out what went on on the job since you last were there?" And (3) "How often do you feel that people from the previous shift left you with unfinished work or problems that they should have handled during their own shift?" The first question provided response alternatives ranging from "it is extremely easy" to "it is hard or difficult," and it was asked of all registered nursing staff respondents in every hospital. The second question provided response alternatives ranging from "it is extremely hard" to "it is extremely easy," and it was asked of nonsupervisory registered nurses. And, the third question provided response alternatives ranging from "I always feel this way" to "I never feel this way," and it was also asked of nonsupervisory registered nurses. Using the distribution of responses to each question, means were computed in the usual manner and separately for each hospital. Before obtaining the means, however, for the purpose of computational convenience and uniformity, we inverted the scales formed by the response alternatives of questions (2) and (3). This procedure ensured correspondence of response alternatives for all three questions, i.e., the most favorable alternative of the first question was assigned the same score as the most favorable alternative of the other two questions, and the least favorable alternative in each case was likewise assigned the same score.

The means of responses to the above questions are here used as three specific measures of nursing department coordination. An overall measure is also used, however. This measure was derived by combining the three specific measures. The ten hospitals were rank-ordered according to their score on each specific measure, and the mean-rank of each hospital on the three measures was obtained to serve as an overall measure of nursing department coordination. This overall measure correlates with the specific measures as follows: .84 with the ease with which one shift can take over from another, .82 with the relative lack of difficulty in finding out what happened on the job since last at work, and .92 with how infrequently personnel feel the previous shift left them with problems that it should have handled. Based on an N of 10 hospitals (or ten nursing departments), these rank-order correlations are statistically significant at better than the .01 level. The specific measures also intercorrelate significantly with one another. The relative ease with which one shift can take over from another correlates .60 with the relative lack of difficulty in finding out what happened on the job, and .67 with how infrequently the previous shift left unhandled problems, while the latter two measures correlate .66.

The above relationships suggest that the four measures of nursing department coordination apparently represent a common phenomenon, as expected. It is also interesting to note that the four measures respectively correlate .73, .25, .72, and .68 with the promptness with which the nursing staff answer the calls of the patients, as judged by registered nurses. Since the timing of activities is an essential aspect of coordination and it could have been used as one indicator of coordination, these relationships enhance our confidence in the measures that were actually employed to represent nursing department coordination.

Nursing Department Coordination in Relation to Hospital Coordination

Since the nursing department is one of the most important departments of the hospital, from the point of view of its participation both in coordination and patient care, we expected that adequacy of coordination in the nursing department would be associated with the adequacy of overall organizational coordination. This expectation was borne out by the data. Table 39 shows that each measure of nursing department coordination correlates positively with the four overall measures of hospital coordination, the specific correlations ranging from a low of .35 to a high of .89. Moreover, three of the four measures of nursing department coordination correlate both positively and significantly with each measure of overall hospital coordination; only the measure "ease with which one shift can take over from another without confusion" does not yield correlations large enough to be statistically significant. The overall measure of nursing department coordination correlates .68, .76, .80, and .62, respectively, with the four overall measures of hospital coordination; it correlates highest with measure #3, which represents general coordination, and lowest with measure #4, which represents programed coordination. These results indicate that good coordination in an organization also filters down to its departments or, perhaps more plausibly in the present case, that good coordination in the nursing department affects coordination for the entire hospital. In any event, hospitals with better overall coordination have nursing departments which also have better coordination, or vice versa.

Factors Affecting Nursing Department Coordination

The relationships between nursing department coordination and overall hospital coordination provide the first empirical indication of support for the proposition that many of the findings about overall coordination are also likely to have their parallels in, or to apply to, nursing department coordination as well. To test this proposition further and in greater detail, several more specific variables were examined in relation to the various measures of nursing department coordination. Most of these independent variables are very similar, and sometimes identical, with independent variables discussed earlier in connection with hospital coordination. Furthermore, these variables were measured in the same manner, i.e., using as measures either data from hospital records or means based on the answers of respondents from each hospital to questions whose response alternatives formed interval scales. Finally, the correlation method of analysis was likewise used here to express the magnitude and direction of relationship between nursing department coordination and each independent variable involved. In short, the methodological procedures used in this part of the study are essentially the same as those described earlier.

The independent variables studied in this section can be grouped into four categories: (1) nursing staff composition variables; (2) variables representing strain within the nursing department; (3) variables concerning overlap or usurpation of functions among different nursing roles; and (4) turnover and absenteeism among nursing staff members. Similar or identical variables representing the first two categories have already been related to overall hospital coordination in the preceding section. The last two categories contain certain

TABLE 39. Relation Between Nursing Department Coordination Measures and the Overall Measures of Hospital Coordination *

Nursing Department Coordination Measures ‡	Measure #1	Measure #2	Measure #3	Measure #4
(1) Ease with which one shift can take over from another without confusion	.40	.49	.55	.35
(2) Relative lack of difficulty in finding out what happened on the job since last at work	.69	.70	.65	.65
(3) How infrequently people feel previous shift left them with unfinished work or problems that it should have handled	.75	.83	.89	.71
(4) Overall measure of nursing department coordination (the mean rank-order of hospitals on the preceding three measures)	.68	.76	.80	.62

Overall Measures of Hospital Coordination †

* All figures are rank-order correlations, based on an N of 10 hospitals in each case. Coefficients larger than .56 are significant at the .05 level, and those .75 or larger are significant at the .01 level.

† These are the same four measures of overall coordination shown in Table 30, Chapter 6.

‡ The rank-order intercorrelations among these four measures of nursing department coordination, based on an N of 10 hospitals, are as follows: .60 between (1) and (2), .67 between (1) and (3), .66 between (2) and (3); and, .84 between (4) and (1), .82 between (4) and (2), and .92 between (4) and (3).

346   FACTORS AFFECTING COORDINATION IN HOSPITALS

variables which are specific to the nursing department, e.g., the extent to which practical nurses are prone to do things that registered nurses should be doing.

The findings about nursing department coordination are presented in Table 40. Considering the variables of nursing staff structure, the results are essentially the same as those obtained in the case of overall hospital coordina-

TABLE 40. Relation Between Coordination in the Nursing Department and Various Independent or Conditioning Variables Representing Certain Aspects of Nursing Activity *

Nursing Department Coordination Measures

Independent or Conditioning Variables	Ease with which one shift can take over from another without confusion	Lack of difficulty in finding out what happened on the job since last at work	How infrequently previous shift left unfinished work or problems it should have handled	Overall measure of nursing department coordination
Proportion of nursing staff members who are registered nurses	.40	.56	.26	.38
Proportion of nursing staff members who are practical nurses	.54	.64	.77	.77
Proportion of nursing staff members who are nurse's aides	−.38	−.72	−.71	−.79
Degree of tension between nursing personnel in different roles (classifications), as perceived by registered nursing staff	−.47	−.36	−.56	−.60
Degree of tension between nursing personnel in different shifts, as perceived by registered nursing staff	−.88	−.37	−.44	−.64
Degree of tension between nursing personnel and hospital administrator, as perceived by registered nursing staff and administrative department heads	−.49	−.30	−.72	−.65
Average level of "unreasonable" pressure for better performance experienced by personnel in the different nursing roles, for all roles combined	−.74	−.67	−.87	−.89

TABLE 40. (Cont.)

Independent or Conditioning Variables	Ease with which one shift can take over from another without confusion	Lack of difficulty in finding out what happened on the job since last at work	How infrequently previous shift left unfinished work or problems it should have handled	Overall measure of nursing department coordination
Extent to which aides are prone to try to do things that practical or registered nurses should be doing, according to registered nurses	—.21	—.16	—.10	—.20
Extent to which practical nurses are prone to try to do things that registered nurses should be doing, according to registered nurses	—.47	—.31	—.54	—.55
Extent to which registered nurses are prone to try to do things that head nurses should be doing, according to registered nurses	—.64	—.20	—.59	—.65
Extent to which registered nurses are prone to try to do things that practical nurses should be doing, according to registered nurses	—.69	—.42	—.66	—.70
Proportion of registered nurses absent twice or more often from regularly scheduled work during the last quarter of 1957 (see Chap. 3 for a description of this measure) †	—.53	—.57	—.52	—.63
Turnover among registered nurses (Measure described in Chap. 3) ‡	.41	.00	.21	.24
Turnover among aides (Measure described in Chap. 3) ‡	.40	.71	.83	.79

* All figures, except those pertaining to absenteeism and turnover, are rank-order correlations, based on an N of 10 hospitals in each case. Coefficients larger than —.56 are significant at the .05 level, and those —.75 or larger are significant at the .01 level.

† These are rank-order correlations, based on an N of 9 hospitals, in each case. A coefficient of —.60 is significant at the .05 level.

‡ These are rank-order correlations, based on an N of 8 hospitals, in each case. A coefficient of —.64 is significant at the .05 level.

tion. The proportion of nursing staff members who are practical nurses is positively related to nursing department coordination, while the proportion of members who are aides is negatively related to coordination. The former correlates .77 and the latter —.79 with the overall measure of nursing department coordination, both producing similar relationships with the specific measures as well. The proportion of members who are registered nurses yields moderate positive correlations with each measure of nursing department coordination, but only one of the four correlations is statistically significant at the .05 level —a correlation of .56 with the relative lack of difficulty in finding out what happened on the job since last at work. As expected, these results replicate the comparable relationships between work force composition and overall hospital coordination which were discussed earlier. The higher the proportion of aides in the nursing staff of a hospital, the poorer the nursing department coordination (and the overall hospital coordination) is likely to be; but, the higher the proportion of practical nurses on the staff the better the coordination, and the same tends to occur for the proportion of staff members who are registered nurses.

Considering next the various measures of strain, we find that internal strain is inversely related to nursing department coordination. For example, Table 40 shows that the degree of tension between nursing personnel in different shifts is negatively related to nursing department coordination; it correlates —.88, —.37, —.44, and —.64, respectively, with the four measures of nursing department coordination, two of the correlations being statistically significant at better than the .05 level. Similarly, the more unreasonable pressure for better performance nursing personnel in the various roles experience, the poorer the coordination in the nursing department. The degree of unreasonable pressure correlates —.74, —.67, —.87, and —.89, respectively, with the four measures of nursing department coordination, all correlations being statistically significant. Comparable patterns of results are produced by the degree of tension among nursing personnel in different classifications, and by the degree of tension between nursing personnel and the hospital administrator. And although not all of the specific correlations are statistically significant, all are negative as predicted. Moreover, the overall measure of nursing department coordination correlates both negatively and significantly with every measure of strain used. Therefore, as hypothesized, the relationships between intradepartmental strain and nursing department coordination are essentially the same as the relationships between intraorganizational strain and overall hospital coordination reported earlier. Internal strain, in the form of tension or excessive pressure, affects coordination adversely.

Even when strain is measured with reference to specific roles in the nursing department, the nature of the above relationships is not altered. For example, additional findings show that the greater the unreasonable pressure for better performance which practical nurses alone feel, the poorer the nursing depart-

Coordination in the Department of Nursing

ment coordination is likely to be. The amount of unreasonable pressure experienced by practical nurses correlates −.75, −.55, −.46, and −.51, respectively, with the measures of nursing department coordination. Similarly, the degree of unreasonable pressure experienced by supervisory registered nurses is found to be inversely related to nursing department coordination, and the same is true for the pressure experienced by nonsupervisory registered nurses, or by nurse's aides. In all cases, the specific correlations are negative and many of them are statistically significant.

Like the hospital, the nursing department brings together in close interaction and interdependence a mixture of professional, semiprofessional, and nonprofessional personnel. The consequent implications for the development of problems and malfunctions with respect to articulating the activities and efforts of these heterogeneous people are many and varied. We have already seen how tension between nursing personnel in different classifications, or different shifts, affects nursing department coordination adversely. Some of the sources of tension within the nursing department, no doubt, stem from professional differences and ambiguities in role functions among nursing personnel. Registered nurses have often resented the intrusion of practical nurses into nursing, being apprehensive lest they lose some of their traditional functions and prerogatives to less qualified personnel. The practical nurse is perceived as a threat to the professional pride and economic security of the registered nurse, despite the shortage of registered nurses experienced by hospitals. This shortage means the influx of more practical nurses in the field, and tensions will continue until their role becomes clearly defined and stabilized. Aides, on the other hand, as Burling and his colleagues (1) point out, often resent the fact that they are always on the receiving end of orders and instructions from other nursing staff. Under these circumstances, the probability of frictions among nursing personnel is relatively high.

A closely related problem concerns the behavior of personnel in different nursing roles with respect to the functions each is performing or tends to perform. In this study, we hypothesized that the extent to which personnel in adjacent roles, or classifications, are prone to attempt to do things that should be done by those in a given role but not by those in another role will be negatively related to nursing department coordination. Accordingly, appropriate data were collected from registered nurses in each hospital to measure the extent to which each nursing group was prone to try to do things that another nursing group should be doing. These measures were then related to nursing department coordination. The findings are presented in Table 40.

On the whole, the results support our expectations. First, we find that the extent to which aides are prone to try to do things that practical nurses should be doing correlates negatively with each measure of nursing department coordination, although the correlations in this case are extremely small. Second, the extent to which practical nurses are prone to try to do things that registered nurses should be doing correlates negatively, though moderately, with every measure of nursing department coordination; two of the four correlations, one with the overall measure of nursing department coordination, being almost significant at the .05 level. Third, the extent to which registered nurses are prone to try to do things that head nurses (i.e., supervisory registered nurses) should be doing correlates —.64, —.20, —.59, and —.65, respectively, with the measures of nursing department coordination, three of the correlations being statistically significant at better than the .05 level. Finally, the extent to which registered nurses are prone to try to do things that practical nurses should be doing similarly correlates —.69, —.42, —.66, and —.70 with the same measures, three of the correlations being significant.

Thus, the tendency for those in a given role to "usurp" functions from those in adjacent roles, or organizational levels, seems to affect nursing department coordination adversely, the effects being most pronounced at the higher levels and least pronounced at the lower levels. In the present case, when registered nurses exhibit this tendency coordination suffers considerably more than when practical nurses do, being almost unaffected by the extent to which aides are prone to do things that practical nurses should be doing. Moreover, the data show that insofar as coordination is concerned, it is irrelevant whether registered nurses tend to appropriate functions of a higher level group such as head nurses, or whether they tend to appropriate functions of a lower group such as practical nurses. In both cases, the findings show that nursing department coordination is adversely affected.

The last three rows of correlations in Table 40 show the relationship between our measures of nursing department coordination and: (1) rate of absenteeism among nonsupervisory registered nurses, (2) rate of turnover among nonsupervisory registered nurses, and (3) rate of turnover among aides in the hospitals studied. The measures of absenteeism and turnover have been discussed in detail in Chapter 3. The results may be summarized as follows:

1. Those hospitals which have higher absenteeism rates among their nonsupervisory registered nurses also have poorer nursing department coordination. More specifically, the higher the proportion of registered nurses who were absent from regularly scheduled work twice or more often during a three-month period (the period of data collection), the poorer the coordination in the nursing department. The former correlates negatively and significantly with the latter (—.63). When, instead of the overall measure of nursing department coordination, the three specific measures are used in the analysis, moreover, similar though somewhat smaller correlations are obtained. And, not shown in Table 40, when, instead of the proportion of nurses absent twice or more often, the proportion absent three or more times during the same period is related to the measures of nursing department coordination, es-

Coordination in the Department of Nursing

sentially the same pattern of relationships emerges. Mere incidence of absenteeism (i.e., the proportion being absent at least once), on the other hand, is unrelated to coordination.

2. Turnover among nonsupervisory registered nurses in the various hospitals is not related to any of the measures of nursing department coordination. The pertinent correlations are all very small and nonsignificant. This finding had not been anticipated. Apparently, a certain amount of turnover among registered nurses, whether high, moderate, or low, is a "normal" experience in each hospital, an experience which is anticipated and predictable, thus making it possible for the nursing department to take precautionary measures which prevent disruptions in coordination.

3. Turnover among aides, on the other hand, is *positively* and significantly related to nursing department coordination. Table 40 shows that, the higher the turnover in this group, the better the coordination. This finding is consistent with earlier results showing a negative relationship between coordination and the proportion of nursing staff members who are aides (hospitals "loaded" with aides tend to have less adequate coordination), as well as with subsequent findings, which will show that the higher the proportion of aides, the poorer the quality of patient care. This finding becomes more meaningful, if viewed in context of the background characteristics of aides discussed in Chapter 3. In brief, the aides constitute a difficult group to integrate in the nursing department and to coordinate its activities with those of other hospital personnel.

The above results pertain to nursing department coordination only, and not to overall hospital coordination. With respect to the latter, we find that neither turnover nor absenteeism among nursing personnel relates significantly to any of our four overall measures of hospital coordination. However, the pattern of correlations is in the same direction as the above patterns concerning nursing department coordination. Specifically, turnover among aides produces moderate positive correlations with each of the four overall measures of hospital coordination; these correlations are all in the fifties, but none is statistically significant. Turnover among registered nurses produces small negative correlations with the same four measures; these correlations range between $-.15$ and $-.43$, but none is significant. The rate of absenteeism among registered nurses yields moderate negative correlations with the overall measures of hospital coordination; some of these approach significance at the .05 level, but none reaches significance. Finally, we find that neither absenteeism among aides, nor absenteeism among practical nurses, is significantly related to coordination in the nursing department or the total hospital, regardless of which measure of absenteeism (see Chap. 3) is used in the analysis.

In summary, nursing department coordination is a function of some of the same independent variables which were found to affect overall hospital coordination. The nature of the composition of the nursing staff is significantly associated with nursing department coordination. The same holds true also for the several variables of internal strain which were examined in the case of nursing department coordination. Parallel variables were earlier found to be similarly related to overall hospital coordination. These results, in conjunction with the fact that nursing department coordination is positively related to overall hospital coordination, lend certain weight to the potential generality of the findings reported in this chapter, although the question of generalization cannot be settled on the basis of the outcome of a single study. Certain other independent variables were examined in relation to nursing department coordination, but not in relation to overall hospital coordination. These variables, which are highly specific to the nursing department, produced results that are congruent with the general pattern of other findings about hospital coordination and nursing department coordination. The variables in question represent the extent to which nursing personnel in a given role tend to perform functions that nursing personnel in another but adjacent role should be performing. This tendency has negative effects for coordination. Finally, absenteeism and turnover among the nursing staff were also examined in relation to coordination and were found to yield rather interesting results.

THE "BEST" vs. THE "POOREST" COORDINATION HOSPITAL: CONTRASTING PROFILES

The results of still another supplementary piece of analysis concerning the relation of organizational coordination to other aspects of hospital functioning are also noteworthy. In this analysis, we contrasted the hospital which scored best among the ten hospitals on overall organizational coordination with the hospital which scored poorest, by examining the relative rank or standing of these two institutions on each of 15 variables. The measurement of these variables has already been discussed. Fourteen of the variables represent different categories of independent variables which were earlier found to be related to coordination, and were selected for further study among many such variables without using any particular system of selection. The remaining variable represents nursing department coordination. The categories of independent variables involved include sharedness and complementarity of expectations among organizational members, cooperation, problem solving, communication, and intraorganizational strain. The analysis itself consists in determining the difference between the ranks of the two hospitals on each variable examined.

The results are summarized in Table 41. As anticipated, the data show that the better coordinated hospital is characterized by considerably more sharedness and complementarity of expectations among its members, higher levels of member cooperation, greater openness in communication channels, more extensive adherence to organizational rules, greater promptness in getting problems settled, lower tension, less "unreasonable" pressure, and better nursing

"Best" vs. "Poorest" Coordination Hospital

department coordination. On every variable, the better coordinated hospital ranks more favorably than the other. Even more importantly, in almost all cases, it ranks more favorably than most of the ten hospitals in the study while the other hospital ranks less favorably than most of the ten hospitals.

TABLE 41. Contrasting Profiles of the "Best" and "Poorest" Coordination Hospitals Showing the Standing of the Two Institutions on Several Other Aspects of Hospital Functioning *

Aspect of Hospital Functioning	The "best" coordination hospital (Hospital #3) ranks: †	The "poorest" coordination hospital (Hospital #1) ranks: †	Difference between ranks
Extent people from different jobs and departments see eye-to-eye on things about the everyday operations of the hospital	2	9.5	7.5
Extent medical staff members understand and appreciate the problems and needs of the nursing staff	3.5	9	5.5
Extent nursing staff members understand and appreciate the problems and needs of the medical staff	2	9	7
Extent trustees understand and appreciate the problems and needs of the medical staff	3	10	7
Degree of willingness of people in related jobs to assist each other when needed	1	10	9
Extent members' work contacts with other departments produce satisfactory results	2	10	8
Extent people from the different departments follow the rules, policies, and regulations of the hospital	1	5.5	4.5
How satisfactorily problems of working together are handled in the hospital	4.5	10	5.5
Promptness with which problems of working together are settled	1	10	9
Ease with which people from interrelated jobs can get together to exchange information and ideas about work	1	10	9
Frequency with which people from interrelated jobs get together to discuss work problems and differences	2	9	7
Intraorganizational strain, or tension among different groups or departments (Tension measure #1)	10	1.5	8.5

TABLE 41. (Cont.)

Aspect of Hospital Functioning	The "best" coordination hospital (Hospital #3) ranks: †	The "poorest" coordination hospital (Hospital #1) ranks: †	Difference between ranks
Average level of "unreasonable" pressure for better performance experienced by nonmedical members (Pressure measure #1)	8	3	5
Degree of tension between the nursing staff and the medical staff	10	4	6
Adequacy of nursing department coordination (Overall measure of nursing department coordination)	3	8	5

Relative Standing Among Ten Hospitals

* According to the data presented in Table 30, Chapter 6, Hospital #3 scored best on overall hospital coordination while Hospital #1 scored poorest among the ten hospitals studied. These two hospitals are referred to here as the highest and lowest coordination hospital, respectively.

† In all cases, smaller ranks correspond to *higher* scores on the variables indicated; accordingly, a low rank on a variable such as tension corresponds to high tension while a high rank represents low tension.

Closer inspection of the data in Table 41 brings the differences between the two hospitals into sharper focus. The hospital which scored best on overall coordination also ranks first or second best among the ten hospitals on 10 of the 15 variables examined. By contrast, the hospital which scored poorest on coordination also ranks poorest or second poorest on 11 of the same 15 variables. Similarly, the former hospital places among the top three hospitals on 14 of the 15 variables, while the latter places among the bottom three hospitals on 13 of the 15 variables. The smallest difference between the ranks of the two hospitals is 4.5 and pertains to the extent to which people from different departments follow the rules and regulations of the hospital. The average discrepancy in the standing of the two institutions among the ten hospitals studied for all 15 variables is almost seven places (6.9) out of a theoretically maximum possible of nine places. This maximum average discrepancy would have occurred if the hospital which scored best on overall coordination also placed best among the ten hospitals on each of the 15 variables, *and* the one which scored poorest on coordination also placed poorest on each of these variables, or if overall coordination were perfectly correlated with each variable involved.

Although the 15 variables examined are not independent of one another since many of them intercorrelate significantly, the discrepancies reported here

Summary and Conclusions 355

illustrate rather graphically how intimately organizational coordination is related to the various aspects of hospital functioning represented by these variables. The above findings take added significance when we consider the fact that some of the variables on which the two hospitals were contrasted correlate negatively with coordination, e.g., the tension variables. These variables do not behave any differently from those which correlate positively with coordination, since in both cases the standing of the two hospitals is in sharp contrast and in the right direction. Finally, it is also worth reiterating that, in most cases, different rather than the same respondent groups provided the data on the basis of which the 15 variables were measured.

SUMMARY AND CONCLUSIONS

The specific relationships between various aspects of hospital operation and coordination have been presented in detail and will not be repeated here. However, the main findings will be summarized and discussed. First, they will be summarized in terms of the particular sets of independent variables which served to organize the results about overall hospital coordination and nursing department coordination. Second, the principal findings will be summarized with reference to different categories and types of coordination which have been distinguished in the preceding chapter. In either case, only the most significant independent variables will be considered here, however. Finally, the findings will be discussed from the point of view of their particular relevance to certain organizational roles and groups in the hospital.

Major Findings about Organizational Coordination

Many different factors were hypothesized to affect organizational coordination and were, therefore, included in the analysis. These factors, representing various aspects of hospital structure and functioning, were viewed as independent social-psychological variables with coordination being viewed as the dependent variable. The specific independent variables investigated were grouped into the following sets, or areas: organizational planning; sharedness and complementarity of expectations among organizational members; cooperation; intraorganizational strain; problem awareness and problem solving; communication; and certain features of hospital structure. Several variables from each set were found to be significantly associated, i.e., to be positively or negatively related, with hospital coordination, consistent with our initial expectations. Furthermore, comparable results were obtained about nursing department coordination.

The data show that such aspects of organizational planning as the definitional clarity of hospital rules and regulations, and the extent to which members conform with established rules are positively and significantly related to coordination. Similarly, the extent of sharedness and complementarity of work-related expectations among organizational members, as measured by (1) the degree to which people from different jobs see eye-to-eye about everyday operations, (2) the degree to which members see one another's viewpoint in their work relations, and (3) the degree to which the medical staff appreciate the problems and needs of the nursing staff, and vice versa, are also highly related to coordination. In the area of cooperation, the data show that the willingness of members in related jobs to assist each other when needed is positively and significantly related to coordination, while the extent to which members do their full share and the extent to which their mutual contacts produce satisfactory results yield moderate but not statistically significant correlations with overall coordination.

Intraorganizational strain is detrimental to coordination, according to the findings. Among different but interdependent groups in the hospital, strain in the form of tension is negatively and significantly related to coordination, and the same is true for strain in the form of experienced unreasonable pressure for better performance on the part of nonmedical personnel. Hospitals with higher levels of tension or pressure have significantly poorer coordination than hospitals characterized with lower levels of tension or pressure.

Concerning problem awareness and problem solving, the results show: (1) The extent to which problems of working together are handled satisfactorily in the hospital, and the promptness with which such problems are settled, are both positively and significantly related to coordination. (2) The combined conflict-solving effectiveness of the administrator and of the director of nursing similarly makes for significantly better hospital coordination, while their individual effectiveness in solving conflicts correlates only moderately with coordination. (3) The extent to which the administrator is aware of problems faced by organizational members produces positive but nonsignificant relationships with coordination, and the same holds true for the problem awareness of the director of nursing; their combined problem awareness, on the other hand, tends to be associated with better coordination.

Such communication variables as the extent to which organizational members feel that decisions which affect their work are explained to them adequately, and the ease with which people in related jobs can meet to exchange information and ideas about work, or the relative openness of communication channels, are positively and significantly related to coordination. The extent to which doctors feel that the communication which they receive from the administrator is adequate also tends to be positively related to coordination. The adequacy with which doctors explain the condition and needs of their patients to nursing personnel produces only moderate positive correlations with coordination. On the other hand, the adequacy of patient charts at nursing stations, as evaluated by registered nurses, is positively and significantly related to coordination. But, the adequacy of charts, as evaluated by doctors, is unrelated to coordination. In this connection, several explanations have been proposed in our earlier discussion.

Summary and Conclusions

When viewing certain aspects of hospital structure as the independent variables, the data show the following results: (1) Organizational size in terms of number of beds, average daily census of patients, or number of paid personnel in the hospital tends to be negatively related to coordination, although only a few of the specific correlations reach statistical significance (partly because the variance in size among the hospitals in the study was limited by the research design). (2) The proportion of medical staff members who are specialty board-certified is unrelated to coordination, and the same holds true for the proportion of staff members who are general practitioners rather than specialists (whether board-certified or not). (3) Certain aspects of the composition of the nursing staff, on the other hand, produce significant relationships with coordination. Specifically, the higher the proportion of nursing staff members who are practical nurses the better the coordination is, and a somewhat similar tendency is suggested by the data for the proportion of nursing staff members who are registered nurses. By contrast, the higher the proportion of nursing staff members who are aides, the poorer the coordination in the hospitals studied.

Additional findings were brought together in a somewhat different form in Table 41. This table presented profiles of the hospital which scored best and the hospital which scored poorest on overall coordination, among the ten hospitals participating in the study. These profiles show that the two hospitals contrast sharply in terms of their standing among the ten hospitals on each of 15 different independent variables—variables such as those indicated above. The average discrepancy in the standing of the two hospitals for all 15 independent variables combined is seven places out of a theoretically maximum possible of nine places. These results amplify and reinforce the corresponding correlational findings between the independent variables examined and coordination, as discussed throughout this chapter.

Essentially similar results to those summarized above were also obtained about nursing department coordination. First, we find that the hospitals which have better overall coordination are also significantly more likely to have better nursing department coordination, or vice versa. Second, the composition of the nursing staff is significantly related to nursing department coordination in precisely the same manner in which it is related to overall hospital coordination; a high proportion of practical nurses on the staff facilitates coordination while a high proportion of aides impedes coordination. Third, such aspects of strain within the nursing department as the degree of tension between nursing personnel in different shifts, or in different classifications, and the level of unreasonable pressure for better performance experienced by the nursing staff are all inversely related to nursing department coordination. These results replicate comparable findings about overall hospital coordination. Finally, the data show that the extent to which registered nurses are prone to do things that head nurses should be doing, or things that practical nurses should be doing, makes for poorer coordination in the nursing department. A similar tendency is also indicated for the extent to which practical nurses are prone to do things that registered nurses should be doing, but no appreciable corresponding relationship exists between the extent to which aides are prone to do things that practical nurses should be doing and nursing department coordination.

These, in brief, are the principal findings of the present study about hospital coordination and about nursing department coordination, summarized here according to the various sets of independent variables with which we have been concerned.

Results about Different Categories and Types of Coordination

In this chapter, we have frequently indicated the relevance of specific findings to categories and types of coordination which were described in the preceding chapter. In this connection, it will be recalled that coordinative activity was divided into two broad categories: programed coordination, and general or nonprogramed coordination. Programed coordination was measured using a set of three items: (1) the extent to which activities in the everyday routine of the hospital are well timed; (2) the extent to which work assignments are well planned; and (3) the extent to which departmental routines are well established. General coordination was measured using a set of four items: (1) how well different jobs and activities fit together; (2) the extent to which patients feel (according to the respondents) that hospital personnel around them work together smoothly; (3) the extent to which organizational members make an effort to avoid creating problems or interference; and (4) the extent to which they perform their work properly without getting in each other's way. The first two items were said to represent the type of promotive coordination, and the last two to represent the preventive type of coordination. The major findings of the study may now be summarized with reference to programed and general coordination, and with reference to promotive and preventive coordination.

The independent variables which were found to relate especially well to preventive coordination are: (1) the degree of clarity of hospital rules, regulations, and policies; (2) the extent of conformity with hospital rules and regulations by organizational members; (3) the extent to which the hospital administrator is aware of problems faced by other organizational members; (4) the effectiveness of the director of nursing in solving conflicts that arise in the organization; (5) the skill of supervisory personnel in planning activities; (6) the frequency with which members get together to exchange ideas and discuss problems arising in their work relationships; and (7) the extent to which decisions that affect their work are explained to members adequately. Each of these variables is positively and significantly related to preventive coordination, at the same time, being related more strongly with preventive than promotive coordination.

The independent variables which were found to relate especially well to pro-

Summary and Conclusions

motive coordination are: (1) the size of the hospital, which is inversely related to promotive coordination; (2) the degree of intraorganizational strain, in the form of tension among interdependent groups, which is also inversely related to promotive coordination; and (3) the adequacy of patient charts at nursing stations, as evaluted by nursing personnel, which is positively related to promotive coordination. Of course, like preventive coordination, promotive coordination is also significantly related to a host of other factors. The variables enumerated here are the ones which appear to be more important to promotive than to preventive coordination.

Promotive and preventive coordination, as measured in the present study, both represent the category of general, or nonprogramed, coordination as against the category of programed coordination. It would, therefore, be of interest to indicate which factors tend to relate better to one rather than the other of these two categories of coordinative activity. In this connection, the findings show that the following variables are especially well related to general coordination: (1) the extent of cooperation among organizational members, particularly willingness to assist one another when needed; (2) good communication practices, in general, and particularly the openness of communication channels, and the adequacy with which decisions are explained to those affected; (3) organizational size, which tends to be negatively related to general coordination; and (4) coordination in the nursing department, which is positively related to general coordination in the total hospital. These variables relate better to general than to programed coordination.

On the other hand, the independent variables which correlate especially well with programed coordination are: (1) the composition of the nursing staff, with high proportions of aides being negatively related to coordination and high proportions of practical nurses being positively related to it; (2) the extent to which members follow established rules and regulations; (3) the degree of complementarity of expectations among members, particularly the extent to which doctors and nurses understand and appreciate each other's problems and needs; and (4) various aspects of problem awareness and problem solving, e.g., the combined problem awareness of the administrator and of the director of nursing, and their combined effectiveness in solving conflicts which arise in the organization. All of these variables tend to relate better to programed than to general coordination, i.e., they relate highly to such aspects of coordination as the timing of activities, the planning of work assignments, and the routinization of functions in interrelated departments.

Some Emerging Implications

The pattern of attitudes and action on the part of trustees, administrator, doctors, and nurses which is conducive to adequate organizational coordination can be readily inferred from the preceding findings. The organizational nature of the community general hospital can likewise be highlighted.

For hospitals, as well as other institutions, the role to be played in the internal affairs of the organization by its board of trustees constitutes an almost classical problem in administration. What precisely should the appropriate role of trustees be, how much should they be directly involved, and how much authority should they exercise over the internal affairs of their organization? According to Parsons, the traditional answer to this problem has been ". . . not so much to tell executives what to do—that is, to exercise 'line authority' over them—as to define broad limits of what they may *legitimately* do and give them relatively broad community support in doing it." (2, p. 14).

It now appears that this pattern of activity is not sufficient for achieving good coordination. The findings clearly show that hospitals whose boards of trustees have a comparatively low understanding and appreciation of the problems and needs of the medical staff, for example, are likely to score poorly on coordination. Limit-setting activity and community support, while important, are not enough. They could easily originate in a partial vacuum, for instance, where the administrator served as the only link between the board and the rest of the organization. This condition can and does occur. One member of the medical staff in the least adequately coordinated hospital spoke on precisely this point: "Actually, we know nothing about the board, or how they operate, and we never see them; there would be a better [mutual] understanding if we had some contact with them." But why is understanding between doctors and trustees so important?

The most common problem between doctors and trustees was summed up by an administrator as follows: "The board of trustees naturally see the management and financial side of a hospital. The board does not understand in detail enough of the professional side; they leave this to the medical staff. The same is true [for the medical staff] in reverse. The medical staff see more and more service but cannot understand the economics of the cost." This role segmentation is not conducive to coordination, which requires that the various interdependent parts of the organization meet one another's needs. Compartmentalization, whether functional or ideological, makes coordination difficult to attain and maintain. If the board makes decisions in comparative isolation from the medical staff, or vice versa, organizational problems are likely to arise rather than be solved. Decisions made out of a parochial frame of reference, which essentially equates the effective attainment of organizational objectives with costs, are likely to engender tensions and pressures which, as the findings show, affect coordination adversely. Operating in the black is only one factor in an equation of many factors which cannot be realized without mutual understanding and sharedness of expectations on the part of the different groups in the hospital. Limit-setting activity may be the primary function of trustees, but from the standpoint of coordination it is not sufficient. A certain amount of involvement, in the form of an active and direct interest in the problems and needs of professional groups of the hospital, is also required.

Summary and Conclusions

The hospital administrator is typically described by the respondents as "liaison" between board and medical staff, as "coordinator" of nonmedical activities, as "director" or "manager" of the organization, and as representing the hospital to the outside world. Obviously, coordination is an essential aspect of his role. In some ways, the hospital administrator occupies a position analogous to that of a business executive or a city manager; yet in other ways his position is quite dissimilar. The hospital administrator is formally responsible to the board of trustees for the day-to-day operations of the hospital but he does not, cannot, and should not disregard the medical staff. His organization, as Smith (3), Wessen (4), and Zugich (5) have pointed out, has multiple seats of power and authority lines. This structural feature of the community general hospital entails a certain insecurity for the administrator, an insecurity which is further accented by his recognized lack of medical expertness. Together, these forces make the administrator's relations with the board and the medical staff a rather delicate affair. An acceptable balance of power among these key parties must be constantly maintained if the organization is to be well coordinated, and the administrator's role is a crucial one in this connection.

The findings show that adequate communication with the medical staff on the part of the administrator is an important factor in relation to coordination, apparently both because the medical staff expects it and because of the administrator's liaison function between doctors and trustees. Adequate explanation of decisions to nonmedical personnel by the administrator and his supervisory staff is likewise important; it too relates positively to coordination. Communication of this kind promotes mutual understanding and sharedness of expectations among diverse but related organizational groups, thus facilitating coordination. The administrator's role is also important with respect to planning and problem solving activities in the organization. The data indicate that high problem awareness and effective problem solving on the part of the administrator and the director of nursing make for better coordination. Last, but not least, the behavior of the administrator is intimately associated with the level of strain prevailing in the organization, and strain is inversely related to coordination. As one doctor put it, "Naturally, the administrator does not handle everything, but he is the key to a smooth-running hospital. Either he builds tension—we do not have tension here, we are relaxed and it is due to our administrator—or [he builds a smooth-running organization]."

The pattern of attitude and action between medical staff and nursing staff which facilitates coordination is also illuminated by the findings. In the earlier, more authoritarian atmosphere which pervaded the quasi-militaristic, quasi-bureaucratic structure of hospitals, doctors ordered, nurses executed the orders, and both understood each other within this framework. The increasing professionalization of nursing and the secularization of the culture within which the modern hospital functions, however, are transforming the older framework into a more equalitarian and less autocratic one. The old norms of duty, strict discipline, and unquestionable subordination no longer characterize correctly the registered nurse of today. "Also I believe, there is disintegration in the former rapport between doctors and nurses, and more and more dissatisfaction on the part of both," observes one of our medical respondents. "Now we have people [nurses] working because they have to supplement family income, rather than being dedicated to the profession [in the traditional framework]; they won't cater to the patient or to the doctor like in former days," observes another.

In this new cultural atmosphere, a mere hierarchical relationship between doctors and nurses is not adequate according to the data. Good coordination demands a certain sharedness of expectations between the two groups, as well as a relatively high degree of understanding and appreciation of each other's problems and needs. And, these requirements cannot be fulfilled solely on the basis of a formal superior-subordinate relationship between these two professional groups. There has to be give and take. The adequacy of patient records—for which both doctors and nurses are responsible—also tends to facilitate coordination, according to the data. Complete patient charts do more than merely satisfy some formally established rules and regulations. Finally, on the negative side, tension between doctors and nurses, as well as between any other interdependent groups in the hospital, impedes organizational coordination.

Within the nursing department, the division of labor among personnel in different classifications also has certain implications for coordination. The tendency by nursing staff in a given category (e.g., registered nurses) to try to do things that staff in another category (e.g., supervisory nurses or practical nurses) should be doing is likely to affect coordination adversely, according to the findings. Role ambiguities of this nature may have their origins in personnel shortages, in definitional inadequacies of the functions ascribed to each nursing role by the organization, in professional and occupational insecurities or differences among different nursing groups, and similar other sources. Regardless of their source, role ambiguities and overlappings are probably detrimental to coordination and would require corrective efforts. The composition of the work force of the nursing department emerges as another important factor affecting coordination. The data show that hospitals whose nursing staff consists of a high proportion of aides in relation to practical and registered nurses tend to have poorer overall coordination and poorer nursing department coordination than hospitals whose nursing staff consists of proportionately fewer aides. Staff imbalances of this kind are apparently dysfunctional from the standpoint of coordination.

Summing Up

Early in this volume questions were raised regarding the essential organizational characteristics of the community general hospital. It was noted that

Summary and Conclusions

there seems to be a good deal of controversy, if not confusion, among both organizational theorists and practicing administrators as to what these characteristics are. Some feel that the hospital should be particularly concerned with primary relationships in which concepts like respect, affection, and loyalty play an important part in welding the different members of the hospital family together into a small, well-integrated community for the care and treatment of the sick. Others believe that the hospital should have more of the characteristics of a quasi-regimented bureaucracy where technical performance is stressed and ensured through a highly impersonal, specialized, task-centered mode of operation that is relatively unconcerned about primary relations and the sentiments of participants. The latter would place great premium upon programed coordination, while the former would correspondingly emphasize general or nonprogramed coordination.

The findings in this chapter argue in favor of an alternate approach. Programed coordination is in part a function of general coordination, and general coordination is in part a function of programed coordination; since the two are highly correlated according to the data, each depends on the other. Programed coordination is indicative of the extent to which the hospital functions as a well-regulated machine. Nonprogramed coordination is indicative of the extent to which motivation, voluntary adjustments and shared expectations on the part of the different participants play an important role in the functioning of the organization. The findings indicate that both programmed and general coordination are important insofar as hospital organization is concerned. The hospital of today is not simply an intricately designed machine whose interlocking parts perform assigned functions mechanically. In addition to programed coordination through the planning, timing, and regulation of activities and departmental routines, general coordination through the development of mutual understanding and shared frames of reference among hospital personnel is required.

Formal organizations typically depend on attaining predictability regarding performance through a structure of explicitly defined and regulated statuses and roles and an elaborate system of programed coordination. The greater the pressure for exact and prompt coordination, moreover, the greater the tendency toward explicit regulation of behavior, hierarchical relationships, impersonality, and ultimately well-defined patterns of deference and social distance. To a large measure, the community general hospital exhibits this structure. Yet, the findings suggest that adequate overall coordination in the hospital also depends upon such things as the willingness of members in related jobs to assist each other when needed, the extent to which members conform with established rules and regulations, the degree to which they understand and appreciate one another's problems and needs, the ease with which they can meet to exchange information and ideas, the pressures and tensions they experience, and the like. The motivations, feelings, and expectations of organizational members that are conducive to adequate coordination cannot be taken for granted. They must be developed and cultivated in the interests of both good general and good programed coordination.

The findings on coordination thus point to an important empirical parameter about the type of social system the community general hospital is today. It appears that the hospital is a complex, formal associational system with many of the characteristics of a bureaucracy, thus requiring a good deal of programed coordination with emphasis on authority relations and task-oriented behavior. At the same time, coordination by advance planning is not enough. In its day-to-day, even minute-by-minute, functioning the hospital is also dependent upon coordination by "feedback," or nonprogramed coordination. In subsequent chapters on communication and superior-subordinate relationships, additional findings should help us pursue the question of the essential characteristic of hospital organization further. The significance of coordination itself for patient care and organizational effectiveness will be shown in the next chapter to which we now turn.

REFERENCES

1. Burling, T., Lentz, E. M., and Wilson, R. N. *The Give and Take in Hospitals.* New York: Putnam, 1956.
2. Parsons, T. "General Theory in Sociology." In Merton, R. K., Broom, L., and Cottrell, Jr., L. S. (eds.). *Sociology Today: Problems and Prospects.* New York: Basic Books, Inc., 1959.
3. Smith, H. L. "The Sociological Study of Hospitals." Doctoral Dissertation. University of Chicago, 1949.
4. Wessen, A. F. "The Social Structure of a Modern Hospital." Doctoral Dissertation. Yale University, 1951.
5. Zugich, J. J. "Influences on Interpersonal Relations in the Hospital Organization." Unpublished M.A. Thesis. Yale University, 1951.

8 FACTORS AFFECTING THE QUALITY OF PATIENT CARE

In Chapter 5, which provides necessary background for the present chapter, we discussed the problem of assessing the quality of care patients received in the various hospitals, and described in detail four measures of care that were developed in this study. The particular measures, it will be recalled, were: a measure of the quality of nursing care given to patients; a parallel measure of the quality of medical care; an overall measure of the quality of total patient care, i.e., a measure taking into account both the medical and nursing aspects of care simultaneously; and a comparative measure of the quality of total care, which indicates the quality of patient care in a hospital as compared to the quality of care rendered in similar other hospitals. All four measures, in view of the evidence amassed in Chapter 5, proved sufficiently valid and reliable, successfully differentiating between the better- and poorer-care hospitals.

Our task in this chapter is to relate the four measures of patient care to certain aspects of hospital structure and functioning, which were also measured in the research, in order to determine some of the major social-psychological variables that affect the quality of care. The main question to be answered by the results in the following pages is this: What particular factors are associated with better patient care in the community general hospital, and which of these factors are the more crucial ones for nursing, medical, and overall patient care? As in the preceding chapter where we showed the correlates and determinants of organizational coordination, we shall here examine a number of independent variables (including coordination) which, on theoretical grounds or according to currently prevailing beliefs in the hospital field, are expected to affect patient care, in order to ascertain their actual empirical relationship to patient care. The familiar correlational method of analysis will again be utilized, with the total hospital serving as the unit of analysis.

Findings will be presented about the relationship of the quality of patient care to each of a number of factors incorporated in the following sets of independent variables: the relative adequacy of various material facilities;

some measures of hospital income and expenditures; certain size-related aspects of hospital structure; the skill composition and distribution of the nursing and medical staffs; absenteeism and turnover among nursing personnel; hospital coordination, and coordination in the nursing department; certain aspects of intraorganizational strain; complementarity of expectations between the medical staff and the nursing staff; medical committee activity and performance; and the individual performance of paramedical departments in the various hospitals.

Many of the independent variables, and their measurement, were discussed previously in the two chapters on coordination, while others were introduced in earlier chapters. Accordingly, instead of repeating our discussion of these variables, in this chapter we shall only indicate where their particular measures are described. In the case of independent variables introduced here for the first time, however, we shall describe the nature of the data by means of which they were measured, before discussing their relationship to patient care. Finally, although the principal results about patient care will be presented in this chapter, not all the relevant findings will be incorporated. Some results concerning patient care and the performance of nursing personnel will be discussed in our chapters about superior-subordinate relationships in the hospital, and about communication practices among nurses, Chapters 9 and 10. These will supplement and, in some instances, amplify some of the findings and conclusions we are about to present here.

ADEQUACY OF MATERIAL FACILITIES AND THE QUALITY OF PATIENT CARE

A hospital, like any other organization, to operate effectively and to produce a high quality product must, among other things, have appropriate and sufficient facilities. Some of these facilities are primarily of a material kind, while others are of a social or psychological kind. In this section, we will be concerned with the relationship between the adequacy of material instrumentalities and the quality of patient care. Is patient care appreciably better in hospitals which have better, or more adequate, facilities of this kind?

To answer this question, we first had to obtain measures of the adequacy of facilities. To get these measures, the doctors, the trustees and the administrator, and the laboratory and x-ray technicians in the hospitals studied were asked the following question:

> Considering what this hospital needs to provide adequate care and high quality service to its patients at reasonable cost, how adequate would you say each of the following [facilities] is?

Respondents answered the question in terms of a five-point scale, with possible choices ranging from "completely adequate" to "inadequate." The par-

Adequacy of Material Facilities

ticular facilities about which data were collected, from one or more of the above respondent groups, are: "the physical plant and layout of the hospital," "space and beds available," "the equipment," "the supplies that are available," and "the general financial condition of the hospital." The data about each facility from each respondent group were converted into arithmetic means to provide us with the desired measures of the adequacy of facilities. These measures were then related to the four measures of patient care. The results are presented in Table 42.

Before reviewing the findings, however, let us briefly consider the data about the adequacy of hospital facilities. First, as might be expected, the data show considerable differences among the ten participating hospitals with respect to how adequate their material facilities are. Using data from doctors, for example, we find that hospital scores on the adequacy of physical plant range from 1.43 to 4.09, on a five-point scale; on the adequacy of space and beds, they range between 1.69 and 4.20; and on the adequacy of equipment, they range between 1.43 and 3.27 (for the remaining facilities, the interhospital ranges are somewhat smaller). Similarly, using data from trustees and the administrator, we find that the corresponding ranges are 1.80 to 3.20, 1.40 to 4.25, and 1.57 to 2.40, respectively. And, when the evaluation of the various facilities by the technicians is used, similar differences across hospitals are found.

Second, the data show that some of the hospitals in the study tend to have generally better facilities than others.[1] The adequacy of the physical plant, for example, correlates positively and significantly with the adequacy of space and beds (.82), with the adequacy of equipment (.85), and the adequacy of supplies (.62) in the ten hospitals, according to data from doctors. The same holds generally true, moreover, when data from the trustees and the administrator, or from the technicians, are analyzed. Not all the intercorrelations regarding the adequacy of the several facilities are statistically significant, however. For instance, we find no significant relationship between the adequacy of space and beds and the adequacy of supplies, or of equipment, as evaluated by the doctors.

Perhaps the most interesting and most important finding concerning facilities is the fact that, surprisingly, there is no relationship between the adequacy of the general financial condition of the hospitals and the adequacy of

[1] Incidentally, it should not be assumed that it is the larger of the institutions that have the more adequate facilities. Examination shows that hospital size (number of beds) is not significantly related to the adequacy of any of the five facilities here discussed, regardless of which respondent group evaluates the adequacy of facilities. In fact, most of the correlations between hospital size and our measures of the adequacy of facilities are negative, though not large enough to be significant. Of all possible correlations only one is significant—a correlation of —.63 between hospital size and the adequacy of equipment, as seen by the doctors. In this one case, it is the smaller hospitals which have the more adequate equipment. It should be remembered, of course, that only medium-size hospitals are involved in the study.

TABLE 42. Relation Between the Adequacy of Certain Hospital Facilities and Patient Care *

Degree of Adequacy of:	Quality of: †			
	Nursing Care	Medical Care	Overall Care	Comparative Overall Care
The general physical plant and layout of the hospital, as seen by:				
Doctors	.20	.02	.24	.12
Administrator and trustees	.49	.50	.51	.50
Lab and x-ray technicians	.35	.24	.55	.49
Space and beds available, as seen by:				
Doctors	−.01	.01	−.03	−.10
Administrator and trustees	.12	.22	.20	.22
Lab and x-ray technicians	.35	.27	.30	.22
The equipment, as seen by:				
Doctors	−.07	−.20	.05	−.04
Administrator and trustees	.39	.25	.35	.30
Lab and x-ray technicians	.57	.28	.64	.54
The supplies that are available, as seen by:				
Doctors	.04	.12	.30	.30
Lab and x-ray technicians	.51	−.15	.55	.42
The general financial condition of the hospital, as seen by:				
Doctors	.42	.03	.35	.24
Administrator and trustees	.29	.20	.15	.18

* All figures are rank-order correlation coefficients, based on an N of 10 hospitals in each case. To be statistically significant at the .05 level, a coefficient must be larger than ±.56.

† The four measures of the quality of patient care are described in detail in Chapter 5.

any of the other material facilities with which we are dealing here. As appraised by the trustees and the administrator, for instance, the adequacy of the financial status of the various hospitals correlates only −.10 with the adequacy of their physical plant, .05 with the adequacy of space and beds, and .18 with the adequacy of equipment. (For all practical purposes, these correlations are equivalent to zero.) As evaluated by the doctors, the adequacy of financial status correlates .41, .49, and .50, respectively, with the adequacy of the same three facilities, and .13 with the adequacy of supplies. None of the correlations is statistically significant although the larger ones are suggestive. Nevertheless, it is clear that the more affluent hospitals are not significantly more likely than the less affluent ones to have better material facilities. This finding may cast aspersions upon the money disposition (and

Adequacy of Material Facilities

financial management?) in the wealthier hospitals and, as we will see in the next section of this chapter, not without good reasons for it. But, let us return to the main issue at hand, for the present, to examine the relationship between the adequacy of material facilities and the quality of patient care.

On the whole, the results in Table 42 indicate that hospitals with more adequate material facilities (the relative adequacy of facilities being evaluated by the groups shown) do not provide significantly better care to their patients than hospitals where facilities are less adequate, as seen by the doctors, the trustees and the administrator, or the technicians from the participating institutions. On the other hand, the former institutions do not provide poorer care than the latter. Actually, with few exceptions, the correlations between adequacy of facilities and the quality of patient care are positive, suggesting a slight tendency for the hospitals with the better facilities to render perhaps somewhat better care. But, since the large majority of the correlations are small and not statistically significant, the hypothesis that patient care is appreciably better in those of the hospitals that have the more adequate material facilities is not substantiated. Of the 52 correlations in Table 42, only two are sufficiently large to be significant at the .05 level. These refer to the adequacy of equipment, as seen by technicians, which correlates .57 with the quality of nursing care and .64 with the quality of overall patient care (but only .28 with the quality of medical care, and .54 with the comparative measure of overall care) in the ten hospitals. However, these two significant relationships are the exception rather than the rule. The pattern is clearly one of small positive but nonsignificant relationships between adequacy of facilities and patient care, regardless of: (1) which of the five facilities is considered, (2) which of the four measures of patient care is considered, or (3) which of the three respondent groups evaluates the adequacy of facilities.[2]

Apparently, having superior material facilities does not necessarily make for better patient care in the hospital, according to the findings. To illustrate this conclusion in specific cases, moreover, we examined the rank-order of the ten hospitals on the measures of the adequacy of their facilities. This analysis is rather revealing. For example, we find that Hospital #3, which ranks among the top three of the ten hospitals on all measures of patient care (see Chap. 5), also ranks among the top three hospitals on the adequacy of its plant, its space, its equipment, its supplies, and its financial condition,

---

[2] In this connection, it may also be pointed out that across hospitals, the adequacy of a given facility, as seen by one of the respondent groups, generally correlates positively, but not always significantly, with the adequacy of the same facility, as seen by the other two respondent groups. Regarding the adequacy of the physical plant, and of space and beds available, the evaluations by the three respondent groups intercorrelate both positively and significantly. The comparable correlations pertaining to the adequacy of the remaining facilities are also positive, but generally not high enough to be significant. Respondents from the three groups apparently evaluate the adequacy of each of these latter facilities from a somewhat different standpoint. For this reason, we have here treated the data from the three groups of respondents separately.

according to the evaluation of these facilities by the medical staff. But, at the same time, Hospital #1, which ranks poorest or second poorest among the ten hospitals on the measures of patient care, ranks best or second best among the ten institutions on the adequacy of four of the above five facilities (on the adequacy of its financial status it ranks seventh). And Hospital #4 which, like Hospital #3, ranks among the top three hospitals on patient care, ranks seventh on the adequacy of its plant, fifth on space and beds, eighth on equipment, third on supplies, and sixth on financial status. Furthermore, if instead of the evaluations furnished by the doctors, we examine those furnished by the trustees and administrator, or by the technicians, we again find patterns similar to those just cited.

The lack of significant relationships between the adequacy of material facilities and the quality of patient care can be interpreted in several ways. One explanation might be that all of the hospitals studied have at least minimally adequate facilities, and that increased adequacy beyond some minimal level has no significant effect upon the quality of patient care. Some of the data about hospital facilities presented earlier in connection with our discussion of the "typical" participating hospital and in the individual hospital profiles (see Chap. 4) suggest that this interpretation is quite plausible. Another explanation might be that the adequacy of physical facilities is entirely irrelevant to patient care, but the findings from this study, as well as common sense, argue against such an interpretation. It is very likely, however, that material facilities *per se* do not play as crucial a role as do social and psychological facilities or the skill and competence of organizational members, insofar as patient care is concerned. Subsequent findings in this chapter provide good support for this proposition. Still another explanation might be that those hospitals which have less adequate facilities manage to make relatively better use of their facilities than the hospitals with superior facilities, with the result that patient care in the former institutions does not suffer perceptibly because of relatively less adequate facilities. This explanation is also tenable. In any event, superior material facilities do not by themselves ensure better patient care in hospitals of the type studied.

FINANCIAL CONSIDERATIONS AND THE QUALITY OF PATIENT CARE

The quantity and quality of the material facilities and human resources of an organization often depend both upon its financial status and the disposition of its income and expenditures. The financial well-being of a hospital may well condition the quality of the patient care it provides, by making it possible to hire and maintain a superior staff, for example, along with adequate equipment. In Chapters 3 and 4, we commented on several different aspects of the financial situation of participating hospitals, and in the pre-

Financial Considerations

ceding section of this chapter we examined the adequacy of the general financial condition of the hospitals, as perceived by doctors, trustees, and administrators, in relation to patient care. In this section, we will investigate the relationship between the quality of patient care and various specific items of hospital income and expenditures. Our measures of these items are based on data from hospital records and cover two time periods: the calendar year 1957 and the last quarter of 1957, i.e., the three months during which data were collected from individual respondents. The question to be answered here is this: What specific aspects of hospital finances, if any, make for better patient care?

Perhaps, we might best begin our discussion by making a few introductory observations about some of the items which we will examine. First, as anticipated, the data show that income (hospital revenues from all sources) and expenditures are a function of hospital size. Hospital size, measured by number of beds, is found to be positively and significantly related to total hospital income (.86), total hospital expenses (.77), and total payroll expenses (.81) in the ten hospitals during 1957; and the same is true for the last quarter of 1957. Similarly, the average daily census (average daily number of patients in the hospital, excluding newborn) correlates very highly with total hospital income (.90), total expenses (.82), and payroll expenses (.82) during 1957. The average daily census, of course, itself correlates very highly with hospital size (.97). Second, the data show that income and expenses in the hospitals studied are highly interrelated. Total hospital income correlates .98 with total expenses; total income per bed correlates .96 with total expenses per bed; and total income per patient (per average daily census) correlates .84 with total expenses per patient. Furthermore, total hospital income correlates an impressive .98 with total payroll expenses, and the sum total of hospital expenses correlates also .98 with total payroll expenses in the ten hospitals. In brief then, the larger hospitals are the hospitals with the higher income and higher total and payroll expenses, the higher-income hospitals also being the higher-expense hospitals.

The high stability and predictability in the financial area implied by the above relationships, however, break down in certain respects. Further analysis of the data indicates, for example, that neither total income, nor total expenses, nor payroll expenses correlate significantly with hospital occupancy, or the proportion of occupied beds in the hospital (i.e., average daily census of patients, excluding newborn, divided by number of beds). The correlation between each of these three items and hospital occupancy is .37, .50, and .48, respectively (significance at the .05 level, for an N of 10 hospitals, requires a correlation of .56 or higher). In other words, the higher-occupancy hospitals are not necessarily more likely than the lower-occupancy hospitals to have a higher total income, higher total expenses, or higher payroll expenses. Similarly, although total payroll expenses are found to correlate positively and significantly with hospital size (.81), average daily census (.82), and total income per bed (.59), they are not significantly related to total expenses per bed (.49), total expenses per patient (.33), or total income per patient (.49). The proportion, or the percentage, of total hospital expenses going into payroll, moreover, is unrelated to hospital size (—.20). These results are, of course, interesting and useful to know but they are only preliminary and incidental to the question of whether the various income and expenditure items bear any relationship to the quality of patient care in the community general hospital, the question to which we now turn.[3]

Table 43 presents our findings about the relationship of income and expenses to the quality of patient care in the participating hospitals. What conclusions can one draw from these findings? First, it is generally obvious from the correlations pertaining to the first three items in the table that the relationship between hospital income, or financial well-being, and the quality of patient care tends to be a negative one, regardless of whether we examine income data for 1957 or for the last quarter of that year. But in most instances, the specific relationships are not sufficiently high to be statistically significant. Total hospital income during 1957, for example, correlates —.57 with the quality of nursing care, —.13 with the quality of medical care, —.52 with the quality of overall care, and —.35 with the comparative measure of overall care, the first of these correlations being significant at the .05 level. Total income per bed yields very similar results, and the same is true for total income per patient (average daily census).

Of the four measures of patient care, the nursing care measure yields the majority of the significant relationships with the income variables, while the medical care measure yields the smallest correlations. Based on data for the year 1957, the quality of nursing care correlates —.57 with total hospital income, —.57 with total income per bed, and —.62 with total income per patient. It also correlates —.57 with total hospital income, and —.65 with total income per bed, based on data for the last quarter of the same year. These relationships are all statistically significant. The remaining measures of patient care also correlate negatively with the income variables in all cases, but the correlations are smaller (one of them is statistically significant, several are suggestive, and the rest are not significant). Considered as a whole, the results indicate that the quality of patient care, especially the quality of nursing care, tends to be lower in the higher-income hospitals. The higher-income hospitals are not the better-care hospitals. On the contrary, the weight of the evidence suggests that it is the lower-income hospitals which tend to have better care in general, and significantly better nursing care in particular.

[3] The above results are based on data for calendar year 1957. But, when data for the last quarter of that year are used in the analysis, the results are essentially the same. For further discussion of financial items, as well as for specific income and expenditure figures, see appropriate sections in Chapters 3 and 4.

Financial Considerations

TABLE 43. Relation of Hospital Income and Expenditures to Patient Care *

First Row: Figures refer to last quarter of 1957
Second Row: Figures refer to calendar year 1957

	Quality of:			
Income or Expenditure Item	Nursing Care	Medical Care	Overall Care	Comparative Overall Care
1. Total hospital income	−.57	−.13	−.52	−.35
	−.57	−.13	−.52	−.35
2. Total income per bed	−.65	−.30	−.58	−.45
	−.57	−.11	−.40	−.29
3. Total income per patient	−.47	−.08	−.38	−.32
or per average daily census (average daily number of patients, excluding newborn)	−.62	−.24	−.53	−.47
4. Total hospital expenses	−.52	−.19	−.49	−.35
	−.55	−.03	−.44	−.26
5. Total expenses per bed	−.54	−.26	−.35	−.25
	−.37	.02	−.21	−.12
6. Total expenses per patient	−.58	−.30	−.43	−.39
or per average daily census	−.25	.04	−.09	−.04
7. Average hospital cost per patient day	−.66	−.30	−.39	−.30
	—	—	—	—
8. Total expenses per paid employee	−.20	−.43	−.13	−.16
	−.28	−.15	−.18	−.14
9. Total payroll expenses	−.60	.12	−.48	−.27
	−.54	.04	−.38	−.19
10. Percentage of all hospital expenses going into payroll	.11	.75	.21	.38
	.01	.37	.16	.27
11. Payroll expenses per employee	−.06	.38	.00	.16
	−.15	.03	−.13	−.01

* All figures are rank-order correlation coefficients, based on an N of 10 hospitals in each case. Coefficients larger than ±.56 are statistically significant at the .05 level. Dashes indicate lack of data.

The correlations referring to items 4, 5, 6, 7, and 8 in Table 43 show the relationship between the quality of patient care and hospital expenses. The emerging pattern is similar, though less clear-cut, with the pattern of correlations showing the relationship of income to patient care, as discussed above. Total hospital expenses during 1957, for example, correlate −.55 with the quality of nursing care, −.03 with the quality of medical care, −.44 with the quality of overall patient care, and −.35 with comparative care. Total hospital expenses per bed, total expenses per patient, and total expenses per employee produce similar relationships with the four measures of care. When expense data for the last quarter of the same year are examined, moreover, the correlations with patient care form a similar pattern. The average cost per patient day during the last quarter of 1957, for instance, correlates —.66 with nursing care, —.30 with medical care, —.39 with overall care, and —.30 with comparative overall care. Of the 36 correlations between the four measures of care, on the one hand, and total hospital expenses, total expenses per bed, total expenses per patient, average cost per patient day, and total expenses per employee, on the other, 34 are negative (and the two positive ones are practically zero).

It would appear from these findings that the higher the expenses, the poorer the patient care in the various hospitals. This conclusion, however, is not quite justified by the evidence. In the first place, although 34 of the 36 correlations are negative, the correlations are not independent of one another, because most of the expenditure items are interrelated among themselves, and because the four measures of care are also interrelated. In the second place, the correlations are generally small (on the average smaller than those between the income items and patient care), only two of them being statistically significant at the .05 level. These two are, a correlation of —.58 between total expenses per patient during the last quarter of 1957 and the quality of nursing care, and one of —.66 between average cost per patient day during the same period and nursing care. With the exception of these two cases, therefore, we cannot conclude that the quality of patient care is significantly poorer in the hospitals with the higher expenses. At the same time, the above findings demonstrate that patient care is not better in the higher-expense hospitals. The results are suggestive of a general tendency for the quality of patient care to be somewhat better in the less expensive hospitals, without establishing conclusively a negative relationship between hospital expenses and patient care.

Table 43 also shows the relationship of patient care to payroll expenses. Correlations are presented with respect to total payroll expenses, the percentage of total hospital expenses going into payroll, and payroll expenses per employee, the last three items in Table 43. The relationship of total payroll expenses to patient care is essentially the same as the relationship between the other expenditure items examined above and patient care. When we recall that total payroll expenses are highly correlated with total hospital expenses, this finding is not surprising. The item "payroll expenses per employee" produces very small correlations with the four measures of patient care. Some of these correlations are positive, others are negative, and none is significant. Apparently, there is no relationship whatsoever between the quality of patient care and how high payroll expenses per employee are in the different hospitals. The only remaining variable to be examined here in relation to patient care is the percentage of hospital expenses going into payroll.

Of the eleven income and expenditure items studied, the percentage of total hospital expenses going into payroll produces the most interesting re-

Financial Considerations

sults. It is the only item that yields positive correlations with all four measures of patient care, whether measured on the basis of data for 1957 or for the last quarter of 1957 alone. Furthermore, it is the only item which produces the single positive significant relationship with any of the measures of patient care, and the only item which produces the single significant relationship with the measure of the quality of medical care. Specifically, the percentage of total hospital expenses going into payroll during the last quarter of 1957 correlates .75 with the quality of medical care in the participating hospitals —a correlation which is statistically significant at the .01 level. This relationship indicates that medical care is of higher quality in the hospitals which apportion a larger part of their total expenses to payroll. There are some problems of interpretation here, however. One problem is that the percentage of expenses going into payroll during the entire year of 1957 correlates only .37 with the quality of medical care, and this relationship is not statistically significant. Another problem is that the percentage of expenses going into payroll does not relate significantly to nursing care—and one would expect it to relate better to nursing care than to medical care, for nurses are on the hospital payroll while doctors are not. In view of these problems, there is a possibility that the correlation of .75 between the proportion of hospital expenses devoted to payroll and medical care could be the result of chance, even though this could occur only once in a hundred times, or it might be the result of some unidentified factor.

In the light of these considerations, we cannot assign too much weight to this one correlation and assert that the quality of medical care is significantly better in the hospitals where a higher percentage of total expenses are assigned to payroll. On the other hand, we cannot discard the possibility of a real relationship here either. If we compare the correlations between the patient care measures and the percentage of hospital expenses going into payroll with the correlations between the patient care measures and total hospital expenses, or total payroll expenses, for example, the comparison reveals strikingly different patterns. For instance, total hospital expenses in the last quarter of 1957 correlate —.60 with nursing care, .12 with medical care, —.48 with overall patient care, and —.27 with comparative care, while the corresponding correlations between the percentage of total expenses going into payroll and the care measures are .11, .75, .21, and .38, respectively. A reversal in the pattern of relationships such as this must certainly be of some importance, perhaps indicating a tendency for the quality of patient care to be associated with the proportion of total hospital expenses going into payroll. If anything, the evidence is suggestive for such a relationship. Certainly, patient care is not better in institutions devoting a relatively smaller proportion of their total expenses to payroll.

The various results concerning the relationship between hospital finances and the quality of patient care in the ten participating hospitals may now be summarized. In general, the quality of nursing care, medical care, overall care, and comparative overall care is not better in the higher-income hospitals, in the higher-expense hospitals, or in the higher-cost hospitals. On balance, the evidence tends to suggest the opposite. It appears that the better-care hospitals are the ones with the lower income and lower expenses, although only a few of the correlations that supply evidence for this relationship are sufficiently high to be statistically significant. It also seems that patient care tends to be somewhat better in those of the hospitals where a higher proportion of the institution's total expenses are assigned to payroll. Therefore, as a group, the findings from relating eleven income and expenditure items to the four measures of patient care provide support for the overall conclusion that the better-care hospitals are also the more efficient (and perhaps better managed), or more economical institutions, from a financial standpoint.

SIZE-RELATED FEATURES OF HOSPITAL STRUCTURE AND THE QUALITY OF PATIENT CARE

It will be recalled that, in this study, hospital size is a rather truncated variable, since only medium-size institutions have been included in the research. This restriction in size does not permit a thorough exploration of the relationship between size and patient care or other aspects of hospital structure and functioning. On the other hand, the range between 100 and 350 beds is not too small to prohibit an examination of the role of hospital size in relation to the quality of patient care. Furthermore, apart from gross size, there are certain other important variables of hospital structure which, while associated with organizational size, are not dependent upon the range of size within which the participating hospitals fall, thus allowing us to study their relationship to patient care, without presenting any serious methodological obstacles.

In addition to size, measured by the number of beds in each hospital, the following size-related variables will be investigated in this section in relation to the patient care measures: total patient admissions, number of admissions per bed, average daily census, occupancy, number of paid personnel per bed, and number of paid personnel per average daily census or per patient. The question to be answered here is whether organizational size, number of patients or patient load, and number of personnel have any relationship, positive or negative, to the quality of patient care rendered in the various hospitals. As with the case of hospital finances, the several independent variables under consideration were measured on the basis of information from hospital records, with data for calendar year 1957 and for the last quarter of the same year. All the variables involved have been introduced in earlier chapters, particularly in Chapter 4 and in Chapter 7. Therefore, they will not be described further in this section.

Theoretically, with reference to size, one could make a good case for a hypothesis predicting either a positive or a negative relationship to patient care and hospital effectiveness. It is frequently maintained, for example, that for given types of groups or organizations some organizations are too big or too small to operate effectively. Coordination would normally be more difficult in very large hospitals, while very small institutions might lack minimally adequate facilities to provide high quality care to their patients, for instance. Along the same lines, some writers suggest specific size limits for optimal hospital functioning. As a case in point, Goldwater feels that "hospitals of from 500 to 600 beds can be satisfactorily supervised and controlled, . . . [but] administrative difficulties are multiplied when the size of a hospital greatly exceeds these figures" (5, p. 16). He also states that "individual clinical departments in a general hospital for acute diseases should not be too large" (5, p. 16).

TABLE 44. Relation Between Certain Size-Related Variables of Hospital Structure and Patient Care *

First Row: Figures refer to last quarter of 1957
Second Row: Figures refer to calendar year 1957

Hospital Structure Variable	Nursing Care	Medical Care	Overall Care	Comparative Overall Care
Number of beds (size)	—.36	—.18	—.48	—.39
	—.36	—.18	—.48	—.39
Average daily census of patients (excluding newborn)	—.32	—.13	—.44	—.36
	—.36	—.15	—.47	—.37
Total patient admissions (excluding newborn)	—.32	—.05	—.28	—.19
	—.42	—.04	—.36	—.21
Occupancy (average daily census divided by number of beds)	—.14	—.02	—.04	.07
	—.06	.18	.10	.24
Number of patient admissions per bed	.17	.10	.37	.35
	.13	—.03	.27	.21
Average number of (full-time) paid personnel per bed	—.38	.09	—.14	—.02
	—.18	.32	.09	.24
Number of paid personnel per average daily census (or, per patient)	—.21	.13	—.03	.03
	—.08	.27	.14	.21

* All figures are rank-order correlation coefficients, based on an N of 10 hospitals in each case. To be statistically significant at the .05 level, a coefficient must be larger than ±.56.

In view of reasonable arguments both in favor and against large, as well as small, size, one might even be tempted to propose a curvilinear relationship between size and the quality of patient care in the community general hospital, asserting that it is in the medium-size, rather than in the larger or the smaller, institutions where patient care is of higher quality. This particular hypothesis is of course untestable in the present study, both because the participating hospitals are of medium size and because we do not have enough hospitals to pursue the investigation of size as far as the hypothesis would require. In the absence of sufficient and conclusive evidence from empirical research about the role of organizational size for organizational effectiveness, we do not prefer to argue in favor of any of the suggested hypotheses. In fact, instead of proposing any particular relationship between hospital size, or size-related variables, and patient care, we simply decided to analyze our data and let the results indicate whether or not there is a relationship, and the nature of the relationship, if there is one. The relevant findings are presented in Table 44 (p. 377).

On the whole, the findings in Table 44 show no statistically significant relationships between the quality of patient care and size, or size-related variables. Directionally, however, the obtained correlations are suggestive in some cases. Hospital size measured by number of beds, for example, correlates —.36 with the quality of nursing care, —.18 with the quality of medical care, —.48 with the quality of overall patient care, and —.39 with comparative care. The average daily census of patients in the various hospitals and the total number of patient admissions, during 1957 or during the last quarter of 1957, produce similar negative correlations with the four measures of patient care.[4] These results indicate that the quality of patient care is not better in those of the hospitals which have more beds, more admissions, or a higher average daily census, without demonstrating that patient care is significantly poorer in these hospitals than in the hospitals with fewer beds, less admissions, or lower daily census. The smaller of the participating hospitals seem to have the edge (and this is in agreement with our earlier findings concerning the relationship of hospital size to coordination, and the findings regarding the relation of patient care to hospital income and expenditures), but the correlations do not show a significant negative relationship between size and care.

Hospital occupancy, or the average daily number of occupied beds during 1957 or during the last quarter of 1957 only, bears no relationship to patient-care quality. The higher-occupancy hospitals are neither more nor less likely than the lower-occupancy hospitals to provide better or poorer care. The number of patient admissions per bed during 1957 or during the last quarter of that year likewise seems to be unrelated to the quality of patient care.

[4] Number of beds, number of admissions, and average daily census in the various hospitals are, of course, significantly related to one another. However, based on 1957 data, the correlation between number of beds and number of admissions is not extremely high; being .71, it accounts for only half of the variance involved. Similarly, the correlation between number of admissions and average daily census is .75. Accordingly, we have used the three variables separately for analysis purposes, even though number of beds and average daily census correlate .97.

However, unlike the other six variables here examined, it generally yields small positive correlations with the care measure. Accordingly, it may be concluded that having more admissions per bed, or a higher patient load, does not make for poorer care in the hospitals studied.

Finally, the number of paid personnel in the hospital, which is a measure of the size of the nonmedical staff, also makes no difference insofar as the quality of patient care is concerned—notwithstanding an assumption to the contrary on the part of many hospital administrators. Both our measures of personnel size show the same pattern of results. The average number of paid personnel per bed during 1957 and during the last quarter of that year yields small and insignificant correlations when related to the care measures, and the same is true for the number of paid personnel per patient (per average daily census). In both cases, moreover, some of the correlations are positive and others are negative, demonstrating the absence of any consistent relationship between staff size and patient care in the participating hospitals.[5] Consequently, any assumption that more personnel per patient, or per bed, makes for improved patient care must be viewed with great suspicion. As we will see in the following section, it is the quality rather than the size of the staff which is the crucial factor.

COMPOSITION AND DISTRIBUTION OF THERAPEUTIC STAFF AND THE QUALITY OF PATIENT CARE

In Chapter 5 we found that, as anticipated, the skill composition of the nursing staff in the ten hospitals is significantly associated with our measure of nursing care. Here, we will test this hypothesis with reference to all of the measures of patient care. In addition, we shall examine the composition of the medical staff in relation to the quality of medical care and in relation to the other three measures of care. The specific independent variables to be examined, as well as the manner in which they were measured, have already been discussed in previous chapters, particularly in Chapters 5 and 7.

First, let us consider the composition and distribution of the medical staff. In this case, four specific variables were studied in relation to patient care: the proportion of attending (active and associate) medical staff members in the various hospitals who are certified "board men"; the number of board men per patient (average daily census); the proportion of attending staff members who are "general practitioners"; and the number of general practitioners per patient. The results are presented in Table 45, the first four rows of correlations being the relevant ones.

[5] The composition of the nonmedical staff in the various hospitals to which the present results refer has been discussed in Chapters 2 and 3. In the latter chapter, we have also shown specific figures indicating the ratio of nonmedical personnel to beds and to average daily census, and the range of participating institutions on these measures.

What do the findings show? In the first place, they show that the proportion of board men correlates .49 with the quality of medical care, while the proportion of general practitioners correlates .15 with medical care. These relationships are in the direction that might be expected—on the assumption that, other things being equal, a greater percentage of board men on the staff is indicative of an overall superior staff—but neither one is statistically significant at the .05 level. In the second place, the number of board men per patient correlates .15, and the number of general practitioners per patient correlates —.03, with the quality of medical care in the participating hospitals, neither of the correlations being significant. It is obvious, therefore, that the quality of medical care is not poorer in hospitals which have a higher percentage of general practitioners on their staff, or a greater number of general practitioners per patient. It is also apparent that hospitals with a greater number of board men per patient are not more likely than other hospitals to have superior medical care. Of the above four correlations, only that between the proportion of staff members who are board men and the quality of medical care is large enough to be suggestive of a slight tendency for medical care to be better in institutions having a greater percentage of board men on their staff.

Had we had more detailed, or purer, measures of the composition of the medical staff, the preceding results might have been more conclusive. While hospital X may have a higher proportion of board men on its staff than hospital Y, for example, most of the board men in the former may be surgeons or internists, by contrast to the latter where the board men may be more evenly distributed among the major services of the hospital. Our measure representing the overall proportion of board men on the staff would obscure the fact that the proportion of board men in surgery is quite different from that in pediatrics or medicine. To the extent to which the board men are unevenly divided among the major services in the various hospitals, to that extent the relationship between the proportion of board men and medical care may be obscured. A similar problem exists, moreover, in the case of the distribution of the medical staff among patients. A better measure than the number of board men per patient might be the number of board men per surgical patient, per medical patient, etc. Until more refined measures become available, therefore, we cannot draw more definitive conclusions regarding the relationship of the quality of medical care to the composition and distribution of the medical staff than the above results permit.

Regarding nursing care, the findings show that only the number of general practitioners per patient correlates positively and significantly (.58) with the quality of nursing care in the participating hospitals. The number of board men per patient also correlates positively with nursing care (.35), but the relationship is not statistically significant. The same is true, moreover, for the proportion of staff members who are board men, and the proportion who

Composition-Distribution of Therapeutic Staff

are general practitioners. The results about the quality of overall care are similar to the results about nursing care, only the number of general practitioners per patient being positively and significantly associated with the quality of overall patient care (.58). And, the results concerning the comparative measure of overall care are similar to those obtained using the noncomparative measure, except that none of the correlations reaches statistical significance in this case. In summary, then, the quality of nursing care and the quality of overall (noncomparative) care are likely to be higher in hospitals having a larger number of general practitioners per patient. The proportion of staff members who are general practitioners, the proportion who are board men, and the number of board men per patient, on the other hand, yield no comparable significant relationships.

The findings concerning the relationship of the composition of the nursing staff to patient care, also shown in Table 45, are more clear-cut. In general, we find that, as in the case of organizational coordination, the quality of pa-

TABLE 45. Relation Between Certain Aspects of the Composition and Distribution of the Medical and Nursing Staffs and Patient Care *

Variable	Nursing Care	Medical Care	Overall Care	Comparative Overall Care
Proportion of medical staff members who are certified "board men"	.12	.49	.05	.07
Number of "board men" per patient or average daily census	.35	.15	.26	.13
Proportion of medical staff members who are "general practitioners"	.45	.15	.48	.48
Number of "general practitioners" per patient or average daily census	.58	—.03	.58	.45
Proportion of nursing staff members who are registered nurses	.71	.71	.54	.53
Number of registered nurses per patient or average daily census	.63	.56	.58	.48
Proportion of nursing staff members who are practical nurses	.65	.38	.71	.62
Number of practical nurses per patient or average daily census	.66	.38	.70	.61
Proportion of nursing staff members who are nurse's aides	—.73	—.44	—.72	—.61
Number of nurse's aides per patient or average daily census	—.63	—.31	—.52	—.42

* All figures are rank-order correlation coefficients, based on an N of 10 hospitals in each case. Coefficients larger than ±.56 are statistically significant at the .05 level.

tient care in the community general hospital depends a great deal upon the skill and training of the nursing staff. The quality of nursing care in the various hospitals correlates positively and significantly (.71) with the proportion of nursing staff members who are registered nurses (both supervisory and non-supervisory), and with the proportion who are practical nurses (.65), while being *negatively* and significantly related to the proportion of nursing staff members who are aides (−.73). The higher the proportion of registered nurses, and of practical nurses, on the staff, the better the quality of nursing care; but, the higher the proportion of aides, the poorer the nursing care. Furthermore, the three proportions produce similar results when related to the quality of overall patient care.

Even more important is the fact that the proportion of nursing staff members who are registered nurses correlates positively and significantly not only with the quality of nursing care, but also with the quality of medical care (.71). Neither the proportion of staff members who are practical nurses, nor the proportion who are aides, shows a significant relationship with medical care (although, consistent with the preceding findings, and disregarding statistical significance, the former measure shows a positive, while the latter shows a negative, correlation with medical care). In fact, the proportion of nursing staff members who are registered nurses is one of the relatively few independent variables in this study that were found to be significantly associated with the medical care measure, attesting to the great importance of the role of the registered nurse in the community general hospital.

When the distribution of the nursing staff among patients is related to the four measures of patient care, the results are practically the same as those involving the composition of the nursing staff. The number of registered nurses per patient, or average daily census, is positively and significantly related to the quality of nursing care, the quality of medical care, and the quality of overall care in the participating hospitals. The number of practical nurses per patient is similarly related to nursing care and overall care, but not to the quality of medical care. And, the number of aides per patient is negatively and significantly related to the quality of nursing care, also yielding negative though not significant correlations with the other measures of care.

Our study, then, shows that the quality of patient care in the community general hospital is a function of the composition and distribution of the nursing staff. Hospitals whose nursing staff consists predominantly of aides, i.e., untrained personnel, have poorer care, while hospitals whose staff contains a high proportion of registered and practical nurses (particularly the former) have generally better care. The same holds true for the distribution of nursing personnel, i.e., when we consider the number of registered nurses, practical nurses, and aides per patient (or average daily census). According to these findings, as well as the earlier findings about coordination, the untrained, low-salaried, and easy-to-hire aides constitute a handicap to high quality care when present in large numbers. Finally, the higher the proportion of nursing personnel who are registered nurses, and the greater the number of registered nurses per patient, the better the medical care in the hospital. High quality medical care requires not only a competent medical staff, but also a competent nursing staff, with the registered nurse playing a central role in this connection.

ABSENTEEISM AND TURNOVER AMONG NURSING PERSONNEL AND THE QUALITY OF PATIENT CARE

In describing the characteristics of the people around the patient in Chapter 3, among other things, we had the opportunity to discuss the phenomena of absenteeism and turnover for certain nursing classifications for which adequate data were available. In the process, we described our measures of absenteeism and of turnover, related these measures to one another, and pointed out that the participating hospitals differ a good deal from one another in the extent of turnover and "unexcused" absenteeism among their nursing personnel. Here, we shall present findings which provide an answer to the question of what relationship there is, if any, between the quality of patient care in the various hospitals and the rates of unexcused absenteeism and turnover among nursing personnel.

On a first thought, one might expect that absenteeism and turnover are disruptive to normal organizational functioning, on the simple assumption that the organization needs a certain number of people working at all times in order to accomplish its objectives, apart from the question of whether these phenomena reflect psychological problems among organizational members. Consequently, it might be hypothesized that absenteeism and turnover will affect individual and organizational performance adversely. Then, by extension, one might be tempted to predict a direct negative relationship between the quality of patient care in the community general hospital and the rate of turnover and absenteeism among nursing personnel.

In reality, however, such an hypothesis is not entirely warranted without proper qualifications. We cannot very well hypothesize a direct relationship between patient care and personnel absenteeism, unless absences represent motivated behavior. Even then, absences will not necessarily affect performance, unless they are related to the motivation to produce, as against the motivation to leave or not to leave the hospital, for example. Similarly, the relationship of absenteeism to patient care may be a complex one, depending on such considerations as the organizational level at which absenteeism prevails, seasonal factors, whether or not absenteeism can be anticipated so as to allow for timely personnel replacements, and the like. Thus, absenteeism may have different consequences for performance and patient care, depending not only upon its extent or rate, but also on a number of intervening factors.

Because of reasons such as these, various previous studies of absences in relation to performance in organizations, some of which have been reviewed by Brayfield and Crockett (2), have produced inconclusive or inconsistent results. More recent studies of organizational effectiveness, such as those by Georgopoulos and Tannenbaum (4), and by Seashore, Indik, and Georgopoulos (7), similarly caution against any hypothesis of a simple relationship between absenteeism and performance. The same caution, moreover, applies with respect to turnover, which is strongly affected by prevailing labor market conditions. Accordingly, in the present research, we decided to explore the question of whether absenteeism and turnover bear any relationship to patient care, without advancing any particular hypotheses. It might be pointed out, however, that our measures of absenteeism (see Chap. 3) are free of some of the above difficulties because: (1) they refer to "unexcused" absenteeism in all cases; (2) they are not affected by sex differences, since they pertain to absences among women only; (3) they refer to the same time period for all personnel groups in all of the hospitals involved—a period which, besides coinciding with the time of data collection from individual respondents, is relatively short, thus circumscribing the issue of seasonal fluctuations; and (4) the measures were computed separately for each organizational level.

With these considerations in mind, we related the four measures of patient care to our measures of absenteeism and turnover, treating each nursing group involved separately. The results of this analysis are summarized below in Table 46 and Table 47. The former table shows the relationship of absenteeism rates to the quality of patient care in the participating hospitals; the latter presents the findings about the relationship between patient care and personnel turnover and stability rates. Our measure of the incidence of absenteeism, i.e., being absent at least once as against not being absent at all during a particular time period (as distinguished from absenteeism rates which indicate the number of times absent), was shown in Chapter 3 to reflect normal, i.e., widespread, rather than deviant behavior, and to represent behavior apparently not determined by organizational forces. Consequently, we expected no relationship whatsoever between mere incidence of absenteeism and the quality of patient care. Subsequent analysis confirmed this expectation, and the measure of absenteeism incidence was excluded from Table 46 to simplify the presentation of the findings.

The results in Table 46 show that the rate of unexcused absenteeism among practical nurses in the participating hospitals has no effect upon the quality of nursing care, medical care, or overall patient care. Similarly, no significant relationship exists between the quality of patient care and the rate of unexcused absenteeism among aides. Hospitals having a higher proportion of practical nurses, or aides, absent from regularly scheduled work twice or more often, and three or more times, during the last quarter of 1957, are not significantly more likely to render poorer patient care. Nor do they render better patient care than other hospitals. By contrast, we find that the rate of unexcused absenteeism among professional nurses is significantly associated with the quality of patient care. (For a discussion of the interrelationship of absenteeism rates among nursing personnel in each classification, and how absenteeism in a given classification relates to absenteeism in others, see Chap. 3.)

TABLE 46. Relation Between Nursing Staff Absenteeism and Patient Care *

	Quality of:			
Personnel Absenteeism †	Nursing Care	Medical Care	Overall Care	Comparative Overall Care
Proportion of nonsupervisory registered nurses absent:				
Twice or more often	−.62	−.55	−.63	−.68
Three or more times	−.53	−.62	−.67	−.67
Proportion of practical nurses absent:				
Twice or more often	.20	.12	.05	−.02
Three or more times	.02	−.17	−.23	−.28
Proportion of nurse's aides absent:				
Twice or more often	−.05	.07	−.13	−.28
Three or more times	−.18	−.22	−.38	−.43

* All figures are rank-order correlation coefficients, based on an N of 9 hospitals in each case (no data were available in the case of one of the ten hospitals in the study). To be statistically significant at the .05 level, a coefficient must be ±.60 or larger.

† The absenteeism rates refer to unexcused absences only, as discussed earlier in Chapter 3, and are for the period of October 1 to December 31, 1957.

The proportion of nonsupervisory registered nurses absent from regularly scheduled work twice or often during the last quarter of 1957, with the result that the job had to remain unfilled or a replacement had to be found, correlates negatively and significantly with the quality of nursing care (−.62). It also correlates negatively and significantly with the quality of overall patient care (−.63) and the quality of comparative care (−.68), and yields a negative, and almost significant, correlation with the quality of medical care (−.55). Similarly, the proportion of professional nurses absent three or more times, reflecting the extent of unexcused chronic absenteeism in the participating hospitals, is negatively and significantly related to the quality of medical care (−.62), the quality of overall care (−.67), and the quality of comparative care (−.67), while also producing a negative, and almost significant, correlation with the quality of nursing care (−.53).

Thus, the more extensive the unexcused absenteeism among professional nurses, the lower the quality of patient care in the community general hospital is likely to be. But, the corresponding rate of absenteeism among practical nurses, or among aides, shows no appreciable relationship to patient care.

This means that whether or not absenteeism will affect patient care adversely depends upon the organizational level within which it occurs. The role of the registered nurse being a crucial one, particularly in the area of coordinative functions and interaction with the medical staff, makes it easy to understand and explain why hospitals with more extensive unexcused absenteeism among their professional nurses are likely to provide not only poorer nursing care, but also poorer medical care.

TABLE 47. Relation of Nursing Personnel Turnover and Stability to Patient Care *

	Quality of:			
Personnel Turnover and Stability †	Nursing Care	Medical Care	Overall Care	Comparative Overall Care
Turnover among nonsupervisory registered nurses	—.16	—.02	—.02	.19
Turnover among nurse's aides	.66	.65	.86	.88
Stability of nonsupervisory registered nurses	.37	.29	.29	.07
Stability of nurse's aides	—.83	—.50	—.75	—.57

* All figures are rank-order correlation coefficients. Correlations for turnover are based on an N of 8 hospitals in each case, and to be significant at the .05 level, they must be ±.64 or higher. Correlations for stability are based on an N of 7 hospitals, and to be significant they must be ±.71 or higher.

† The measures of turnover and stability are for the period between October 1 and December 31, 1957, and have been discussed in detail in Chapter 3.

The results concerning the relationship of nursing personnel turnover and stability to patient care are shown in Table 47. It should be noted that the measures of turnover and stability are significantly, but far from perfectly, interrelated. For registered nurses, turnover and stability correlate —.75; for aides, they correlate —.68. As discussed in Chapter 3, the turnover measure represents the proportion of personnel terminations during the last quarter of 1957, while the stability measure represents the proportion of personnel on the hospital payroll as of October 1 who were still on the payroll as of December 31, 1957. It is also useful to recall here, from our discussion in Chapter 3, the absence of a significant relationship between turnover among registered nurses and turnover among aides, as well as between the stability of the former group and the stability of the latter. In that same chapter, moreover, we pointed out that, for each nursing group involved, there is no relationship between turnover or stability, on the one hand, and absenteeism, on the other.

The results appearing in Table 47 demonstrate that the turnover rate among nonsupervisory registered nurses in the participating hospitals is unrelated to the quality of patient care, regardless of which measure of care we consider. The stability measure for the same group is likewise unrelated to patient care. In both cases, the obtained correlations are too small even to be suggestive of a tendency. The rate of turnover among aides, on the other hand, correlates significantly with all four measures of patient care, and the direction of the relationship is positive in all cases. In other words, patient care, including nursing care and medical care, is better in hospitals having a *higher* turnover rate among their aides. Consistent with this relationship, moreover, we find that the higher the stability of aides, the poorer the nursing care and the poorer the overall care in the various hospitals. The quality of medical care and the comparative measure of overall care also correlate negatively with the stability of aides, but the correlations are not statistically significant.

The lack of a relationship between the turnover, or the stability, of professional nurses and the quality of patient care may be due to a number of factors. One interpretation might be, for example, that our measures of turnover and stability cover too short a period of time to reflect these phenomena realistically and yield significant results. Such an interpretation, however, is not likely to be correct, for in the case of aides the stability and turnover measures yielded very significant results, even though referring to the same period of time. Another interpretation might be that the phenomena of turnover and stability are totally irrelevant to patient care. This is also unlikely. Our own interpretation is that, on the basis of past experience, individual hospitals are probably capable of predicting, fairly accurately, that a certain amount of turnover will occur among their professional nurses. Consequently, they expect so much turnover for a given period of time and take appropriate precautions to make allowance for the number of people they expect to lose and the number they expect to acquire. If hospitals with more turnover actually tend to hire proportionately more nurses than hospitals with less turnover, the danger of being seriously understaffed is lessened or alleviated in the higher turnover institutions. Since, in addition, the newly hired registered nurse, unlike the aide, is not likely to require much on-the-job training upon entering the hospital—she is already trained in the essential aspects of her role and can assume her duties more or less immediately—nurse turnover of the magnitude that prevails in the hospitals studied turns out to have no appreciable adverse effect upon the quality of patient care. The finding that turnover among aides is beneficial, while stability is harmful, insofar as the quality of patient care is concerned, is entirely congruent with our earlier findings concerning the composition of the nursing staff in relation to patient care, the findings about coordination, and the findings about the characteristics of aides.

ORGANIZATIONAL COORDINATION AND THE QUALITY OF PATIENT CARE

In Chapter 6, we discussed the nature of organizational coordination, the theoretical importance of coordination for the functioning of organizations, and a number of specific and overall measures which were developed in this study to distinguish the better coordinated from the less adequately coordinated institutions. Then, in Chapter 7, we related the measures of coordination to certain aspects of hospital structure and functioning, in order to identify some of the major social-psychological factors which affect coordination in the community general hospital. One of the underlying theoretical themes in those two chapters was that complex organizations, such as the hospital, cannot operate effectively without adequate coordination. The efforts, skills, and roles of organizational members, and the different specialized, but interdependent, activities of the various segments and departments which make up the organization must be coordinated, if the system is to function as a unified structure and accomplish its objectives. Successful mobilization of concerted action, it was asserted, will depend on whether or not the various parts of the organization function each according to the needs of the others and according to the needs of the entire organizational system, i.e., on the degree to which the organization is well coordinated.

The relevant literature cited in Chapter 6 overwhelmingly suggests that coordination should be positively related to organizational effectiveness. And the few relevant empirical studies that are available to date provide good support for this hypothesis. For example, Torrence (9) reports results from survival research which show that better coordinated crews in earlier test situations were subsequently more effective under simulated survival conditions. Similarly, Andrews (1) concludes that, in general, groups which have greater coordination are more effective than less well-coordinated groups. Elsewhere, Simon (8) observes that cooperation is impossible without coordination, while Deutsch (3) presents experimental evidence which shows that cooperation facilitates coordination in group situations.

In a recent study of problems of measuring patient care in hospital outpatient departments, Klein and his associates (6) also obtained some interesting results which are pertinent here. They interviewed 24 administrative officials (medical directors, directors of nursing, supervisors, and directors of social services) in six metropolitan hospitals in an attempt to find out what constitutes "good" patient care in the outpatient departments. The respondents mentioned some 80 specific criteria of good patient care. The investigators were then able to allocate these into a total of 13 different criterion categories, and to order these categories according to the number of interviewees who had mentioned criteria in each and according to the number of times criteria belonging to each category had been mentioned. In the ordered set of the 13 categories, the category "interrole, interdepartmental coordination" placed second. Coordination was mentioned as a criterion of good patient care by 17 of the 24 interviewees (only one other category, called "attitudes of personnel," was mentioned by more respondents—by 19 persons), and it was mentioned as a criterion a total of 40 times (the highest number of times that any of the 13 criterion categories was mentioned by the

Organizational Coordination

respondents). Incidentally, the five most frequently mentioned categories of criteria of good patient care were: "attitudes of personnel—towards patients, doctors, *et cetera*," "interrole, interdepartmental coordination," "case loads, amounts of contact with patients," "patient satisfaction and convenience," and "medical skills and facilities."

The available evidence, then, leads us to expect that organizational coordination is an important requirement for effective organizational functioning or group performance. Here, we shall examine our own data to find out whether hospital effectiveness depends on coordination or, more precisely, whether the quality of patient care in the hospitals studied is in fact related to hospital coordination. The main purpose of this section, therefore, is to present empirical results which provide a test for this hypothesis. The relevant findings were obtained by relating the four measures of patient care to: (1) the four overall measures of hospital coordination and the seven specific measures from which they were derived, as discussed in Chapter 6, and (2) the four measures of nursing department coordination which were discussed in Chapter 7.

Viewed as a whole, the results in Table 48 provide rather strong support in favor of the hypothesis under examination. With certain exceptions, most of the relationships between the various measures of coordination and the measures of patient care are not only positive, i.e., in the expected direction, but also high and significant. The exception to this pattern concerns the relationship between the quality of medical care and the coordination measures. In this case, all of the correlations are likewise positive, but they are not large enough to be statistically significant. Let us review the results a little more closely, however, considering first the four overall measures of hospital coordination in relation to the four measures of patient care.

It is clearly evident from the findings that the quality of nursing care is strongly related to overall hospital coordination, regardless of whether we consider measure #1, measure #2, measure #3, or measure #4 of coordination. (The first two measures, it may be recalled, are alternate measures of total coordination in the hospital, not differentiating between programed and nonprogramed coordination, and were computed by combining the seven specific measures of coordination shown in Table 48 into an index. Measure #3 represents what we have termed in Chapter 6 as general or nonprogramed coordination, and was computed by combining the first four specific measures shown in Table 48 into an index. And measure #4 represents what we have referred to as programed coordination, and was obtained by combining the last three specific measures shown in Table 48 into an index. For a detailed discussion, see Chap. 6.) Hospitals having better overall coordination (measure #1, measure #2), better nonprogramed coordination (measure #3), and/or better programed coordination (measure #4) are also significantly more likely to have better nursing care. In short, the more adequate

TABLE 48. Relation Between Organizational Coordination and Patient Care *

Coordination Measure †	Quality of: Nursing Care	Medical Care	Overall Care	Comparative Overall Care
Overall coordination in the hospital (Measure #1 of coordination)	.73	.17	.68	.53
Overall coordination in the hospital (Measure #2 of coordination)	.78	.21	.78	.64
Nonprogramed or general coordination (Measure #3 of coordination)	.76	.17	.78	.65
Programed coordination (Measure #4 of coordination)	.75	.22	.66	.50
How well the different jobs and activties in the hospital fit together	.80	.51	.91	.86
Extent members make an effort to avoid creating problems or interference	.20	.03	.28	.22
Extent members do their jobs properly without getting in each other's way	.60	.14	.60	.46
Extent patients feel the personnel around them work together smoothly	.77	.20	.82	.70
How well timed activities are in the everyday routine	.81	.26	.84	.67
Extent work assignments are well planned	.56	.03	.41	.27
How well established are the routines of interdependent departments	.65	.42	.64	.53

* All figures are rank-order correlation coefficients, based on an N of 10 hospitals in each case. Coefficients larger than .56 are statistically significant at the .05 level, and those .75 or larger are significant at the .01 level.

† The four overall measures of organizational coordination, as well as the seven specific measures on which they are based, are discussed in detail in Chapter 6.

the coordination, the higher the quality of nursing care in the participating hospitals.

Unlike nursing care, the quality of medical care is not significantly related to any of the four overall measures of coordination; the correlations are positive but very small, ranging from .17 to .22. The quality of overall patient care, like the quality of nursing care, is highly associated with the four measures of overall coordination, the relevant correlations ranging between .66 and .78. And, the comparative measure of the quality of total patient care correlates .53 with coordination measure #1, .64 with coordination measure #2, .65 with coordination measure #3, or nonprogramed coordination, and

Organizational Coordination

.50 with coordination measure #4, or programed coordination. The larger two of these correlations are statistically significant at better than the .05 level, with the other two approaching significance at this level.

In general, then, Table 48 shows that the better coordinated hospitals are also likely to have better nursing care, better overall patient care, and better comparative care. However, they are not more likely than hospitals with less adequate coordination to have appreciably better medical care (nor are they more likely to have poorer medical care, of course). The results from relating the seven specific measures of coordination to the four measures of care, also shown in Table 48, lead to the same conclusions. The quality of medical care correlates positively with all seven measures, the specific correlations ranging from a low of .03 to a high of .51. These correlations are all in the right direction but, since they are not statistically significant, we cannot definitely assert the presence of a relationship here, even though the results may be suggestive from the standpoint of direction. The quality of nursing care correlates positively with each of the seven specific measures of coordination, and positively and significantly with six of them. Excluding the single non-significant case, these correlations range from a low of .56 to a high of .81, leaving no doubt of the existence of a strong relationship between nursing care and hospital coordination. Similarly, the quality of overall patient care correlates positively with all of the specific measures of coordination, with all but two of the correlations being statistically significant. And the comparative measure of overall care correlates positively with all of the specific measures of coordination, and positively and significantly with three of them.

Further analysis of the findings leads to certain conclusions regarding the relative importance of the categories and types of coordination discussed in Chapter 6. Of the seven specific items, or measures, of coordination listed in Table 48, the last three, it will be recalled, pertain to programed coordination. These are "how well timed activities are," the extent to which "work assignments are well planned," and "how well established are the routines" in the hospital. The first four specific items in the same table pertain to non-programed coordination. Of these items, two represent the promotive type of coordination, while the other two refer to what we have termed as the preventive type of coordination. The promotive coordination items are "how well the different jobs and activities in the hospital fit together," and the extent to which "patients feel that the personnel around them work together smoothly"; the preventive coordination items are the extent to which organizational members "make an effort to avoid creating problems or interference," and the extent to which members "do their job properly without getting in each other's way."

What conclusions can one draw regarding the relative importance of the different kinds of coordination for patient care? First, it is obvious from the results in Table 48 that it is the promotive rather than the preventive type of coordination which relates best to the quality of patient care in the hospitals studied. The degree to which the various jobs and activities fit well together, for example, correlates .80 with the quality of nursing care, .91 with the quality of overall care, .86 with the comparative measure of overall care, and .51 with the quality of medical care. The corresponding correlations between how smoothly personnel work together and the four measures of care are .77, .82, .70, and .20, respectively. By contrast, the extent to which hospital members make an effort to avoid creating problems does not produce a single significant relationship with the four measures of care, being the only one of the seven specific items of coordination in this respect. The second preventive coordination item, the extent to which members do their job without getting in each other's way, correlates positively and significantly with nursing care (.60) and overall care (.60), but not with medical care (.14) or with the comparative measure of care (.46). Apparently, positive attempts toward better coordination are much more crucial for effective organizational functioning than the efforts of members toward avoiding disruptive behavior in the system. Preventive coordination is not enough.

Of the three programed coordination items, the timing of activities is the most important in relation to patient care (the timing of activities also constituting the most troublesome aspect of programed coordination for the hospitals studied, as we have shown earlier in Chap. 7). How well timed the activities are in the everyday routine of the hospital correlates .81 with nursing care, .26 with medical care, .84 with overall care, and .67 with the comparative measure of overall care. The least crucial of the three programed coordination items in relation to patient care is the extent to which work assignments are well planned, which correlates .56, .03, .41, and .27, respectively, with the four measures of care. The item about how well established departmental routines in the hospital are occupies an intermediate position, according to the findings. Finally, if one compares the results between our measures of programed coordination and patient care with the results between our measures of nonprogramed or general coordination and patient care, shown in Table 48, one finds that both programed and nonprogramed, or more informal, coordination are important for patient care. But, they are about equally important according to the obtained results and, consequently, neither can be recommended as the superior kind of coordination from the standpoint of the quality of patient care.

At this point a question might also be raised as to why the quality of medical care, unlike the other three measures of care, is not significantly associated with the quality of hospital coordination. Before attempting to answer this question, however, it would be useful to know whether the measures of patient care, including that of medical care, bear any relationship to the measures of nursing department coordination that were discussed in Chapter 7. Theoretically, it was pointed out in that chapter, one would ex-

Organizational Coordination

pect that coordination in the nursing department will show similar relationships to a variety of dependent variables, including patient care, as coordination in the entire hospital because of the central role of the nursing department for hospital functioning and patient care, because of the close interaction between medical and nursing staff, and because, as we have seen in Chapter 7, nursing department coordination is positively and significantly related to overall hospital coordination. Still, we could not exclude the possibility that the quality of medical care, or any other measure of patient care, may be related to nursing department coordination, regardless of the above findings concerning patient care and hospital coordination. For these reasons, the four measures of patient care were also studied in relation to our measures of coordination in the nursing department. The results are presented in Table 49.

TABLE 49. Relation Between Nursing Department Coordination and Patient Care *

Coordination Measure †	Nursing Care	Medical Care	Overall Care	Comparative Overall Care
Overall measure of coordination in the nursing department	.80	.42	.88	.82
Ease with which one shift can take over from another without confusion	.69	.18	.64	.55
Relative lack of difficulty in finding out what occurred on the job since last at work	.71	.52	.74	.70
How infrequently personnel feel the previous shift left them with unfinished work or problems that it should have handled	.78	.42	.91	.85

(Quality of:)

* All figures are rank-order correlation coefficients, based on an N of 10 hospitals in each case. Coefficients larger than .56 are statistically significant at the .05 level, and those .75 or larger are significant at the .01 level.

† The overall measure of nursing department coordination, as well as the three specific measures, are discussed in Chapter 7.

The results in Table 49 confirm the expectation that patient care is related to nursing department coordination in a manner consistent with the obtained relationships between patient care and hospital coordination. The quality of nursing care, the quality of overall patient care, and the comparative measure of overall care are positively and significantly related both to the overall measure of nursing department coordination and to the three specific measures on which it is based—the ease with which one shift can take over from another without confusion, the degree to which nursing personnel can find out without difficulty what occurred on the job since last at work, and how infrequently the previous shift left the succeeding shift with unfinished work or problems that it should have handled. Of the twelve correlations between the four measures of nursing department coordination and the measures of nursing, overall, and comparative overall care, eleven are statistically significant at better than the .05 level, ranging in size from a low of .64 to a high of .91 (the remaining correlation is .55, with a correlation of .56 required for significance at the .05 level). The quality of medical care, on the other hand, correlates .42 with the overall measure of nursing department coordination, and .18, .52, and .42 with the three specific measures. These correlations are in the expected direction and, very probably, suggestive of a slight tendency for the quality of medical care to be associated with the adequacy of nursing department coordination, but the association is weak and rather tenuous since the correlations are not statistically significant.

In summary, then, we find that good coordination plays a very important role in hospital functioning. Hospitals having better organizational coordination in general, as well as better coordination within their nursing department alone, are significantly more likely than hospitals with poorer coordination to provide better nursing care, better overall patient care, and better comparative care. They do not, however, render appreciably better medical care, even though their medical care is in no way inferior to that provided in the less well-coordinated institutions. Furthermore, we find that nonprogramed coordination does not behave differently from programed coordination in relation to patient care. In the community general hospital, programed and nonprogramed coordination appear to be equally important. On the other hand, the promotive type of coordination is more crucial than the preventive type. Mere efforts to avoid disruptions in the system do not make for better organizational functioning, unless accompanied by positive efforts to improve coordination. Finally, of the several aspects of programed coordination that were investigated, the most important aspect insofar as patient care is concerned is good activity timing.

The preceding empirical results confirm our earlier theoretical expectations, except that there still remains the question of the absence of a significant relationship between the quality of medical care and coordination. The absence of a direct relationship here can best be attributed to several interrelated factors concerning the functions and place of the medical staff in hospital organization. For one thing, the medical staff in the community general hospital, unlike the nursing staff, carries very few coordinative functions and responsibilities. These are primarily concerned with the relationship of the medical staff to the hospital rather than with patient care. For the implementation of day-to-day coordinative functions necessitated by doctor-nurse-patient interaction, i.e., functions directly relevant to patient care, both the hospital and the medical staff rely heavily on the nursing staff, as previously indicated.

In the second place, however crucial a component it may be, the medical staff is not too well integrated with the rest of the organization. The doctors are not employees of the hospital, and the hospital, as an organization, has very limited authority over the medical staff. Doctors are subject to few hospital rules and regulations, and even in those instances that they are, the hospital relies on medical self-discipline to ensure compliance rather than on organizational authority, sanctions, and rewards. The doctors are allowed to practice medicine in the hospital on the basis of their own constitution and bylaws, and in accordance with the standards and rules of the medical profession and its various associations, being responsible mainly to themselves and their own staff organization for all aspects of medical practice. The hospital constitution defines only very broadly the limits of medical activity, the limits themselves dealing primarily with ethical issues and minimum requirements established by outside accrediting institutions. And although the doctors are no longer as prone—as many would have us believe—to view the hospital merely as their workshop (actually, our data show that, very frequently, doctors take considerable interest in the problems of the hospital, even though their organizational sophistication may be low), the fact remains that, by comparison to the various other groups in the hospital, they constitute an anomalous group from the standpoint of their organizational integration.

In addition, the medical staff organization within the hospital is essentially an organization of professional peers and specialists, relying more on its individual members rather than on sustained group activity, insofar as the process of medical care is concerned. The doctor-patient relationship is more of a personalized than an organizational character. It tends to be insulated, if not isolated, from other activities required by the flow of work, and depends most immediately on what the individual doctor, and the individual patient, does or does not do. Of course, this is not to imply that the doctor can function effectively without nursing help or without adequate paramedical services; it is only intended to point out that the doctors in the hospital tend to render their services to their individual patients unilaterally rather than on a group basis.

Under these circumstances, it might perhaps be too much to expect a direct significant relationship between the quality of medical care in the various hospitals and organizational coordination. Yet, if anything, the obtained results are directionally suggestive of a possibility that hospitals with better coordination may tend to have somewhat better medical care. This is only a possibility, however, and further research will be necessary before a definitive conclusion can be reached. It may be that good hospital coordination does not necessarily make for superior medical care, but if coordination is poor (e.g., poorer than in any of the ten hospitals studied) medical care will suffer, regardless of the competence of the medical staff. It may also be that coordination within the medical staff, rather than the entire hospital or the nursing department, will prove to be a decisive factor in relation to medical care. In any event, what is clear from the available findings is that the better coordination hospitals, apart from rendering better nursing care and better overall patient care, render no poorer medical care than the poorer coordination institutions.

INTRAORGANIZATIONAL STRAIN AND THE QUALITY OF PATIENT CARE

Because hospital organization is made up of a large number of people whose backgrounds, attitudes, positions, and functions vary a great deal, because of the highly rational character of the system and its requirements for strict adherence to formal rules and regulations that are often ambiguous, incomplete, or insufficiently understood by the members, and because the flow of work is not always even and cannot be anticipated with a great degree of predictability, stress and strain are likely to arise in the system. The presence of the element of emergency in the patient care process, moreover, is likely to accentuate rather than reduce the prevailing tensions and pressures experienced by organizational members. The rapid turnover of patients, and frequently of personnel, also necessitates adjustments and contributes to uncertainties and tensions. Similar other factors such as personnel shortages, the presence of inadequately qualified personnel, professional competition, breakdowns in communications, lack of supplies or facilities, unclear procedures, poor interpersonal relationships, poor administration, and a host of other factors often constitute sources of tension, pressure, and even conflict. Since many of these factors are likely to be present in every hospital, at any given time, one would correspondingly expect a certain amount of intraorganizational strain to exist in the system at all times. In addition, the mere fact of organizational membership automatically implies certain restrictions in behavior, and these restrictions frequently translate themselves into tensions, pressures, and counterpressures among organizational members. The hospital is not exempt in this respect.

A minimum amount of intraorganizational strain, therefore, is always likely to be present in the organization in the form of tension and pressure. However, because of imperfections in organizational coordination, because of imperfections in integration between the organization and its members, because of deficiencies in the areas of communication, supervision, and administration, and because of various deficiencies in the work relationships and performance of individuals and departments, the degree of prevailing tension and pressure in the system is likely to lie somewhere beyond the minimum level. We have already discovered in the preceding chapter that the poorer the coordination, the greater the strain in the hospital. And, although a relatively small amount of intraorganizational strain may produce no adverse effects for organizational functioning, it is certain that high strain will be dysfunctional. We may recall

Intraorganizational Strain

here, for example, the findings of Georgopoulos and Tannenbaum (4), from their study of an industrial organization, showing an inverse relationship between the performance of similar organizational units and the degree of prevailing tension between workers and supervisors in the various units studied. Moreover, tension will be more likely to affect organizational performance adversely, if it exists between directly interacting and interdependent organizational members and parts. Since work in the hospital is highly dependent upon the cooperation and concerted efforts of many people, who perform different things, but who depend in the process upon the work of others, intraorganizational strain is particularly likely to have dysfunctional consequences for hospital effectiveness and patient care.

In the light of these considerations, as in the case of coordination, we hypothesized that the degree of prevailing tension among interacting groups and departments will be negatively related to the quality of patient care in the community general hospital. Similarly, we hypothesized a negative relationship between patient care and the degree of "unreasonable" pressure for better performance experienced by nonmedical hospital personnel. In other words, the higher the intraorganizational strain, in the form of either tension among interdependent members or "unreasonable" organizational pressure upon members, the poorer the patient care in the various hospitals.

To test this hypothesis, we related the same four measures of strain described in the preceding chapter about coordination to our measures of patient care. Two of the measures of strain, it will be remembered, refer to tension, while the other two refer to pressure. One measure of tension represents the average level of overall tension in each participating hospital, and was derived by taking into account the degree of tension characterizing each of 26 pairs of interacting groups in the organization (tension measure #1). The other measure of tension (tension measure #2) represents the average level of tension in each hospital which characterizes each of ten pairs of key groups, e.g., tension between doctors and nurses, tension between administrator and department heads, tension between doctors and trustees, etc. (see Chap. 7). The two measures of pressure both represent the average amount of "unreasonable" pressure for better performance experienced by nonmedical personnel in each hospital, but were computed by different methods. More specifically, they represent the pressure experienced by the hospital administrator, the administrative department heads, the supervisory and nonsupervisory registered nurses, the practical nurses, the aides and orderlies, and the laboratory and x-ray technicians. For a detailed description of the four measures of strain, and their interrelationships, see Chapter 7.

The empirical results which show the relationship between intraorganizational strain and patient care in the ten participating hospitals are presented in Table 50. As predicted, we find that all 16 correlations between the four measures of strain and the four measures of patient care are negative. In addition, the correlations between the quality of nursing care, the quality of overall patient care, and the quality of comparative overall care, on the one hand, and each of the measures of strain, on the other, are both sizable and statistically significant at better than the .05 level. Their size ranges between a low of —.60 and a high of —.84. The correlations between the quality of medical care and the four measures of strain also follow the same pattern, in the sense that they are negative, but they are rather small. Their size ranges between —.30 and —.36.

TABLE 50. Relation Between Intraorganizational Strain and Patient Care *

Measures of Strain †	Quality of:			
	Nursing Care	Medical Care	Overall Care	Comparative Overall Care
Degree of prevailing tension among various interacting groups in the hospital (or tension measure #1)	—.83	—.34	—.74	—.60
Degree of prevailing tension among interacting key groups in the hospital (or tension measure #2)	—.62	—.30	—.64	—.60
Degree of unreasonable pressure for better performance experienced by nonmedical personnel (or pressure measure #1)	—.75	—.36	—.83	—.75
Degree of unreasonable pressure for better performance experienced by nonmedical personnel (or pressure measure #2)	—.62	—.30	—.84	—.79

* All figures are rank-order correlation coefficients, based on an N of 10 hospitals in each case. Coefficients larger than —.56 are statistically significant at the .05 level, and those —.75 or larger are significant at the .01 level.

† The measures of tension and pressure listed here, and their interrelationships, are discussed in detail in Chapter 7.

Clearly, hospitals with a higher level of tension among their various interacting (interdependent) groups and departments are significantly more likely than the lower tension institutions to provide poorer nursing care, poorer overall patient care, and poorer comparative care. Stated differently, we find that the lower the tension among the various interdependent parts of the organization, the better the care. The same is true, moreover, when we consider only the level of tension among the key interacting groups in the hospital. Similarly, hospitals whose nonmedical staff experience a higher amount of unreasonable pressure for better performance—pressure over and above what they consider reasonable—are more likely than other hospitals to provide poorer nursing care and poorer overall care for their patients. Regarding medical care, the results are not statistically significant—very prob-

Complementarity of Work-Related Expectations

ably for the same reasons discussed in the preceding section in connection with the relationship of coordination to medical care, and for the additional reason that our two measures of pressure do not include pressure experienced by doctors. They too, however, suggest a directionally negative relationship between the degree of intraorganizational strain and the quality of medical care. Intraorganizational strain among interdependent groups is thus found to be negatively related to organizational effectiveness in the community general hospital. Moreover, it is inversely related to organizational coordination, as the results of the preceding chapter demonstrate, and coordination itself is a prerequisite to effective hospital functioning. High strain and inadequate coordination seem to go hand in hand, each reinforcing the other, and both affecting patient care adversely.

COMPLEMENTARITY OF WORK-RELATED EXPECTATIONS BETWEEN MEDICAL AND NURSING STAFF AND THE QUALITY OF PATIENT CARE

The negative relationship between intraorganizational strain and the quality of patient care may be partly accounted for by the fact that strain is inversely related to coordination. As shown in the preceding chapter, high strain impedes good coordination in the hospital, while, as we have also seen, coordination is positively related to the quality of nursing and overall patient care. In addition, and apart from whatever independent effects it may have upon patient care, however, strain among organizational members whose work is interdependent results in (as well as from) unsatisfactory mutual expectations among the members. In turn, unsatisfactory expectations among members lead to inadequate understanding of one another's problems and needs in the work situation, and inadequate understanding obstructs effective performance.

When members who work interdependently, e.g., doctors and nurses, do not share the same or complementary expectations in their interaction, the understanding which they come to have of each other's problems is likely to be poor. And, when the members of one group fail to understand and appreciate the problems and needs of the members of the other group, high-quality performance on the part of all concerned is unlikely. For one thing, organizational members will not be able to anticipate correctly each other's behavior or act according to each other's needs, and coordination will be poor; for another, poor understanding is likely to lead to strain or to accentuate already existing strain. Conversely, complementarity of expectations is likely to facilitate mutual understanding of work problems and needs, and good understanding is likely to facilitate performance through, among other things, better predictability, better coordination, and lower strain.

In Chapter 6, we discussed the theoretical importance of complementarity of expectations for organizational coordination and hospital functioning, and in Chapter 7 we showed the empirical relationship of complementarity to coordination. In the present section, using the same measures of complementarity as previously, and focusing again on the medical and the nursing staff, we will present our findings which test the hypothesis that the quality of patient care in the community general hospital will be positively related to the extent to which the expectations of doctors and nurses about each other's work problems and needs are complementary. As in Chapter 7, the extent to which doctor-nurse expectations are complementary is here represented by the degree to which the nursing staff understand and appreciate the work problems and needs of the medical staff, and vice versa.

TABLE 51. Degree of Understanding of Each Other's Work Problems and Needs, on the Part of the Medical and Nursing Staffs, as Related to Patient Care *

	Quality of:			
Variable	Nursing Care	Medical Care	Overall Care	Comparative Overall Care
Extent to which the *nursing staff* understand and appreciate the work problems and needs of the medical staff, as seen by:				
Doctors	.90	.62	.76	.65
Registered nurses	.25	.46	.15	.20
Doctors and nurses combined	.85	.72	.73	.69
Extent to which the *medical staff* understand and appreciate the work problems and needs of the nursing staff, as seen by:				
Registered nurses	.68	.41	.65	.61
Doctors	.25	.55	.33	.42
Nurses and doctors combined	.68	.34	.56	.46

* All figures are rank-order correlation coefficients, based on an N of 10 hospitals in each case. Coefficients larger than .56 are statistically significant at the .05 level, and those .75 or larger are significant at the .01 level.

The results in Table 51 show that in hospitals where greater complementarity of expectations between doctors and nurses prevails, patient care is of higher quality. First, the extent to which the nursing staff understand and appreciate the work problems and needs of the medical staff, as doctors see it, correlates .90 with the quality of nursing care, .62 with the quality of medical care, .76 with the quality of overall patient care, and .65 with the quality of comparative care in the participating hospitals. All these relationships are statistically significant beyond the .05 level. Second, the extent to which the medical staff understand and appreciate the problems and needs of the nursing staff, as registered nurses see it, correlates .68, .41, .65, and .61,

Complementarity of Work-Related Expectations 401

respectively, with the four measures of patient care. Three of the four correlations are again significant. In short, the greater the complementarity of work-related expectations between doctors and nurses, the better the patient care; hospitals scoring higher on complementarity are significantly more likely to provide better patient care than hospitals scoring lower.

Other results in Table 51 show that the extent to which nurses understand the problems of doctors, or vice versa, as seen by both doctors and nurses, also correlates positively with the four measures of care, with most of the correlations being significant. However, neither the extent to which nurses understand the problems of doctors, as nurses themselves see it, nor the extent to which doctors understand the problems of nurses, as doctors themselves see it, correlates significantly with the patient-care measures, although all of the specific correlations are again positive. In other words, what is important for patient care is complementarity of understanding, i.e., when doctors feel that their problems are well understood by nurses, and vice versa, or joint understanding, i.e., when both doctors and nurses feel that nurses understand the problems of doctors and that doctors understand the problems of nurses, rather than the all too frequently observed condition where the members of one group feel that they have a good understanding of the problems and needs of the members of the other group. Being convinced that you understand and appreciate the problems and needs of the members of the other group is generally less important than when the members of the other group are convinced that you understand their problems, or when you are both convinced.

It is also interesting to note in examining the results in Table 51 that the extent to which the nursing staff understand the problems and needs of the medical staff, as seen by the latter, produces appreciably stronger relationships with each measure of patient care than the extent to which the medical staff understand the problems and needs of the nursing staff, as seen by the latter. This is apparently due to the fact that, in their work, the medical staff rely much more on the performance of the nursing staff than the nursing staff rely on the performance of the medical staff. Doctors depend more on nurses than the other way around, insofar as their hospital activities are concerned, partly because the former spend much less time with the patient or in the hospital, and partly because of the coordinative functions which nurses carry out in relation to both medical and nonmedical activities in the hospital.

Finally, of special interest is the relationship between complementarity and medical care. Table 51 shows that the better the nursing staff understand and appreciate the problems and needs of the medical staff, as seen by doctor respondents, or by both doctor and nurse respondents, the better the quality of medical care in the various hospitals (as seen by doctors, the degree of understanding correlates .62 with the quality of medical care, and as seen by both doctors and nurses it correlates .72). Complementarity of understanding is thus one of the relatively few independent social-psychological variables that were found in this study to be significantly associated with the quality of medical care. When we also recall, in this connection, that complementarity, measured by the extent to which nurses understand the problems and needs of the medical staff as seen by the latter, was earlier found to be highly and significantly related to coordination, while coordination was not found to correlate significantly with the medical care measure, the results about complementarity and medical care assume added importance.

Similarly, we have earlier found that intraorganizational strain correlates negatively and significantly with all our measures of patient care, except the medical care measure (also being negatively related to our measures of coordination). It so happens, that the measures of strain are also negatively and significantly related to complementarity, e.g., the degree of tension among interacting groups in the hospital (earlier referred to as tension measure #1) correlates —.87 with the extent to which the nursing staff understand the problems and needs of the medical staff, as seen by the latter. Yet, while none of the measures of strain produced a statistically significant relationship with the measure of medical care, we find that complementarity yields certain highly significant relationships with the quality of medical care. It, therefore, appears that (1) complementarity of expectations between doctors and nurses is more important in relation to the quality of medical care than either strain or coordination, and (2) the importance of complementarity for medical care seems to be independent both of its importance for coordination and its connection with intraorganizational strain. Like coordination and strain, however, complementarity is found to be significantly related to the quality of nursing care and the quality of overall patient care.

MEDICAL COMMITTEE BEHAVIOR AND THE QUALITY OF PATIENT CARE

It is often assumed by hospital people, as well as others, that, if each of the individual specialized parts of the hospital would do an effective job, the quality of patient care would necessarily be high. Furthermore, this assumption is made about all kinds of "parts"—including departments, organizational groups, subgroups, committees, and even individual members. Applied to the specific case of medical committees, the assumption leads to predictions such as this one: "The quality of medical care will be better in hospitals having more effectively functioning records committees (or executive committees, or tissue committees, etc.)." The relative effectiveness of the various committees is usually judged in terms of how active the committees are, and in terms of the extent to which each committee accomplishes its particular tasks.

In its general form, the assumption in question is of course unjustified. Those who make it perpetrate the well-known, still often committed, fallacy of composition (to use the logician's terminology)—if the various parts of the system function adequately, then the total system will presumably also operate adequately. Thus, the "whole" is viewed as, and equated with, the "sum of its parts." In more concrete terms, the problem is that the assumption disregards, or sidesteps, such important considerations as the need for, and requirements of, concerted effort and coordination, the consequences of the fact that the individual parts are interrelated and functionally interdependent, i.e., they interact rather than merely acting independently of one another, and the fact that the final product of the system is the result of both individual and joint activity. In short, "it takes two to tango."

Yet a prediction that "the quality of medical care will be positively related to the performance of the tissue committee," for example, may prove true because the tissue committee is one of the key committees of medical staff organization, and because its work is directly concerned with the review and evaluation of medical care; because its activities may affect the practice of medicine by both individual doctors and medical services; or because its actions may produce consequences for the actions of other committees (e.g., the executive committee of the staff), other departments (e.g., the laboratory), other personnel, etc. A similar case may be made, moreover, with reference to other important medical committees. Accordingly, it would be useful to know whether, and to what extent, the quality of medical care in the community general hospital is related to the behavior of major medical committees.

To accomplish this task, it was necessary to obtain data which would provide us with a measure of the level of activity and a measure of the quality of performance of principal medical committees whose work might affect the quality of patient care, particularly medical care. The measures were derived from information supplied by medical respondents (the general medical staff subgroup) from each hospital in response to two questions: (1) "In general, how active would you say each of the following committees is?" and (2) "On the whole, what kind of a job would you say each of the following committees does?" The respondents were requested to answer the first question on a five-point scale indicating varying levels of activity, from "rather inactive" to "extremely active," and to answer the second question in terms of a similar scale whose alternatives, indicating quality of performance, ranged from "excellent" to "poor." Data were thus obtained about the performance and activity of each of the following medical committees in each hospital: the executive committee, the tissue committee, the records committee, and the credentials committee. The data from the individual doctors representing each hospital were then combined and converted into means, separately for the variables of activity and performance, and separately for each committee involved. These hospital means constitute our measures of committee behavior.

These measures show that, as might be expected, a particular committee may be very active in some hospitals and less active in others. Similarly, a given committee may be doing a very good job in some institutions and a poorer job in others. Thus, interhospital differences exist both with respect to activity and performance.[6] Moreover, within the same hospital, some committees may be more active than others, and the same may be said with reference to performance. For example, the data show that Hospital #5 has the most active credentials committee of all the hospitals studied, while it also has the least active records committee. In general, however, we find that the hospitals differ more from one another in how active their tissue and records committees are, and less in how active their executive and credentials committees are. And the same applies to committee performance. Furthermore, regarding both activity and performance, interhospital differences are the smallest in the case of the executive committee, i.e., the medical executive committees in the ten hospitals tend to be more uniform than the other committees, both with respect to how active they are and how good a job they are doing.

Concerning the relationship between the variables of activity and performance, an analysis of the data reveals that, for each of the four committees involved, the higher the activity of the committee the better its performance. Stated differently, hospitals that have more active medical committees are also likely to have better performing committees. The correlation between the activity measure and the performance measure is .58 in the case of the executive committee, .72 for the tissue committee, .80 for the records committee, and .70 for the credentials committee. These rank-order correlations, based on an N of 10 hospitals in each case, are all significant at the .05 level or better. The relative size of the correlations, moreover, indicates that level of activity and quality of performance are most closely related in the case of the records committee, and least closely related in the case of the executive committee.

Concerning the relationship between the performance, or activity, of one committee and the performance, or activity, of the other committees in the participating hospitals, the data show even more interesting results. We find,

---

[6] With respect to how active the various committees are across the ten hospitals, the range in hospital scores, computed on a five-point scale, is as follows: for the executive committee, 3.36 to 4.27; for the tissue committee, 2.81 to 4.13; for the records committee, 2.80 to 4.00; and for the credentials committee, 2.94 to 4.00. The higher the score, the more active the committee. With respect to how good a job the various committees do, the range in hospital scores, also based on a five-point scale, is as follows: for the executive committee, 1.69 to 2.36; for the tissue committee, 1.70 to 2.88; for the records committee, 1.62 to 3.00; and for the credentials committee, 1.82 to 2.67. The lower the score, the better the performance.

in the case of committee performance, that only the performance of the tissue committee correlates significantly with the performance of each of the other three committees: .60 with the performance of the executive committee, .56 with the performance of the records committee, and .76 with the performance of the credentials committee. The performance of the executive committee is significantly related to the performance of the tissue (.60) and records (.81) committees, but not to the performance of the credentials committee (.35). The performance of the records committee is significantly related to the performance of the executive and tissue committees, as already shown, but not to the performance of the credentials committee (.18). And the performance of the credentials committee is significantly related only to the performance of the tissue committee, as can be seen from the above correlations. Finally, the comparable results about the activity of the various committees show only two significant relationships—a correlation of .65 between how active the tissue committee is and how active the records committee is in the various hospitals, and a correlation of .71 between the activity of the tissue committee and the activity of the executive committee. It would, therefore, appear that of the four medical committees involved, the most central is the tissue committee, in the sense that the work of this committee (in contrast to the other committees) is more closely related to the work of each of the remaining committees.

Returning now to the question of whether the quality of patient care, and especially the quality of medical care, is related to the behavior of the above medical committees, we find the results shown in Table 52. These results were obtained by correlating our measures of committee activity and committee performance, discussed above, with the four measures of patient care developed in this study. The findings may be summarized as follows:

1. The quality of nursing care in the participating hospitals is entirely unrelated to how active each of the four medical committees is, or to how good a job each of these committees does, as appraised by the medical staff. This is shown by the first column of correlations in Table 52. The specific correlations range between —.28, through .00, to .12, all being nonsignificant.

2. Similarly, the quality of overall patient care in the various hospitals is not significantly related to the activity or performance of the executive, tissue, records, and credentials committees of the medical staff. This is shown by the third column of correlations in Table 52. The specific correlations range between —.11 and .33, none being statistically significant.

3. The comparative measure of the quality of overall care is similarly unrelated to the activity and performance of the various committees, as shown by the fourth column of correlations in the same table. Although all eight of the relevant correlations are positive, their size is too small (ranging between .02 and .44) for statistical significance.

4. The results about the relationship of the quality of medical care to medical committee activity and performance, shown by the second column of correlations in Table 52, are again not statistically significant, but they are a little more suggestive of a possible positive relationship.

TABLE 52. Relation of Medical Committee Activity and Performance to Patient Care *

Committee Activity and Committee Performance as Evaluated by the Medical Staff	Nursing Care	Medical Care	Overall Care	Comparative Overall Care
How active the medical executive committee is	.00	.33	.00	.19
How good a job it does for the hospital	−.08	.50	.33	.44
How active the tissue committee is	.01	.53	.12	.25
How good a job it does for the hospital	−.16	.31	−.07	.02
How active the records committee is	−.03	.25	.02	.08
How good a job it does for the hospital	.05	.10	.10	.12
How active the credentials committee is	.12	.35	.19	.31
How good a job it does for the hospital	−.28	.37	−.11	.08

* All figures are rank-order correlation coefficients, based on an N of 10 hospitals in each case. To be statistically significant at the .05 level, a coefficient must be ±.56 or more.

In connection with this last statement, we find that the correlations between the quality of medical care and how active each of the four medical committees is range from a low of .25 to a high of .53. The correlations between the quality of medical care and how good a job each of the four committees does range from a low of .10 to a high of .50. The average correlation between the activity of the four committees and medical care quality is about .38, and the average correlation between how good a job the four committees do and medical care quality is about .35. Directionally, the relationships are positive in all cases, as one might have expected, but in terms of size they are very modest, failing to reach statistical significance at the .05 level. However, two relationships approach significance at this level rather closely. These are, a correlation of .53 between how active the tissue committee is and the quality of medical care, and a correlation of .50 between how good a job the executive committee does and the quality of medical care (significance requires a correlation of .56). These two correlations are probably indicative of a connection between the quality of medical care and the work of the two committees. They are also congruent with the above cited results about the centrality of the tissue committee. In addition, these two correlations, together with the other correlations between medical care and committee activity and performance (second column in Table 52), exhibit a pattern which, by comparison to the correlational patterns between the other measures of patient care and committee activity and performance, is more clear-cut and more in the direction that one might have predicted. For these reasons, we cannot discard the possibility of a small relationship between the quality of medical care and the activity and performance of the medical committees, particularly of the executive and tissue committees.[7]

In summary, it may be concluded that hospitals with relatively more active, or better performing, major medical committees do not provide lower quality medical care (or nursing care, and overall patient care) than hospitals with less active, or less well-performing committees. On the other hand, the former institutions do not provide appreciably superior medical care than the latter, although a slight tendency in this direction seems to exist, particularly in connection with the work of the tissue committee and the executive committee. Further research in this area (especially research that would cover a larger number of hospitals than we did) is indicated, in the hope of supplying more conclusive evidence concerning the role of medical committees.

If future research fails to establish significant relationships between the quality of medical care and the quality of the work of the principal medical committees, a highly probable explanation may be that it is not the work of individual committees that is the important factor in relation to medical care. Rather, it is the final product of the concerted efforts of all these committees considered jointly and simultaneously which is the decisive factor. (The latter cannot be demonstrated analytically here, because we are dealing with a relatively small number of hospitals, and because the data show both significant and nonsignificant relationships between the activity-performance of each committee and the activity-performance of the remaining committees.) A second explanation, though not exclusive of the first, may be that the crucial factor is the skill and performance of the total medical staff and of the individual doctors rather than the work of medical committees. Still another explanation may be that the work of medical committees has in fact no consequences at all for the quality of medical care, however untenable this explanation may appear to be on *a priori* grounds. Additional explanations are, of course, also possible, but this takes us beyond the scope of the present study.

THE PERFORMANCE OF PARAMEDICAL DEPARTMENTS AND THE QUALITY OF PATIENT CARE

The theoretical statements in the preceding section on the role of individual medical committees in relation to the quality of patient care in the hospital are also relevant to the role of individual departments in relation to patient

---

[7] Parenthetically, we might also point out here that when a measure of the activity (and of the performance) of the executive committee of the board of trustees was examined in relation to the four measures of patient care, it yielded no significant relationships.

care. Empirically, however, the individual performance of departments must itself be examined in order to ascertain its relationship to patient care. As we have already seen, in addition to its major medical services and various committees, the community general hospital has a number of paramedical and nonmedical departments. Some of these departments perform primarily therapeutic functions (nursing), others perform diagnostic functions (laboratory), or both therapeutic and diagnostic functions (x-ray), while others perform service and educational functions (records), or purely service functions (maintenance, laundry). Obviously, the work of some departments is more directly relevant to the care process, and it is these paramedical departments with which we are mainly concerned here. The question in which we are interested is whether, and to what extent, the performance of individual departments is related to the quality of patient care, and whether some of the departments are more crucial in this connection than others, as one might hypothesize on *a priori* grounds.

The five departments with which we will be concerned are: the laboratory, x-ray, nursing, admissions, and records (the records department is not, of course, the same as the medical records committee). The performance of each department, in each hospital, was measured on the basis of data obtained by means of this question: "On the whole, what kind of a job would you say each of the following [departments] does for this hospital?" The response alternatives offered by the question ranged from "an excellent job" to "a rather poor job," forming the familiar five-point scale. The question was asked of these groups of respondents in every hospital: the doctors, supervisory registered nurses, including the director of nursing, laboratory and x-ray technicians, and the trustees and administrator (the supervisory nurses were asked the question in a slightly modified form, however, while the trustees and the administrator were treated as one respondent group in this case). The respondents answered the question separately for each of the five departments.

The data collected from each respondent group, about each department, were properly combined and averaged to yield a mean-score representing each group's evaluation of departmental performance in the individual hospitals. In the end, for each of the five departments under examination, we derived and used two measures of performance: one measure based exclusively on the evaluations given by the doctors representing each hospital, the other based on the evaluations given by all of the respondent groups combined (including the doctors). However, the two measures correlate very highly, regardless of the department being evaluated. Specifically, if we rank-order the ten hospitals according to each measure, and with reference to each specific department involved, the two rank-orders are nearly identical in every case. Thus, we find that how good a job the laboratory does for the hospital, as evaluated by doctors only, correlates .97 with the performance of the laboratory, as evaluated by all of the relevant groups of respondents. Similarly, for x-ray, the two measures of departmental performance correlate .90 in our group of ten hospitals; for admissions, they correlate .95; for the records department, they correlate .96; and for nursing, they correlate .97. Therefore, for all practical purposes, the two measures are interchangeable in every case, although we have retained them both in the analysis.

The interhospital range in performance scores varies, however, depending upon the department being considered, but regardless of which of the two measures is used as a basis. This suggests that, across hospitals, some of the departments are performing more uniformly than others. Using the measure based on the evaluations of all of the respondent groups, the mean-scores on departmental performance range as follows across the ten hospitals: for the laboratory, they range between 1.44 and 3.38 (in all cases the scores are based on a five-point scale, with smaller scores corresponding to a more favorable evaluation of departmental performance); for x-ray, they range between 1.44 and 2.83; for admissions, they range between 1.86 and 3.11; for the records department, they range between 1.52 and 2.38; and for nursing, they range between 1.83 and 2.67. Hence, the range in performance is highest for the laboratory and lowest for nursing, there being considerably more variance among hospitals with respect to how good a job their laboratory does as compared to how good a job nursing does.

The five departments vary not only in performance range, but also with respect to whether the performance of a given department is associated with the performance of the remaining departments. In this connection, using again the performance scores based on the data from all respondent groups involved, we find that, in the ten participating hospitals, only the performance of nursing is positively and significantly related to the performance of admissions, the correlation between the two being .88. No comparable significant relationship is found for any other possible pair of departments, although the performance of the laboratory correlates almost significantly with the performance of x-ray (.55). (The performance of nursing in the various hospitals correlates only .24 with that of records, .07 with that of the laboratory, and —.13 with that of x-ray; the performance of admissions correlates only .04 with that of records, .15 with that of the laboratory, and .05 with that of x-ray; and the performance of the records department correlates .39 with that of the laboratory, and —.08 with that of x-ray.) In other words, hospitals having better performing nursing departments are also likely to have better performing admissions departments, or vice versa; and, to an extent, the same tendency probably applies in the case of the laboratory and x-ray pair of departments. Apart from this exception, however, the quality of performance of a given department is almost completely unrelated to the quality of performance of the remaining departments here considered. This, of course, means that in any given hospital some of these departments may be doing an excellent job while others may be performing less adequately, and that the better performing individual departments are not likely to be concentrated in only a few of the hospitals. (Incidentally, these conclusions remain unaltered if the performance measure which is based solely on data from doctors is used.)

According to these results, one cannot expect the performance of every individual department to be related to the quality of patient care, and this actually proves to be the case. When the measures of departmental performance are examined in relation to our measures of patient care, we find the results presented in Table 53, which may be summarized rather quickly. First, how good a job the records department does is not directly related to the quality of patient care in the participating hospitals, irrespective of which measure of patient care and departmental performance is utilized. Hospitals having better performing records departments are not more likely than other

TABLE 53. Relation Between the Performance of Paramedical Departments and Patient Care *

How Good a Job Each of the Following Departments Does for the Hospital	Nursing Care	Medical Care	Overall Care	Comparative Overall Care
Nursing,† according to				
Doctors	.93	.48	.88	.76
Doctors and others	.94	.47	.82	.66
Admissions, according to				
Doctors	.81	.41	.77	.65
Doctors and others	.87	.43	.75	.62
The Records Department, according to				
Doctors	.04	.12	.15	.16
Doctors and others ‡	.08	.15	.19	.20
The Laboratory, according to				
Doctors	−.13	.14	−.12	−.15
Doctors and others	−.11	−.02	−.12	−.21
X-ray, according to				
Doctors	.13	.13	.22	.20
Doctors and others	−.18	−.13	−.03	−.07

* All figures are rank-order correlation coefficients, based on an N of 10 hospitals in each case. Coefficients larger than .56 are statistically significant at the .05 level or better.

† In this case, respondents were asked about the "nursing staff" rather than the "nursing department." Consequently, the corresponding correlations are not completely comparable with those for the other departments. However, additional relevant data yield essentially the same results. For example, "How well the nursing department is doing in relation to what it should be accomplishing," as evaluated by both supervisory and nonsupervisory registered nurses, correlates .73 with nursing care, .27 with medical care, .78 with overall care, and .71 with the comparative measure of overall care.

‡ In addition to the doctors, this includes the supervisory registered nursing staff, the laboratory and x-ray technicians, and the trustees and administrator.

hospitals to provide better nursing care, better medical care, or better overall patient care. Second, it is equally evident from the results that patient care in hospitals having better performing laboratories is not significantly superior, or inferior, from patient care in hospitals having less well performing laboratories. Third, the same may be said regarding the performance of x-ray. In all these cases, the correlations between departmental performance and patient care quality are extremely small and nonsignificant. These findings, it will be noted, are similar to those in the preceding section concerning the relationship between the behavior of medical committees and the quality of patient care.

By contrast, Table 53 shows that the quality of performance of the admissions department is positively and significantly related to the quality of nursing care, the quality of overall patient care, and the comparative measure of overall care. It also tends to correlate positively with the quality of medical care, but here the relationship is not statistically significant. Similarly, though even more strongly, the quality of the performance of the nursing department is positively and significantly related with all patient-care measures, except the quality of medical care. In this latter case, the relationship is not significant, but it is sufficiently large to be suggestive. More specifically, we find that how good a job nursing does in the various hospitals, as seen by doctors, correlates .93 with the quality of nursing care given to the patients, .48 with the quality of medical care, .88 with the quality of overall care, and .76 with comparative overall care. Thus, on the average, the hospitals with the better performing nursing departments, and also admissions departments, tend to be the better-care hospitals. On the other hand, the individual performance of laboratories, x-ray, and records departments in the hospitals studied does not produce a significant relationship with the measures of patient care.

These differential relationships cannot be attributed to a restricted interhospital range in departmental performance scores. Nor can they be attributed to variations in the range that characterizes the different departments studied. It will be noted, for example, that the interhospital range in departmental performance was greatest in the case of the laboratory (1.44 to 3.38). Certainly this range is wide enough to have yielded significant relationships with the patient care measures, if such relationships actually existed. Similarly, while the interhospital range in the case of the records department is almost identical with that obtained in the case of nursing (1.52 to 2.38 compared with 1.83 to 2.67), the results show that the performance of nursing is significantly associated with the quality of patient care, while the performance of records is not. Furthermore, to take two departments whose interhospital range is very similar but greater than that of nursing, namely, the admissions and x-ray departments, we again find significant relationships between the quality of departmental performance and the quality of patient care in the case of admissions but not in the case of x-ray. Apparently, the quality of patient care is related to the performance of some of the individual departments but not others, apart from any issues regarding the range of departmental performance.

In the case of nursing, of course, it is not difficult to explain the obtained relationships, in view of the crucial place of the nursing department and the nursing staff in the broader hospital organization, and in view of the therapeutic and coordinative functions carried out by the nursing department, as repeatedly demonstrated throughout this volume. (In Chapter 10, we shall also discuss a number of specific aspects of nursing performance, as well as some of the factors which make for better nursing performance at different levels.) But why should the performance of admissions be significantly related to the quality of patient care, unlike the performance of, for example, records or x-ray? This is almost an impossible question to answer on the basis of the available data. It is not unlikely, however, that the performance of admissions is related to the quality of patient care because it happens to correlate highly (.88) with the performance of nursing. In other words, the relationship between how good a job admissions does and the quality of patient care may be a spurious one, being largely accounted for by the variable of nursing performance (or even some other factor). But, we cannot test this interpretation because the application of partial and multiple correlation techniques when dealing with only ten hospitals, i.e., cases, is inappropriate. It could also happen that future studies will show the relationship in question to be a "real" one, rather than spurious, in which case some other explanation would be the correct one.

Finally, as regards the lack of significant relationships between the quality of patient care and the performance of records, x-ray, and the laboratory, the interpretations advanced earlier in connection with a similar lack of direct relationships between the quality of care and the performance of individual medical committees are equally applicable here. It seems that the quality of patient care is more a function of the performance of all the various departments taken together and considered jointly and simultaneously than a matter of how good a job the several departments (or committees) do individually. (Unfortunately, no satisfactory measure of the joint performance of the five departments is available to investigate this matter further, partly because we have no way of weighting the relative importance of the performance, or contribution, of the different departments, and partly because how well a given department performs is in most, yet not all, cases unrelated to how well the remaining departments perform in the participating hospitals.) The quality of performance of individual paramedical departments will probably affect the quality of patient care directly in cases where departmental performance falls below some minimum, but unknown, required level (perhaps, if it is poorer than in any of the hospitals in this study), in the few cases where the department is a central and crucial one to many other organizational parts, like the nursing department, or if the performance of a given department happened to reflect accurately the quality of the joint performance of several departments.

SUMMARY AND RESTATEMENT

In this chapter we have been concerned with the problem of identifying among a large number of variables those of the variables that relate significantly to the quality of patient care. Previously, the reader was introduced to the theoretical and operational problems of assessing the quality of patient care in the community general hospital, and of obtaining relevant measures of certain important aspects of hospital structure and functioning that might relate to one or more of the measures of patient care which have already been described. The latter measures were a measure of the quality of nursing care patients receive, a parallel measure of the quality of medical care, a measure of the quality of total patient care, and a comparative measure of overall care. It has been the task of this chapter to present the results of the study which show the specific empirical relationships between these four measures of care and a number of independent variables representing different aspects of the hospital situation.

Stated in their most general (and of necessity least precise) form, the principal findings from this part of the study show that the quality of patient care in the participating hospitals is

not higher in institutions having
    superior material facilities
    better financial status or higher income
    higher costs or higher expenses
    more personnel or a larger paid staff
    larger size in terms of number of beds and patient admissions
    medical committees individually performing at a high level
but *is inversely* (*negatively*) related to
    the level of prevailing tension among interacting groups and departments in the organization
    the rate of unexcused absenteeism among professional nurses
    the degree of experienced "unreasonable" pressure for better performance by nonmedical personnel
and *positively* related to
    the quality of organizational coordination in the hospital
    coordination within the nursing department alone
    certain aspects of the composition and distribution of the therapeutic staff (medical and nursing staff)
    the performance of the nursing department (but not the individual performance of the records, laboratory, and x-ray departments)
    complementarity of work-related expectations between doctors and nurses
    the rate of turnover among nurse's aides.

Each of these findings is, of course, much more complex than might be implied by this brief résumé or the somewhat more detailed review which follows below. For the complete story, reference should be made to the main body of the chapter.

While we find considerable differences among the ten participating hospitals with respect to how adequate their material facilities are, hospitals having more adequate facilities are not significantly more likely to provide superior care to their patients than hospitals whose facilities are comparatively less adequate. Nor do the hospitals with the superior facilities provide poorer care than those with the less adequate facilities, according to the data. The obtained relationships between the patient-care measures and adequacy of physical plant, space and beds, equipment, and supplies are generally positive but not large enough to be statistically significant. Only the adequacy of equipment, as evaluated by laboratory and x-ray technicians (but not as evaluated by doctors or by trustees and the administrator), is positively and significantly related to the quality of nursing and overall patient care. It is not, however, significantly related to the quality of medical care or the comparative measure of overall care. In brief, then, having superior material facilities does not necessarily assure better patient care. In the appropriate section of the chapter, we proposed several reasons to account for this finding.

Concerning the financial status of the hospitals and various measures of hospital income, expenditures, and costs, the results are a good deal different from what they might have been supposed to be. The quality of nursing care, medical care, overall patient care, and comparative care is in no way better in the higher-income, higher-expense, or higher-cost institutions. Actually, the better-care hospitals tend to be the ones with lower income, expenses, and costs. The quality of nursing care is significantly higher in hospitals having lower total income, lower income per bed, lower income per patient, and lower expenses per patient. The same tends to be also true for the quality of overall patient care and, to a lesser extent, for the quality of medical care, although the majority of the relationships are not statistically significant in these cases. There is some evidence, however, that the quality of medical care is better in those hospitals where a higher proportion of the institution's total expenses are going into payroll. While only a few of the correlations between the four measures of care and some eleven different measures of hospital income and expenditures are sufficiently high to be statistically significant, the total pattern of the obtained relationships clearly suggests that the quality of patient care, especially the quality of nursing care, tends to be better in the less affluent institutions. The evidence from this series of findings supports the conclusion that the better-care hospitals are also the more efficient, or more economical, organizations from a financial point of view.

Other findings from the study directionally suggest that the relationship between the quality of care and hospital size might be a negative one. Hospital size, as measured by number of beds, average daily census of patients, and total number of patient admissions, generally produces small negative correlations with the patient care measures. The number of patient admissions per bed, however, does not—indicating that a higher patient load does not make for poorer care. Since none of the relationships in this area is statistically significant, however, the only conclusion that can be properly drawn is that, for medium-sized hospitals, the quality of patient care rendered by the larger institutions is not superior to the care provided by the smaller institutions. It is, of course, important to remember here that the study has covered hospitals of a certain size-range only, i.e., hospitals having between 100 and 350 beds.

A number of findings concerning the relationship of the quality of patient care to the composition and distribution of the medical staff are in the expected direction, but comparable results involving the distribution and composition of the nursing staff are both more clear-cut and more provocative. The correlation between the proportion of medical staff members who are certified "board men" and the quality of medical care in the various hospitals (.49) is in the right direction, but falls short of being statistically significant. The number of "general practitioners" per patient correlates positively and significantly with the quality of nursing care and overall patient care, but not with the quality of medical care. The proportion of nursing staff members who are registered nurses correlates positively and significantly both with the quality of nursing care and the quality of medical care; and the same is true for the number of registered nurses per patient. The proportion of nursing staff members who are practical nurses correlates significantly with the quality of nursing care, but not with the quality of medical care. And the proportion of nursing staff members who are aides is *negatively* and significantly related to the quality of nursing and overall care; the higher the proportion of aides—unskilled staff—the poorer the care. These findings demonstrate not only that the quality of patient care in the community general hospital is a function of the composition and distribution of the nursing staff, but also that the role of the registered nurse is a crucial one in this connection.

Confirmation of the key role of the registered nurse in relation to patient care is also supplied by a series of findings regarding the connection between patient care quality and absenteeism among nursing personnel. We find that the quality of patient care is lower in hospitals having more extensive unexcused absenteeism among their professional nurses. At the same time, corresponding rates of absenteeism among practical nurses, or among aides, yield no significant relationships with the measures of patient care. These results underscore once more the centrality of the registered nurse in the hospital system, reflecting the fact that hers is the task of interrelating and making continuously operational the specialized activities necessary to the care of the specific patient. In the last analysis, it is she who must maintain a technical-organizational-social environment that will support the patient toward recovery; it is she who constitutes the psychological center of the doctor-nurse-patient-hospital relationship.

That the skill of the registered nurse is an essential requirement for high quality care also receives indirect support from a rather unanticipated source—certain findings regarding turnover among registered nurses and among aides. First, we find no relationship between the rate of turnover among nonsupervisory registered nurses in the participating hospitals and the measures of patient care. Apparently, the responsible administrative staff, recognizing the organizational centrality of the registered nurse, has prepared for the contingency of relatively high turnover among their professional nurses through such devices as employing, when possible, a relatively larger number of nurses (both registered and practical) than they may immediately need. Potential losses and additions to this group are planned for more carefully, and new arrivals of professional nurses in the community are followed up rather assiduously in preparation for the time when the hospital will need more registered nurses. Careful planning, coupled with a relatively high ability to predict the likely turnover among their professional nurses, enables the administrators to avoid the condition of serious understaffing in this group. The fact that the members of this group have been trained almost without regard to the specific institutional setting in which they will practice enables them to assume their duties immediately upon entering the hospital, thus ensuring the continuity of care without any adverse consequences. These and other related factors combine to explain why registered nurse turnover of the magnitude prevailing in the hospitals studied does not result in poorer patient care.

The rate of turnover among nurse's aides, unlike the above findings, correlates *positively* and significantly with all four measures of patient care. The higher the turnover, the *better* the care in this case. If we take into account the fact that aides are untrained and unskilled personnel, the fact that their activities have to be constantly supervised and coordinated by nurses, and the fact that some hospitals tend to have on their staff a disproportionately large number of aides because of nurse shortages and because aide help is inexpensive, it is not difficult to understand why turnover among aides is beneficial for the hospital insofar as the quality of patient care is concerned.

When the quality of performance of individual paramedical departments in the hospital is examined in relation to the quality of patient care, we find that the quality of care is not related to how good a job the laboratory, x-ray, or the records department is individually doing for the hospital. By contrast, and consistent with the above findings, how good a job the nursing department does for the hospital is positively and significantly related to the quality of nursing and overall patient care. A similar finding is obtained regarding the performance of the admissions department. When the quality of patient care in the participating hospitals is examined in relation to how active the major medical committees of these institutions are, or to how good a job they are doing individually, we again find no significant relationships between committee performance and patient-care quality. In this connection, we have proposed cer-

Summary and Restatement

tain explanations to account for these clusters of findings in the main body of this chapter, where the results are discussed more fully.

An important series of findings concerns the relationship between organizational coordination and the quality of patient care in the participating hospitals. On the aggregate, these findings clearly demonstrate that good coordination is a *sine qua non* to the functioning of the community general hospital. In this area, the four measures of patient care were related to four overall and seven specific measures that represent different categories and types of hospital coordination, as well as to an overall and three specific measures of coordination within the nursing department. The results from this analysis provide strong support for the conclusion that hospitals with better coordination are significantly more likely to provide better care to their patients than hospitals where coordination is less adequate. This conclusion applies with reference to all measures of patient care, except the medical care measure. This last measure also produces positive correlations with the various measures of coordination, but the individual correlations are generally small and nonsignificant. Apparently, the quality of medical care is more dependent upon the skill and competence of doctors than on coordination.

The principal conclusions which emerge from our analysis of the role of organizational coordination for patient care include the following:

1. Good coordination is essential to the effectiveness of the community general hospital.
2. The quality of nursing care and the quality of total patient care are significantly higher in hospitals having better coordination.
3. The quality of medical care is not appreciably better in the more adequately coordinated institutions. Although all pertinent correlations between medical care and various coordination measures are positive—indicating that medical care in the better coordinated hospitals is in no way inferior to that provided in the less adequately coordinated institutions—none is statistically significant.
4. The adequacy of coordination within the nursing department relates to patient care as the adequacy of coordination in the entire hospital does.
5. Our measure of programed coordination, involving such things as the timing of activities and how well established the routines of interdependent departments are, relates to the various measures of patient care as our measure of nonprogramed, or more informal, coordination does. Programed and nonprogramed coordination, in other words, appear to be equally important in relation to patient care in the hospitals studied.
6. The promotive type of coordination, implying a more perfect articulation of interdependent activities in the organization through positive efforts, is better related to patient care than the preventive type of coordination, which implies efforts to avoid creating problems of interference in the work structure. Mere

avoidance of disruptions in the hospital system is not enough to ensure effective functioning.

7. Of a number of different aspects of coordination, the timing of activities emerges as the single most important aspect in relation to patient care. The better the timing, the better the care.

Perhaps no other set of findings, from among the results of this study, entails greater practical significance or more implications for hospital administration than the findings in the area of coordination.

Closely associated with the phenomenon of coordination in large-scale organizations is the phenomenon of intraorganizational strain. Less than perfect coordination, communication, supervision, administration, and subunit performance, all contribute to tensions and pressures in the system. The study shows that hospitals with higher levels of tension among their various interacting groups and departments are significantly more likely than hospitals with lower levels of tension to provide poorer nursing care, poorer overall patient care, and poorer comparative care. Similarly, hospitals whose nonmedical personnel feel that they are working under a higher amount of unreasonable pressure for better performance are more likely than other hospitals to provide poorer care to their patients. Intraorganizational strain, in the form of intergroup tension or unreasonable pressure upon members for better performance, is thus inversely related to the quality of patient care in the community general hospital. Equally important in this connection is the additional fact that the adequacy of organizational coordination itself is negatively related to the degree of prevailing intraorganizational strain in the hospital. Poor coordination and high strain both affect patient care adversely.

Finally, another interesting series of findings in the present chapter underscores the importance of complementarity of expectations between the two therapeutic groups in the hospital—doctors and nurses—for patient care. The results show that the quality of patient care in the participating hospitals varies with the extent to which doctors feel that the nursing staff understand and appreciate the work problems and needs of the medical staff, the extent to which nurses feel that doctors understand the problems of the nursing staff, and the extent to which both doctors and nurses jointly have a good understanding of each other's work problems and needs. The results also show that complementary understanding and joint understanding only are related to patient care; it is not enough that the members of one staff merely feel that they have a good understanding of the problems of the other staff. That complementarity of expectations between doctors and nurses is essential to patient care stems from the fact that it is these two groups that are most directly concerned with the patient and with the care process, the fact that doctor and nurse activities are highly interdependent, the fact that the entire work structure of the hospital is geared to the activities of these two key staffs, and the fact that doctors and nurses constitute the two largest groups in the organization.

Of special significance, in this last series of results, is the finding that the degree of complementarity of work-related expectations between doctors and nurses, unlike the variables of coordination and intraorganizational strain (with which complementarity also happens to be significantly related), is positively and significantly related not only to the quality of nursing care, overall care, and comparative overall care but also to the quality of medical care. More specifically, hospitals in which the nursing staff has a good understanding of the problems and needs of the medical staff, as seen by the latter, are significantly more likely than other hospitals to provide better medical care to their patients, in addition to providing better nursing and overall care—the better the understanding, the better the care. A comparison of the relative strength of the obtained relationships between the measures of complementarity and the patient care measures, moreover, indicates that the quality of patient care is more dependent on the extent to which the nursing staff understand the problems of the medical staff, as seen by the latter, than on the extent to which the medical staff understand the problems of the nursing staff, as seen by the latter. This can, of course, be accounted for by the fact that the medical staff rely much more on the performance of the nursing staff in their work than the nursing staff rely on the performance of the medical staff.

In brief, these are our major findings about the quality of patient care in the community general hospital. Before concluding the chapter, however, it might be worth while also to attempt a quick review of the results from the standpoint of what appear to be the variables to which the quality of nursing care relates best, and the variables to which the quality of medical care relates best, or most closely. The emerging pattern of findings indicates that the quality of nursing care given to patients in the ten participating hospitals relates most strongly to the following variables:

1. The quality of organizational coordination in the hospital, and the adequacy of nursing department coordination (positive relationship).

2. The degree of prevailing intraorganizational strain among interdependent groups and departments in the hospital (negative relationship).

3. The degree of complementarity of expectations between the medical staff and the nursing staff (positive relationship).

4. The proportion of nursing staff members in the various hospitals who are registered nurses (positive relationship).

5. The proportion of nursing staff members who are aides (negative relationship).

6. The performance of the nursing department (positive relationship).

7. The rate of turnover among aides (positive relationship).

The quality of nursing care is, of course, also significantly related to a host of other variables, but somewhat less strongly. Included among these variables are: the rate of unexcused absenteeism among registered nurses (negative relationship); the number of registered nurses per patient (positive relationship); the proportion of nursing staff members who are practical nurses, and the number of practical nurses per patient (positive relationships); the number of aides per patient (negative relationship); the number of general practitioners per patient (positive relationship); and certain measures of hospital income, costs, and expenses (negative relationship). In addition, suggestive evidence indicates a tendency for the quality of nursing care to be related, although not significantly, to such things as the adequacy of hospital facilities (positive tendency), and hospital size and certain size-related variables (negative tendency).

The quality of medical care in the participating hospitals is best related to the following variables:

1. Complementarity of expectations between doctors and nurses, as measured by the extent to which the nursing staff understand and appreciate the work problems and needs of the medical staff, as seen by the latter, and as jointly seen by both doctors and nurses (positive relationship).

2. The proportion of nursing staff members in the hospital who are registered nurses, and the number of registered nurses per patient (positive relationships).

3. Unexcused absenteeism among registered nurses (negative relationship).

4. The rate of turnover among aides (positive relationship).

5. The percentage of the hospital's total expenses going into payroll (positive relationship).

A number of additional results, though not statistically significant, are highly suggestive of a tendency for the quality of medical care also to be associated with such variables as: the proportion of medical staff members who are certified "board men" (positive tendency); the performance of the medical executive committee (positive tendency); the activity of the tissue committee (positive tendency); the performance of the nursing department (positive tendency); the quality of coordination in the nursing department (positive tendency); and a few other variables. In general, however, considering all the independent variables studied, we find that the quality of medical care in the participating hospitals relates to considerably fewer variables than does the quality of nursing care, and that the size of obtained relationships is generally greater in the latter case. (The quality of medical care, it should be recalled, is also related to certain variables, presented in Chap. 5, which were used there for the purpose of validating the measure of medical care.)

The quality of overall patient care in the hospitals studied and the quality of overall patient care as compared to the care rendered at similar other institutions, i.e., the comparative measure of overall care, on the whole, relate significantly to the same variables to which the quality of nursing and/or medical care relates, as might be expected. It is also of interest to note here that, generally, all four of our measures of patient care yield better relationships with those of the independent variables which represent either purely social-psychological aspects of the hospital situation or aspects of the composition, distribution, and skill of the therapeutic staff than with variables representing such things as material facilities, financial matters, or size and size-related factors.

Finally, not included among the above cited findings, there is a series of relationships between each of the four measures of patient care and certain variables which were also investigated in this study, but which were earlier used for the purpose of validating the patient care measures. These variables, and their particular empirical relationship to the quality of medical, nursing, and overall patient care, have been discussed in detail in Chapter 5. Similarly, the next two chapters to which we now turn, respectively dealing with problems of supervision and communication, also contain certain supplementary findings regarding the quality of patient care in the community general hospital.

REFERENCES

1. Andrews, R. E. *Leadership and Supervision: A Survey of Research Findings.* U.S. Civil Service Commission, Personnel Management Series, No. 9, 1955.
2. Brayfield, A. H., and Crockett, W. H. "Employee Attitudes and Employee Performance," *Psychological Bulletin,* 52:396–424, 1955.
3. Deutsch, M. "An Experimental Study of the Effects of Cooperation and Competition upon Group Process," *Human Relations,* 2:199–232, 1949.
4. Georgopoulos, B. S., and Tannenbaum, A. S. "A Study of Organizational Effectiveness," *Amer. Sociol. Rev.,* 22:534–40, 1957.
5. Goldwater, S. S. *On Hospitals.* New York: Macmillan, 1947.
6. Klein, M. W., Malone, M. F., Bennis, W. G., and Berkowitz, N. H. "Problems of Measuring Patient Care in the Out-Patient Department," *J. Health & Human Behav.,* 2:138–44, (Summer) 1961.
7. Seashore, S. E., Indik, B. P., and Georgopoulos, B. S. "Relationships Among Criteria of Job Performance," *J. Applied Psych.,* 44:195–202, 1960.
8. Simon, H. A. *Administrative Behavior.* New York: Macmillan, 1947.
9. Torrence, E. P. Survival Research. HRRL *Memo.,* Report No. 29, 1952.

9 SUPERVISORY AND ADMINISTRATIVE BEHAVIOR

One of the objectives of the study was to examine the role of supervision in relation to satisfaction with supervision, patient care, and coordination in the hospital, in an attempt to provide some answers to a number of frequently raised questions which have both practical and theoretical significance. What are the styles or patterns of leadership, for example, that prevail in today's community general hospital? What is the relationship between supervisory practices and the attitudes and satisfactions of subordinates? How is supervisory and administrative behavior related to organizational effectiveness? What specific aspects of the behavior of supervisors are likely to affect the performance of subordinates? Or, more generally, what patterns of supervision and administrative behavior would be most appropriate, or most desirable, in hospital organization? Does directive leadership or the "human relations" approach provide the answer, and, in either case, what are the limiting conditions? Obviously, these are complex and difficult questions, and an entire program of research could be devoted to this area alone, instead of the present limited examination. In view of the paucity of systematic empirical research, however, even a limited treatment does much to complement our understanding of hospital organization and hospital functioning.

In task-centered organizational systems, like the hospital, formal leadership constitutes an important mechanism for ensuring the channeling and integration of specialized performances. As we have seen in previous chapters, specialization places a premium on organizational coordination. The performance of specific tasks by specialized groups working interdependently toward shared or common, but complex, goals requires an elaborate system of coordination. Coordination can be attained through detailed organizational planning, and through formal rules and regulations concerning activities and operating procedures; through the informal system of shared expectations, norms, and understandings among organizational members; and through the more formal system of hierarchical and directive roles—supervisory, administrative, and liaison-coordinative roles—provided by the organizational structure of the hospital. The problem of leadership and supervision is, thus, intimately related to the problem of organizational coordination.

The hospital, unlike many other large-scale organizations, however, is also an organization that mobilizes the efforts and competences of widely divergent professional and nonprofessional members to provide a highly personalized service to individual patients. Care must be provided in a manner that is seen by the patient as tailored to him as a unique human being and aimed at satisfying his own personal needs. But, at the same time, patient care must be rendered at a level of relative emotional detachment that promotes maximum technical efficiency and allows for the continued performance of organizational roles that are emotionally taxing. A degree of impersonality in the performance of various roles in the hospital is thus required institutionally.

Moreover, the hospital is an organization designed to handle crises and emergencies, which involve matters of human life, and whose outcome is often uncertain and unpredictable. Under these circumstances, it is important that organizational lines of authority and responsibility be clearly drawn and discipline be maintained. Consequently, a good deal of regimented behavior is required by the system, and coordination of activities must in part be achieved in a highly directive manner, through formal hierarchical relationships. This reliance on authority, moreover, is accentuated because of financial considerations. To an extent, individualized service and the factor of unpredictability contribute to inefficiency. Regardless of cost, frequency of need, and frequency of actual use, for example, the hospital must have available equipment, supplies, and medicines which are costly, but which may be rarely used. Formal supervision and administration are, therefore, relied upon to keep the level of this inherent inefficiency at a minimum.

Since supervisors, administrators, and other formal leaders are expected to coordinate, direct, and even control the activities and working relationships of organizational members, without particularly great concern for the attitudes and sentiments of the participants, prescriptions for supervisory behavior in the hospital typically call for a great deal of impersonality, deference, and social distance. Under these conditions, the problem of motivating the participants toward effective attainment of organizational objectives is a difficult one to handle. In view of the formal requirements of the organization, individually rewarding activities involved in informal social behavior, independence of action, autonomy, and self-expression are not easy to satisfy for a large number of organizational members. The role of supervision and administration is, therefore, a crucial one in reconciling the impersonal demands of the situation with the personal needs of the members, in order to maintain sufficient motivation for high-level performance. The medical staff is, of course, virtually exempt from lay-supervisory-administrative authority, but all other professional and nonprofessional personnel are subject to such authority (some being subject to medical authority, in addition). Herein lies the problem of maintaining adequate motivation—a problem, which, in all probability, is most difficult to handle in the case of such nonmedical, but professional, personnel as x-ray and laboratory technicians, registered nurses, and some administrative department heads. It is a well-known fact that professionals are reluctant to submit to regimentation.

The preceding considerations combine to suggest that a directive type of superior-subordinate relationship would, perhaps, be most appropriate in hospitals. On the other hand, a variety of studies in industry have in recent years demonstrated the importance of a different type of leadership, which emphasizes a less directive and more permissive kind of superior-subordinate relationship. Under the impact of industrial research, many people in the hospital field have come to believe that the "human relations" approach is more likely to be effective, and that approximately the same supervisory practices would be related to hospital effectiveness as have been found to be related to organizational effectiveness in industrial situations. In the light of this belief, and perhaps somewhat uncritically in view of the lack of adequate comparable research in hospitals, many hospital administrators have begun to invest heavily in programs designed to develop the human relations skills of their supervisory personnel. The present research was partly designed to explore these issues, and to uncover possible limiting conditions that are relevant to the application of the human relations approach in the community general hospital.

Our main objective in this chapter is an initial attempt to study supervision in the hospital setting, in the hope of eventually providing an answer to the question of what kinds of administrative leadership and supervision are most appropriate for effective hospital functioning. More specifically, the purpose of this chapter is fourfold. First, we will examine the kinds of supervisory skills, or competences, that are required at different organizational levels in the hospital, and then study their relationship to satisfaction with supervision on the part of subordinates. Second, we will show some of the supervisory practices that prevail at different levels in the participating hospitals and examine their relationship to both supervisory skills and satisfaction with supervision. Third, we will investigate the relationship between supervisory skills and practices and the quality of patient care in the various hospitals. And fourth, we will similarly examine the relationship between supervisory skills and practices and organizational coordination.

In all cases, we shall be concerned with superior-subordinate relationships among nonmedical personnel, including the nursing staff, the technicians, and the administrative staff. In the case of nursing personnel, an additional examination of superior-subordinate relationships in the area of communication has been reserved for the next chapter, Chapter 10, where we will be concerned with the communication practices prevailing among professional nurses and their relation to certain aspects of nursing activity and performance. Before we begin the presentation of our empirical findings in the present chapter, however, let us briefly consider the concept of supervision to provide the theoretical background against which the findings may be viewed.

THEORETICAL CONSIDERATIONS

Complex organizations are made up of a large number of relatively small work groups or organizational families. Each of these units has its own objectives, responsibilities, and tasks to perform. At the same time, the objectives and activities of each unit are a part of the total organizational complex, and must contribute to the attainment of system-wide objectives. Formally, the different organizational units are related to one another, and coordinated through the office of supervisors. The activities within each organizational unit are also related to one another under the direction of a supervisor. In turn, the work of a number of supervisors is coordinated and directed by a supervisor in the next higher level of the organization, and this cycle is repeated up to the point where a few individuals in the top supervisory and administrative positions of the organization have the responsibility of integrating the work of the understructure, so that the total organization is capable of unified activity. Structurally, then, the organizational role of the supervisor, at any level, is primarily one of linking together different parts of the organizational structure and integrating their specialized performances.

Specifically, in addition to whatever technical aspects it may involve, the role of the supervisor entails the following functions: (1) the direction and coordination of the activities of his own subordinates and work group; (2) the relating of these to those of other work groups at the same organizational level with which his group interacts; and (3) the relating of the activities of his group, and his own activities, to those of other organizational units operating at the next higher, as well as the next lower, level in the organization. In short, the organizational role of the supervisor is to link his own organizational family, i.e., the unit consisting of himself and his immediate subordinates, with other organizational families, so that the entire system may achieve and maintain unity and coherence. In the process of performing the above functions, the supervisor has still another important task to accomplish, however. As the leader of his organizational family, he must deal with the motivational problem of reconciling and integrating the impersonal requirements and objectives of the organization with the personal needs and goals of his immediate subordinates.

The *raison d'être* of every organization is to accomplish some objective. The physical and mental capacities and energies of men are among the principal means and resources through which the objectives of organizations can be attained. But, men also have their own goals which they want to accomplish through their working in the organization. The interests of the individual members of the organization, and the goals they are trying to attain, may or may not be the same as, or compatible with, those of the organization. The degree of congruence between the objectives of the organization and the goals of its members will, in all probability, vary among organizations. In voluntary organizations there will probably be more congruence than in contractual ones; in primary groups, like the family, we will also expect more congruence than in large-scale organizations such as industrial firms; and, among large-scale organizations, we will expect greater congruence in some than in others, depending upon such things as the purposes of the organization, its standing in the community, and the values of society—we will probably find more congruence in hospitals than in factories, for example. In any case, those organizations which are best able to tap all of the relevant energies of their members, and to meet their members' personal needs, aspirations, and goals, will presumably be more likely to attain their institutional purpose.

One of the basic problems of organizations, then, is how to reconcile and integrate member needs and goals with organizational requirements and objectives; and the role of supervisors is of key importance in this connection. The magnitude of this problem for supervisors varies directly according to the actual and potential discrepancy between organizational and individual goals. It, of course, also varies across different organizations, and within the same organization it may vary over time, as the organization changes and moves from one stage of its development to another. Furthermore, at any given time, it varies from one organizational-supervisory level to another. The principal executive of an organization, working closely with the heads of major departments who, along with him, have a great deal to say about setting organizational objectives and prescribing means for their accomplishment, virtually faces no problem motivationally. At the other extreme, the first-line supervisor is constantly confronted with the task of making organizational objectives compatible with the needs and goals of his subordinates. Intermediate levels of supervision also have to reconcile the two sets of goals, but the problem becomes increasingly less severe at successively higher levels. It is the first-line supervisor who has the biggest job in this respect. He ordinarily has had the least to say about the objectives of the organization, yet he is expected to understand these objectives fully and to make them meaningful imperatives for those under his supervision, which of course also requires that he understand the needs and goals of his subordinates.

There is little discrepancy, and practically no conflict, between individual goals and organizational aims for those occupying the top-echelon offices in the organization. These individuals have either established the objectives of the organization, and/or determined the means of attaining the objectives, or have been selected to fill these positions because their needs and values were congruent with organizational aims. The potential discrepancy becomes greater for

Theoretical Considerations

each succeeding lower level. Nonsupervisory employees have generally little or no say about organizational means and objectives. Their relationship with the organization is characteristically more contractual, and their identification with it much more tenuous. Since only some of their needs and goals—comparatively, a smaller proportion than is the case for higher level personnel—can be met through the performance of their organizational roles, they may give only that proportion of their energies that is necessary to remain in the organization, i.e., to keep employed. The extent to which the bond between the individual member and his organizational office, or position, is contractually and economically based, rather than psychologically and intrinsically rewarding, is evidenced by the frequency with which many individuals at the lowest levels in organizations seen simply to be trading hours of their life, doing personally unsatisfying tasks, for security or money that they hope to use to "buy" fuller lives off the job.

Supervisory Skills: Administrative, Human Relations, and Technical Skills

The preceding discussion of the concept of supervision has direct implications concerning the essential skills that an occupant of the generic office of supervisor must have. To perform the functions required to coordinate the activities of one organizational family with another, the supervisor must have *administrative competence*. To integrate organizational objectives with individual member needs, he must have *human relations competence*. And to accomplish his other assigned tasks, including the performance of concrete day-to-day work functions and specialized subobjectives, he must possess *technical competence*.

The marked division of labor and high degree of specialization that characterize hospitals, as well as other large-scale organizations, require that the occupants of supervisory positions have at least the minimum technical competence necessary to understand and direct the work being done within their respective organizational units. The higher the degree of specialization and differentiation, moreover, the greater the need for supervisors with technical competence is likely to be. *Technical skill,* or competence, as used here, refers to the ability to use pertinent knowledge, methods, techniques, and equipment necessary for the performance of specific tasks and activities, and for the direction of such performance. Fundamentally, it involves an understanding of, and proficiency in, a specific class of functions in the organization. This includes not only concrete motoric skills of doing things, however, but also the abstract orientations and basic frames of reference that are normally associated with particular professional roles and affiliations. The technical skills of a head nurse, for example, would encompass such highly specialized activities as giving intravenous injections, and such value orientations as implied in continuing to read, study, master new techniques, and generally keep up with the profession and improve her standing as a professional nurse. Technical skills are acquired through formal training in professional schools, informal on-the-job training, and combinations of academic and internship or apprenticeship programs. Once acquired, moreover, they tend to remain stable and are seldom lost.

Just as technical skills are primarily concerned with task-centered competence, human relations skills are concerned with the ability to work with other people effectively. In the case of supervisors, the other people involved are one's subordinates, superiors, and colleagues at the same organizational level, i.e., other supervisors. *Human relations skill,* then, refers to the ability to use pertinent knowledge and methods of working with people or through people. It includes an understanding of general principles of human behavior, particularly those principles which involve the regulation of interpersonal relations and human motivation, and the skillful utilization of this understanding in day-to-day interaction with others in the work situation.

The supervisor with human relations skills not only understands how the principles of behavior affect others but himself as well. Furthermore, these skills involve not only consideration and support for others and their problems, but also the ability of the supervisor to motivate his subordinates sufficiently so that they may perform their assigned tasks effectively, and the ability to integrate the goals of individuals with the objectives of the organization. The supervisor must be able to identify those needs of others which are central to their self-concept, and to relate these to organizational objectives in a manner that is psychologically meaningful and rewarding to them. At times, this will mean coordinating the goals of one's subordinates with those of people in higher levels; at other times, it will mean creating, modifying, or shifting either organizational or individual goals so that a balance or integration between the two may be attained. Basically, the present class of skills involves managing the emotional and motivational dimensions of interpersonal relations in an organization.

The human relations skills of a head nurse, for example, would include getting members of the nursing team to work together cooperatively; getting them to do the best they can as individuals; being available to discuss their problems; and helping them with their work when necessary or requested. They would also involve, on occasion, the development of the aspirations of her subordinates regarding the contribution they might make to the hospital and the larger community. The head nurse might also on occasion find herself in the position of vigorously defending the behavior of her subordinates before others, or trying to modify the actions of her superiors for the benefit of her work group. In general, it would be her function to build and maintain the loyalty and commitment of her subordinates to the hospital and its goals.

The third class of basic supervisory skills deals with administrative competence. *Administrative skill,* or competence, refers to the ability of the supervisor to think and act in terms of the total organizational system within which he operates—in terms of the organization as a system of people and physical objects, with its own image, structure, and process, which functions as a complex problem-solving arrangement for the purpose of attaining particular objectives. The emphasis here is on understanding and acting according to the objectives of the total organizational system, rather than on the basis of the goals and needs of one's immediate work group only. Administrative skills include such things as planning, programing, and organizing the work; assigning the right tasks to the right people; giving people the right amount of responsibility and authority; and coordinating the efforts and activities of different organizational members, levels, and departments. In short, administrative skill requires an ability to conceptualize and comprehend the organizational system as a whole, and to fit individual parts in the overall organizational frame. The administrative skills of a head nurse, for example, would involve an ability to organize effectively the work of the members of her nursing team, to relate nursing functions to medical activities, and even to coordinate work among different groups and shifts. They would also involve the ability to translate broad organizational aims into sets of specific tasks and processes that are capable of being implemented, and the ability to allocate resources and distribute people and work properly.

In summary, we have suggested three classes of essential skills that are normally required of supervisors and those in administrative positions in the organization—technical skills, human relations skills, and administrative skills.[1] Technical skills pertain to "know-how" competence regarding particular tasks for which the supervisor is responsible. Human relations skills concern the understanding of organizational members as people with their own problems and needs, or the understanding of the emotional and motivational dimensions in interpersonal relations. Administrative skills deal with the demands of the organization for unified activity and integration. Thus, the three kinds of skills respectively concern tasks, people, and organization.

The Supervisory Skill-Mix

While all supervisors, regardless of their level in the organization, must have some minimum technical skill, some minimum human relations skill, and some minimum administrative skill, not all of them are likely to be equally strong in these different skills. More importantly, what may be an effective combination of skills for supervisors at one organizational level may not be an effective skill-mix for supervisors at another level. The relative importance of

[1] As early as 1953-54, Mann and Dent (21) found it necessary to distinguish between technical competence and human relations competence in a study of supervision. In subsequent studies, dealing with problems of supervision and automation, Mann and Hoffman (23) and Mann and Williams (24) found the distinction among technical, human relations, and administrative competence a fruitful one. Katz (19), in a study of the skills of effective administrators, also made a distinction among technical, human relations, and, what he terms, conceptual skills.

each kind of supervisory skill is likely to vary markedly across organizational levels. At the lower levels of the organization, for example, we expect that technical and human relations skills are the most important. At intermediate levels, technical skills are likely to be less important and administrative skills more important. And at the top managerial and administrative levels, administrative skills are likely to be the most important. Human relations skills are probably important for supervisors at all levels but, in view of our earlier suggestion that the motivational problem is not as acute at the higher levels, they are likely to become comparatively less important as one moves up the hierarchy. Certainly, they are no substitute for either administrative competence at the top or technical competence at the bottom levels of the organization.

Theoretically, therefore, one may suggest a paradigm in which technical skills become less important and administrative skills more important for supervisors at each succeeding higher level in the organization, with human relations skills being about equally important for supervisors at all levels, but somewhat less crucial at the very top level. Figure 1 presents schematically our conception of the relative importance of the three kinds of supervisory skills for different levels of supervision. Elsewhere, Katz (19) has proposed a similar view concerning the relativity of the supervisory skill-mix at different levels in an organization.

In addition to the variations in skill-mix required at different organizational levels, there is typically a good deal of variation in skill requirements at different times. Early in the life of an organization, technical and human relations skills are probably essential; later, as the organization becomes more complex, administrative skills become increasingly crucial. Similarly, during periods of rapid change, technical skills are likely to become very important at higher organizational levels. With the initiation of reorganization, or when new technology is introduced in the system, upper-level supervisory personnel have to draw more heavily on their technical competence at the early stages. During such a period of transition, the problems faced by the organization are basically of a technical character, and their solution depends very greatly on thorough command of specialized knowledge and technical-analytical ability. But, in the later stages of reorganization and change, human relations skills assume greater importance once again; after the technical difficulties have been overcome, the remaining organizational problems are frequently of the human relations variety.

Thus, it is not enough to think in terms of the combination of the three kinds of supervisory skills required at different organizational levels. It is also necessary to consider the time dimension—how their combination, for a particular level, must vary over time. In this connection, on the basis of their findings from a study of the introduction of electronic data-processing equipment in an organization, Mann and Williams (24) point out that, over an extended

Figure 1.

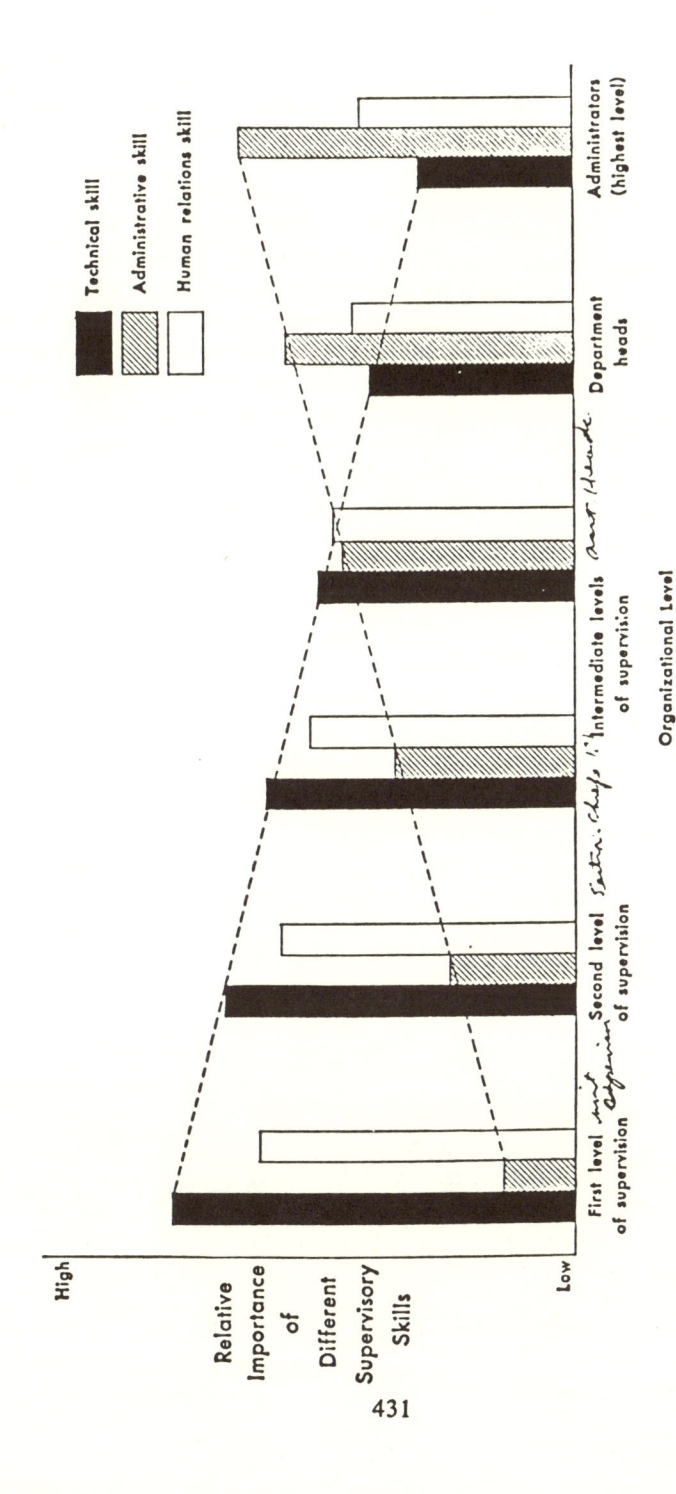

Schematic Representation of Supervisory Skill-Mix Required at Different Levels in Hierarchical Organizations

period of change, different combinations of the three basic supervisory skills were required of different supervisory levels at the same time, and of the same supervisory level at different times.

The Relativity of "Effective" Supervision

In view of the preceding theoretical considerations, the question of what effective supervision requires is a highly relative one, defying any single pat answer that is applicable to all organizations, to all levels within the same organization, or at all times. As Likert (20) has pointed out, supervision is "always an adaptive process," meaning that the supervisor, or leader, to be effective, must always adapt his behavior to fit the expectations, needs, and values of those with whom he is interacting, as well as to fit the particular demands of the situation. Several other social psychologists have arrived at a similar conclusion on the basis of their research in this area. Among them, Argyris has perhaps best captured the essence of this position:

> Effective leadership depends upon a multitude of conditions. There is no one predetermined, correct way to behave as a leader. The choice of leadership patterns should be based upon an accurate diagnosis of the reality of the situation in which the leader is imbedded. If one must have a title for effective leadership, it might be called *reality-centered leadership* (1, p. 207).

However, as he indicates, the concept of "reality-centered leadership" does little to further our understanding of the role of the leader.

To understand the role of the supervisor, or leader, we need to have some guiding concepts and principles which, while taking into account the relativity of supervision and noting the issue of potential conflict between organizational objectives and member goals, help us unravel the complexity of the problem of the effective supervisor. We need to sift what may be more essential and more permanent and general requirements of effective supervision from the more trivial, more ephemeral, and more circumscribed aspects. The approach we have outlined in the preceding pages constitutes one step in this direction that we have explored in the hospital setting. Our conception of leadership underscores the relativity of supervision, but also helps us make some statements as to what effective supervision will require under certain conditions. The technical, human relations, and administrative skill requirements, as discussed in this section, for example, suggest that the effective supervisor is reality-centered and adaptive if he possesses the appropriate skill-mix that enables him to meet the needs of the place, i.e., organizational level and position, and time in which he finds himself—requirements that are researchable and specifiable, and that we have tried to outline above.

Before concluding this section, we might also note that there have been a number of studies, in a variety of organizations, which indicate that supervisors and other leaders must have skills of the kind here proposed, including the ability to reconcile organizational objectives and individual member goals. Hemphill (16), for example, reports that, in a study of college departments, those of the departments with the best reputation had chairmen who were described as above average in both "consideration" (i.e., human relations skills) for others and in "initiating structure" (i.e., technical and administrative skills). Halpin (14, 15), in a study of airplane commanders, reports that the more respected commanders were concerned both with developing warm relationships with members of their units and with initiating new ways of solving organizational problems. Similarly, based on their review of several studies in this area, Kahn and Katz (18) conclude that the effective supervisor in industrial organizations is both "employee-centered" and "production-centered." And Roethlisberger (27) points out that, all too often, persons in positions of organizational responsibility are trying hard to be employee-centered, group-centered, subordinate-centered, and person-centered (i.e., to emphasize human relations skills), while being in situations where they also need to be production-centered and task-centered (i.e., require technical skills), as well as superior-centered and organization-centered (i.e., require administrative skills).

In short, technical, human relations, and administrative skills are all important. The problem is to identify the combinations of the three classes of skills most appropriate in given organizational settings, for given organizational levels, and at given times, and to gear specific supervisory practices to the requirements of the situation. With these considerations in mind, let us now examine the problem of supervision in the community general hospital, beginning with the presentation of certain data concerning supervisory skills at different organizational levels, and a discussion of the interrelationship among the supervisory skills.

SUPERVISORY SKILLS, AND THE RELATIONSHIP AMONG SUPERVISORY SKILLS AT DIFFERENT LEVELS OF SUPERVISION

Apart from certain aspects of administrative behavior discussed earlier in relation to internal coordination, and those aspects of superior-subordinate relationships which will be discussed in the next chapter in relation to communication patterns, the measures of supervisory behavior in this study were geared to the three classes of supervisory skills just described—technical, administrative, and human relations skills. Most of the measures, however, are concerned with human relations competence. Our measures of supervision were designed primarily for two purposes: first, to provide an indication of the extent to which the three classes of supervisory skills are present at different levels of supervision in the community general hospital; and second, to allow an investigation of the relationship between supervisory skills and characteristics, on the one hand, and measures of (1) the satisfaction of subordinates with their superiors, (2) organizational coordination, and (3) patient care, or hospital effectiveness, on the other.

The measures of coordination and patient care are from among those studied in previous chapters. The measure of satisfaction with supervision, to be described later, is based on data from a question asked of respondents at different levels in each hospital. The measures of supervisory skills and characteristics are also based on questionnaire data obtained from department heads, nursing personnel in different classifications, and laboratory and x-ray technicians with reference to their respective immediate superiors in the hospital. Before discussing the particular measures, however, we will briefly comment on the units and method of analysis employed in this part of the study.

As in previous chapters, our measures and analyses in the area of supervision will typically be based on group data; only occasionally will data be presented about individual respondents. Similarly, most of the findings will refer either to particular groups of hospital personnel at various levels—like the department heads or the supervisory nurses—or to the total hospital, in which case data from several groups of respondents combined will be involved. In short, the unit of analysis will again be the group or the organization, rather than individuals, and the N will be 10 (i.e., equal to the number of participating hospitals) in all but a few instances, which will be pointed out.

Relationships between variables will be presented in the familiar form of correlations. The correlations will, of course, be based on group or hospital measures, namely on group-hospital means. In general, the same techniques of analysis will be employed here as in previous chapters, with one notable deviation which concerns the kinds of correlations used. In this part of the study, two kinds of correlation will be used: the conventional rank-order correlation, and a correlation which is known as the tau-correlation. Simple tau-correlations are not much different from simple rank-order correlations (except that they are computed differently and tend to be smaller in size) and may be interpreted in a similar manner. The reason for using tau-correlations will become evident below. For the moment, it is sufficient to say that, if we have simple tau-correlations, it is possible to compute what are known as partial tau-correlations. The latter are very useful for certain purposes, and may be properly utilized even though based on as small an N as 10, which is the N in our case. Partial rank-order correlations, on the other hand, are not statistically appropriate for an N of 10—they require a larger N, unlike simple rank-order correlations which may be used legitimately even when the N is smaller than 10.

The Measures of Supervisory Skills

A set of three questions was asked of respondents in each hospital concerning the technical, administrative, and human relations skill of their respective superiors. The response alternatives offered by each question are

Supervisory Skills at Different Levels

shown in Table 54. The exact wording of the stem of each question, as it appeared on the questionnaires, was as follows:

Regarding human relations skill:

> On the whole, how does your immediate superior handle the *human relations side* of the job? (This includes such things as getting people to work together, getting them to do the best they can, giving recognition and expressing appreciation for good work done, letting people know where they stand, and the like.)

Regarding administrative skill:

> On the whole, how well does your immediate superior handle the *administrative side* of the job? (This includes such things as assigning the right job to the right people, indicating clearly when work is to be finished or what is to be done first, giving people the right amount of responsibility and authority they need to do their job, inspecting and following up the work, organizing, making overall plans about the work, and the like.)

Regarding technical skill:

> On the whole, how well does your immediate superior handle the *purely technical side* of the job? (This includes *other than* "human relations" and "administrative" aspects of the job; for example, it includes such things as knowledge of the job, technical skills needed by his profession, the operation of equipment, and the like.)

The three questions were asked of five groups of respondents in each hospital: administrative department heads (nonmedical), supervisory nurses, nonsupervisory registered nurses, practical nurses, and laboratory and x-ray technicians. (They were not asked of aides and orderlies because of the relative difficulty of the questions; aides and orderlies were not considered as having the ability required to comprehend and make meaningful distinctions among the three concepts.) The respondents answered the questions, along with other questions about supervision, with reference to their immediate superior in the hospital. They were first asked to indicate the name of their *immediate superior,* and then to answer the questions with reference to him. Therefore, the supervisory skills and characteristics under consideration in this chapter are not those of the respondents, but those of the respondents' immediate superiors.

Different groups of respondents in the individual hospitals, of course, tend to have different immediate superiors, and the same group of respondents in the same hospital may name a number of persons as their superiors. For all participating hospitals combined, 86 percent of the administrative department heads named the hospital administrator as their immediate superior (thus, the data concerning supervisory skills and characteristics in this case refer to the administrator). Of the supervisory nurses (including head nurses) in the various hospitals, about half (49 percent) named the director of nursing as their immediate superior, 3 percent named the assistant-associate director of nursing, 36 percent named one of the top nursing supervisors, and the remaining named others. Of the nonsupervisory registered nurses, 69 percent named some nursing supervisor as their immediate superior, and 12 percent named a head nurse (i.e., 81 percent named a person belonging to the supervisory nurses group of respondents); another 5 percent named the director or the assistant director, and the rest named other individuals as their immediate superior. Of the laboratory and x-ray technicians, 42 percent named the director of the laboratory or x-ray (i.e., a doctor), 33 percent named a head technician or chief technician, and the rest named some other persons. And of the practical nurses, 37 percent named a nursing supervisor, 14 percent named a head nurse, 23 percent named a staff nurse (nonsupervisory registered nurse), 11 percent named the associate or assistant director of nursing, 3 percent named the director of nursing, and the rest named others. It is clear, therefore, that supervision is most concentrated in the smallest number of persons in the case of department head respondents, while being most diffuse in the case of the practical nurses group of respondents. (In the case of aides and orderlies diffusion is also great.) Keeping this point in mind will facilitate understanding of the findings.

Returning now to the three questions on supervisory skills, Table 54 shows how the nonsupervisory registered nurses from the ten hospitals combined answered each question. The data show that about eight out of every ten registered nurses (81 percent) perceive their immediate superior as handling the technical side of the job extremely well or very well, 72 percent perceive him as handling the administrative side equally well, and 68 percent perceive him as handling the human relations side equally well. At the same time, 9 percent of these respondents perceive their immediate superior as handling the human relations side inadequately (compared to 6 percent for the administrative side, and 3 percent for the technical side). On the whole, then, the immediate superiors of nonsupervisory registered nurses are seen as doing best in technical skill and least well in human relations skill, with administrative skill occupying the middle position. (The difference between technical and human relations skills, based on the data shown in Table 54, is statistically significant at the .01 level.)

The pattern of responses given by the nonsupervisory registered nurses, as it appears in Table 54, moreover, is very similar to that which we find for the remaining respondents. Every group of respondents evaluates its superiors higher on technical skill *than* on administrative skill, and higher on administrative skill *than* on human relations skill. As with the case of nonsupervisory registered nurses, however, the differences among the evaluations of the supervisory skills are not extremely great, except in the case of technician respondents. The technicians' evaluation of their immediate superiors' admin-

TABLE 54. Nonsupervisory Registered Nurses' Evaluation of Their Immediate Superior's Technical, Administrative, and Human Relations Skills

	Respondents from All Hospitals Combined (N = 196)
	(percent)
On the whole, how well does your immediate superior handle the *human relations side* of the job? (This includes....) *	
My immediate superior handles the human relations side of the job	
Extremely well	32 ⎫ 68
Very well	36 ⎭
Fairly well	22
Not so well	8
Not at all well	1
Not ascertained	1
	100
On the whole, how well does your immediate superior handle the *administrative side* of the job? (This includes....) *	
My immediate superior handles the administrative side of the job	
Extremely well	30 ⎫ 72
Very well	42 ⎭
Fairly well	21
Not so well	5
Not at all well	1
Not ascertained	1
	100
On the whole, how well does your immediate superior handle the *purely technical side* of the job? (This includes....) *	
My immediate superior handles the technical side of the job	
Extremely well	43 ⎫ 81
Very well	38 ⎭
Fairly well	15
Not so well	3
Not at all well	0
Not ascertained	1
	100

* The material contained in the parentheses after each question was designed to illustrate and briefly define for the respondents each particular skill (see p. 435).

istrative and human relations skills is perceptibly less favorable by comparison to the evaluations of the other respondent groups: about three-fourths of the laboratory and x-ray technicians (76 percent) in the ten hospitals perceive their immediate superiors as handling the technical side of the job extremely well or very well, but less than half see their superiors as handling the administrative side (49 percent) or the human relations side (45 percent) equally well. Thus, as compared to the other groups of respondents, the technicians are a good deal more critical about the administrative and human relations skills of their immediate superiors.

The Relationship Among Supervisory Skills

According to the above data, people in supervisory-administrative positions in the participating hospitals are generally seen by their immediate subordinates as "strongest" on technical skill and "weakest" on human relations skill, but there is also some variation from one group of respondents to another. The next question that arises logically is whether there is a relationship among the three supervisory skills in the community general hospital. How closely are the three skills interrelated, or how independent are they of each other? Table 55 helps us answer this question. It presents the interrelationships among the technical, administrative, and human relations skills of supervisory personnel at different organizational levels in the ten participating hospitals. The simple rank-order correlations in the upper third part of Table 55 show that, across hospitals, the three supervisory skills are highly and significantly related to one another, regardless of which supervisory level we examine, and in spite of the fact that subordinates at each level tend to evaluate their superior's technical and administrative skills more favorably than his human relations skill. Stated differently, these correlations indicate that hospitals where supervisory personnel are seen by their subordinates as strong on one of the three skills also tend to be seen as strong on each of the other two skills, particularly with respect to technical and administrative skills (rather than any other pair of skills).

Considering the data from supervisory nurses, for example, we find that technical and administrative skills are highly and significantly correlated (.82). Human relations and administrative skills are likewise significantly related (.79). And, the same is true for technical and human relations skills, but to a smaller extent (.61). Considering the data from registered nurses, or the data from practical nurses, we again find that the three skills are significantly interrelated. There are two exceptions to this general pattern, however. First, when the data from department heads (whose immediate superior is the hospital administrator in most cases) are examined, we find that technical and human relations skills correlate only .54, i.e., again they tend to be positively related, but this relationship is not quite significant at the .05 level. Second, when the data from technicians are examined, we find a small positive, but nonsignificant, correlation of .32 between the technical and human relations skills of the technicians' superiors. If, instead of the simple rank-order correlations, we consider the simple tau-correlations (the two sets of correlations refer to the same skills, are based on the same data, and are equivalent expressions of the same interrelationships among the three skills), shown in the middle part of Table 55, the same patterns of findings emerge, as might be expected.

TABLE 55. The Interrelationship Among the Technical, Administrative, and Human Relations Skills of Supervisory Personnel in the Participating Hospitals, Based on Data from Each of Five Groups of Respondents (Subordinates) Who Evaluated the Skills of Their Immediate Superiors *

	Correlations Among the Skills of Their Superiors Based on Data from:			
	Depart- ment Heads	Super- visory Nurses	Nonsuper- visory Registered Nurses	Practical Nurses	Lab and X-ray Technicians
Rank-Order Correlation Between:					
Technical and human relations skills	.54	.61	.73	.85	.32
Technical and administrative skills	.88	.82	.84	.91	.69
Human relations and administrative skills	.61	.79	.67	.94	.61
Tau-Correlation Between:					
Technical and human relations skills	.37	.51	.57	.73	.18
Technical and administrative skills	.76	.71	.73	.76	.49
Human relations and administrative skills	.37	.67	.52	.81	.39
Partial Tau-Correlation Between:					
Technical and human relations (administrative) †	.15	.07	.33	.30	—.01
Technical and administrative (human relations)	.72	.58	.62	.42	.46
Human relations and administrative (technical)	.15	.51	.19	.57	.35

* All correlations are based on an N of 10 hospitals in each case. Rank-order correlations larger than .56 are significant at the .05 level, and those .75 or larger are significant at the .01 level. In general, tau-correlations greater than .39 are significant at the .05 level. No tests of significance exist for partial tau-correlations.

† The expression, "technical and human relations (administrative)," is used to indicate the correlation between technical skill and human relations skill, with the effect of administrative skill being held constant, or with administrative skill having been removed. In the other two sets of partial correlations, human relations skill and, then, technical skill are held constant.

On the whole, apart from the two exceptions noted, the results in Table 55 indicate a rather close association among the three supervisory skills. However, the same results show that technical and administrative skills are the most closely correlated, while technical and human relations skills are the least closely related, with administrative and human relations skills occupying the intermediate position. Furthermore, the relationship among the three skills, taken two at a time, tends to vary from one level of supervision to another. It is clear from the simple rank-order and simple tau-correlations, for example, that the three skills are most highly interrelated when using data from the practical nurses group of respondents about their superiors, and least highly related when using data from the technicians about their superiors. The data from department heads show almost the same pattern as the data from the technicians, in this respect; and the data from supervisory nurses and from registered nurses show an intermediate relational pattern—intermediate to that produced by data from practical nurses, on the one hand, and data from technicians or from department heads, on the other. The simple correlations in Table 55 are also interesting from another point of view: looking at the relationships among the three skills based on data from the three nursing groups, we can see that the relationship between technical and human relations skills decreases as we move up the hierarchy, i.e., going from practical, through registered, to supervisory nurses, and the same tends to be true for the relationship between technical and administrative skills.

The above results are consistent with our earlier theoretical suggestion that the combination of skills (skill-mix) appropriate, or required, at one organizational level is expected to differ from its counterpart at other levels. At the same time, however, the relationships obtained among the three skills are rather high in most cases. This raises a question of whether the superiors who are doing an effective job (in terms of the three skills) in the eyes of their subordinates in the various hospitals are actually competent in all three skills, or whether the respondents did not differentiate sufficiently among the three supervisory skills in their evaluations of them.

Respondent Discrimination Among the Three Supervisory Skills

While it is not possible, within the limitations of a sample of only ten hospitals, to answer the question of how discriminating the respondents were in their separate evaluations of the three supervisory skills precisely and definitively, certain evidence suggests that most of the respondents differentiated fairly well among the three skills. First, the simple correlations in Table 55 show that for two of the five groups of respondents—department heads and technicians—the relationships among the three skills, taken two at a time, are neither unexpectedly high (in two cases they are not even statistically significant, as earlier noted) nor consistently high. This indicates that department heads and technicians from the participating hospitals discriminated among the three skills of their respective superiors. Second, the patterns of correlations based on data from supervisory nurses and from registered nurses indicate that these two groups also discriminated among the three supervisory skills, although not to the same extent as department heads or technicians did.

In the case of the practical nurses group, however, the pertinent correlations appear to show little discrimination by the respondents; here the correlations among the three skills are both high and of about the same size. This relative lack of discrimination may in part be due to our earlier finding that supervision for the practical nurses group is considerably more diffuse and heterogeneous (practical nurses named people from several different levels as their immediate superiors), and in part to the inability of these respondents to comprehend the questions about the three skills of their superiors adequately (this being consistent with the educational level and other characteristics of these respondents, as presented in Chap. 3). At any rate, whatever the reason for the absence of discrimination in this case, the results suggest that the data about supervisory skills from practical nurses should be viewed with caution and treated accordingly. As a matter of fact, in this chapter we shall not present the results of all analyses which involve the evaluation of the three skills by practical nurses because of this problem of conceptual discrimination. (In this connection, the reader may also recall that most analyses in previous chapters do not involve data from practical nurses, partly because of the same reasons discussed here.)

On the whole, the preceding evidence suggests that interskill discrimination is not a serious issue, since department heads, supervisory nurses, registered nurses, and technicians apparently distinguished quite well among the technical, administrative, and human relations skills of their superiors (seemingly, only practical nurses did not distinguish sufficiently). These results, moreover, are in line with similar findings from a study of supervision in power plants, where Mann and Hoffman (23) found that workers could distinguish among the three supervisory skills under consideration, as well as with findings from a study of supervision in an office situation, where Mann and Williams (25) found that subordinates could distinguish among the technical, administrative, and human relations skills of their superiors (the measures of supervisory skills used in these two studies are very similar to those in the present study).

Certain additional evidence from the present study reinforces the conclusion that respondents discriminated sufficiently among the three supervisory skills in their evaluations. This evidence derives from an analysis of the answers of individual respondents to our three questions about the supervisory skills of their superiors. In this analysis, we intercorrelated the answers to the three questions given by all individual respondents belonging to each of the five groups, regardless of the hospitals involved, i.e., for each respondent group separately, but using data from all individual respondents and all hospitals combined. Instead of using the hospital as the unit of analysis, here we used the individual respondent as the unit of analysis (we also used product-moment correlations rather than rank-order correlations, since the N was quite large in every case, but this is immaterial for the purpose at hand).

This individual-level analysis yielded results that are comparable to the results shown in Table 55, insofar as interskill discrimination on the part of respondents is concerned. For example, using data from department heads, we find that the correlation between their evaluations of technical and human relations skills is .30; between technical and administrative skills it is .27; and between human relations and administrative skills it is .54. Similarly, using data from nonsupervisory registered nurses, the corresponding correlations are .53, .62, and .66, respectively. The corresponding correlations based on data from technicians and from supervisory nurses are similar to the ones based on data from department heads and from registered nurses. But, the relevant correlations based on data from practical nurses are higher on the average (respectively being .65, .70, and .82). These results provide added support for the interpretation that four of the five respondent groups involved discriminate quite well among the three supervisory skills, while practical nurses—the fifth group—may not be discriminating sufficiently.

Finally, the partial tau-correlations among the three supervisory skills that are shown in the lower third part of Table 55, provide some more supportive evidence. But, before reviewing these correlations, let us briefly discuss their meaning and the reasons for using them here. First, having found direct and significant relationships among the three supervisory skills, examined two at a time and with reference to different levels of supervision in the participating hospitals (these relationships are shown by the simple rank-order and tau-correlations in Table 55), we would also like to know how the relationship between any two of the three skills is affected, or influenced, by the third skill at each supervisory level. This may be ascertained through the use of partial correlation techniques. When the interrelationship among three variables (in the present case, skills) is known in the form of simple correlations, then, by computing partial correlations, it is possible to isolate the influence that any one of the three variables has upon the simple relationship between the other two variables. In effect, we can ascertain the relationship between two variables (e.g., between technical and human relations skills), with the effects of the third variable (e.g., the effects of administrative skill) being eliminated or, in technical terms, "partialled out" statistically.

Now, while it is not appropriate to compute partial correlations from simple rank-order correlations when dealing with a small N (in the present case the N being equal to 10 hospitals), it is feasible to use partial tau-correlations, i.e., to compute partial correlations from the simple tau-correlations available, as we have done. (For a relevant discussion of the appropriateness of this technique, see Siegel [29].) The lower third of Table 55

Supervisory Skills at Different Levels

presents the partial tau-correlations relevant to each pair of supervisory skills, based on data from each of the five groups of respondents involved. These partial correlations serve two purposes: (1) they provide some pertinent evidence about the issue of interskill discrimination on the part of respondents, and (2) they show, for each supervisory level, the relationship characterizing each pair of supervisory skills when the effects of the third skill are removed. This latter relationship provides us with a clue as to the skill-mix which prevails at each supervisory level in the community general hospital.

Concerning interskill discrimination, and other things being equal, the smaller the partial correlations are, the more they suggest that respondents distinguish among the three supervisory skills—technical, administrative, and human relations skills. Examining Table 55, we note, in this connection, that the partial correlation between technical and human relations skills, with the effects of administrative skill removed, is .33 when using data from registered nurses (the corresponding simple tau-correlation between technical and human relations skills is, of course, much higher—as shown in Table 55, it is .57). Similarly, using data from the same respondents, we note that the partial correlation between human relations and administrative skills, with the effects of technical skill eliminated, is only .19 (again, considerably smaller than the corresponding simple tau-correlation, which is .52). These two partial tau-correlations indicate that the human relations skills of the registered nurses' superiors are relatively independent of both the technical and the administrative skills of these superiors. In addition, they suggest that the registered nurses in the participating hospitals distinguish very well between the two skills in each of the two pairs of skills to which the partial correlations refer, i.e., between the technical and human relations skills, and between the administrative and human relations skills of their superiors. On the other hand, the moderately high partial correlation of .62 between technical and administrative skills (with human relations skills partialled out), which is also based on data from registered nurses, suggests that registered nurses do not discriminate as highly between the technical and administrative skills of their superiors as they do between the technical and human relations skills or between the administrative and human relations skills of their superiors.

This pattern of interskill discrimination on the part of registered nurses, suggested by the partial correlations in Table 55, moreover, is very similar to the corresponding pattern obtained in connection with each of the other groups of respondents except the practical nurses group. Respondents from each group seem to distinguish fairly well among the three supervisory skills; but they distinguish least well between the technical and administrative skills of their superiors (except for practical nurses, who distinguish least well between the administrative and human relations skills of their superiors).

The partial correlations among the three supervisory skills in Table 55 also show the relationship for each pair of supervisory skills, at different levels of supervision, with the effects of the third skill statistically removed. These relationships may now be summarized. First, when the effects of administrative skill are held constant, the relationship between technical and human relations skills in the participating hospitals is *very small* at each supervisory level (.15 based on data from department heads, .07 based on data from supervisory nurses, .33 based on data from registered nurses, .30 based on data from practical nurses, and —.01 based on data from technicians), indicating that human relations skills are independent of technical skills, and vice versa. There is, of course, some variation across supervisory levels in this connection, as the above partial correlations show.

Second, when the effects of technical skill are eliminated, the relationship between human relations and administrative skills in the participating hospitals is *small to moderate*, depending upon the supervisory level considered: based on data from department heads, for example, the partial correlation is only .15, while based on data from supervisory nurses it is .51; in the former case, human relations and administrative skills are fairly independent of each other, while in the latter case they are interrelated to a moderate degree. And third, when the effects of human relations skill are removed, the relationship between technical and administrative skills in the participating hospitals is *moderate to high* (ranging between .42 and .72), again depending upon the supervisory level considered; the relationship is highest when we consider the data from department heads, whose immediate superiors are the hospital administrators. Even in this latter case, however, the correlation is not so high as to suggest that technical and administrative skills are the same (the correlation of .72 explains only half of the variance involved). At the same time, of course, technical and administrative skills are much more closely interrelated than are technical and human relations skills, or administrative and human relations skills, according to the obtained results.[2]

SUPERVISORY SKILLS AND THE SATISFACTION OF SUBORDINATES WITH THEIR SUPERIORS AT DIFFERENT LEVELS OF SUPERVISION

In the preceding section we found that human relations skills at different levels of supervision are generally independent from both technical and administrative skills, and that the respondents discriminated rather well among the three skills (except for practical nurses), this discrimination being highest between technical and human relations skills. Based on these findings, it

[2] The conclusions stated in this paragraph are based on a comparative examination of the relative size of the partial tau-correlations involved, and not on the statistical significance of these correlations or of the differences among them. Unfortunately, the sampling distribution of partial tau-correlations is unknown and, consequently, no tests of significance are available in this case. For a detailed discussion of this problem, see Siegel (29).

Supervisory Skills and Subordinate Satisfaction

is now possible to ascertain how each of the three skills of supervisory personnel in the hospitals studied relates to the satisfaction of subordinates with supervision. Is the employees' satisfaction with supervision dependent upon any of the three supervisory skills, and, if so, is it more dependent upon technical, administrative, or human relations skills? Furthermore, are there any differences across supervisory levels in this connection?

To answer these questions, in addition to the measures of the three supervisory skills, we need a measure of subordinate satisfaction with supervision. The latter measure was derived from questionnaire data, separately for each of the five groups of respondents involved (department heads, supervisory nurses, nonsupervisory registered nurses, practical nurses, and technicians), and separately for each participating hospital. Specifically, we used the arithmetic mean of the answers each group of respondents, from each hospital, gave to this question: "Taking all things into consideration, how satisfied are you with your *immediate superior?*" The response alternatives offered by the question form the familiar five-point scale and are shown below, together with the percentage distribution of the answers of nonsupervisory registered nurses from the ten hospitals combined.

Taking all things into consideration, how satisfied are you with your *immediate superior?* (Check one.)

	(percent)
I am completely satisfied with my immediate superior	39 ⎫ 72
I am very well satisfied	33 ⎭
I am fairly well satisfied	20
I am somewhat dissatisfied	7
I am dissatisfied with my immediate superior	1
Not ascertained	0
	100
	($N = 196$)

It can be seen from this tabulation that almost four out of every ten nonsupervisory registered nurses in the participating hospitals are completely satisfied with their respective immediate superior, and another three in ten are very well satisfied. At the same time, however, 8 percent of these professional nurses express some dissatisfaction. Across individual hospitals, of course, there are considerable differences in subordinate satisfaction with supervision. But, for all hospitals combined, 72 percent of the nonsupervisory registered nurses are very well or completely satisfied with their immediate superiors. The corresponding percentage figure for the remaining groups of respondents is 91 percent for department heads, 82 percent for practical nurses, 74 percent for supervisory nurses, and 60 percent for technicians. These results, as in many other instances reported in previous chapters, also indicate that, as a group, the technicians are the most critical of their immediate superiors, followed by the nonsupervisory registered nurses. The department heads are the least critical (or most favorable), followed by the practical nurses in this respect.

Concerning the relationship between the satisfaction of respondents with their immediate superiors in the participating hospitals and the three supervisory skills studied, Table 56 provides the answer. The simple rank-order and simple tau-correlations in Table 56 show the relationship between each supervisory skill and subordinate satisfaction with supervision for each group of respondents, or at each supervisory level, in the ten hospitals. The partial tau-correlations show the relationship between satisfaction with supervision and each supervisory skill, when the effects of the other two supervisory skills have been removed (partialled out) from it, i.e., they show the relationship in a "purer" form.

It is clear from the simple correlations in Table 56 that: (1) The higher the technical skill of supervisory personnel, the higher the satisfaction of subordinates with supervision in the various hospitals; this relationship obtains at all supervisory levels, except for the case of practical nurses, who are not significantly more satisfied with their superiors in hospitals where they evaluate their superiors more highly on technical skill. (2) The higher the human relations skill of supervisory personnel at different levels, the higher the satisfaction of subordinates with their superior in the various hospitals, excepting again the case of practical nurses. (3) A similar significant relationship exists between the administrative skill of supervisors and the satisfaction of their subordinates with supervision, based on data from department heads, supervisory nurses, and nonsupervisory registered nurses, but not according to data from practical nurses or technicians.

In general, then, apart from the case of practical nurses (the group that was earlier found to distinguish least well among the three supervisory skills), we find, without much surprise, that each of the three supervisory skills relates positively and significantly to the satisfaction of subordinates with their immediate superiors in the hospitals studied. As we are about to see from the partial tau-correlations in Table 56, however, the three supervisory skills do not contribute equally to the satisfaction of subordinates with supervision. And satisfaction with supervision is not determined to the same degree by the same supervisory skill at all organizational levels. These, of course, are the most interesting of the findings concerning the relationship between supervisory skills and subordinate satisfaction with supervision, consistent with our earlier theoretical expectations.

When the relationship between technical skill and satisfaction is analyzed with the effects of administrative and human relations skills removed from it, we find that it becomes drastically reduced for all levels of supervision, ex-

TABLE 56. The Relationship Between the Skills of Supervisory Personnel, as Evaluated by Immediate Subordinates and the Satisfaction of Subordinates with Their Immediate Superior, Based on Data from Each of Five Groups of Respondents (Subordinates) in the Participating Hospitals *

Correlations between Supervisory Skills and the Satisfaction of Subordinates with Their Superior Based on Data from:

	Department Heads	Supervisory Nurses	Nonsupervisory Registered Nurses	Practical Nurses	Lab and X-ray Technicians
Rank-Order Correlation Between:					
Technical skill and satisfaction	.82	.66	.68	.44	.68
Administrative skill and satisfaction	.93	.74	.62	.22	.50
Human relations skill and satisfaction	.66	.93	.67	.29	.76
Tau-Correlation Between:					
Technical skill and satisfaction	.64	.51	.58	.29	.54
Administrative skill and satisfaction	.85	.58	.49	.13	.33
Human relations skill and satisfaction	.48	.82	.58	.20	.57
Partial Tau-Correlation Between:					
Technical skill and satisfaction (administrative and human relations) †	—.07	.18	.27	.26	.54
Administrative skill and satisfaction (technical and human relations)	.73	—.04	.06	.17	.15
Human relations skill and satisfaction (technical and administrative)	.34	.71	.36	.11	.56

* All correlations are based on an N of 10 hospitals in each case. Rank-order correlations larger than .56 are significant at the .05 level, and those .75 or larger are significant at the .01 level. In general, tau-correlations greater than .39 are significant at the .05 level. No tests of significance exist for partial tau-correlations.

† The expression, "technical skill and satisfaction (administrative and human relations)" is used to indicate the correlation between the technical skill of superiors and the satisfaction of subordinates, when the administrative and human relations skills of superiors are held constant. The other two sets of partial correlations show the relationship between administrative skill and satisfaction when technical and human relations skills are held constant, and the relationship between human relations skill and satisfaction when technical and administrative skills are held constant.

cept the level to which data from the technicians refer. According to the partial tau-correlations in the lower third of Table 56, for example, we find that the correlation between the satisfaction of department heads with their immediate superiors (administrators) in the participating hospitals and the technical skill of their superiors becomes —.07, when the effects of administrative and human relations skills are partialled out. For all practical purposes, this relationship is equivalent to zero. At the other extreme, the comparable partial correlation when we consider data from the technicians is .54, which indicates that the satisfaction of technicians with their immediate superiors in the participating hospitals depends a great deal upon the technical skill of their superiors (as evaluated by the technicians themselves). The comparable findings based on data from supervisory nurses, nonsupervisory registered nurses, and practical nurses occupy an intermediate position. They show some relationship between technical supervisory skill and subordinate satisfaction with supervision, when the influence of human relations and administrative skills is controlled, but the relationship is very small.

Similarly, when the relationship between administrative skill and satisfaction is further analyzed, with the effects of technical and human relations skills removed from it, it also is sharply reduced at all levels of supervision, with the rather outstanding exception of the very top level. When we consider the data from department heads, we find a strong partial correlation of .73 between the administrative skill of the department heads' superior (the administrator) and department head satisfaction with supervision in the hospitals studied. This means that satisfaction with supervision at this top level is determined substantially by the administrative skill of the hospital administrators involved. But this finding constitutes the exception rather than the rule, when all of the supervisory levels are examined. For the remaining levels, there is practically no relationship between administrative skill and satisfaction when the effects of technical and human relations skills are controlled.

Finally, when the relationship between human relations skill and satisfaction with supervision is similarly analyzed, with the effects of technical and administrative skills removed from it, the pattern of findings is different from the above patterns. For three of the five supervisory levels involved, the partial correlations in Table 56 show that human relations skill primarily determines the satisfaction of subordinates with their immediate superior in the participating hospitals—supervisory nurses, nonsupervisory registered nurses, and technicians being the relevant groups of subordinates. However, the degree to which subordinate satisfaction with supervision in the hospitals studied is determined by the human relations skill of supervisory personnel (with administrative and technical skills controlled) varies considerably from one level of supervision to another: the appropriate partial correlation between human relations skill and satisfaction is .71 based on data from supervisory nurses,

.56 based on data from technicians, and only .36 based on data from registered nurses. The corresponding correlations based on data from department heads and from practical nurses—the two groups for which human relations skill is not the primary determinant of satisfaction with supervision—are .34 and .11, respectively. The primary determinant of satisfaction with supervision in the case of department heads is the administrative skill of their superiors. In the case of practical nurses, none of the three skills shows an appreciable relationship to satisfaction when the effects of the other two skills are partialled out. Perhaps this is due to the fact that, of the five respondent groups, practical nurses discriminated the least among the three skills.

Supervisory Skills as Determinants of Subordinate Satisfaction with Supervision at Different Levels

As anticipated, the findings from this part of the study have shown that the technical, administrative, and human relations skills of supervisory-administrative personnel in the ten hospitals are related, in certain ways, to the overall satisfaction of subordinates with supervision. In general, employees are more satisfied with their immediate superiors in hospitals where they evaluate their superiors as more highly skilled in the human relations, administrative, and technical areas. Also, as expected, however, the findings have shown that the extent to which each of the three supervisory skills contributes to the satisfaction of subordinates with supervision varies considerably from one organizational level to another. This variation indicates that, from the standpoint of the criterion of satisfaction with supervision, a different supervisory skill-mix is important, or required, for different levels of supervision in the hospitals studied.

The findings from the data supplied by administrative department heads in the ten hospitals clearly show that the overall satisfaction of department heads with the administrator (their immediate superior) is mainly dependent upon their estimate of the latter's administrative skill. The administrator's technical skill has no bearing whatsoever upon the satisfaction of the department heads, if the effects of administrative and human relations skills are controlled for. The human relations skill of the administrator accounts for only a small portion of the satisfaction of his subordinates with him, when his administrative and technical skills are held constant. Thus, insofar as subordinate satisfaction with supervision is concerned, the most important element in the skill-mix of hospital administrators is administrative competence and not technical or human relations competence. The satisfaction of department heads with the administrator, in other words, depends upon the administrator's ability to plan, organize, and coordinate, and his ability to assign the right people to the proper job, and give them the right authority and responsibility to do their job. But, administrative skill is the primary determinant of subordinate satisfaction with supervision only at this top level in the hospital organization.

For supervisory nurses, general satisfaction with supervision is mainly determined by the human relations skill of their respective superiors, according to the findings. (In this connection, it will be recalled that half the supervisory nurses named the director of nursing as their immediate superior, and the rest named other nursing personnel in top positions.) Administrative skill is totally unrelated to satisfaction at this level, when technical and human relations skills are held constant. And technical skill accounts for only a negligible portion of subordinate satisfaction, when human relations and administrative skills are controlled for. In short, supervisory nurses are more satisfied with their immediate superiors in hospitals where they evaluate their immediate superior highly on human relations skill. At this level, the superior's competence in getting people to work together and do the best they can, in giving recognition and appreciation for good work done, in letting people know where they stand, and the like is the most important element in the supervisory skill-mix, from the point of subordinate satisfaction with supervision.

In the case of nonsupervisory registered nurses, none of the three supervisory skills accounts for a high portion of their general satisfaction with their immediate superior (a member of the above group of supervisory nurses) in the participating hospitals, when the influence of the other two skills has been partialled out. Human relations skill appears as the most important determinant of subordinate satisfaction with supervision at this level (as in the case of supervisory nurses), but the relevant partial correlation is rather small (.36); administrative skill, as in the case of supervisory nurses, shows no relationship at all (.06) to subordinate satisfaction; and technical skill is of intermediate importance (.27). Apparently, the satisfaction of nonsupervisory registered nurses with their immediate superiors in the various hospitals depends only to a moderate degree upon the supervisory skills investigated.

In the case of practical nurses (for which the findings must be viewed with caution for the reasons discussed earlier), we again find only a very small relationship between each of the three supervisory skills and satisfaction with supervision (even smaller than in the case of registered nurses), when the other two skills are partialled out. Among the three supervisory skills, the dominant skill at this level, from the standpoint of satisfaction with supervision, seems to be technical skill; but the relationship between technical skill and satisfaction is still a very weak one (.26). The emphasis on technical skill at this level is, of course, consistent with what might have been anticipated. For practical nurses, the immediate superiors are the highly trained professional nurses (either nonsupervisory registered nurses or supervisory nurses). The gap in technical skill between supervisory nurses and nonsupervisory registered nurses is minimal (if any), while the gap between professional nurses and practical nurses is very great. Apparently, practical nurses are quite cognizant of their technical limitations vis-à-vis professional nurses, and not only are they sensitive on this but are probably also anxious to learn and improve their own technical skill. Consequently, it is not surprising that technical competence—more than administrative or human relations competence—is the type of leadership skill that practical nurses may want most in their immediate superiors.

Finally, the relationship between supervisory skills and satisfaction with supervision in the case of laboratory and x-ray technicians in the ten hospitals shows a rather interesting pattern. First, it may be recalled that, of the five groups of respondents, technicians constitute the group least satisfied with supervision (as well as with other aspects of their job). Second, it will also be remembered that the simple correlations in Table 56 showed a significant relationship between the satisfaction of technicians with their immediate superiors and their superiors' technical and human relations skills, but not with their superiors' administrative skill. Third, and perhaps most interestingly, the partial correlations in Table 56 clearly confirmed this same relational pattern. According to this pattern, the satisfaction of technicians with their immediate superior is unaffected by the latter's administrative skill, when the effects of the other two skills are removed by partial correlations—even though over 40 percent of the technicians named the director of the laboratory or of x-ray as their immediate superior, i.e., they named a doctor who also has a good deal of administrative responsibility. By contrast, the satisfaction of technicians is very much affected by both the human relations skill and the technical skill of their superior (when each skill is related to satisfaction with the effects of the other two skills removed), but it is affected almost equally by each, unlike what we have found above for the other groups of respondents.

Thus, the supervisory skill-mix most conducive to the overall satisfaction of technicians with their immediate superior in the community general hospital is human relations skill plus technical skill. The fact that satisfaction with supervision at this level is determined a good deal by the human relations skill of superiors is entirely consistent with the findings concerning the relationship between human relations skill and subordinate satisfaction for supervisory nurses, nonsupervisory nurses, and, to an extent, department heads also. Furthermore, it is in agreement with our earlier theoretical expectation that human relations skill, among the three supervisory skills, is probably of importance at all, or nearly all, supervisory levels. The fact that satisfaction with supervision on the part of technicians is also importantly (and about equally) affected by the technical skill of their superiors can be explained by taking into account the role of technicians in the community general hospital, and the nature of the superior-subordinate relationship in the laboratory and x-ray.

Technicians work in the laboratory or in x-ray, both of which are typically isolated geographically from most other units of the hospital. As their title suggests, the technicians' role is mainly a technical one, and the tasks they perform tend to be more routine, more specifically prescribed, and more predictable than is the case for the other groups of respondents. At the same time, technicians are supervised either directly by the heads of the laboratory and x-ray, who are medical specialists (doctors) in pathology and radiology, or by a chief technician (or senior technician) to whom supervisory responsibility is delegated by the head of the department or by the hospital. Under these circumstances, the emphasis is upon the technical requirements of the job in these departments. In addition, the laboratory and the x-ray are relatively small departments, and the technical competence of each individual member—subordinate as well as superior—is highly visible to all, apart from the fact that it can also be, and usually is, regularly tested in the day-to-day work. The importance of supervisory technical skill as a determinant of the satisfaction of technicians with their supervisors becomes very clear and very meaningful in this context.

SPECIFIC SUPERVISORY PRACTICES, AS THEY RELATE TO SUPERVISORY SKILLS AND TO THE SATISFACTION OF SUBORDINATES WITH SUPERVISION AT DIFFERENT ORGANIZATIONAL LEVELS

We have seen how the technical, administrative, and human relations skills of supervisory personnel at various levels relate (1) to each other, and (2) to the general satisfaction of subordinates with their immediate superior in the hospitals studied. The next question we wish to consider is whether, and to what extent, certain specific aspects of the behavior of supervisory personnel, as perceived by subordinates, relate to the three supervisory skills and the satisfaction of subordinates with supervision. The specific supervisory practices and characteristics to be examined in this connection concern the nature of the superior-subordinate relationship which prevails at each supervisory level in the participating hospitals.

Much previous research in industrial settings has shown that the degree to which supervisors are meeting the needs of employees, as perceived by the latter, is related to the satisfaction of employees with their supervisors and the organization, and, under certain conditions, to performance as well. To determine whether this might be also true of the hospital situation, we obtained data about certain supervisory practices and characteristics that provide an indication of how well supervisory personnel in the hospitals studied are meeting some of the needs of their subordinates. These data were then related to the skills of supervisory personnel and the satisfaction of subordinates with supervision, in the present section, and to patient care and organizational coordination, in subsequent sections.

Nine questions were used to collect relevant data for the measurement of as many specific supervisory practices or characteristics. The questions were asked of department heads, supervisory nurses, nonsupervisory registered nurses, practical nurses, nurse's aides, and laboratory and x-ray technicians from each hospital about their respective superiors. The questions were:

1. How well do you think your immediate superior understands the employees' viewpoint? (Check one.)
   _____(1) Has complete understanding of how employees think and feel
   _____(2) A very good understanding
   _____(3) A good understanding
   _____(4) A fair understanding
   _____(5) Has a rather poor understanding of how employees think or feel.

2. How good is your immediate superior in dealing with people? (Check one.)
   _____(1) Excellent in dealing with people
   _____(2) Very good
   _____(3) Good
   _____(4) Fair
   _____(5) Rather poor
   _____(6) Poor
   _____(7) Very poor in dealing with people.

3. How free do you feel to discuss personal problems with your immediate superior? (Check one.)
   _____(1) I always feel free to discuss personal problems with my immediate superior
   _____(2) I usually feel free
   _____(3) Sometimes I feel free
   _____(4) Only once in a while I feel free
   _____(5) I never feel free to discuss personal problems with my immediate superior.

4. How often does your immediate superior express appreciation for your work? (Check one.)
   _____(1) Always or nearly always expresses appreciation for my work
   _____(2) Very often
   _____(3) Often
   _____(4) Sometimes
   _____(5) Seldom or never expresses appreciation for my work.

5. Does your immediate superior ask your opinion when a problem comes up that involves your work? (Check one.)
   _____(1) Always or nearly always asks my opinion
   _____(2) Very often
   _____(3) Often
   _____(4) Sometimes
   _____(5) Seldom or never asks my opinion.

6. How often does your immediate superior tell you in advance about any changes that affect your work? (Check one.)
    _____(1) Always or nearly always tells me in advance about any changes that affect me or my work
    _____(2) More often than not
    _____(3) Sometimes
    _____(4) Seldom
    _____(5) Never tells me in advance about any changes that affect me or my work.

7. How good is your immediate superior in planning, organizing, and scheduling the work? (Check one.)
    _____(1) Excellent in planning, organizing, and scheduling the work
    _____(2) Very good
    _____(3) Good
    _____(4) Fair
    _____(5) Rather poor
    _____(6) Poor
    _____(7) Very poor in planning, organizing, and scheduling the work.

8. How sure are you of what your immediate superior thinks of you and your work? (Check one.)
    _____(1) I am very sure of what my immediate superior thinks of me and my work
    _____(2) Quite sure
    _____(3) Fairly sure
    _____(4) Not too sure
    _____(5) I am not sure at all of what my immediate superior thinks of me and my work.

9. If you have a suggestion for improving the job or changing the setup in some way, how easy is it for you to get your ideas across to your superiors? (Check one.)
    _____(1) It is very difficult to get my ideas across to my superiors
    _____(2) It is rather difficult
    _____(3) It is not too easy
    _____(4) It is fairly easy
    _____(5) It is very easy to get my ideas across to my superiors.

The nine questions were not all asked consecutively, or in the order indicated above, in the different questionnaire forms. The first question, designed to ascertain how adequately supervisory personnel at each level understand the viewpoint of their subordinates, was worded somewhat differently for department heads: "How well do you think your immediate superior understands the viewpoint of people at your level?" The second question asked respondents to evaluate their superior's skill in dealing with people. It was a "check question" expected to yield data that should correlate highly with our earlier measure of supervisory skill in human relations—which proved to be the case (see Tables 57, 58, 59, and 60). The seventh question in the series, about how good the immediate superior is in planning, organizing, and scheduling the work, was also a "check question" expected to provide data that would correlate highly with our earlier measures of technical and administrative skills, depending upon the supervisory level involved. The remaining six questions were all designed to yield information about different aspects of the communication climate between superior and subordinates at each level (for additional aspects of communication investigated in the research, see Chap. 10).

The third and the ninth of the above questions deal with the ease with which subordinates feel they can discuss their problems with their superiors, including ideas that they may have about changing or improving the work situation. The fourth, fifth, and sixth questions—about expressing appreciation, asking subordinates their opinion on work problems, and informing subordinates in advance of changes that affect their work—all deal with communication initiated by the superior. The eighth question—about how sure the respondent is of what his superior thinks about him or his work—also presupposes communication that is probably initiated by the superior, but it asks the respondent to estimate how sure he is of where he stands vis-à-vis his superior, rather than how frequently his superior tells him where he stands. This particular question was not asked of department heads, since it was felt that people at this top organizational level would generally know where they stand with their immediate superior (i.e., the hospital administrator) in each hospital; they are in close and frequent contact with him.

As with previous questions in the area of supervision, all except the last of the nine questions concerning supervisory practices and characteristics refer to the respondent's immediate superior in every case. The last question, however, has as its referent all individuals whom the respondent considers as his superiors, for there are usually no restrictions as to what supervisory personnel are appropriate when a respondent is attempting to get his ideas across. This question is also different from the other eight in that the response alternatives which it provides form an inverted scale (from unfavorable to more favorable alternatives) by comparison. This was taken into account in computing our measures by inverting the scale for this question, so that all measures as finally derived from the data are comparable. Finally, with reference to each of the nine questions, each group of respondents, and each hospital involved, the arithmetic mean was computed from the data to serve as the measure of each supervisory practice or characteristic studied.

How each of the nine supervisory practices and characteristics relates to (1) the technical, administrative, and human relations skills of supervisory personnel, and (2) the overall satisfaction of subordinates with supervision, at each level in the ten participating hospitals, is shown in Tables 57, 58, 59, and 60, below. (The measures of the three supervisory skills and of subordinate satisfaction with supervision are the same as those discussed in the preceding sections of this chapter.) Table 57 presents the relevant findings based on data from department heads in the ten hospitals; Table 58 presents corresponding results based on data from supervisory nurses; Table 59 presents the results based on data from nonsupervisory registered nurses; and Table 60 presents the results based on data from the technicians. The data from practical nurses and aides are not presented in tabular form, but are discussed later in this section. Most of the findings in this series, because of their rather repetitive and detailed nature, have been summarized at the end of the section, and the reader may first wish to read this integrative summary, and then return to consider the results in greater detail.

Results Concerning Supervision of Department Heads

As shown in Table 57, using data from department heads, we find that some supervisory characteristics are significantly related to the three supervisory skills of the hospital administrators (who are the immediate superiors of department heads), and to the satisfaction of department heads with their administrator, while others are not. Furthermore, the specific characteristics which are related most highly to the human relations, technical, and administrative skills of the administrators are not the same for all three skills. Of the eight supervisory practices and characteristics examined at this level, five are significantly related to the human relations skill of administrators, three are significantly related to the technical skill of administrators, and three are related to the administrative skill of administrators. Similarly, four of the eight supervisory characteristics are significantly related to the satisfaction of department heads with their respective administrators in the various hospitals.

The two supervisory practices or characteristics that relate most closely to the human relations skill of administrators are: how good the administrator is in dealing with people (.87), and how often the administrator expresses appreciation to department heads for their work (.87). The two that relate most closely to the technical skill of administrators are: how good the administrator is in planning and organizing (.88), and the extent to which the administrator understands the viewpoint of his department heads (.69). And the two that relate most highly to the administrative skill of administrators are: the extent to which the administrator understands the viewpoint of his department heads (.84), and the ease with which the department heads can get their ideas across to the administrator (.79). Finally, the two supervisory practices or characteristics of administrators that relate most highly to the overall satisfaction of department heads with supervision (with the administrator) in the various hospitals are: the extent to which the administrator understands the viewpoint of department heads (.89), and the ease with which department heads can get their ideas across to the administrator (.72)—the same two items that relate most highly to the administrative skill of the hospital administrators. This finding is, of course, completely consistent with the earlier finding that of the three supervisory skills—technical, administrative, and human relations —the superior's administrative skill is the primary determinant of satisfaction with supervision at the department-head level.

TABLE 57. **The Relationship of Specific Supervisory Characteristics, as Perceived by** *Administrative Department Heads* **About Their Superior, to Certain Supervisory Skills and to the Satisfaction of Department Heads with Their Immediate Superior in the Participating Hospitals** *

(Correlations Are Based on Data from Administrative Department Heads in Each Hospital)

Specific Characteristics of Immediate Superior	Human Relations	Technical	Administrative	Overall Satisfaction of Department Heads with Their Immediate Superior
Superior understands the viewpoint of his subordinates	.82	.69	.84	.89
Superior is good in dealing with people	.87	.40	.43	.58
Subordinates feel free to discuss personal problems with superior	.69	.15	.32	.50
Superior expresses appreciation	.87	.24	.31	.42
Superior asks subordinates' opinion about work problems	.31	.09	.17	.22
Superior tells subordinates in advance about changes	.45	.28	.33	.42
Superior is good at planning, organizing, and scheduling work	.16	.88	.74	.67
Superior lets subordinates know where they stand	—not asked—			
Superior makes it easy for subordinates to get their ideas across	.71	.68	.79	.72

* All figures are rank-order correlations, based on an N of 10 hospitals in each case. Correlations larger than .56 are significant at the .05 level, and those .75 or larger are significant at the .01 level.

Of the eight practices and characteristics of hospital administrators appearing in Table 57, the one that relates most highly and significantly to all three supervisory skills, and to the satisfaction of department heads with supervision, is the extent to which the administrators in the various hospitals understand the viewpoint of their respective department heads. Only one more of the eight items relates significantly both to the three supervisory skills of administrators and to the satisfaction of department heads with the administrator —the ease with which department heads feel that they can get their ideas and suggestions across to their respective superiors, i.e., the administrators. It is also worth noting that, with one exception, the three items that reflect direct initiation of communication on the part of administrators toward the department heads—expressing appreciation for good work, asking subordinates their opinion about work problems, and informing subordinates in advance of changes that affect their work—do not relate significantly to the three supervisory skills of administrators nor to the satisfaction of department heads with supervision. Communication practices such as these are probably taken for granted at this top level in the hospital organization. The one exception is that expressing appreciation is highly related to human relations skill.

Finally, it can be seen from the results in Table 57 that the satisfaction of department heads with their respective administrators is not significantly related to how frequently the administrator expresses appreciation, asks opinion, or informs department heads of changes in advance, or to how free department heads feel to discuss personal problems with the administrator. On the other hand, department heads are significantly more satisfied with the administrator in hospitals where the administrator understands their viewpoint, is good in dealing with people, and is good at planning and organizing, and where department heads feel that it is easy for them to get their ideas and suggestions across to the administrator (their superiors).

Results Concerning Supervision of Supervisory Nurses

The counterpart of the above findings for the top nursing level in the community general hospital is presented in Table 58, which contains results based on data from the supervisory nurses in the participating hospitals. It is clear from these results that:

1. All but two (superior lets subordinates know where they stand, and superior expresses appreciation) of the nine specific supervisory practices and characteristics, perceived by supervisory nurses in their respective immediate superiors in the hospitals studied, are significantly related to the human relations skill of their superiors.

2. By contrast, only two of the same nine characteristics—the extent to which supervisory nurses feel it is easy for them to get their ideas across to their superiors, and the extent to which their superiors understand their viewpoint—are significantly related to the technical skill of their superiors in the hospitals studied.

3. Of the nine supervisory practices and characteristics attributed by supervisory nurses to their immediate superiors in the various hospitals, five are significantly related to the administrative skill of their superiors, as it is appraised by the supervisory nurses: superior understands the viewpoint of subordinates, superior is good in dealing with people, superior informs subordinates of changes in advance, subordinates feel free to discuss personal

problems with their superior, and subordinates find it easy to get their ideas across to their superiors.

4. All but one (superior lets subordinates know where they stand) of the nine practices and characteristics attributed by supervisory nurses to their immediate superior (or their relationship with him) are positively and significantly related to the overall satisfaction of supervisory nurses with their respective immediate superior in the participating hospitals. The item "superior lets subordinates know where they stand" is totally unrelated to the three supervisory skills at this level.

Of the nine supervisory practices and characteristics, two are significantly related to each of the three supervisory skills and to the satisfaction of supervisory nurses with supervision. These are: the extent to which the superior understands the viewpoint of the supervisory nurses, and the extent to which

TABLE 58. The Relationship of Specific Supervisory Characteristics, as Perceived by *Supervisory Nurses* About Their Superior, to Certain Supervisory Skills and to the Satisfaction of Supervisory Nurses with Their Immediate Superior in the Participating Hosptals *

(Correlations Are Based on Data from Supervisory Nurses in Each Hospital)

Specific Characteristics of Immediate Superior	Immediate Superior's Skills			Overall Satisfaction of Supervisory Nurses with Their Immediate Superior
	Human Relations	Technical	Administrative	
Superior understands the viewpoint of his subordinates	.94	.56	.76	92
Superior is good in dealing with people	.92	.45	.74	.87
Subordinates feel free to discuss personal problems with superior	.83	.38	.68	.70
Superior expresses appreciation	.52	.45	.49	.61
Superior asks subordinates' opinion about work problems	.79	.38	.48	.84
Superior tells subordinates in advance about changes	.93	.44	.69	.85
Superior is good at planning, organizing, and scheduling work	.74	.47	.55	.90
Superior lets subordinates know where they stand	−.08	−.35	−.27	.02
Superior makes it easy for subordinates to get their ideas across	.87	.61	.88	.83

* All figures are rank-order correlations, based on an *N* of 10 hospitals in each case. Correlations larger than .56 are significant at the .05 level, and those .75 or larger are significant at the .01 level.

supervisory nurses feel it is easy for them to get their ideas across to their superiors (the director of nursing, top supervisory nursing staff, and perhaps also the administrator). It is interesting to note, in this connection, that this identical pattern of results was also obtained at the department-head level (see Table 57). Other findings, however, point to contrasting patterns that reflect the relativity of supervision at these two levels. Based on data from supervisory nurses (Table 58), for example, we find that the satisfaction of supervisory nurses with their immediate superior in the various hospitals is positively and significantly related to each of the three specific supervisory practices that imply direct initiation of communication from their superior—superior expresses appreciation, asks opinion, and tells subordinates in advance about changes. None of these three items, it will be recalled, was found to be related to the satisfaction of department heads with their superiors. Of the same three practices, moreover, only the one concerning expression of appreciation is not significantly related to the human relations skill of the supervisory nurses' immediate superior; by contrast, this is the only one among these three practices that relates significantly to the human relations skill of the department heads' superior.

Other comparisons and contrasts between the results in Table 58, concerning the supervision of supervisory nurses, and Table 57, concerning the supervision of department heads, may be readily made. In the case of supervisory nurses, for example, the human relations skill of their immediate superior in the hospitals studied is most highly related to the extent to which their superior understands their viewpoint, and the extent to which their superior informs them of changes in advance. In the case of department heads, on the other hand, it is most highly related to how good their immediate superior is in dealing with people, and to how frequently he expresses appreciation. By contrast, for both supervisory nurses and department heads, the administrative skill of their immediate superiors is most highly related to the same two items: the extent to which their superior understands their viewpoint, and how easy they feel it is for them to get their ideas across to their superiors. The reader may wish to pursue this comparative examination between the department head level and the supervisory nurses level further (and also compare and contrast each of these with the nonsupervisory registered nurses level, data for which are shown in Table 59).

At this point, we would only like to indicate the two supervisory practices or characteristics that are most highly related, according to the findings, to the technical, administrative, and human relations skill of those supervising the supervisory nurses, and to the general satisfaction of supervisory nurses with their immediate superior in the participating hospitals. The two items most highly related to technical skill—in fact the only two of the nine items that are significantly related to technical skill—are: how easy supervisory nurses find it to get their ideas across to their superiors, and how well their superiors understand their viewpoint. These same two items are also the ones that are most highly related to the administrative skill of the supervisory nurses' superiors. The two items most highly related to human relations skill are: how well the superior understands the viewpoint of supervisory nurses, and whether he informs them of changes in advance. And the two items that are most highly related to the satisfaction of supervisory nurses with their respective immediate superiors in the hospitals studied are: how well their superior understands their viewpoint, and how good their superior is in planning and organizing. Thus, the superior's understanding of the viewpoint of his subordinates is a crucial aspect of supervision (relates both to the three supervisory skills and to the satisfaction of subordinates with supervision) for supervisory nurses, and also for department heads, as the results in Table 58 and Table 57 indicate. When viewed in the context of our earlier findings concerning the relationship between the mutual understanding of hospital people whose work is interdependent and various measures of coordination and patient care, this finding assumes even greater importance.

Results Concerning Supervision of Nonsupervisory Registered Nurses

Comparable findings to those presented above concerning supervisory nurses and department heads, and their superiors, are shown in Table 59 for the nonsupervisory registered nurses and their superiors (the supervisory nurses group) in the ten participating hospitals. Table 59 shows, in other words, how the technical, administrative, and human relations skills of those who supervise the nonsupervisory registered nurses in the various hospitals relate to the nine specific supervisory practices and characteristics with which we have been dealing in this section, as well as how the overall satisfaction of nonsupervisory registered nurses with their respective immediate superiors relates to each of the same nine characteristics. Let us review some of these relational findings, with emphasis on how they differ from the corresponding findings reported for supervisory nurses.

First, it is clear from the results in Table 59 that the item concerning the ease with which registered nurses can get their ideas across to their superiors is not related either to the human relations, technical, and administrative skill of their superiors, or to their own satisfaction with supervision. These results contrast very sharply with the comparable results reported above for the supervisory nurses level, and also for the department heads level, for which the same item was highly and significantly related to each of the three supervisory skills and to subordinate satisfaction with supervision. Second, the extent to which nonsupervisory registered nurses feel free to discuss personal problems with their immediate superior is highly and significantly related to their satisfaction with their superior and to their superior's technical, administrative, and human relations skills. For administrative department heads, this same item related only to the human relations skill of their superior; for supervisory nurses, it did not relate to the technical skill of their superior. Third, the item superior lets subordinates know where they stand is highly and significantly related to the satisfaction of nonsupervisory registered nurses with their immediate superior, and to the administrative and technical skills of their superior. But, the same item was earlier found to bear no relationship to the satisfaction of supervisory nurses with supervision or to the technical, administrative, and human relations skills of those supervising the supervisory nurses in the various hospitals.

TABLE 59. The Relationship of Specific Supervisory Characteristics, as Perceived by *Nonsupervisory Registered Nurses* About Their Superior, to Certain Supervisory Skills and to the Satisfaction of Registered Nurses with Their Immediate Superior in the Participating Hospitals [*]

(Correlations Based on Data from Registered Nurses in Each Hospital)

Specific Characteristics of Immediate Superior	Immediate Superior's Skills			Overall Satisfaction of Registered Nurses with Their Immediate Superior
	Human Relations	Technical	Administrative	
Superior understands the viewpoint of his subordinates	.72	.60	.64	.70
Superior is good in dealing with people	.73	.65	.53	.89
Subordinates feel free to discuss personal problems with superior	.83	.70	.59	.64
Superior expresses appreciation	.40	.22	.22	.62
Superior asks subordinates' opinion about work problems	.34	.49	.68	.71
Superior tells subordinates in advance about changes	.24	.75	.61	.61
Superior is good at planning, organizing, and scheduling work	.69	.64	.59	.90
Superior lets subordinates know where they stand	.48	.56	.68	.81
Superior makes it easy for subordinates to get their ideas across	.34	.41	.39	.36

[*] All figures are rank-order correlations, based on an N of 10 hospitals in each case. Correlations larger than .56 are significant at the .05 level, and those .75 or larger are significant at the .01 level.

On the other hand, the extent to which the superior understands the viewpoint of his subordinates is significantly related to the satisfaction of nonsupervisory registered nurses with their immediate superior and to the technical, administrative, and human relations skills of their superior—a finding obtained also at the supervisory nurses level, and at the department heads level. Similarly, all but one of the nine items examined (ease with which nurses can get their ideas across to their superiors) relate positively and significantly to how satisfied registered nurses are with their immediate superior in the participating hospitals. The same was true for supervisory nurses, except that the one item which did not relate significantly to satisfaction with supervision was different (superior lets subordinates know where they stand).

Of the nine supervisory practices and characteristics shown in Table 59, the two that relate most closely to the satisfaction of nonsupervisory registered nurses with their immediate superior in the participating hospitals are: how good the superior is in planning and organizing, and in dealing with people. Both of these items are also among the three most highly related items to the satisfaction of supervisory nurses with their immediate superior. The two items that relate most highly to the administrative skill of those who supervise the nonsupervisory registered nurses in the hospitals studied are: the extent to which the superior lets his subordinates know where they stand, and the extent to which he asks their opinion about work problems. Asking subordinates their opinion was earlier found not to be related to the administrative skill of those who supervise the supervisory nurses or the department heads; letting subordinates know where they stand was likewise unrelated to the administrative skill of those who supervise the supervisory nurses (this item was not asked of department heads).

Of the nine items concerning different supervisory skills and characteristics, the two that are most closely associated with the technical skill of those supervising the nonsupervisory registered nurses are: the extent to which the superior informs his subordinates in advance about changes, and how free subordinates feel to discuss personal problems with their immediate superior. Neither of these two items was significantly related to the technical skill of those supervising the supervisory nurses, or those supervising the department heads in the participating hospitals. The two items that relate most highly to the human relations skill of those supervising the nonsupervisory registered nurses are: the extent to which nurses feel free to discuss personal problems with their immediate superior, and how good their immediate superior is in dealing with people. Both these items were also significantly related to the human relations skill of those supervising the supervisory nurses and those supervising the department heads, but not both of them constituted the two items most closely associated with human relations skill at these levels.

Finally, of the nine supervisory practices and characteristics of those supervising the nonsupervisory registered nurses in the participating hospitals, three are related significantly both to the satisfaction of these nurses with supervision and to the technical, administrative, and human relations skill of their superiors. These items are: the extent to which the superior understands the viewpoint of his subordinates, how free subordinates feel to discuss personal problems with their immediate superior, and how good their immediate superior is at planning, organizing, and scheduling the work. Concerning the supervisory nurses level and the department head level, two items were earlier found to behave in this manner, i.e., to produce the same results. For both department heads and supervisory nurses, the two items were the same: the extent to which the superior understands the viewpoint of his subordinates (like the case of nonsupervisory registered nurses), and how easy subordinates feel it is for them to get their ideas across to their superiors (unlike the case of nonsupervisory registered nurses).

Results Concerning Supervision of Practical Nurses and of Aides

The next level below that of nonsupervisory registered nurses is the practical nurses level, which is followed in turn by the aides level—the lowest level of nursing personnel in the community general hospital. Unfortunately, we do not have a complete set of findings for these two levels comparable to the findings discussed in connection with department heads, supervisory nurses, and nonsupervisory registered nurses. In the case of aides, as earlier mentioned, no data were obtained about the technical, administrative, and human relations skill of their immediate superior because of the difficulty of the appropriate questions for this personnel. Only data concerning the satisfaction of aides with their immediate superior in the various hospitals and the nine specific supervisory practices and characteristics were obtained from the aides. In the case of practical nurses, data were obtained about the three supervisory skills but, as pointed out earlier, it is very doubtful that practical nurses distinguished sufficiently among the technical, administrative, and human relations skills of their immediate superior. Consequently, we choose not to risk here a discussion about the relationship between these three skills and specific supervisory practices and characteristics on the basis of the rather suspect data from practical nurses. As a result of these methodological difficulties, we shall only consider the relationship between the satisfaction of practical nurses with their immediate superiors in the participating hospitals and the nine supervisory practices and characteristics with which we have been concerned in this section of the chapter. The same will be done in the case of aides.

The relevant findings can be summarized very quickly for both practical nurses and aides. In the case of practical nurses, our analysis of the pertinent data shows that none of the nine specific supervisory practices and characteristics (perceived by practical nurses in their immediate superiors) is significantly related to the satisfaction of practical nurses with their respective immediate superior in the hospitals studied. The specific rank-order correlations between satisfaction with supervision and the various supervisory characteristics (the same nine characteristics shown in Table 59) range from a low of .25 to a high of .52. Based on an N of 10 hospitals, none of these correlations is statistically significant at the .05 level. Furthermore, only the largest two of the nine correlations involved are sufficiently high to be even suggestive

Supervisory Practices at Different Levels

of a relationship between the satisfaction of practical nurses with supervision and the specific practices and characteristics of those who supervise the practical nurses. These two correlations are: a correlation of .52 between the item of how good the superior is in dealing with people and the satisfaction of practical nurses with their superior, and a correlation of .50 between the extent to which the superior expresses appreciation and the satisfaction of practical nurses with their immediate superior.

The lack of significant findings at the practical nurses level contrasts very sharply with the results obtained about department heads, supervisory nurses, and nonsupervisory registered nurses. It is probably due to (1) the earlier mentioned fact that the supervision of practical nurses in the various hospitals is quite diffuse (it is scattered among a large number of supervisory and nonsupervisory registered nurses), and (2) the often-commented-upon fact that practical nurses tend to evaluate things extremely favorably which, in effect, restricts the interhospital range of the measures involved very severely. Both these considerations are capable of obscuring any empirical relationships that might exist between supervisory characteristics and the satisfaction of practical nurses with supervision.

The results concerning the aides, as might be expected, are much more similar to those for practical nurses than to those obtained for any of the other groups studied. At this bottom level, we find that only two of the various specific supervisory practices and characteristics of those who supervise the aides are significantly related to the satisfaction of aides with their immediate superior. How good their superior is in planning, organizing, and scheduling the work correlates .91 with how satisfied aides are with their immediate superior in the participating hospitals. And similarly, how good their immediate superior is in dealing with people correlates .82 with how satisfied aides are with supervision. The particular correlations between the other supervisory practices and characteristics studied and the satisfaction of aides with supervision vary between —.28 and .48, none being statistically significant at the .05 level. Again, the fact that aides, being at the lowest level, are supervised by most everyone else in the nursing department is in part responsible for not obtaining findings comparable to those for professional nurses, and for obtaining findings similar to those for practical nurses.

Results Concerning Supervision of Technicians

The last set of findings in the present series pertains to the supervision of laboratory and x-ray technicians, and is shown in Table 60. Let us review some of these findings, with special emphasis on how they compare, or contrast, with the results pertaining to the nonsupervisory registered nurses, as earlier shown in Table 59. Judging from the findings in Chapter 3, where the characteristics of the people around the patient were described and discussed, the technicians are much more similar to nonsupervisory registered nurses than to any of the other hospital groups included in the study. This similarity, indicated by data concerning the background characteristics of the various groups of respondents, their attitudes and outlook in the hospital situation, and their organizational stability, suggests that nonsupervisory registered nurses and technicians in the community general hospital are approximately at the same organizational level, or an equivalent level, even though registered nurses may enjoy a somewhat higher status-prestige than the technicians. Consequently, a comparison of the results obtained for registered nurses with the results concerning the technicians would be both appropriate and instructive.

TABLE 60. The Relationship of Specific Supervisory Characteristics, as Perceived by *Laboratory and X-ray Technicians* About Their Superior, to Certain Supervisory Skills and to the Satisfaction of Technicians with Their Immediate Superior in the Participating Hospitals *

(Correlations Are Based on Data from Technicians in Each Hospital)

Specific Characteristics of Immediate Superior	Human Relations	Technical	Administrative	Overall Satisfaction of Technicians with Their Immediate Superior
Superior understands the viewpoint of his subordinates	.78	.18	.67	.52
Superior is good in dealing with people	.65	.35	.42	.52
Subordinates feel free to discuss personal problems with superior	.91	.40	.38	.81
Superior expresses appreciation	.08	−.08	.02	.25
Superior asks subordinates' opinion about work problems	.40	.75	.60	.74
Superior tells subordinates in advance about changes	.71	.62	.56	.80
Superior is good at planning, organizing, and scheduling work	.38	.76	.70	.39
Superior lets subordinates know where they stand	.28	.23	.06	.55
Superior makes it easy for subordinates to get their ideas across	.72	.26	.66	.43

* All figures are rank-order correlations, based on an N of 10 hospitals in each case. Correlations larger than .56 are significant at the .05 level, and those .75 or larger are significant at the .01 level.

First, the results in Table 60 show that, of the nine supervisory practices and characteristics of those who supervise the technicians in the hospitals studied, only three are significantly related to the satisfaction of technicians with their immediate superiors—the extent to which technicians feel free to discuss personal problems with their superior, the extent to which their superior informs them of changes in advance, and the extent to which he asks their opinion about work problems. In the case of nonsupervisory registered nurses (see Table 59), these three items are also significantly related to satisfaction with supervision, but they are not the three items that are most closely related to satisfaction. In addition, of course, in the case of registered nurses, all but one of the nine supervisory characteristics examined relate significantly to the satisfaction of nurses with their immediate superior.

Second, in the case of technicians, of the nine items representing different supervisory practices and characteristics, only one item is significantly related both to the satisfaction of technicians with their immediate superior and to the technical, administrative, and human relations skill of their superior. This item is the extent to which immediate superiors inform the technicians of changes that affect their work in advance. By contrast, in the case of nonsupervisory registered nurses, three of the nine items behave in this same manner, and these do not include the item concerning advance information about changes.

Third, of the nine items studied, three relate significantly to the technical skill of those who supervise the technicians in the participating hospitals, five relate significantly to human relations skill, and five relate significantly to administrative skill. The corresponding numbers of items in the case of registered nurses are six, four, and six, respectively. Furthermore, the two items that relate most highly to the technical skill of those who supervise the technicians—superior is good in planning and organizing, and superior asks subordinates their opinion—are not the same as the corresponding two items in the case of registered nurses (in fact, asking opinion is not even significantly related to the technical skill of those supervising the registered nurses). The two items that relate most highly to the administrative skill of those who supervise the technicians are: how good the superior is in planning and organizing, and the extent to which the superior understands the viewpoint of his subordinates; in the case of nurses, the two items are: superior lets subordinates know where they stand, and superior asks subordinates their opinion (although how good the superior is in planning, and his understanding of the subordinates' viewpoint also relates significantly to administrative skill at this level). On the other hand, the two items that relate most closely to the human relations skill of those who supervise the technicians are: the extent to which subordinates feel free to discuss personal problems with their immediate superior, and the extent to which their immediate superior understands their viewpoint. The former item is also the one, among all nine items, that relates most closely to the administrative skill of those supervising the nurses, while the latter is the third most closely related item to administrative skill at this level.

Finally, of the nine items studied, the one concerning the ease with which respondents can get their ideas and suggestions across to their superiors is of some importance in the case of technicians (relates significantly to the human relations and administrative skills of their superiors), but it is of little, if any, consequence in the case of registered nurses in this connection. By contrast, the extent to which the superior lets subordinates know where they stand is of little significance in the case of technicians, while being rather important in the case of nurses. The above findings, among other things, demonstrate that the specific supervisory practices and characteristics that appear crucial with respect to the supervision of technicians are not necessarily the crucial ones with respect to the supervision of nonsupervisory registered nurses in the community general hospital, irrespective of the similarities between registered nurses and technicians shown in Chapter 3. Once more, as expected, supervision is relative to the immediate situation that characterizes the various groups. And the requirements of the immediate supervisory situation apparently vary for different groups, as do supervision skills and requirements across organizational levels.

Summary: The Relative Importance of Particular Supervisory Practices to the Satisfaction of Subordinates with Supervision at Different Levels

A review of the findings relating to the satisfaction of subordinates with their respective immediate superiors in the participating hospitals, as presented in this section, reveals certain interesting patterns, from the standpoint of which specific supervisory practices, among the nine studied, are the most important ones for supervising personnel at different levels. If we consider the relative level to which each personnel group involved belongs, it is possible to indicate these patterns and, at the same time, condense and systematize the numerous discrete and specific findings reported in the preceding pages. In this connection, the department heads undoubtedly constitute the highest-level, while the aides constitute the lowest-level personnel. The supervisory nurses follow the department heads and are followed by the nonsupervisory registered nurses and the technicians, at about the same level, and then the practical nurses. In other words, the two high-level groups are the department heads and the supervisory nurses; the two middle-level groups are the nonsupervisory registered nurses and the technicians; and the two low-level groups are the practical nurses and aides.

Now, a comparative analysis of all the findings presented in this section shows the following major patterns of results:

1. The extent to which the superior is good in dealing with people, as perceived by his subordinates, seems to be increasingly more important for the satisfaction of subordinates with their immediate superior as one moves from the higher toward the lower levels of personnel. Among the nine items studied, how good the superior is in dealing with people is the fourth highest related item to the satisfaction of department heads with their superior; but, it is the third highest in the case of supervisory nurses, the second highest in the case

of nonsupervisory registered nurses, and the highest in the case of practical nurses (in the case of aides it is the second highest, while in the case of technicians this item is of little importance to satisfaction). These results are consistent with the view that human relations skills on the part of supervisors are more important at the lower levels of the organization.

2. How good the superior is in planning, organizing, and scheduling the work also appears to be increasingly important for the satisfaction of subordinates with supervision as one moves toward the lower levels of personnel. This item is the third highest related item to the satisfaction of department heads with their superior, the second highest in the case of supervisory nurses, and the highest in the case of nonsupervisory registered nurses and in the case of aides (in the case of practical nurses and technicians, this item is not related to satisfaction with supervision). Apparently, the lower-level personnel expect their superiors to do most of the necessary planning, organizing, and scheduling as part of the technical requirements of their job, while the higher-level personnel perform many of these activities themselves or jointly with their superiors.

3. Insofar as the satisfaction of subordinates with supervision is concerned, the extent to which subordinates feel it is easy for them to get their ideas and suggestions across to their superiors is more important at the higher levels. Of the nine items studied, the ease of getting ideas across is the second most highly related item to the satisfaction of department heads with their superiors (administrators) in the various hospitals. The same item is also significantly related to the satisfaction of supervisory nurses with their respective immediate superiors, but it is not related to satisfaction in the case of the other personnel groups studied. This pattern of results is consistent with the relatively higher opportunity for information exchange and joint planning and decision making by subordinates and superiors at the higher levels of organizations. It is likewise consistent with the widely held expectation in organizations that top personnel ought to have and exchange ideas and suggestions. This expectation, on the other hand, tends not to be one of the role requirements of personnel at lower levels, and personnel at these levels undoubtedly have adjusted to these realities of the organizational situation.

4. The extent to which the superior understands the viewpoint of his immediate subordinates is also more important at the higher levels, from the standpoint of the satisfaction of subordinates with supervision, probably for the same reasons concerning ideas and suggestions. Among all nine items, understanding the subordinates' viewpoint is the item that relates most highly to the satisfaction of department heads and of supervisory nurses with their respective immediate superiors in the participating hospitals. It also relates significantly to satisfaction in the case of nonsupervisory registered nurses, but not in the case of technicians, practical nurses, or aides.

5. With respect to subordinate satisfaction with supervision, the extent to

which the superior informs his subordinates of changes in advance is more important at the middle and higher levels (but not at the highest level, i.e., for department heads). This is also true, moreover, for the extent to which subordinates feel free to discuss personal problems with their immediate superiors, and the extent to which the superior asks subordinates their opinion about work problems. In other words, these three items are more important in the case of supervisory nurses, nonsupervisory registered nurses, and technicians. Apparently, adequate communication between superior and subordinates about both work-related problems and personal problems constitutes an important aspect (at least with respect to subordinate satisfaction) of the superior-subordinate relationship at the middle and higher (but not highest) levels of hospital organization.

6. Finally, the remaining two of the nine items—the extent to which the superior expresses appreciation to subordinates for good work, and how sure subordinates are of what their superior thinks of them and their work—did not yield very consistent results in relation to the satisfaction of subordinates with supervision in the hospitals studied. Expressing appreciation was found to be significantly related to satisfaction only in the case of supervisory nurses and nonsupervisory registered nurses (it also produced the second highest correlation with satisfaction, among all items, in the case of practical nurses, but this correlation is not statistically significant). The extent to which subordinates know where they stand vis-à-vis their respective superiors produced only one significant relationship to satisfaction (in the case of nonsupervisory registered nurses it was found to correlate .81 with satisfaction) and one almost significant relationship (in the case of technicians it produced a correlation of .55 with satisfaction). These results tend to suggest, however, that expressing appreciation is probably more important to personnel at the middle levels in the community general hospital.

In addition to showing how each of the nine supervisory characteristics studied relates to the satisfaction of subordinates with their superior at different levels in the participating hospitals, in the present section we examined the relation between the nine supervisory characteristics and the technical, administrative, and human relations skills of supervisory personnel at various levels. These latter relationships have been pointed out for each group of hospital personnel involved. Here, we might only add that the supervisory practices and characteristics studied were found to produce different patterns of results in relation to the three supervisory skills at different levels of supervision. These patterns, however, are not as clear-cut as those concerning the relationships between supervisory practices and subordinate satisfaction with supervision just discussed.

Nevertheless, a comparative examination of the relevant findings shows that, for most levels of supervision, the following patterns seem to emerge: (1) The

Supervision and Patient Care 471

human relations skill of supervisory personnel is, generally, most closely related to how well the superior understands the viewpoint of his subordinates, to how good he is in dealing with people, and to how free subordinates feel to discuss personal problems with him. (2) The technical skill of supervisory personnel is most closely related to how good the superior is in planning, organizing, and scheduling the work, and to how well he understands the viewpoint of his subordinates. (3) The administrative skill of supervisory personnel is most closely related to the same two items that are related to technical skill and, in addition, to the ease with which subordinates can get their ideas and suggestions across to their superiors, and the extent to which the superior informs his subordinates of changes in advance. In view of these results, it may be concluded that, of the nine supervisory practices and characteristics, one is highly relevant to all three supervisory skills: the extent to which supervisory personnel understand the viewpoint of their subordinates reflects technical, administrative, and human relations skill at almost every supervisory level considered. Moreover, this same item is highly and significantly related to the satisfaction of professional nurses and of department heads with their respective superiors in the hospitals studied.

SUPERVISORY SKILLS AND CHARACTERISTICS AND THE QUALITY OF PATIENT CARE

Thus far, in this chapter, we have considered: (1) the technical, administrative, and human relations skills of supervisory personnel at different levels in the hospital; (2) the interrelationship among these three skills; (3) the relationship between the three skills and nine specific supervisory practices or characteristics; (4) the relationship between the three supervisory skills and the satisfaction of subordinates with supervision at different organizational levels; and (5) the relationship between each of the nine supervisory characteristics and the satisfaction of subordinates with supervision. We will now examine the relationship between these same supervisory skills and characteristics and the quality of patient care in the participating hospitals.

The degree of satisfaction of subordinates with their respective immediate superiors obviously constitutes one criterion of the effectiveness of supervision in organizations. But, the fact that certain supervisory skills and characteristics were shown to be related to subordinate satisfaction at different levels is only one indicator of the effectiveness of supervision in the various hospitals (and of the relative importance of the different supervisory skills and characteristics investigated). The question, therefore, arises whether the supervisory skills and characteristics studied are also related to criteria other than satisfaction with supervision. For example, are they related to the organizational effectiveness of the hospitals, as measured by the quality of patient care rendered? Similarly, are they related to the adequacy of organizational coordination, which is an essential requisite to effective hospital functioning as we have already demonstrated?

In the remaining part of this chapter, we shall attempt to answer these two questions, both because they are important questions in themselves, and also because the finding that certain supervisory skills and characteristics are related to satisfaction with supervision does not necessarily imply that they will also be related either to the quality of care or to coordination. Satisfaction with supervision and satisfaction with organizational performance, whether in the form of patient-care quality or in the form of good coordination, are quite different things. In fact, it so happens that satisfaction with supervision (whether considered separately for each organizational level or for all levels combined) in the hospitals studied relates neither to the quality of patient care, as represented by the four measures of care discussed in Chapter 5, nor to organizational coordination, as represented by the overall measures of hospital coordination discussed in Chapter 6 and the overall measure of nursing department coordination discussed in Chapter 7. Analysis of the relevant data shows, for example, that the extent to which the several groups of subordinates involved are satisfied with their immediate superiors in the ten participating hospitals correlates only —.15 with the quality of overall patient care (noncomparative measure), and only .28 with hospital coordination (measure #1 of coordination).

In short, it is essential to ascertain whether the various supervisory skills and characteristics are related to patient care and to coordination, independently and regardless of their relationship to satisfaction with supervision. In this section, we will be concerned with the question of the relationship of supervisory skills and characteristics to the quality of patient care, leaving the question of their relationship to coordination for the next section. Before presenting any findings, however, it might be helpful to review briefly some of the more important results of previous research concerning the relationship between supervision and organizational effectiveness—the quality of patient care being considered here as a criterion of the organizational effectiveness of hospitals.

Supervision and Organizational Effectiveness

Much of the research which has been conducted in large-scale organizations, especially industrial organizations, since World War II was designed to determine the relationship between leadership patterns and supervisory practices, on the one hand, and various criteria of organizational effectiveness, on the other. In numerous studies, researchers have attempted to demonstrate that organizational effectiveness, as measured by such things as actual productivity figures, rated individual and group performance, organizational member satisfactions, costs, employee turnover, absences, accidents, and various less direct measures, is markedly affected by the kind of leadership and supervision prevailing in the organization. But, while a rather impressive array of empirical findings demonstrating the importance of supervision in this connection is now available from this research, there is no simple answer—much less a definitive or final answer—to the question of what precisely is the relationship between supervisory behavior and organizational effectiveness.

It appears that different styles and practices of supervision affect the attitudes and satisfaction of organizational members differently and significantly. In general, supervisory practices of the human relations kind are associated with favorable attitudes and high employee satisfaction, while more directive and more autocratic or authoritarian supervisory behavior is associated with less favorable attitudes and lower employee satisfaction. The findings in the preceding section are in line with this general picture. It also appears that different practices and styles of supervision affect the behavior, including performance behavior, of organizational members significantly, but in rather complex ways. No single, unqualified answer can be given at present as to the exact relationship between a particular style of supervision, e.g., directive supervision, and organizational effectiveness that would be applicable to all or nearly all organizations, in all situations, at all times, or even to different levels or parts of the same organization. In short, there are limiting conditions and "intervening" variables which must be taken into account in each case.

The particular effects of supervision for organizational effectiveness depend upon a host of different factors and conditions, including the type of organization being studied, the tasks and objectives to be accomplished, the particular division of labor and accompanying specialization and interdependence in the work structure, the needs, goals, expectations, and characteristics of organizational members, and other similar considerations. Many research findings are now available that show us certain principles and guides for effective supervision (see below), but each principle may apply much more to some situations than others, or with reference to some criteria of organizational effectiveness and not to others, and it should be modified accordingly. It is for these reasons that, early in this chapter, we emphasized the relative character of supervision. As Likert (20) and Argyris (1), among others, have suggested, there is no single, specific, and correct way in which to supervise that has universal applicability. There are only general principles.

The generality or applicability of a given principle can, of course, be ascertained only through research in different organizational settings, including the hospital, for in the absence of empirical evidence there is no guarantee that a principle which, for example, was established in industrial settings will also hold equally well in the hospital situation, or vice versa. In a sense, what we have tried to do in the present study of supervision in the community general hospital is to subject to empirical testing (1) our conception of supervision, as already outlined, which emphasizes the relativity of "effective" supervision, and

(2) some of the more important and more general findings of previous research concerning leadership and supervision in industrial and other organizations. What are some of these findings?

Kahn and Katz (18), summarizing a good deal of the early work of the Survey Research Center in this area, concluded that there are four classes of supervisory characteristics or variables which were found to relate rather consistently to various measures of organizational effectiveness including measures of productivity and member satisfaction, in several different organizations. These are: (1) the supervisor's ability to play a role that is clearly different from that of his subordinates—to plan, organize, and coordinate the work, to train people, and to handle the resources required by the group to do its work; (2) the degree to which the supervisor delegates authority and grants autonomy to his subordinates in their work—whether he supervises more or less closely; (3) the extent to which the supervisor tends to be supportive of his subordinates and employee-oriented, rather than being concerned only with productivity or being identified mainly with management—whether he is concerned with the needs of his subordinates; and (4) the extent to which his subordinates take pride in the work and standing of their work group. The first two of the above principles correspond rather closely to our concepts of administrative and technical skills required of supervisors, while the third corresponds to our concept of human relations—all three skills presumably being important. As Cartwright and Zander observe, "Apparently, the good supervisors possess both the technological skills needed to perform the group tasks and the ability to help members satisfy the needs that are important to them" (3, p. 549).

Similarly, Comrey, High, and Wilson (5, 6), in a study of organizational effectiveness in an aircraft plant, found that supervisory practices much like the above were related to organizational effectiveness. The effectiveness of work groups under first-line supervisors was related to such things as the supervisor's helpfulness, his concern for human relations rather than pressure for production, and his availability for discussing the various problems of his subordinates. In a study of factors associated with the effectiveness of more than 30 operating units (groups) of a nation-wide organization engaged in the transportation business, Georgopoulos and Seashore (10, 11) likewise found that the more effective units, in terms of both actual productivity figures and management-rated effectiveness, had supervisors who were seen by their men as more supportive and considerate than their counterparts in the less effective units. In turn, the supervisors in the more effective units perceived their own superiors as more supportive than the supervisors in the less effective units.

In a study of supervision in a utilities company, Metzner and Mann (26) found that absence rates among the employees were lower where supervisors emphasized human relations practices. In another study by Mann and Dent (21), both the superiors and subordinates of supervisors agreed well in their evaluations of the most effective and least effective supervisors, but while

superiors emphasized production and technical skill in rating the supervisors as effective, subordinates emphasized human relations skill. In a study concerned with the impact of the introduction of electronic data-processing equipment in the accounting departments of a large organization, Mann and Williams (25) obtained results comparable to those of the above studies. Supervisors who were evaluated by their superiors as the most effective in managing the introduction of this major change were also seen by their subordinates as having both technical and human relations skills, although technical skill was seen as the more important for the period of change.

The above studies, in the company of many others, lead to the conclusion that supervisory skills and practices such as those with which we have been concerned in the present research affect organizational effectiveness rather significantly, and that the human relations skill of supervisors constitutes an important factor in this connection. However, not all the available research is entirely supportive of these conclusions. Fiedler (7, 8), and Cleven and Fiedler (4), for example, in studies of both industrial and military settings, did not find the supervisors or leaders of the more effective groups more accepting, approachable, supportive, or considerate of their subordinates. Apparently, the leaders of the more effective units tended to perceive and maintain greater psychological distance from their subordinates, and to be more analytical and critical in their relationships with them, compared to the leaders of the less effective units. In other words, while human relations practices on the part of supervisors did not relate to performance in this research, psychological distance did. These results raise the important issue of limiting conditions and intervening variables regarding the relationship between supervisory behavior and organizational effectiveness.

A number of leadership studies conducted in recent years by researchers associated with Ohio State University have brought this issue into sharper focus. These investigators first attempted to describe and measure leadership behavior systematically, and then to relate their measures of leadership and supervision to measures of performance and effectiveness in different situations. Based on the results of several exploratory projects, Hemphill (17), Stogdill (30), and their associates were able to identify empirically two important general dimensions of leadership—"consideration" and "initiating structure." "Consideration" refers to the extent to which the leader or supervisor is considerate of the feelings, attitudes, and needs of his subordinates, and can be inferred from behaviors that are indicative of friendship, mutual trust, supportiveness, and respect between the leader and his group. Essentially, consideration may be viewed as equivalent to the concept of human relations skill. "Initiating structure," on the other hand, represents the extent to which the supervisor defines the situation for his subordinates to facilitate interaction toward goal attainment. It would include clarification and definition of what the supervisor expects of his men, establishing routines and procedures of work, and prescribing ways for getting the job done. Administrative and technical skills could be probably brought under this dimension of initiating structure.

What are some of the results of research where these two dimensions—consideration, and initiating structure—have been used? In one study of 22 departments in a liberal arts college, Hemphill (16) found that departments that achieved a reputation for good administration were those led by chairmen who emphasized both consideration and initiating structure. Furthermore, a minimal amount of each of the two dimensions was required for achieving good reputation, and an excess of consideration behavior did not compensate for lack of initiating structure, and vice versa. In other words, both dimensions related to departmental performance, the latter as judged on the basis of reputation. Along the same lines, in a study of the behavior of aircraft commanders in relation to the effectiveness of crews in combat missions over Korea, Halpin (14, 15) found that high initiating structure on the part of leaders was generally associated with more favorable performance ratings by their superiors, and high consideration was related to the acceptance of the leaders by their crews and to the satisfaction of crew members. Aircraft commanders who were rated high by their superiors on overall performance tended to score about average on both consideration and initiating structure, whereas those rated low by their superiors tended to score below the mean on both dimensions. Effective leadership required both consideration and initiating structure.

On the other hand, in a study of 72 production departments of a manufacturing organization, Fleishman (9) found that the proficiency ratings of foremen by their superiors on "doing the better job" were positively related to initiating structure and negatively related to consideration. At the same time, however, he found no significant relationships between similar proficiency ratings and the two leadership dimensions in the case of 23 nonproduction departments. Finally, when using criteria of effectiveness other than proficiency ratings, he obtained a different pattern of results. Foremen in production departments who were evaluated high on consideration by their subordinates had lower absenteeism among their men; those evaluated high on initiating structure had higher absenteeism. The number of formal grievances was also higher in the case of foremen emphasizing initiating structure. In the nonproduction departments, turnover was higher where supervisors stressed initiating structure, and accident rates were lower where foremen stressed consideration.

Very clearly, Fleishman's findings are consistent with the notion of relativity of supervision, while also pointing to some of the complexities encountered in attempting to relate supervisory practices and behavior to criteria of organizational effectiveness. These findings suggest that consideration has different consequences for effectiveness, depending on whether production or nonproduction units are involved and on what criteria of effectiveness are employed, and the same is true for initiating structure. In the case of production units, high initiating structure is associated with high performance, but also with high absenteeism and more grievances, or subordinate dissatisfaction, while high consideration is associated with low performance, but also low absences and grievances. In the case of nonproduction departments, neither consideration nor initiating structure affects performance, but high consideration is associated with low turnover and high initiating structure is associated with high accident rates. Thus, it appears that high initiating structure affects performance favorably in production units, while high consideration minimizes withdrawal behavior (absences and turnover), accidents, and grievances, apparently in both production and nonproduction departments.

In a review of the literature concerning the relationship between employee attitudes and satisfactions, on the one hand, and individual and group performance, as measured by productivity, absenteeism, turnover, and the like, on the other, Brayfield and Crockett (2) arrived at a similar conclusion. Their review suggests that high employee satisfaction (including satisfaction with supervision) is generally associated with low withdrawal behavior, but it is not consistently related to productivity behavior. Absences, accidents, and turnover on the part of employees apparently have different motivational bases than does performance behavior. We can largely account for the former in terms of employee satisfaction and dissatisfaction, but this is not true for the latter. The motivation to leave or to remain in the organization depends upon the satisfaction of the members with the organizational situation and the opportunities that it offers, but the motivation to produce high or low depends on many additional considerations. In this connection, Georgopoulos, Mahoney, and Jones (12), for example, have shown that whether or not workers will produce high (or low) depends, among other things, upon their path-goal perceptions, i.e., upon the extent to which they perceive high (or low) productivity as potentially instrumental to attaining their particular personal goals.

The dependence of the relationship between a given dimension of supervision and organizational effectiveness upon intervening factors, and upon the kinds of criteria used to represent effectiveness, obviously constitutes a very important and very complex problem. Currently, this problem is of great concern to many researchers, along with the problems of what criteria of effectiveness, other than conventional measures of production, satisfaction, absences, turnover, etc., might be usefully employed in future research in this area. For a recent study concerned with the former problem, see Seashore, Indik, and Georgopoulos (28), and for a study concerned with the latter problem, see Georgopoulos and Tannenbaum (13). Here, we can only sensitize the reader to some of the difficulties with which one is faced in attempting to study the relationship between different supervisory practices and different measures of organizational effectiveness.

In summary, the preceding review of representative research concerning supervision and organizational effectiveness suggests that: (1) the behavior of those in leadership and supervisory positions in organizations can typically be related to various measures of organizational effectiveness, but the relationships that can be expected may vary depending on what aspects of supervision are involved and what criteria of effectiveness are used; (2) depending on the nature and requirements of the organizational situation, and the needs, goals, and expectations of organizational members, a particular style of supervision, or a particular supervisory skill or characteristic, may have different consequences for organizational effectiveness and for different aspects of effectiveness; and (3) the combination of the technical, administrative, and human relations skills and practices of supervisory personnel that is most effective from the standpoint of organizational effectiveness will probably be different for different types of organizations, and even for different levels within the same organization.

With these considerations in mind, and having established the relationship between certain supervisory skills and characteristics and the satisfaction of subordinates with supervision at different levels in the hospitals participating in the present study, we are ready to present our findings regarding the relationship between the same skills and characteristics and the quality of overall patient care in the various hospitals. Subordinate satisfaction with supervision, it should be reiterated, represents one criterion of hospital effectiveness, while the quality of patient care represents another.

Results Regarding the Relationship of Supervisory Skills and Practices to the Quality of Patient Care in the Participating Hospitals

Table 61 presents the main findings from our analysis of the relationship between supervisory behavior and the quality of overall patient care rendered in the hospitals studied. (Certain supplementary results will be presented in the next section of this chapter, in Table 63.) Supervisory behavior is represented here by the same measures of the three supervisory skills—technical, administrative, and human relations—and by the nine specific supervisory practices and characteristics with which we have been dealing throughout this chapter. The quality of patient care is represented by the noncomparative, overall measure which has been used in previous analyses and which was fully discussed in Chapter 5. Correlational findings are shown with reference to each of the several levels of supervision included in this part of the study, and for all levels combined. All correlations are rank-order correlations, based on an N of 10 hospitals in each case, since the unit of analysis is, again, the hospital and not the individuals who provided the data.

On the whole, the results in Table 61 show no direct relationship between the quality of patient care in the various hospitals and the supervisory skills and characteristics investigated. Hospitals where supervisory and administrative personnel are evaluated by their subordinates as more technically skilled, for example, are neither more nor less likely than other hospitals to render better

Supervision and Patient Care

patient care—regardless of whether we consider the several levels of supervision separately or together. Furthermore, the same conclusion applies with reference to administrative skill and to human relations skill. Of the 21 correlations between the three supervisory skills and the quality of overall patient care shown in Table 61 (the first three rows of correlations) not a single one is statistically significant. These correlations practically vary randomly around zero, between —.45 and +.43, indicating that the quality of patient care in the hospitals studied is not directly affected by any of the three supervisory skills.

The remaining correlations in Table 61 similarly show no direct relationship between the quality of patient care in the participating hospitals and any of the nine specific supervisory practices and characteristics studied. Of the 71 pertinent correlations only four are large enough to be statistically significant at the .05 level, i.e., larger than $\pm.56$. Of these four, which are produced by three different measures, one (the largest) is positive and three are negative: there is a correlation of .71 between the quality of care and the extent to which practical nurses in the various hospitals feel that their respective immediate superiors are good in planning, organizing, and scheduling the work; a correlation of —.62 between the quality of care and the extent to which laboratory and x-ray technicians evaluate their immediate superiors as good in dealing with people, as well as a correlation of —.58 between the quality of care and the extent to which technicians feel free to discuss personal problems with their superiors; and a correlation of —.64 between the quality of care in the various hospitals and the extent to which department heads, supervisory nurses, nonsupervisory registered nurses, practical nurses, aides, and technicians combined evaluate their immediate superiors as good in dealing with people (but, when the data are examined separately for each of these groups, only the correlation based on data from the technicians is statistically significant).

Thus, of the total of 92 correlations between supervisory skills and characteristics and the quality of patient care appearing in Table 61 (77 of which are smaller than $\pm.40$, some being positive and others negative), only 4 are statistically significant. These 4, moreover, are very probably the result of chance rather than indicative of actual relationships. By chance alone, more than 4 of the 92 correlations would be expected to be as large as the 4 correlations in question, i.e., they could be large enough to be statistically significant without reflecting social reality. The only conclusion that could be properly drawn from the results in Table 61, therefore, is that, in this study, we find no *direct* relationship between supervisory behavior, as represented by the measures of the three supervisory skills and the nine specific supervisory characteristics, and the organizational effectiveness of the participating hospitals, as represented by the measure of the quality of overall patient care.

It should also be pointed out here that, as we have demonstrated in Chapter 5, the measure of the quality of patient care used in the above analysis corre-

TABLE 61. The Relationship of Particular Supervisory Skills and Characteristics, as Evaluated by Immediate Subordinates, to the Quality of Overall Patient Care in the Participating Hospitals *

(Correlation Between Each Skill or Characteristic and the Quality of Care) †
Subordinates Evaluating Supervisory Skills-Characteristics in Each Hospital

Skill or Characteristic of Immediate Superior	Department Heads	Supervisory Nurses	Nonsupervisory Registered Nurses	Practical Nurses	Aides	All Nursing Groups	Lab and X-ray Technicians	All Groups Combined
Technical skill	−.29	.43	−.03	.16	NA ‡	.29	−.12	.09
Administrative skill	−.12	.06	−.17	.40	NA	.20	−.30	.31
Human relations skill	.07	.18	−.12	.33	NA	.23	−.45	.03
Superior understands the viewpoint of his subordinates	.04	.27	.13	.19	−.35	.28	−.43	−.18
Superior is good in dealing with people	−.03	.10	−.26	.21	−.49	−.26	−.62	−.64
Subordinates feel free to discuss personal problems with superior	.21	.04	−.29	.13	−.15	−.07	−.58	−.17
Superior expresses appreciation	−.03	.20	−.09	.01	.52	.07	−.15	.20
Superior asks subordinates' opinion about work problems	.46	.43	−.22	.03	.09	.02	.06	.16
Superior tells subordinates in advance about changes	−.31	.18	−.02	.11	.02	.13	−.12	.10
Superior is good at planning, organizing, and scheduling work	−.14	.39	−.12	.71	−.32	.44	−.27	−.31

Superior lets subordinates know where they stand	NA	.46	−.54	.14	.13	−.09	.02	.25
Superior makes it easy for subordinates to get their ideas across	.23	−.14	.26	.36	.14	−.09	−.38	.11

* The measures of supervisory skills and characteristics were computed separately for each hospital, and are based on data from the specified groups of respondents. The measure of the quality of care has been discussed earlier and is fully described in Chapter 5; it is the noncomparative measure of overall patient care.

† All correlations are rank-order correlations based on an N of 10 hospitals in each case. Correlations larger than ±.56 are significant at the .05 level, and those ±.75 or larger are significant at the .01 level.

‡ NA indicates that these questions were not asked of these groups.

lates highly with the other three measures of care used in the study. More specifically, it correlates .96 with the comparative measure of the quality of overall patient care, .67 with the measure of the quality of medical care, and .91 with the measure of the quality of nursing care rendered in the different participating hospitals. Accordingly, one might suspect that the supervisory skills and characteristics investigated would also be unrelated to these other three measures of patient care, or hospital effectiveness. Upon further examination of the pertinent data, this suspicion also turned out to be true. Briefly, further analysis confirms that there is no direct relationship between the various supervisory skills and characteristics and the quality of patient care in the hospitals studied, irrespective of which of the four measures of care is employed in the analysis. Furthermore, this conclusion holds true whether or not we examine the several levels of supervision separately, as well as when the supervisory skills and characteristics of personnel in the nursing department only are studied in relation to the quality of nursing care.

This lack of direct relationships between supervisory behavior and the criterion of quality of patient care, of course, contrasts very sharply with the results obtained earlier (Tables 56 through 60) regarding the relationship between supervisory skills and behavior and the criterion of subordinate satisfaction with supervision. It likewise contrasts sharply with the previously reported findings on the relationship between patient care and different aspects of hospital structure and functioning, including the important variable of organizational coordination. At the same time, when viewed in the context of the present state of our knowledge regarding the relationship between supervisory behavior and organizational effectiveness, as shown above in our review of the relevant literature, the obtained results on supervision in relation to patient care cannot be considered too surprising. The relationship between supervisory behavior and organizational effectiveness depends upon the kind of criteria of effectiveness used, is affected by many intervening factors and conditions, and is generally very complex rather than simple and direct.

In short, that supervision is important to organizational functioning cannot be doubted. But, the consequences of particular supervisory skills and behaviors may be more or less pronounced or direct for different types of organizations, different organizational levels, and different criteria of organizational effectiveness. Several of the supervisory skills and characteristics studied in this research, for instance, were found to be directly and significantly related to subordinate satisfaction with supervision in the participating hospitals, but not to the quality of patient care. Similarly, the particular consequences of particular supervisory skills and practices for different aspects of organizational functioning may or may not be simple and direct; they may be conditioned, modified, or mediated through other factors in the situation.

In the present study, for example, since coordination proved to be crucial to patient care and effective hospital functioning, and since certain aspects of

Supervision and Coordination

supervisory and administrative activity were earlier found to affect coordination, it is not unlikely that some supervisory skills or characteristics may be found to be *indirectly* related to the quality of patient care through the medium of coordination, i.e., by making for good coordination. We shall investigate this possibility, and actually show certain relationships of this kind, but not before we study the relationship of supervisory skills and characteristics to organizational coordination. Furthermore, in the next chapter, we will discover that certain aspects of work-relevant communication between supervisory and nonsupervisory nursing personnel in the hospitals studied also relate to the quality of patient care, suggesting that some relationships between supervision and patient care are mediated through certain communication factors. First, however, we will consider the question of what relationship, if any, is there between supervisory skills and characteristics and coordination.

SUPERVISORY SKILLS AND CHARACTERISTICS IN RELATION TO COORDINATON

Having found no simple direct relationship between supervisory behavior and the quality of patient care in the hospitals studied, the principal question that remains is whether any of the supervisory skills and characteristics with which we have been concerned are related to coordination. In the event that they are related to some of the measures of organizational coordination which were previously found to be positively and significantly associated with the quality of patient care (see Chap. 8), we would tentatively conclude that the relationship between supervisory behavior and the quality of patient care in the community general hospital is an indirect one—one mediated through, among other things, coordination variables. What do the data show?

When the three skills and nine specific characteristics of supervisory personnel at all levels combined (i.e., when using measures of supervisory behavior based on data from all the groups of subordinates representing each hospital) are examined in relation to the four overall measures of hospital coordination developed in this study (see Chap. 6), we find the results presented in Table 62. Most of these results are not statistically significant. Even though all but 4 of the 48 correlations involved are positive, i.e., directionally "right," and even though the 4 negative correlations are very small, nonsignificant, and produced by a single supervisory characteristic—superior is good in dealing with people, the majority of the correlations fail to reach statistical significance at the .05 level. For example, the 12 correlations between the technical, administrative, and human relations skills of supervisory personnel in the participating hospitals, on the one hand, and each of the 4 measures of hospital coordination, on the other, range in size from a low of .16 to a high of .37, all being statistically nonsignificant. In other words, hospitals whose supervisory personnel is more highly evaluated by subordinates with respect to technical, administrative, or human relations skill are not significantly more likely than other hospitals to have better overall coordination. Furthermore, what is true with reference to the three skills is also true for most of the nine specific supervisory practices or characteristics investigated. It is not, however, true for all of them; some are related to hospital coordination.

TABLE 62. **The Relationship of Particular Supervisory Skills and Characteristics to Organizational Coordination in the Participating Hospitals** *

Skill or Characteristic of Immediate Superior ‡	Overall Measures of Coordination †			
	Measure #1	Measure #2	Measure #3	Measure #4
Technical skill	.29	.31	.28	.27
Administrative skill	.23	.19	.17	.19
Human relations skill	.24	.28	.37	.16
Superior understands the viewpoint of his subordinates	.16	.09	.09	.10
Superior is good in dealing with people	−.13	−.19	−.14	−.19
Subordinates feel free to discuss personal problems with superior	.13	.15	.19	.01
Superior expresses appreciation	.61	.55	.52	.56
Superior asks subordinates' opinion about work problems	.62	.60	.57	.52
Superior makes it easy for subordinates to get their ideas across	.50	.40	.40	.43
Superior tells subordinates in advance about changes	.27	.26	.17	.32
Superior is good at planning, organizing, and scheduling work	.27	.18	.17	.30
Superior lets subordinates know where they stand	.44	.43	.41	.36

* All figures are rank-order correlations, based on an N of 10 hospitals in each case. Correlations larger than .56 are significant at the .05 level.
† The four measures of coordination have been discussed earlier, and are fully described in Chapter 6.
‡ The measures of supervisory skills and characteristics were computed separately for each hospital, and are based on data from administrative department heads, supervisory nurses, nonsupervisory registered nurses, practical nurses, and laboratory and x-ray technicians in each hospital.

Table 62 shows that two supervisory items are significantly related to two or more of the overall measures of coordination, while another two produce correlations that are suggestive of a probable relationship to coordination. More specifically, the extent to which supervisory personnel in the various hospitals ask subordinates their opinion about work problems correlates .62

Supervision and Coordination 485

with measure #1 of coordination, .60 with measure #2, .57 with measure #3 (the overall measure of general or nonprogramed coordination), and .52 with measure #4 (the overall measure of programed coordination). Similarly, the extent to which supervisory personnel express appreciation to subordinates for their work correlates .61, .55, .52, and .56, respectively, with the four measures of hospital coordination. Parenthetically, these results also show that the former item relates better to general than to programed coordination, while the converse is true for the latter item. But, what is important here, of course, is that most of the obtained correlations between these two items and the measures of coordination are statistically significant, indicating that the better-coordinated hospitals are those where supervisory personnel ask subordinates their opinion about work problems, and express appreciation to subordinates for their work, more frequently. Finally, the two items that produce correlations that are probably suggestive of a relationship to coordination are: the extent to which subordinates feel free to get their ideas and suggestions about work improvements across to superiors, and how sure subordinates are of what their superiors think of them and their work—whether superiors let their subordinates know where they stand.[3]

Thus, it appears that the items regarding the supervisors' behavior with respect to asking subordinates their opinion, expressing appreciation for their work, and facilitating the exchange of work-relevant information, while not directly related to the quality of patient care in the hospitals studied, are related to hospital coordination. By contrast to these items, all of which pertain to superior-subordinate communication that is work-relevant, the purely human relations items (how good the superior is in dealing with people, and how free subordinates feel to discuss personal problems with their superior) are related neither to patient care nor to coordination. Could it be that, whereas hospital personnel, as a group, may not expect their superiors to be particularly concerned with the purely human relations side of the superior-subordinate relationship, when they feel that they are treated by their superiors as capable employees who are contributing importantly to the functioning of the organization, they are more likely to act so as to facilitate coordination, thereby making for better overall patient care? The answer is probably yes, in view of the results presented above and the results immediately following, but it must be

---

[3] Another two of the nine supervisory characteristics shown in Table 62 are significantly related to nursing department coordination, but not to overall hospital coordination. When the overall measure of nursing department coordination, described in Chapter 7, is related to the characteristics of supervisory personnel in the nursing department (using data from the principal nursing groups—supervisory nurses, nonsupervisory registered nurses, and practical nurses—only), it is found to correlate .63 with how good superiors are in planning, organizing, and scheduling the work, and .59 with how well superiors understand the viewpoint of their subordinates. Supervisory planning and supervisory understanding of the point of view of subordinates facilitate coordination within the nursing department.

considered as tentative rather than conclusive. A good deal more research will be required before a definitive answer can be given.

Supervisory Behavior, Coordination, and Patient Care

Because of the importance of the above question, the four supervisory items which were found to be related (in the manner indicated above) to the overall measures of hospital coordination were subjected to more detailed study. Each item was examined in relation to the various specific measures of coordination which were introduced and described in Chapter 6. The significant findings from this analysis are presented in Table 63. (In the interests of clarity and economy, only the significant relationships obtained from this analysis are shown in Table 63.) This table shows, both quantitatively and schematically, the following information: (1) how the selected supervisory items are related to certain specific measures of coordination; (2) how these specific measures of coordination are, in turn, related to measure #1 of overall coordination, based on previous findings; and (3) how this overall measure of coordination is, in its turn, related to the noncomparative measure of the quality of overall patient care, also based on findings reported earlier.

In composite, the results in Table 63 suggest that organizational coordination constitutes an important intervening variable between the kind of supervisory practices prevailing in the hospitals studied and the quality of patient care. First, it will be recalled, none of the four supervisory items involved—superior asks subordinates their opinion about work problems, superior expresses appreciation to subordinates for their work, it is easy for subordinates to get their ideas about work across to their superiors, and superior lets subordinates know where they stand—was found to be directly related to the quality of patient care, while all of them showed a tendency to relate to the overall measures of coordination. Table 63 specifies this tendency further. For example, according to the findings, the extent to which supervisory personnel in the participating hospitals ask subordinates their opinion about work problems is significantly related to each of three specific measures of coordination, as follows: it correlates .69 with the extent to which organizational members do their job without getting in each other's way, .67 with the extent to which organizational members make an effort to avoid creating problems or interference in their work relationships, and .67 with the extent to which work assignments in the everyday routine of the hospital are well planned. The first two of these measures represent what we have previously designated as preventive coordination, while the third is a measure of programed coordination.

The frequency with which supervisors express appreciation to subordinates for their work is also significantly related to each of the same three specific measures of coordination as shown in Table 63. The ease with which subordinates can get their ideas about work across to their superiors is significantly related to two of the specific measures of coordination—the preventive co-

TABLE 63. Some Indirect Relationships Between Selected Supervisory Practices and the Quality of Overall Patient Care in the Participating Hospitals—Relationships Mediated Through Coordination Variables *

Selected Supervisory Practices ‡	Coordination Variables †		Quality of Overall Patient Care §
	Specific Measures of Coordination	Overall Measure of Coordination	

Immediate Superior:

Expresses appreciation —.73 ⎫
Asks subordinates' opinion —.69 ⎬ Extent organizational members do their job without getting in each other's way —.96 ⎫
Makes it easy for subordinates to get their ideas across —.69 ⎪
Lets subordinates know where they stand —.58 ⎭

Expresses appreciation —.67 ⎫
Asks subordinates' opinion —.67 ⎬ Extent organizational members make effort to avoid creating problems or interference in their work relationships —.73 ⎬ Measure #1 of overall coordination —.68 Quality of overall patient care (noncomparative measure)
Makes it easy for subordinates to get their ideas across —.85 ⎭

Expresses appreciation —.79 ⎫
Asks subordinates' opinion —.67 ⎬ Extent work assignments are well planned in the everyday routine of the hospital —.83 ⎭
Lets subordinates know where they stand —.69 ⎭

* All figures are rank-order correlations, based on an N of 10 hospitals in each case. Correlations larger than .56 are significant at the .05 level, and those larger than .75 at the .01 level.
† The measures of coordination have been discussed earlier, and are fully described in Chapter 6.
‡ The measures of these supervisory practices were computed separately for each hospital, and are based on data from department heads, supervisory nurses, nonsupervisory registered nurses, practical nurses, and laboratory and x-ray technicians.
§ The measure of the quality of care has been discussed earlier, and is fully described in Chapter 5; it is the noncomparative measure of overall patient care.

ordination measures. And the extent to which superiors let their subordinates know where they stand, as reflected in how sure subordinates are of what their superiors think of them and their work, is significantly related to one measure of preventive coordination (the extent to which organizational members do their job without getting in each other's way) and one measure of programed coordination (how well planned the work assignments are in the everyday routine of the hospital).

Briefly, then, the above four supervisory practices contribute to organizational coordination in the community general hospital. Especially, they contribute to preventive coordination—the type of coordination where organizational members make those adjustments in their behavior that are required to prevent or avoid disruptions in normal organizational functioning, but which cannot be effected through organizational planning, or advance programing, alone. To an extent, moreover, the same supervisory practices seem to contribute to the kind of coordination which is attained through the planning of work assignments in the organization, i.e., to programed coordination. In turn, of course, we already know from previously reported findings that organizational coordination contributes to the quality of patient care. This linkage between supervisory behavior and the quality of patient care through the mediation of coordination may be further clarified at this point.

Thus far, we have seen that: (1) the four supervisory practices under consideration are associated with one or more of the overall measures of hospital coordination, with two of the four practices yielding statistically significant relationships and the other two showing a tendency to relate to overall coordination; and (2) each of the same four supervisory practices is significantly related to at least two of the three specific measures of coordination shown in Table 63—the extent to which organizational members do their job without getting in each other's way, the extent to which they make an effort to avoid creating problems or interference in their work relationships, and how well planned the work assignments in the hospital are. Now, we also know that, as demonstrated in Chapter 6, these three specific measures of coordination are highly and significantly related to the overall measures of coordination; for example, they correlate .96, .73, and .83, respectively, with measure #1 of overall coordination. And, finally, we similarly know that, as demonstrated in Chapter 8, coordination is significantly related to the quality of patient care in the hospitals studied.

In connection with this last statement, for instance, we know that measure #1 of overall coordination was found to correlate .68 with the noncomparative measure of the quality of overall patient care in the participating hospitals, and .73 with the measure of the quality of nursing care. And the other three measures of overall coordination were found to produce similar relationships with the measures of patient care. In addition, two of the three specific measures of coordination with which we are dealing here, and to which the four supervisory practices (superior asks subordinates their opinion regarding work problems, expresses appreciation for their work, makes it easy for them to get their ideas across, and lets them know where they stand) were found to relate, are also significantly related to some of the measures of patient care. Specifically, the extent to which organizational members do their job without getting in each other's way correlates .60 with the quality of nursing care, and also .60 with the quality of overall patient care (the noncomparative measure) in the various hospitals; and the extent to which work assignments in the everyday routine of the hospital are well planned correlates .56 with the quality of nursing care.

In view of the preceding interrelationships among the specified measures of supervisory behavior, organizational coordination, and patient care quality in the hospitals studied, partly summarized in Table 63, it appears that in the community general hospital supervision relates to patient care only indirectly through the mediation of coordination variables. The better-care hospitals are those that have more adequate coordination, and the better-coordination hospitals are those where supervisory practices of the kind specified prevail, but the quality of patient care is not directly related to these supervisory practices. Apparently, in hospitals where supervisory personnel (1) ask subordinates their opinion about work problems, (2) express appreciation to subordinates for their work, (3) are receptive to the ideas and suggestions of subordinates, and (4) keep subordinates well informed of what is expected of them organizationally, supervisors successfully motivate their subordinates to behave in ways that are consistent with, or an aid to, good coordination, and particularly preventive coordination, thereby facilitating the attainment of organizational objectives.

Certain results from two additional analyses (not shown here) reinforce the conclusion that organizational coordination constitutes an important intervening variable between the supervisory practices investigated in the present section and the quality of patient care, or organizational effectiveness. One of these analyses shows that the above supervisory practices are positively and significantly related to the extent to which hospital personnel working interdependently (including, but not limited to, personnel in superior-subordinate relationships) see each other's viewpoint in their work relationships. This latter item, indicative of the sharedness of work-related expectations among organizational members whose jobs are interrelated, was earlier found also to be an important correlate of coordination (see Chap. 7). And, as we know, coordination is positively related both to the supervisory practices in question and to the quality of patient care in the ten participating hospitals.

The other, and last, analysis which has a bearing on the problem of the present section concerns the clarity of formal organizational specifications. In

Chapter 7, we found that the more clearly defined hospital rules, regulations, and policies are, the better the coordination. Now, it also happens that the four supervisory practices with which we have been dealing here are more evident in hospitals where rules and regulations are more clearly defined. The clarity of organizational rules is significantly related to: (1) the frequency with which supervisory personnel ask subordinates their opinion about work problems (.91); (2) the frequency with which supervisory personnel express appreciation to subordinates for their work (.78); (3) the ease with which subordinates can get their ideas and suggestions about work across to superiors (.88); and (4) the extent to which superiors let their subordinates know what is expected of them, or where they stand (.60). (And, incidentally, the clarity of rules and regulations in the various hospitals also correlates highly and significantly, .90, with how well satisfied subordinates are with their respective immediate superiors.) The four supervisory practices, of course, are also significantly related to coordination, while coordination is significantly related to the quality of patient care. These results suggest that patient care, or hospital effectiveness, is dependent upon the relative adequacy of organizational coordination; good coordination is associated with the clarity of organizational rules and regulations, and the four specific supervisory practices are significantly related both to the clarity of rules and to coordination. In short, we have here one more indication of the linkage between supervisory behavior and the quality of patient care through the mediation of coordination.

In summary, the preceding analyses show that most of the supervisory skills and practices investigated in this study relate neither to the quality of patient care nor to coordination in the hospitals studied, even though they relate significantly to satisfaction with supervision. However, four of the specific supervisory practices are associated with different aspects of hospital coordination—without being directly related to the quality of patient care. In turn, coordination is significantly related to patient care or organizational effectiveness. Tentatively, and taking into consideration the methodological limitations of our research (see Chap. 2), it may be concluded that the relationship between supervisory behavior and organizational effectiveness, or the quality of patient care, in the community general hospital is an indirect one—one that becomes evident only when the intervening variable of coordination is taken into account. Moreover, this indirect relationship between supervisory behavior and patient care occurs only in the case of four of the supervisory practices investigated (superior asks opinion, expresses appreciation, is receptive to ideas and suggestions from subordinates, and keeps subordinates well informed of what is organizationally expected of them). These particular practices share in common the fact that they pertain to those aspects of the superior-subordinate relationship which involve the communication and exchange of information about work-related matters, i.e., which involve task-relevant communication.

SUMMARY

In this chapter we have explored the role of supervisory and administrative behavior in the community general hospital with emphasis on the relationship between certain supervisory skills and practices, on the one hand, and the satisfaction of subordinates with supervision, organizational coordination, and patient care or organizational effectiveness, on the other. While the ultimate question to which the chapter is addressed has been what type of supervision is likely to be the most appropriate or the most effective in hospitals of the kind studied, an attempt was also made to outline and partially test a new theoretical approach to the study of leadership and supervision in formal organizations. In part, this approach stems from an effort to reconcile certain findings from previous research in this area that are inconsistent with one another or theoretically incompatible, and in part from an attempt to begin to explore and specify heretofore untackled limiting conditions, which intervene to influence the relationship between particular styles of supervisory behavior and organizational effectiveness.

The approach here employed is partly based on results from previous studies (as reviewed in this chapter) which suggest that a type of supervision which is effective in some organizations, for some levels in the same organization, at particular times or under certain circumstances, and with reference to given criteria of effectiveness, is not necessarily equally effective or most appropriate for other organizations, other organizational levels, other times and circumstances, or other criteria of effectiveness. In short, this approach emphasizes the relativity of "effective" supervision. It then proposes that differential combinations of supervisory-leadership skills, practices, and characteristics would be required by different types of organizations, different levels of supervision in the same organization, and at different times in the life cycle of an organization.

The role of supervisors is viewed in both structural and functional terms. Structurally, in the hospital and other large-scale organizations, the role of the supervisor is one of linking his organizational family—the unit consisting of himself and his immediate subordinates—with other relevant organizational units, so that the entire system may achieve certain unity and coherence of action. Functionally, the role of the supervisor is one of interrelating organizational objectives and requirements with the needs, goals, and behaviors of the members of his unit. The physical and mental energies of members must be made as congruent as possible with the expectations of the organization, if the latter is to function effectively. Such congruence depends a good deal on how successful the supervisor is in motivating his subordinates toward institutional purposes. In addition, of course, the role of the supervisor presupposes certain technical qualifications that are appropriate to the position he occupies in the organizational system.

The proposed approach has direct implications for the kinds of basic skills, or competences that are required, if not indeed essential, of an occupant of the office of supervisor. In this connection, we pointed out that a supervisor must at least have some minimum technical skill, some minimum administrative skill, and some minimum skill in human relations in order to perform his role, as viewed above, successfully. We also pointed out, however, that these three skills are not equally important for different levels of supervision in the same organization, or for the same level of supervision in different organizations, or at different times. One major problem in this area, then, is to ascertain the relative importance of the three skills and the combination of skills that is most appropriate for given levels of supervision in given types of organizations, such as the hospital. Specific supervisory practices and characteristics also can be viewed in the manner that supervisory skills are viewed.

One important implication of the present approach is that the kind of supervisory behavior which has been found effective in various other organizational settings need not be the most appropriate or effective in the hospital setting. The hospital, like many other organizations, is a purposeful, task-oriented organization in which many specialized groups work, in a coordinated fashion, toward certain ends. But, unlike other organizations, it is an organization that deals mainly with human resources and human life rather than raw materials or physical objects. Moreover, the hospital aims to produce not a uniform, but a highly personalized product—to provide individualized patient care, and to do so with precision and predictability, even though it lacks such simple organizational supports as physical-mechanical systems or standardized workflows that would serve to coordinate and integrate its operations. A hospital must be able to handle the problem of giving adequate and continuing care to anxious and self-oriented patients whose recovery is often slow or in doubt, while being able to adapt successfully to internal and external changes, and while being flexible enough to meet the demands posed by the frequent emergencies that it must also handle.

Under circumstances such as these, the problem of achieving and maintaining adequate organizational coordination is of paramount importance. To solve this problem, the hospital tends to rely rather heavily on formal authority and formal prescriptions for behavior. However, as we have earlier seen, formal planning and programed coordination are not enough; informal supports and nonprogramed coordination are also indispensable. Reliance on formal authority and programed coordination, of course, implies that supervisory behavior in the hospital is often highly directive, and relationships among organizational members, including superior-subordinate relationships, are likely to be characterized by a good deal of impersonality, deference, and social and psychological distance. But, it is just this type of situation in which successful solution of the motivational problem is difficult to accomplish, and in which one of the most important functions of supervisors is to balance effectively the

Summary

formal and impersonal requirements of the situation with the personal needs and goals of their subordinates. However (and fortunately for the hospital), the motivational problem is substantially mitigated by the fact that there is considerably more initial congruence between the goals of people working in the hospital and the objectives of the organization than is the case in many other formal organizations, e.g., factories. (In turn, other things being equal, this happenstance facilitates coordination.) As it turns out, the results from this and previous chapters suggest that, in the community general hospital the problem of organizational coordination is even more crucial than the problem of motivating members toward organizational objectives.

The principal findings of the present chapter may now be summarized, after a brief summary concerning our measures of supervisory behavior. Data about the skills and behavior of supervisory personnel in the participating hospitals were obtained from the following groups of respondents: administrative department heads, supervisory nurses, nonsupervisory registered nurses, practical nurses, aides, and laboratory and x-ray technicians. Respondents at each level, except aides, evaluated the technical, administrative, and human relations skills of their respective immediate superiors, and provided information for the measurement of nine specific supervisory practices and characteristics also attributable to their immediate superiors. These measures of the three supervisory skills and the nine supervisory practices were then examined in relation to each other and, more important, in relation to (1) the general satisfaction of subordinates with their immediate superior at each level of supervision, (2) the quality of patient care rendered in the participating hospitals, and (3) certain measures of organizational coordination. What are some of the main results?

First, for most levels of supervision, we find a marked interrelationship among the technical, administrative, and human relations skills of supervisory personnel in the hospitals studied. In other words, hospitals where supervisory personnel are evaluated highly on one of the three skills, by their subordinates, are also significantly more likely than other hospitals to have supervisory personnel evaluated highly on each of the remaining skills. However, as anticipated on theoretical grounds, the obtained relationship between any two of the three skills varies considerably from one level of supervision to another, according to the findings. This suggests that the skill-mix which characterizes supervisory personnel at a particular organizational level is different from that which prevails in other levels.

Second, we find that each of the three supervisory skills relates significantly only to some of the nine specific supervisory practices studied and not to others. For most levels of supervision, for example, supervisory skill in human relations correlates significantly with: how good an understanding the supervisor has of the viewpoint of his subordinates, as perceived by the latter; how good the supervisor is in dealing with people; and how free subordinates feel to discuss personal problems with their supervisor. Technical skill correlates, in most cases, with two items: how good the superior is in planning, organizing, and scheduling the work, and how well be understands the viewpoint of his subordinates. And administrative skill correlates significantly with the same two items with which technical skill does and, in addition, with the extent to which subordinates are sure of what their supervisor expects of them, and the ease with which subordinates can get their ideas and suggestions regarding work across to their superiors.

The particular correlational patterns obtained between each of the three supervisory skills and the various supervisory practices and characteristics studied, however, are not identical for all levels of supervision. Different levels of supervision have different patterns of supervisory practices related to the same supervisory skills. Similarly, of the nine supervisory practices and characteristics investigated, only one is significantly and consistently (i.e., in most levels of supervision) related to all three supervisory skills. Specifically, the extent to which subordinates feel that their immediate superior has a good understanding of their point of view correlates highly with the technical, administrative, and human relations skills of supervisory personnel, as evaluated by immediate subordinates. These results are, of course, consistent with our emphasis on the relative character of supervision.

A third set of findings concerns the relationship between supervisory skills and practices and the satisfaction of subordinates with supervision at different levels in the hospitals studied. Considering first the three supervisory skills, we find a positive and significant relationship between each skill and the overall satisfaction of subordinates with their respective immediate superiors. In general, subordinates are more satisfied with supervision in hospitals where supervisors are evaluated more highly on technical, administrative, or human relations skill. This relationship was obtained for all levels of supervision studied, except where practical nurses constitute the appropriate group of subordinates. At the same time, however, we also find that the extent to which each of the three supervisory skills contributes to subordinate satisfaction with supervision varies substantially from one organizational level to another. And the same is true when each of the three skills is examined in relation to satisfaction, but with the effects of the other two skills having been removed. In this connection, the results show that the satisfaction of department heads with their immediate superiors (hospital administrators) in the various hospitals is mainly determined by the administrative skill of their superiors, while the satisfaction of supervisory nurses is primarily determined by the human relations skill of their superiors, and the satisfaction of laboratory and x-ray technicians is about equally determined by the human relations and technical skills of their superiors. Briefly, then, from the standpoint of subordinate satisfaction with supervision, the three supervisory skills are not equally important. The contribution that a particular skill makes to subordinate satisfaction with supervision varies markedly across organizational levels, as was anticipated.

Summary

Considering next the nine specific supervisory practices and characteristics studied in relation to the satisfaction of subordinates with supervision at each level in the participating hospitals, we find that (1) different practices contribute differentially to subordinate satisfaction, and (2) the relationship between a particular practice, or characteristic, and satisfaction varies from one organizational or supervisory level to another. Insofar as the overall satisfaction of subordinates with their respective immediate superior is concerned, we find the following patterns of results:

1. The extent to which the superior is seen as good in dealing with people, and the extent to which he is evaluated highly on his ability to plan, organize, and schedule the work are more important to the satisfaction of lower than higher level personnel in the hospital, i.e., at the lower levels of supervision in the hospitals studied.

2. By contrast, the ease with which subordinates can get their ideas and suggestions about work across to their superiors, and how good an understanding superiors have of the viewpoints of their subordinates are more important at higher than lower levels.

3. The extent to which the superior informs his subordinates of changes affecting their work in advance, the frequency with which he asks subordinates their opinion about work problems, and how free subordinates feel to discuss personal problems with their superior are more important to satisfaction with supervision at the middle levels (i.e., they are more important to the satisfaction of supervisory nurses, nonsupervisory registered nurses, and technicians than to the satisfaction of either department heads or practical nurses and aides).

4. The remaining two of the nine items examined—how often the superior expresses appreciation to his subordinates for their work, and how sure subordinates are of what their superior thinks of them and their work—produce no consistent relationships to the satisfaction of subordinates with supervision.

A fourth set of findings shows that neither the three supervisory skills nor the nine specific supervisory practices and characteristics studied are directly related to the quality of patient care rendered in the participating hospitals. Moreover, this lack of a direct significant relationship between the various aspects of supervision and patient care quality, or hospital effectiveness, is confirmed regardless of (1) which of our measures of patient care is used in the analysis, and (2) whether the skills and practices of supervisory personnel at all levels combined, or at each individual level separately, are examined in relation to patient care. These results contrast sharply with the results concerning the relationship between supervisory behavior and the overall satisfaction of subordinates with supervision.

Another set of findings, dealing with the relationship between supervisory behavior and organizational coordination in the participating hospitals, shows that some of the specific supervisory practices and characteristics are related to coordination, particularly to preventive coordination. These practices and characteristics share in common the fact that they pertain to work-relevant communication between superiors and subordinates. Specifically, the frequency with which superiors in the various hospitals ask subordinates their opinion about work problems, and the extent to which they express appreciation to subordinates for their work are positively and significantly related to overall coordination and to several of the specific measures of coordination, especially the preventive coordination measures. (Interestingly enough, expressing appreciation was earlier found to be one of the two supervisory items, among a total of nine, that yielded no consistent relationships to satisfaction with supervision.) In addition to these two supervisory practices, the ease with which subordinates can get their ideas and suggestions about work across to their superiors, and how sure subordinates are of what their superior expects of them also relate to preventive coordination. In short, in the better coordinated hospitals superiors more frequently ask subordinates their opinion and express appreciation to subordinates for their work, while subordinates find it easier to get their ideas across to their superiors and have a better knowledge of what is expected of them.

Moreover, the same superior-subordinate communication practices that were here found to relate to coordination in the hospital also happen to relate to the clarity of hospital rules and regulations, while clarity itself was earlier found to facilitate coordination. And similarly, like clarity of rules, the extent to which people from the different jobs and departments in the hospital see each other's viewpoint in connection with their work relationships is significantly related both to coordination and to the four items with which we are concerned here—how frequently superiors ask subordinates their opinion about work problems, how often they express appreciation to subordinates for their work, how easy subordinates find it to get their ideas about work changes or improvements across to their superiors, and how sure subordinates are of what is expected of them or where they stand with their respective superiors. These results suggest that, where there is free and frequent communication about the work and work problems between superiors and subordinates, each member of the organization can make a contribution to coordination by being better able to make the hour-to-hour, and even minute-by-minute, adjustments in his behavior that are required in the daily operation of the organization, but which can seldom be handled through advance planning or programed coordination. (For further discussion and findings regarding the importance of other aspects of superior-subordinate communication for organizational coordination and performance in the hospital, see Chap. 10.)

In summary, we find that purely emotional-supportive behavior on the part of supervisory personnel in the hospitals studied (e.g., superior is good in dealing with people, subordinates feel free to discuss personal problems with

Summary

their supervisor) relates neither to coordination nor to patient care, although it relates to the satisfaction of subordinates with their respective immediate superior. On the other hand, coordination in the hospital (particularly general coordination of the preventive type) is apparently facilitated by frequent exchange of certain kinds of work-relevant communication between superiors and subordinates. These aspects of supervisory behavior are related to organizational coordination, but they are not directly related to the quality of patient care. However, we know from earlier reported findings that coordination is positively and significantly related to the quality of patient care. Consequently, supervisory behavior of the kind specified above might relate to the quality of patient care indirectly, by making for better coordination (any direct relationship between supervision and patient care having been ruled out, since none of the supervisory skills and practices investigated produced a direct significant relationship with the measures of patient care).

The last, and final, set of results reported in this chapter derive from an analysis designed to examine and tentatively test this interesting proposition that supervisory behavior in the hospitals studied relates to the quality of patient care only indirectly, through the mediation of coordination variables. The pertinent findings are supportive of this proposition, and suggest that additional research in this connection would be warranted. Certain supervisory practices involving superior-subordinate communication that is work relevant, as specified above, are more evident in the better coordinated hospitals, while the quality of patient care is also higher in the better coordinated institutions. It appears that coordination is an important intervening variable between supervisory behavior and patient care in the community general hospital. Supervision affects coordination which, in turn, affects patient care. There are several reasons for the presence of such an indirect relationship between supervisory behavior and organizational effectiveness.

Hospital effectiveness, like the effectiveness of other complex organizations, is dependent upon good coordination. But, unlike many other organizations, the hospital is in large measure dependent upon the actions of its personnel for the attainment and maintenance of adequate coordination. There are no assembly lines, and few precisely repetitious flows of work are available in the hospital to serve as mechanisms of coordination. Under these conditions, the role of supervision, through the kinds of superior-subordinate relationships we have specified, can be very instrumental to ensuring adequate coordination. Advance planning and formal organizational rules and regulations are essential to organizational functioning and coordination, but they are not enough in and of themselves. Effective day-to-day communication between superiors and subordinates about the work process and work problems provides an additional key mechanism for coordination. Among other things, an open and frequently used channel of communication between superiors and subordinates accomplishes the following:

1. Lays the groundwork for understanding and accepting the rules and regulations set up by the organization;

2. Helps identify and bring into the open problems arising in the everyday operations of the organization, especially problems that cannot be fully anticipated but which require solution, with continuity and regularity;

3. Facilitates the development of common understandings and shared expectations regarding the work on the part of organizational members who have to work with one another; and

4. Allows individual members to contribute further to the coordination of the organization by being better able to make adjustments in their behavior so as to avoid creating problems or interference in their work relationships, and by being able to transmit their ideas and suggestions about the work situation to those with formal authority to act.

In conclusion, supervisory behavior that facilitates work-relevant communication between supervisory and nonsupervisory personnel in the hospitals studied contributes to coordination, and coordination allows the hospital as an organization to accomplish its objectives effectively. In the community general hospital, the supervisory practices that make a difference contribute directly to the fundamental task of organizational coordination. And while the human relations skills of supervisors are important to subordinate satisfaction with supervision, it is the pattern of superior-subordinate communications regarding work and work arrangements that is directly related to coordination and indirectly to patient care—the principal objective of the organization.

REFERENCES

1. Argyris, C. *Personality and Organization*. New York: Harper, 1957.
2. Brayfield, A. H., and Crockett, W. H. "Employee Attitudes and Employee Performance," *Psychol. Bull.*, 52:396–424, 1955.
3. Cartwright, D., and Zander, A. (eds.). *Group Dynamics: Research and Theory*. Evanston, Ill.: Row, Peterson, 1953.
4. Cleven, W. A., and Fiedler, F. E. "Interpersonal Perceptions of Open-Hearth Foremen and Steel Production," *J. Applied Psychol.*, 40:312–14, 1956.
5. Comrey, A. L., High, W. S., and Wilson, R. C. "Factors Influencing Organizational Effectiveness VI: A Survey of Aircraft Workers," *Personnel Psychol.*, 8:79–99, 1955.
6. ——— "Factors Influencing Organizational Effectiveness VII: A Survey of Aircraft Supervisors," *Personnel Psychol.*, 8:245–57, 1955.
7. Fiedler, F. E. "Assumed Similarity Measures as Predictors of Team Effectiveness," *J. Abnorm. & Social Psychol.*, 48:381–87, 1954.
8. ——— "The Influence of Leader-Key Man Relations on Combat Crew Effectiveness," *J. Abnorm. & Social Psychol.*, 51:227–35, 1955.
9. Fleishman, E. A. "A Leader Behavior Description for Industry." In Stogdill, R. M., and Coons, A. E. (eds.). *Leadership Behavior: Its Description and Measurement*. Columbus, Ohio: Ohio State University, 1957.

References

10. Georgopoulos, B. S., and Seashore, S. E. "Comparison of Men in (Groups) Stations of High and Low Overall Effectiveness." Survey Research Center, 1956.
11. ———— "Comparison of Supervisors in (Groups) Stations of High and Low Overall Effectiveness." Survey Research Center, 1956.
12. Georgopoulos, B. S., Mahoney, G. M., and Jones, N. W., Jr. "A Path-Goal Approach to Productivity," *J. Applied Psychol.*, **41**:345–53, 1957.
13. Georgopoulos, B. S., and Tannenbaum, A. S. "A Study of Organizational Effectiveness," *Am. Sociol. Rev.*, **22**:534–40, 1957.
14. Halpin, A. W. "The Leadership Behavior and Combat Performance of Airplane Commanders," *J. Abnorm. & Social Psychol.*, **49**:15–22, 1954.
15. ———— "The Leader Behavior and Effectiveness of Aircraft Commanders." In Stogdill, R. M., and Coons, A. E. (eds.). *Leadership Behavior: Its Description and Measurement*. Columbus, Ohio: Ohio State University, 1957.
16. Hemphill, J. K. "Leadership Behavior Associated with the Administrative Reputations of College Departments," *J. Ed. Psychol.*, **46**:385–402, 1955.
17. Hemphill, J. K., and Coons, A. E. "Development of the Leader Behavior Description Questionnaire." In Stogdill, R. M., and Coons, A. E. (eds.). *Leadership Behavior: Its Description and Measurement*. Columbus, Ohio: Ohio State University, 1957.
18. Kahn, R. L., and Katz, D. "Leadership Practices in Relation to Productivity and Morale." In Cartwright, D., and Zander, A. (eds.). *Group Dynamics: Research and Theory*. Evanston, Ill.: Row, Peterson, 1953.
19. Katz, R. L. "Skills of the Effective Administrator," *Harvard Business Rev.*, **33**:33–43, 1955.
20. Likert, R. "Effective Supervision: An Adaptive and Relative Process," *Personnel Psychol.*, **11**:317–32, 1958.
21. Mann, F. C., and Dent, J. K. "Appraisals of Supervisors and the Attitudes of their Employees in an Electric Power Company." Survey Research Center. 1954.
22. ———— "The Supervisor: Member of Two Organizational Families," *Harvard Business Rev.*, **32**:103–12, 1954.
23. Mann, F. C., and Hoffman, L. R. *Automation and the Worker: A Study of Social Change in Power Plants*. New York: Holt, 1960.
24. Mann, F. C., and Williams, L. K. "Organizational Impact of White Collar Automation." In *Proceedings of Eleventh Annual Meeting of Industrial Relations Research Association*, Chicago, December 1958. Publication No. 22, 1959, 55–69.
25. ———— *Automation in the Office*. (In preparation.)
26. Metzner, H., and Mann, F. C. Employee Attitudes and Absences. *Personnel Psychol.*, **6**:467–85, 1953.
27. Roethlisberger, F. J. *Training for Human Relations*. Boston: Harvard University, Graduate School of Business Administration, 1954.
28. Seashore, S. E., Indik, B. P., and Georgopoulos, B. S. "Relationships among Criteria of Job Performance," *J. Applied Psychol.*, **44**:195–202, 1960.
29. Siegel, S. *Nonparametric Statistics for the Behavioral Sciences*. New York: McGraw-Hill, 1956.
30. Stogdill, R. M., and Coons, A. E. (eds.). *Leadership Behavior: Its Description and Measurement*. Columbus, Ohio: Ohio State University, 1957.

10 THE COMMUNICATION PATTERNS OF REGISTERED NURSES IN RELATION TO NURSING ACTIVITY AND PERFORMANCE[1]

The literature on organization, decision making, and administration is replete with reference to the organizational significance of communication phenomena. In describing the role of management, for example, Drucker (3) lists "motivating and communicating" as one of the fundamental tasks of management. Moore (6), in discussing executive functions, also asserts the importance of "establishing and maintaining lines of communication." And, Burling (2), speaking of internal communication in hospitals, concludes that extensive communication is necessary in the hospital because of the irregularity of workflow and because of the needs of personnel with related jobs to coordinate their everyday work relationships. One might add that adequate patient care requires both high performance standards and successful coordination, and one of the means for setting and maintaining high standards and coordinating activities is communication.

The organizational function of communication is to transmit enough relevant information accurately and efficiently so as to reduce or prevent incompatibility, irrationality, and unwanted diversity in the behavior and attitudes of those involved. To this effect, organizations usually establish and maintain

---

[1] We are indebted to Dr. Ruth E. Searles, Ph.D., former Assistant Study Director on our research staff, for her contribution to this part of the study. As a member of the staff, she played a major role in the development, analysis, and interpretation of the data about communication, and she wrote a preliminary draft of this chapter.

formal channels of communication along organizational authority lines, linking the various jobs and positions in the system. Not all communication proceeds along formally prescribed channels, however. Because organizational members frequently interact with one another on an informal basis, informal channels of communication are also likely to be established and exist along with formal ones. Most if not all organizations, therefore, have both a formal and an informal network of communication. More importantly, the two networks may often work at odds instead of complementing or supplementing each other, and this may result in organizationally undesirable outcomes. Ideally, therefore, it is important for studies of communication in organizations to take into account both the formal and the informal aspects of the communication process. Results from previous research clearly point in this direction.

In a study of communication in informal groups, Festinger, Schachter, and Back (4) found that various aspects of communication related to interpersonal attraction and friendship among members, on the one hand, and to uniformity of attitudes and behavior, on the other. They concluded that where people have friendship relationships with one another active channels of communication are likely to be established between them, and a considerable volume of diverse information is likely to be exchanged through these channels, with the result that people come to develop increasingly shared opinions and attitudes. In addition, the more cohesive a group is (i.e., the more friendship ties and the greater the interpersonal attraction among group members), the more active the communication process is, and the higher the chances are for producing uniformity in group standards and conformity to such standards. In the absence of physical barriers such as distance, social barriers such as status, or psychological barriers such as antagonism, people who share some socially relevant characteristic—e.g., membership in a profession, residence in a neighborhood, or employment in an organization—tend to develop channels for the flow of information and ideas among themselves. In turn, through the exchange of information and ideas, group members tend to develop similar frames of reference and outlooks which come to color their interaction with other people.

Additional support for the above position is provided by Newcomb. He suggests that "communication among humans performs the essential function of enabling two or more individuals to maintain simultaneous orientation toward one another as communicators *and* toward objects of communication" (7, p. 149). For example, a nurse and her supervisor, talking about ways to improve patient care, constitute a communicative system in which the orientation or attitude of the nurse toward her supervisor and toward patient care, and the orientation of the supervisor toward the nurse and toward patient care are interdependent. According to Newcomb's theory, the greater the interpersonal attraction between the nurse and the supervisor in this system, the more they will both strive toward symmetry in their attitudes about patient care. Conversely, the less the attraction between them, the more limited this symmetry is likely to be; symmetry will tend to be limited to those objects in the situation about which the nurse and the supervisor are forced to have consensus due to the conditions of their association. In turn, lack of symmetry in their orientations toward different objects, together with the lack of interpersonal attraction, will result in lack of communication, or insufficient communication, about these objects. Such lack of communication will then tend to perpetuate the divergence in their orientations toward the objects involved. Under these conditions, achievement of consensus becomes difficult, if not impossible. Since a certain amount of consensus is essential to the continuity of the system, moreover, such a situation will ultimately create organizational problems.

Studying communication processes in more formalized experimental situations, Bales (1) was able to observe various aspects of the dynamics involved when communicators, acting as a group, attempted to solve certain assigned problems. Working with small, problem-solving groups, under controlled laboratory conditions, he found that these groups would generally go through certain phases before completing a task, in each phase concentrating on a certain aspect of communication. He calls these phases orientation, evaluation, and control. "Orientation" refers to the process of arriving at a shared definition of what the problem is; "evaluation" refers to the process of deciding what attitudes toward the problem are appropriate; and "control" refers to the process of influencing group decision about ways to resolve the problem. At the same time that the group had to handle these communication problems, moreover, it also had to maintain itself as a group and to prevent or mend cleavages that might hinder its work. In this connection, both leadership with respect to accomplishing the task involved and leadership with respect to providing social and emotional support to group members were observed to develop in the group. On the basis of these findings, if we can conceive of a work group or a superior-subordinate relationship in a real life situation as a problem-solving system, we can infer that the participants involved will have to solve problems related both to the performance of their tasks and to the maintainance of the group itself. Aspects of communication that are task relevant include such things as giving or requesting information, opinions, and suggestions about the problem at hand; aspects that are relevant to group maintenance include such things as the expression of appreciation, approval, and disapproval. In this study, we will be concerned both with the former and with the latter.

Although the preceding studies point to certain important aspects of communication and their relation to attitudes and behavior concerning task performance and group maintenance, they do not actually confront the complexity of communication problems found in large-scale organizations such as hospitals. With extensive division of labor, extensive specialization, and extensive status and skill differentiation, the exchange of information is an important means of adjusting, regulating, and coordinating many interdependent tasks and activities in work relationships. Moreover, the less routinized and mechanized an organization is, the more complicated this situation becomes. Under these conditions, one of the most important problems of administration is to establish and keep open whatever communication channels are needed for making available information and facts which are necessary to sound decision making by organizational members.

This problem has been studied in some detail by Jaques (5), in an industrial plant in Great Britain. On the basis of his findings, he concludes that, among other things, successful fact finding—a necessary condition to problem solving—requires that the relationship between superior and subordinates permit free talk on all matters, whether they pertain to technical problems, questions of policy, interpersonal relations, or the attitudes and behavior of the superior himself. If the superior can establish in his subordinates the expectation that he will be constructive and helpful, relevant information will be transmitted and problems will be identified and solved; if not, information will probably be concentrated in informal channels, and this may result in undesirable consequences such as "by-passing" those in positions of decision making and formal responsibility. Jaques recognizes, however, that openness of communication may create problems if the content of communication is irrelevant to the problems at hand, and he makes a distinction between barriers which inhibit necessary information and barriers which screen out unnecessary information. In the present study, we will be concerned with both kinds of barriers.

The Problem of This Chapter

The studies cited above have suggested the importance of certain aspects of communication to the attitudes and behavior of group members in various settings. In the hospital, communication is potentially a medium by which people in different jobs and departments can be informed about organizational goals and standards of patient care and about the rules and conditions governing their jobs and work relationships; it is a medium for exchanging ideas about hospital routines, schedules, and procedures. It is also a powerful means for developing shared points of view among different people with strikingly diverse backgrounds, and for establishing shared or uniform standards of behavior and, then, effecting conformity to them. From an organizational standpoint, communication is needed to coordinate different roles and activities that are necessary to the continuous provision of adequate patient care, and to achieve a certain amount of consensus about the work situation on the part of a large and heterogeneous membership.

Not all communication in a hospital, or any other organization, is functional for the system or its members, however. Under some circumstances, communication—too little, too much, or of the wrong kind—may also be dysfunctional. In general, the consequences for an organization of prevailing communication practices among its members will depend on such specific considerations as who talks with whom, about what, in what way, and for how long. Both qualitative and quantitative factors are important; both formal and informal channels and their relative availability and use are important; and both relevant and irrelevant information passing through these channels are important to the solution of problems and to successful role performance on the part of organizational members. The problem of this chapter is to relate these aspects of the communication process to certain aspects of nursing activity and performance across hospitals. Because of the centrality of the role of the registered nurse in hospital organization, the focus of this part of the study will be on registered nurses. Furthermore, our discussion will be mainly based on data collected through questionnaires from nonsupervisory registered nurses in each of the ten hospitals studied.

The contents of this chapter have been organized, and will be presented, in four major sections. The first section, immediately following, deals with certain theoretical considerations about communication among hospital nurses and presents a number of ideas and hypotheses that were investigated in this study. These hypotheses propose certain relationships between various aspects of communication and various aspects of nursing activity and performance. The second section presents a discussion of the methods and procedures used to obtain the necessary data in order to test the several ideas and hypotheses in a systematic manner. This discussion answers such questions as how and from whom the relevant data were collected, what kinds of data were used to measure communication and nursing performance, i.e., the independent and dependent variables in the study, and in what manner these data were analyzed to test the hypotheses involved. The third section presents the findings in detail, together with a discussion of these findings. And the fourth, and final, section summarizes the main results appearing in the chapter and presents a number of conclusions based on these results.

COMMUNICATION AMONG NURSES: SOME THEORETICAL CONSIDERATIONS AND HYPOTHESES

Perhaps the best way to introduce this section is to begin with some relatively simple but actual difficulties in communication encountered in the various hospitals participating in the study. Such concrete problems of communication among nursing personnel are suggested by the comments of nurses to certain questions asked of them, as shown below.

> Q: How clearly defined are the policies and the various rules and regulations of the hospital that affect your job?

A: I have never been informed as to hospital rules and regulations.
Q: How frequently do you talk with your immediate superior about ways of improving patient care?
A: Seldom allowed to present your views. Usually [the superior] objects before you more than start.
Q: If you have a suggestion for improving the job or changing the setup in some way, how easy is it for you to get your ideas across to your superiors?
A: Not given the opportunity.
Q: When decisions that affect your work are made, how adequately are such decisions explained to you?
A: When things are changed on our floor and it is explained one day—if you are off that day, you miss it. It is told to all who are there never giving a thought to the ones who are off that day. . . .

Written by the respondents to explain their answers to the corresponding questionnaire items, the above comments illustrate some of the problems that can and do arise from inadequate opportunity to exchange information, or from the existence of barriers along communication channels. Although these comments may not be representative of the situation in any single hospital, they serve to indicate both possible failures in the communication process and possible connections between such failures and other organizational problems involving nursing personnel. The fact, for example, that a nurse was not informed of hospital rules and regulations will likely have significant implications for her work as well as for others in related jobs. Similarly, the fact that another nurse experiences difficulty in communicating with her supervisor about ways to improve patient care is likely to have important repercussions both for her own behavior and for patient care in the hospital. These connections become more apparent if one keeps in mind the nature of the work situation, or the action structure, within which nurses function.

The organization of nursing personnel, both in terms of division of work among them and in terms of the articulation of their activities, frequently varies from one nursing section or shift to another in the same hospital, and from hospital to hospital. Sometimes each member of the nursing staff in a particular section is given a set of specific assignments, although both the section and the assignments are subject to change over time. Sometimes, groups or teams of nursing personnel, e.g., a registered nurse, two practical nurses, and four aides, may be assigned a certain number of patients, the ranking member of the team, usually the professional nurse, having responsibility for distributing tasks among team members. Other variations in the pattern of organizing nursing roles and activities may also occur. Whatever the particular pattern may be, however, nursing tasks are not mechanized as in an assembly line. Consequently, specifications for their performance, distribution, and coordination cannot be automatically controlled. The same is true, to an even greater degree, for the work relationships between nursing personnel, on the one hand, and other staffs and groups, including the patients, on the other. Accordingly, interaction and communication, both among nursing personnel and between nursing personnel and others, is necessary for allocating work responsibilities, prescribing and implementing procedures, setting and following standards of care and performance, establishing and modifying schedules and routines, and resolving existing problems or avoiding new ones. In this connection, the role of the registered nurse is a particularly crucial one since registered nurses, more than any other personnel in the hospital, come in frequent contact with other nursing personnel, with doctors, and with people in most of the other roles in the hospital, including the patients.

The accomplishment of all these activities with a minimum of strain on the part of those involved depends, to a large extent, upon consensus and mutual understanding of the role each is to play within the nursing staff, and between nursing personnel and others. The ability of the nursing staff to provide excellent care to the patient depends not only on their skill—which is clearly of great importance—but also upon a web of relationships among them which facilitates the establishment of shared expectations about their own activities and work relationships and about the day-to-day operations of the hospital. Ease of communication among those whose jobs are related should facilitate the development of such a web. This, in turn, should facilitate nursing performance.

One of the tasks of supervision and administration is the development and maintenance of shared expectations and consensus among organizational members. Another is that of making decisions and solving problems arising in the work situation. But successful problem solving, or sound decision making, depends in part upon whether or not relevant information is channeled from those who are in a position to see a problem to those who are in a position to act on it. It depends, for example, on whether or not the nurse on duty will pass relevant information to her supervisor, or to the doctor, as well as to others with whom she works. In this connection, we can think of the available formal communication channels as relatively open or closed to the transmission of adequate relevant information. Both the relevance of information exchanged and the openness of the organizational channels through which it should pass will have an effect on whether problems are solved and decisions are taken when needed, thus affecting the role performance of those involved. Thus, amount of communication, ease of communication, relevance of communicated material, and openness of the prescribed channels of communication ultimately have implications for successful task completion and role performance. These ideas will all be tested later in the chapter in the form of more specific hypotheses.

Another important class of variables concerns the referents of communication. Specifically, communication about certain topics, e.g., patient care, working conditions, etc., may or may not be concentrated in formally pre-

scribed channels. If communication about task-relevant topics is concentrated in informal rather than formal channels, it is likely that organizational problems will arise. On the other hand, if formal channels are blocked with regard to information which is irrelevant, the consequences will either have no bearing on the role performance of those involved or they will be beneficial. By relevant information we mean information which is concerned with the identification and solution of task problems and the carrying out of the work responsibilities of the communicators, or information which, although not directly related to task and role performance, tends to establish a relationship among communicators which keeps channels open for task-relevant communication. A certain amount of general conversation between a nurse and her supervisor, for example, may be instrumental in establishing the "custom" of talking out problems.

There are two kinds of openness of communication channels to task-relevant information, one of a quantitative and the other of a qualitative character. Frequent use of a channel is not in itself sufficient to ensure that adequate relevant information will be transmitted. The style which characterizes the communication of those using the channel is also a determining factor. There must be an expectation on the part of the prospective communicators that talking with one another will be useful or rewarding, or at least as rewarding as not talking. Expectations on the part of either communicator that communication will be a waste of time, unpleasant, or threatening will result either in the creation of barriers along the channel or in selective, and perhaps distorted, transmission of information. Under these conditions, moreover, the very information which may be necessary to the performance of their jobs might encounter considerably greater difficulties in transmission than any other kinds of information, if it is not actually withheld altogether. Discussion of ways to improve existing work arrangements, for example, if it implies criticism from the point of view of either communicator, or if interpreted as punitive, will be likely to be cut short if it is initiated at all.

Free exchange of enough task-relevant information between a superior and subordinate requires that each feel relatively secure in his relationship and respective position. And, as far as the subordinate is concerned, one of the most important kinds of security-enhancing communication is that which tends to increase or affirm his competence. Accordingly, if the superior employs a style of communication which is supportive and permissive rather than threatening or punitive in character, he or she is likely to structure the situation in a manner that makes for free exchange of relevant information. And, this is probably applicable not only to persons in superior-subordinate relationships, but also to persons on the same organizational level.

The structure of the superior-subordinate relationship itself may vary at different organizational levels, being affected by the nature of the roles of the participants. In the hospital situation, for example, since the nonsupervisory registered nurse is more similar to her immediate superior in terms of position, training, skill, and work activity than is an aide to her immediate superior, the topics and style of communication that are appropriate to the former relationship may not necessarily be appropriate to the latter. For a nursing supervisor to ask a registered nurse, or for one registered nurse to ask another, about the condition or needs of a patient may be entirely fitting, if not indeed required. But for a nurse, whether supervisory or nonsupervisory, to ask the same question of an aide may be inappropriate or useless, and it may even be disconcerting to the aide. Accordingly, what is applicable in the case of registered nurses, insofar as communication is concerned, need not always apply to other nursing classifications.

In general, however, the freer the exchange of task-relevant information between superiors and subordinates, or among persons whose jobs are related, the greater the probabilities are for rational planning, efficient articulation of effort, and adequate coordination of activity. Conversely, the more limited the exchange of adequate relevant information is, the greater the probabilities are for the development of tensions and conflicts among organizational members. Similarly, the more adequate the communication among work group members is, in terms of amount as well as of quality, the better the possibility for developing shared expectations and consensus about the work and commitment to the group and its standards. In turn, the higher the consensus about work standards, the more likely it is that the performance of members will consistently conform to such standards; and, assuming that high standards of performance have been set for the group, the better the performance of group members should be.

In summary, both the qualitative and the quantitative aspects of communication here discussed should be taken into consideration in attempting to relate communication phenomena to other aspects of organizational functioning. They are both important for achieving adequate coordination in the work structure and maintaining satisfactory work relationships among the participants. With whom nurses communicate, whether formally or informally, the extent to which they communicate, the style of their communication, the topics of their communication, and the direction of their communication with respect to organizational position and organizational level will all have an effect on their attitudes and behavior toward the objects of communication and toward the work situation in general. They will affect not only their perception and evaluation of their own role and the role of those with related jobs in the system, but also their ability to carry out their responsibilities and, therefore, their contributions to the organization.

If the preceding views about communication phenomena in general and communication among registered nurses in the hospital in particular are correct, the relevant data collected from the ten hospitals studied should support the following hypotheses:

Some Theoretical Considerations

1. The extent to which the superior's communication is seen by subordinates as adequate, or as involving explanation, suggestion, or the expression of appreciation will be positively related to the nurses' evaluation of how well their superior performs her role and to their satisfaction with supervision.

2. The extent to which the superior's communication is seen by subordinates as involving unnecessary information or the expression of criticism will be negatively related to the nurses' evaluation of how well their superior performs her role and to their satisfaction with supervision.

3. The extent to which the superior's communication is seen by subordinates as adequate, or as involving explanation, suggestion, or the expression of appreciation will be positively related to the extent to which task-relevant communication in the system tends to be concentrated in formal rather than informal channels.

4. The extent to which the superior's communication is seen by subordinates as involving unnecessary information or the expression of criticism will be negatively related to the extent to which task-relevant communication in the system tends to be concentrated in formal rather than informal channels.

5. The degree to which task-relevant communication (e.g., communication about ways to improve patient care) among nurses tends to be concentrated in formal rather than informal channels will be positively related to nursing performance (e.g., the kind of job each of the various nursing groups does).

6. The greater the amount of task-relevant communication passing through formal organizational channels (i.e., between superiors and subordinates), the better the nursing performances.

7. The greater the amount of task-relevant communication passing through formal organizational channels (i.e., between superiors and subordinates), the higher the commitment of nurses to their work group.

8. The extent to which nurses are likely to communicate more with people at their own level rather than across levels will be negatively related to nurses' commitment to their work group.

9. The extent to which nurses are likely to communicate more with people at their own level rather than across levels will be negatively related to nursing performance in the hospital.

10. The extent to which task-relevant communication among registered nurses tends to be concentrated in formal rather than informal organizational channels will be positively related to nursing department coordination and negatively related to tension among people in different nursing roles.

The first two hypotheses pertain to the style of communication and suggest that, other things being equal, if the communication which nurses receive from their superior is characterized by aspects that may be relevant to the identification and solution of problems or to the maintenance of satisfactory work relationships, then nurses will be likely both to evaluate their superior as doing a good job and to be satisfied with their superior. Conversely, if the communication from their superior is seen as irrelevant or threatening, nurses will be likely to feel that their superior is not performing her role well. The next two hypotheses state that if the superior's communication is similarly perceived by subordinates as positive, or negative, then the subordinates will tend to communicate with her more, or less, about task-related topics such as patient care, supervision, and the like. According to the fifth hypothesis, if communication about task-relevant topics tends to follow superior-subordinate lines, rather than informal channels, the greater the chances will be that both nurses and their supervisors will be able to do an effective job, since, as the tenth hypothesis states, better coordination of activities and less tension among personnel will prevail. According to the sixth and seventh hypotheses, the greater the amount of task-relevant communication in the formal channels, the higher the commitment of nurses to their work group, and the better the nursing performance is expected to be. The eighth and ninth hypotheses suggest that, because of the centrality of the role of the registered nurse in the system, if nurses tend to communicate more within their own level rather than with persons in higher or lower positions whose jobs are related to theirs, commitment to the work group is likely to be low and nursing performance is likely to suffer. The tenth, and last, hypothesis predicts better coordination and less tension in nursing departments where task-relevant communication among registered nurses tends to be concentrated in formal rather than informal channels.

These are the hypotheses through which, in this part of the study, we will attempt to investigate the significance of communication to other organizational phenomena. These hypotheses were designed to permit study of the relationship between various communication patterns among nurses and certain aspects of nursing role performance in the hospital. All hypotheses were especially formulated with the role of the registered nurse in mind, although they are probably applicable to other nursing groups as well; accordingly, they will be tested mainly on the basis of data from registered nurses. Because of the centrality of the role of the registered nurse, both within the nursing department and within the total hospital organization (registered nurses being expected to coordinate the work of other nursing groups and to relate nursing activities of people in other departments), because of the relatively heavy reliance on formal authority lines in the work structure, and because of the relatively high emphasis on task orientation in the hospital (everything being focused on the patient and patient care), the above hypotheses were deliberately formulated to emphasize these important characteristics of our research site. We next turn to the methods and procedures used to measure the several variables which are indicated in the above hypotheses and which will permit us to test these hypotheses.

METHODOLOGICAL CONSIDERATIONS: MEASUREMENT OF COMMUNICATION AND ROLE PERFORMANCE

This section of the chapter will be concerned with a discussion of the procedures used in collecting and analyzing the data on communication and role performance among nurses. In more technical terms, it will be concerned with a discussion of (1) the respondents involved, (2) the measurement of the various independent (communication) and dependent (role performance) variables contained in the hypotheses discussed in the preceding section, and (3) the method used to analyze the data and to study the relationships between the independent and dependent variables.

Data for this part of the study were for the most part collected from nonsupervisory registered nurses in the ten hospitals studied. For each hospital separately, a sample of nurses was drawn (see Chap. 2 regarding sampling, questionnaires used, response rates, and respondent reaction). The sample was drawn in such a manner as to represent the entire group of nonsupervisory registered nurses in each hospital, regardless of work shift or whether working full-time or part-time. In seven of the ten hospitals, one out of every three nurses was thus selected; in the remaining three hospitals, one out of every two was selected because the total group was relatively small. In all cases, however, an individual nurse in a given hospital had the same chance of being selected in the sample as any other member of her group. In all hospitals combined, of a grand total of 213 individual nurses initially selected to participate in the study and still working for the hospital during data collection, 196 finally completed appropriate questionnaires. Thus, the overall questionnaire completion rate was 92 percent. The number of nonsupervisory registered nurses who were selected and completed questionnaires in each hospital ranges across hospitals from a low of 14 persons in one hospital to a high of 27 in another, the average being almost 20 per hospital. In each hospital, the nurses in the sample provided the pertinent data about communication. The background characteristics of nonsupervisory registered nurses have been discussed in Chapter 3.

In the analysis of the data, for each hospital and for most of the questions involved, the nonsupervisory registered nurse group of respondents will be represented by its mean response to each questionnaire item, i.e., it will be represented by the "average" of the answers its members gave to each of the several items about communication and role performance. Where some other measure instead of the mean is used, explicit reference will be made when discussing the particular measure involved. The unit of analysis in all cases will be the group of respondents in each hospital, i.e., all nonsupervisory registered nurses in each hospital separately, rather than the individual group member across hospitals. In short, in analyzing the data, our number of cases will always be ten—the number of hospitals in the study. Finally, as for most other analyses in the study, the statistical tool used here to express the magnitude and direction of association between communication and role performance variables will be the rank-order correlation coefficient.

The Independent Variables: Aspects of Communication Studied

The several questions which were used to obtain data that would permit us to measure those aspects of communication among nurses about which hypotheses were proposed will now be presented. First, to obtain a measure of the adequacy of communication between superior and subordinates, the following question was used:

> In general, how do you feel about the kind of communication which you receive from your *immediate superior?* (Check one.)
> _____(1) The kind of communication I receive from my immediate superior is completely adequate
> _____(2) Very adequate
> _____(3) Fairly adequate
> _____(4) Rather inadequate
> _____(5) The kind of communication I receive from my immediate superior is inadequate

Using the five-point scale formed by the response alternatives in this question, hospital means were computed based on the responses supplied by the nurses. The range of the obtained means was from 1.69 signifying the hospital where communication between nonsupervisory registered nurses and their superiors is most adequate, to 2.36 signifying the hospital where such communication is least adequate according to the respondents. The other eight hospitals fall between these two extremes.

Next, in order to measure the amount of communication between nurses and their superiors, the following question was used:

> On the whole, what is the average amount of time per week you talk with your *immediate superior* in the hospital? (Check one.)
> _____(1) I usually talk with my immediate superior less than ¼ hour per week
> _____(2) Between ¼ and ½ hour per week
> _____(3) Between ½ and 1 hour per week
> _____(4) Between 1 and 2 hours per week
> _____(5) Between 2 and 4 hours per week
> _____(6) I usually talk with my immediate superior more than 4 hours per week

Using the six-point scale formed by the response alternatives in this question, hospital means were again computed. The range of the obtained means was from 2.79 for the hospital where nonsupervisory registered nurses talk least

Methodological Considerations

with their immediate superiors, to 3.73 for the hospital where they talk most. The other eight hospitals fall between these two extremes.

Then, to determine the frequency with which nurses communicate with their immediate superior, or to measure the amount of time they spend communicating about certain topics of varying task relevance, this question was used: "How often do you usually talk with your immediate superior about each of the following things?" The items about which this information was obtained were, in order: "about ways in which patient care could be improved"; "about ways in which nursing supervision could be improved"; "about work"; "about employee wages, hours, or benefits"; "about ways in which working relations between departments could be improved"; "about ways in which satisfaction or morale among nursing personnel could be improved"; and "about things, people, or happenings outside the hospital." The response alternatives provided were identical for all seven items: (1) "once a month or less often," (2) "two or three times a month," (3) "about once a week," (4) "several times a week," and (5) "once a day or more often."

Using the five-point scale formed by these response alternatives, hospital means were separately computed with respect to each of the seven items involved. The obtained hospital means ranged as follows: from 2.00 to 2.86 concerning communication about patient care; 1.25 to 2.06 concerning nursing supervision; 2.83 to 3.71 concerning work; 1.07 to 1.81 concerning employee wages and hours; 1.31 to 1.87 concerning relations between departments; 1.57 to 2.18 concerning satisfaction and morale; and from 2.47 to 3.58 concerning things outside the organization. The particular hospital means obtained with respect to these seven items also show that, on the average, nurses talk most frequently about work and next most frequently about things outside the hospital. The next most frequently talked about item is ways to improve patient care followed, in order, by personnel satisfaction and morale, relations between departments, and nursing supervision. The least talked about item is employee wages, hours, or benefits.

To measure various qualitative aspects of communication between superiors and subordinates, two questions were asked of the respondents. First, one question was asked to obtain a measure of the extent to which communication from the superior involves the expression of appreciation about the work of the subordinates:

> How often does your immediate superior express appreciation for your work? (Check one.)
>
> _____(1) Always or nearly always expresses appreciation for my work
> _____(2) Very often
> _____(3) Often
> _____(4) Sometimes
> _____(5) Seldom or never expresses appreciation for my work

The obtained hospital means from responses to this question ranged from 2.50 to 3.65.

The second question designed to obtain data for the measurement of qualitative aspects of communication was a multiple-item question instructing the respondent to: "Check in the appropriate column . . . how often your *immediate superior* talks to you in each of the following ways: (Check one for each item)." Among the items involved were: "explains things or gives information or suggestions"; "asks you for suggestions or opinions"; "asks you for information, explanation, or clarification"; "criticizes you, refuses to help, or is unnecessarily formal"; and "gives excess, unnecessary information or comments." For each of these items, the respondents could choose one of the following response alternatives: (1) "always or nearly always"; (2) "most of the time"; (3) "sometimes"; (4) "a few times"; and (5) "seldom or never."

On the basis of the five-point scale corresponding to the response alternatives in this question, hospital means again were computed with respect to each item in the question. The obtained hospital means ranged across hospitals as follows: from 2.06 to 2.86 for the item about explaining things; 2.46 to 3.35 for the item about asking for suggestions; 2.29 to 3.45 for the item about asking for information; 4.50 to 4.89 for the item about criticism; and 4.39 to 4.94 for the item about unnecessary information or comments. These data show a good deal of variation in communication practices across hospitals. They also show, however, that on the whole communication between nonsupervisory registered nurses and their immediate superiors involves relatively infrequent criticism or unnecessary commentary (the last two of the above items).

All of the preceding questions elicited data concerning communication between nurses and their immediate superior. Therefore, these data represent communication in formal organizational channels. To represent communication through informal channels, respondents were also asked identical or similar questions about their communication with that person in the hospital with whom they talk most, in the majority of cases this person being someone other than the respondent's superior. With reference to the person in the hospital with whom they communicate most, nurses were asked about the following things: (1) the average amount of time they spend talking with this person per week; (2) the frequency with which they talk with this person about ways to improve patient care, about improving nursing supervision, etc.—exactly the same items asked about communication with their superior; and (3) the position of the person with whom they talk most, i.e., whether this is a person at a higher level, at the same level, at a lower level, or whether it happens to be the immediate superior.

In most cases, the data obtained from this last set of questions, compared with the data obtained about communication with the immediate superior, show that nurses talk more frequently about each of the several specific topics

Methodological Considerations 515

with the person with whom they talk most in the hospital rather than with their immediate superior. The specific disparities between the average frequency of talking with the most-talked-to person and talking with the immediate superior, of course, vary by hospital and topic. What is more relevant to our hypotheses, however, is that the arithmetic difference between the mean frequency of talking with the immediate superior and the mean frequency of talking with the most-talked-to person provides us with an indicator of the relative degree of concentration of communication, or centralization of communication, in the formal channels. The greater the frequency of talking about a given topic with the immediate superior in relation to talking with the most-talked-to person, the more concentrated the communication is in the formal channels. This measure, rather than straight frequency measures, often will be used in presenting findings in the next major section of this chapter.

A final communication variable about which data were also obtained has to do with the direction of communication among nurses. We can think of communication in an organization such as the hospital, or in an organizational unit such as the nursing department, as being primarily horizontal, i.e., as taking place among persons of the same or an equivalent organizational position, or as being primarily vertical, i.e., as taking place across positions or levels. To measure the direction of communication between nurses and persons other than their immediate superior, the following question was asked of the respondents.

> What position in the hospital does this person with whom you talk most frequently have? (Check one.)
> _____(1) This person has a position lower than mine
> _____(2) This person has a position at the same level as mine
> _____(3) This person is my immediate superior
> _____(4) This person has a position higher than mine (but is not my immediate superior)

Since the response alternatives in this question do not form a scale, unlike the case with the previous questions, percentages instead of means were used to indicate direction of communication in the various hospitals. The data obtained from this question show that, of all nonsupervisory registered nurses in all hospitals combined, 51 percent say that the person with whom they talk most is at the same level as they are; 20 percent say that this person is at a lower level; 22 percent say that this person is their immediate superior; and the remaining 7 percent say that this person is at a higher level but not their immediate superior. The corresponding percentage figures for the individual hospitals range, respectively, as follows: from 24 percent to 70 percent; from 0 percent to 36 percent; from 4 percent to 48 percent; and from 0 percent to 21 percent. These data show considerable variation from hospital to hospital with respect to the direction of communication among nurses, and the importance of this phenomenon will be discussed in the next section. They also show that, as might be expected, the person with whom nurses talk most in the hospital is someone other than their immediate superior, and that this person, as might not be expected, is most frequently one at their own level.

Thus far, we have discussed the measures of the communication variables studied, i.e., the data which provide us with measures for the independent variables contained in the hypotheses presented earlier in the chapter. We next turn to a similar discussion of measures for the dependent variables in the study, i.e., the variables about nursing activity and performance. The objective is eventually to relate the various independent variables to the various dependent variables, in order that we may test the several hypotheses which we have proposed.

The Dependent Variables: Aspects of Nursing Activity and Role Performance

Three questions were asked of the nurses to provide data for the measurement of certain aspects of the role performance of their immediate superior. The first of these questions was:

> How good is your immediate superior in planning, organizing, and scheduling the work? (Check one.)
> _____(1) Excellent
> _____(2) Very good
> _____(3) Good
> _____(4) Fair
> _____(5) Rather poor
> _____(6) Poor
> _____(7) Very poor

On the basis of the responses of nonsupervisory registered nurses in each hospital, and using the seven-point scale formed by the response alternatives in this question, hospital means were computed. For the ten hospitals in the study, these means range from 1.85 to 2.55.

The second question in this set was a multiple-item question asking the respondents to: "Check in the appropriate column . . . how much you agree with each statement as it applies to your *immediate superior*. (Check one for each item.)" The response alternatives provided were: (1) "strongly agree"; (2) "agree"; (3) "I cannot decide"; (4) "disagree"; and (5) "strongly disagree." Among the items about which this information was requested were the following: "is helpful . . ."; "does the things which are right for someone in her position"; "is personally likable . . ."; and "is an expert in her field. . . ." These are items designed to measure different aspects of the role performance of the superior, as seen by the subordinates. The percentage of

Methodological Considerations

respondents in each hospital who answered "agree" or "strongly agree" with respect to a given item was then used as the measure for that particular item. For the nonsupervisory registered nurses group of respondents, the obtained range of percentage figures across hospitals was: from 64 percent to 92 percent for the item "is helpful;" 64 percent to 96 percent for the item "does the things which are right . . ."; 68 percent to 90 percent for the item "is personally likable"; and from 50 percent to 83 percent for the item "is an expert in her field. . . ." Interestingly enough, these figures show that nurses are likely to feel that expertness on the part of their superior is a scarcer characteristic than is helpfulness or any other of the above characteristics.

The last question asked about the role performance of the immediate superior was: "Taking all things into consideration, how satisfied are you with your *immediate superior?*" Respondents could choose any one of the following alternatives: (1) "I am completely satisfied . . ."; (2) "I am very well satisfied"; (3) "I am fairly well satisfied"; (4) "I am somewhat dissatisfied"; and (5) "I am dissatisfied with my immediate superior." Using the five-point scale, formed by the response alternatives in this question, hospital means were computed about satisfaction with the superior. The obtained hospital means range from 1.63, signifying the hospital where nurses are most satisfied with their immediate superior, to 2.50, signifying the hospital where they are least satisfied.

Some of the hypotheses in this chapter have proposed certain relationships between aspects of communication and the commitment of nurses to their work group. To measure commitment to the work group, as well as to other aspects of the hospital situation, the following question was asked: "How strongly identified do you feel (how much do you feel that you *really* belong) with each of the following?" Among the objects of identification were: "my immediate work group"; "this hospital and its goals"; "my profession or occupation"; and "the team that treats the patients." In all cases, respondents were asked to answer along the following four-point scale: (1) "very strongly," (2) "quite strongly," (3) "fairly strongly," and (4) "a little." On the basis of this scale, the data were again transformed into hospital means. The obtained hospital means range as follows: from 1.36 to 1.86 concerning commitment to the work group; from 1.82 to 2.42 concerning commitment to the hospital; from 1.33 to 1.73 concerning commitment to the profession; and from 1.43 to 1.83 concerning commitment to the team that treats the patients. These data show a certain amount of variation across hospitals. They also show that nonsupervisory registered nurses feel less committed to the organization, i.e., the hospital and its goals, than to any of the other groups mentioned.

The final set of measures for nursing activity and role performance, i.e., for the dependent variables of the study, is somewhat different from the preceding sets in that it makes use of the combined responses of registered nurses and of doctors to the same items. Instead of using hospital means based on the responses of nurses only, composite measures are used based on means from more than one group. The particular groups involved in each case will be specified below. At this point, it is sufficient to note that, because of our interest in the consequences of different communication patterns among nursing personnel in the ten hospitals, this deviation in our method was made so that we might take advantage of the responses of all groups whose professional training permits them to be competent judges of nursing performance.

The first measure in this final set was based on the following question: "On the whole, what kind of a job would you say each of the following does for this hospital?" The term "following" referred to various nursing groups, including registered nurses, practical nurses, and nurse's aides. The response alternatives offered by this question were: (1) "an excellent job," (2) "a very good job," (3) "a good job," (4) "a fair job," and (5) "a rather poor job." Again, in the usual manner, hospital means were computed on the basis of the five-point scale formed by these alternatives, for each of the nursing groups to which the question refers. However, in the present case, our final measures of the performance of these nursing groups are based on responses from doctors and nonsupervisory registered nurses in each hospital. Members of these two groups were considered both competent and relevant judges in making the evaluation requested by the question here discussed. In terms of procedure, for each hospital, means were computed separately on the data from registered nurses and on the data from doctors; then these means were properly combined and averaged to yield the final hospital mean that was used in each case to measure the performance of the various groups involved. These hospital means range across hospitals as follows: from 1.88 to 2.51 concerning the job done by registered nurses; from 2.10 to 2.70 concerning the job done by practical nurses; and from 2.28 to 3.11 concerning the job done by aides.

Another similar measure of nursing performance was obtained by asking an analogous question about "what kind of a job does the nursing staff as a whole do" rather than specifying particular groups within the nursing staff. Hospital means obtained in connection with this question are based on the responses of supervisory nursing personnel and doctors in each hospital. On this measure, the hospitals in the study range from a mean of 1.87 to one of 2.62, the means being based on response alternatives identical to those used in the immediately preceding question.

Finally, three more measures of nursing activity and performance that are used in the present chapter have already been discussed in previous chapters. Therefore, they will only be mentioned at this point. First, one of these measures was designed to measure the quality of nursing care patients receive in each hospital; this measure was discussed in Chapter 5. Second, another meas-

Findings 519

ure was designed to measure the adequacy of coordination in the nursing department; this measure was discussed in Chapter 7. And, third, a final measure was designed to measure the level of tension among nursing personnel in the different nursing roles; this measure was also discussed in Chapter 7. These measures will be referred to in the present chapter, respectively, as "quality of nursing care," "nursing department coordination," and "tension between nursing classifications."

In summary, it will be recalled that the ten hospitals in the study were rank-ordered according to their score (a hospital mean or a percentage figure) on each of the several communication (i.e., independent) variables and on each of the several nursing activity and performance (i.e., dependent) variables which have been discussed in this section. On the basis of the obtained rank-orders, correlations were then computed to measure the magnitude and direction of relationships between the independent and dependent variables. It is these correlational findings that will enable us to test the several hypotheses discussed earlier in this chapter, and that will be presented in the various tables in the following section. We now turn to the presentation of the findings.

FINDINGS

For purposes of convenience and economy of presentation, the results will be presented in tabular form. In all, eight tables have been used to summarize the various correlational findings which are relevant to the hypotheses under investigation. This section of the chapter has been organized into four, smaller parts. The first part will present findings relating qualitative aspects of communication to nursing activity and performance. The second part will present findings relating quantitative aspects of communication to nursing activity and performance. The third part will present findings relating the direction of communication to nursing role performance. And the fourth part will present findings relating certain aspects of communication among nurses to the adequacy of coordination in the nursing department and to the level of tension among nursing personnel in different roles. In all cases, the findings will be discussed in relation to the particular hypothesis to which they are appropriate.

The Importance of Qualitative Aspects of Communication

It was earlier stated, in the form of specific hypotheses, that the style of communication superiors employ toward their subordinates will be related to certain aspects of their performance and to the relative concentration of communication in formal organizational channels. The first two tables, below, present findings relevant to these relationships. Specifically, the correlational findings shown in Table 64 pertain to hypothesis #1 and hypothesis #2; those shown in Table 65 pertain to hypothesis #3 and hypothesis #4.

According to hypothesis #1, the extent to which their superior's communication is seen by nurses as "adequate" or as involving explanation, suggestion, or the expression of appreciation will be positively related to the nurses' evaluation of their superior's performance and to their satisfaction with their superior. The findings in Table 64, based on data from nonsupervisory registered nurses in the ten hospitals studied, show that this hypothesis is supported. For example, the first row of correlation figures in this table shows that, across hospitals, the more adequate nurses feel the communication they receive from their immediate superior is, the more highly they evaluate different aspects of the performance of the superior, and the more satisfied they are with their superior. Specifically, adequacy of communication from the immediate superior correlates .93 with how good the superior is seen at planning and organizing the work, .90 with the extent to which the superior is seen as doing the "right things" for someone in that position, .71 with the extent to which the superior is seen as an expert in the field, and .68 with the extent to which the superior is seen as helpful, and as likable. Similarly, adequacy of communication correlates .95 with the degree to which nurses express general satisfaction with their immediate superior. All of these rank-order correlations, based on data from ten hospitals, are in the predicted direction and statistically significant at the .05 level—i.e., the probability that any of these relationships could be due to chance factors rather than to the association between the variables involved is smaller than 5 percent in each case.

The second row of correlations in Table 64 shows that essentially the same results obtain when, instead of adequacy of communication, the variable "explains things or gives information and suggestions" is considered. That is, the extent to which the communication nurses receive from their immediate superior involves explanation and suggestions is positively related to how satisfied they are with their superior, and to how they evaluate different aspects of supervisory role performance, such as planning and organizing, expertness, and helpfulness. Other correlations in Table 64 similarly show that these same aspects of supervisory role performance, as well as overall satisfaction with the immediate superior, are related to the extent to which the superior asks for information, asks for suggestions, and expresses appreciation in communicating with subordinates.

According to the results in Table 64, of the specific qualitative characteristics of the superior's communication just discussed, excluding adequacy, the one which generally correlates most with the nurses' evaluation of the different aspects of their superior's role performance is the item "superior explains things. . . ." The one that correlates least is the item [superior] "asks for suggestions or opinions." On the other hand, of the various items about supervisory role performance, the one which produces the fewest significant correlations with the different characteristics of communication is

Findings

the item "superior is likable." This is not surprising, however, since from the point of view of a registered nurse liking is probably the least relevant of all aspects of supervisory role performance shown in the table. Apart from such details as these, on the whole, the data provide strong support for the proposition that in hospitals where nurses feel that the communication they receive from their superior is of a positive nature—in the sense of being adequate or being relevant to the identification and solution of problems or to the maintenance of satisfactory work relationships—they also are likely both to evaluate their superior as doing a good job and to be satisfied with supervision. In short, hypothesis #1 is borne out in this study.

Table 64 also presents findings relevant to hypothesis #2 which states that "the extent to which the superior's communication is seen by subordinates

TABLE 64. Relation Between Certain Qualitative Aspects of the Immediate Superior's Communication and Certain Aspects of the Superior's Role Performance, As Seen by Nonsupervisory Registered Nurses *

Qualitative Aspects of Communication from Immediate Superior	Superior Is Good at Planning, Organizing	Superior Does Right Things	Superior Is Expert	Superior Is Helpful	Superior Is Likable	Satisfied with Immediate Superior
Adequacy of communication from superior †	.93	.90	.71	.68	.68	.95
Superior explains things or gives information and suggestions	.90	.78	.75	.59	.75	.90
Asks for information, explanation or clarification	.74	.74	.63	.68	.39	.73
Asks for suggestions or opinions	.51	.62	.43	.56	.19	.65
Expresses appreciation	.72	.80	.53	.75	.21	.62
Gives excess, unnecessary information or comments	−.11	−.07	.00	−.05	.16	.07
Criticizes, refuses to help, or is unnecessarily formal	.09	−.09	.02	.16	−.22	.26

* All figures are rank-order correlation coefficients, based on an N of 10 hospitals in each case. Coefficients larger than .56 are significant at the .05 level, and those .75 or larger are significant at the .01 level.
† "Adequacy" of communication correlates .95 with "superior explains," .82 with "asks for information," .65 with "asks for suggestions," .72 with "expresses appreciation," −.04 with "gives excess, unnecessary information," and .07 with "criticizes." These are also rank-order correlation coefficients, based on an N of 10 hospitals in each case.

as involving unnecessary information or the expression of criticism will be negatively related to the nurses' evaluation of how well their superior performs her role and to their satisfaction with supervision." The last two rows of correlations in Table 64 pertain to this hypothesis. None of these correlations is statistically significant, however, and not all of them are negative; in fact, they all tend to be close to zero, some being positive and others negative, and each could have occurred by chance. The conclusion to be drawn from these findings is that, in the case of nonsupervisory registered nurses, there is no necessary relationship between giving excess or unnecessary information, or between criticizing on the part of their superior, and supervisory role performance or satisfaction with supervision. Apparently, in superior-subordinate communication among registered nurses a certain amount of irrelevant information, and a certain amount of criticism is something to be expected, and it does not have a significant impact on how subordinates evaluate their superiors.

With respect to hypothesis #2, and not shown in Table 64, supplementary data from practical nurses and aides yielded essentially the same results concerning the characteristic of giving excess or unnecessary information. Regarding the item "criticizes, refuses to help, or is unnecessarily formal," however, data from these two groups tend to support the hypothesis, at least partially. In the case of practical nurses, this item was found to correlate −.76 with "superior does right things," −.68 with "superior is expert," and −.42 with how satisfied they are with their immediate superior. In the case of aides and orderlies, criticism on the part of their superior similarly correlates −.59 with satisfaction with supervision, −.70 with "superior is likable," −.59 with "superior does right things," and −.59 with "superior is good at planning." These findings, when compared to the corresponding findings obtained for registered nurses, suggest that criticism is probably seen as more threatening by persons in the nonprofessional nursing groups, thus having a significant impact on how these persons evaluate their superiors. As suggested earlier, the organizational level of the respondent appears to be acting as an intervening factor here and, therefore, it should be taken into account by hypothesis #2.

Differences in organizational level among nursing groups in the hospital reflect corresponding differences in training, work activities, and status vis-à-vis the immediate superior. Such differences, in turn, may account for the results obtained in the case of hypothesis #2, since psychologically and socially the gap between superior and subordinate is greater or smaller depending on the particular group compared. In a superior-subordinate relationship, the difference between a nonsupervisory and a supervisory registered nurse is not as great as the difference between a practical nurse, or an aide, and a registered nurse. In the former case, the difference is primarily one of function; education, professional training, skills, and organizational status are

Findings

likely to be very similar. In the latter case, however, in addition to differences in function there are considerable differences in education, training, skills, and status. Similarly, supervisory and nonsupervisory registered nurses both have considerable responsibility for patient care and for directing the work of other nursing personnel. As a consequence, a nonsupervisory registered nurse is not likely to feel very "subordinate" in relation to her supervisor, while practical nurses and aides are clearly subordinate. This may make practical nurses and aides more sensitive to and less tolerant of supervisory criticism, thus accounting for the differences in the results obtained for nonsupervisory registered nurses in contrast to those obtained for practical nurses and aides.

In addition to the above hypotheses relating the style of superior's communication to various aspects of the superior's role performance, it was hypothesized that the style of communication will also be associated with the relative openness of communication between superiors and subordinates. Hypothesis #3 and hypothesis #4 stated that the various qualitative aspects of the superior's communication, presented above, will affect the extent to which subordinates tend to communicate with their superiors about task-relevant subjects and, thus, will affect the relative concentration of communication in formal organizational channels. Subordinates whose superiors employ communication of a positive style, such that it increases or affirms the competence and security of subordinates or contributes to problem solution and group maintenance, will exchange comparatively more information with their superiors than subordinates whose superiors use communication that is seen as ego deflating or unnecessary. As a result, in the former case as against the latter, communication among registered nurses about task-relevant topics is likely to be concentrated in formal rather than informal channels. Table 65, below, presents the correlational findings which test these hypotheses.

Hypothesis #3 specifically states that "the extent to which the superior's communication is seen by subordinates as adequate, or as involving explanation, suggestion, or the expression of appreciation, will be positively related to the extent to which task-relevant communication in the system tends to be concentrated in formal rather than informal organizational channels." The relevant correlations presented in Table 65 support this hypothesis. First, the findings show that the frequency with which registered nurses talk to their immediate superior (formal communication) about ways to improve patient care, relative to talking to the most-talked-to person in the hospital (informal communication), increases with the extent to which the communication they receive from their superior is seen by them as adequate or as involving explanation, suggestions, or the expression of appreciation. Second, similar results obtain with respect to talking about ways to improve nursing supervision. Although not all the specific correlations between each of these two task-relevant topics, i.e., patient care and nursing supervision, and each of the various "positive" qualitative aspects of the superior's communication are statistically significant, the pattern of results shown by these correlations clearly supports the present hypothesis. In the hospitals where their superiors employ positive communication, nurses are likely to engage in more communication with their superior about patient care and about nursing supervision; thus, task-relevant communication among nurses in the system tends to be concentrated in formal rather than informal channels.

TABLE 65. Relation Between Certain Qualitative Aspects of the Immediate Superior's Communication, as Seen by Nonsupervisory Registered Nurses, and the Frequency of Talking to Immediate Superior Relative to Talking with the Most-talked-to Person in the Hospital *

Qualitative Aspects of Immediate Superior's Communication	Ways to Improve Patient Care	Ways to Improve Nursing Supervision	Employee Benefits	Things Outside the Hospital
Adequacy of communication from superior	.56	.70	—.27	.48
Superior explains things or gives information and suggestions	.50	.62	—.24	.44
Asks for information, explanation, or clarification	.67	.53	—.43	.68
Asks for suggestions or opinions	.71	.51	—.71	.77
Expresses appreciation	.54	.36	—.54	.44
Gives excess, unnecessary information or comments	—.19	.00	.00	—.18
Criticizes, refuses to help, or is unnecessarily formal	—.04	.10	.10	.08

* All figures are rank-order correlation coefficients, based on an N of 10 hospitals in each case. Coefficients larger than ±.56 are significant at the .05 level, and those ±.75 or larger are significant at the .01 level.

Comparable findings appearing in Table 65 also show that with respect to talking about employee benefits—which is not a task-relevant topic—the opposite situation is true: the frequency of talking about employee benefits with one's superior, relative to talking with the most-talked-to person, decreases with the extent to which supervisory communication is of a positive nature. This topic, which in the case of hospital nurses is outside the jurisdiction of either the superior or the subordinate, is discussed relatively less frequently with the superior whose communication is seen as positive by subordinates and relatively more frequently with others, i.e., in informal channels. On the other hand, the findings concerning another topic which is also not task relevant, namely, "things outside the hospital," are similar to the findings

Findings

obtained for the task-relevant topics "ways to improve patient care," and "ways to improve nursing supervision," and opposite to the findings obtained for the topic "employee benefits." Perhaps a tendency for some talk with the superior whose style of communication is positive about things outside the organization enhances the likelihood for talking about task-relevant things within the organization, and vice versa. This does not hold true, however, for things and events within the organization that are not task relevant. In short, while communication among nurses about task-relevant topics proceeds according to hypothesis #3, as the findings in Table 65 show, communication about topics that are not relevant does not operate consistently across such topics. This suggests that our initial decision to confine hypothesis #3 only to task-relevant topics was correct.

The last two rows of correlations appearing in Table 65 are relevant to hypothesis #4: "The extent to which the superior's communication is seen by subordinates as involving unnecessary information or the expression of criticism will be negatively related to the extent to which task-relevant communication in the system tends to be concentrated in formal rather than informal channels." The findings show that, whether we consider task-relevant topics (patient care and nursing supervision) or topics which are not task-relevant (employee benefits and things outside the hospital), instead of the present hypothesis an alternative proposition is supported: There is no relationship at all between the frequency with which subordinates talk with their immediate superior, relative to talking with others in the system, and the extent to which the superior's communication involves criticism or unnecessary information. The specific correlations obtained vary around zero, ranging from $-.19$ to $+.10$.

These findings, in conjunction with the findings discussed with respect to hypothesis #3 in the present section, suggest that only certain qualitative aspects of the superior's communication have an effect on the extent to which communication among registered nurses in the system is likely to be concentrated in formal rather than informal organizational channels. Only those aspects of the superior's style of communication which we have termed positive (e.g., adequacy, superior explains things, superior asks for suggestions, superior expresses appreciation) relate to the relative concentration of communication in formal channels. They relate positively for topics that are task relevant, and they relate either positively or negatively, depending on the subject involved, for topics that are not task relevant. Those aspects of the superior's communication which we have termed negative (i.e., gives excess, unnecessary information, and criticizes, refuses to help . . .) produce no significant relationships in either direction.

The Importance of Quantitative Aspects of Communication

We have just discussed various relationships between several qualitative aspects of the superior's communication toward subordinates, on the one hand, and several aspects of the superior's role performance on the other (Table 64). Similarly, we have discussed the relationship between the same qualitative aspects and the extent of relative concentration of task-relevant communication in formal rather than informal channels (Table 65), based on data from ten hospitals. Granted, now, that the extent to which communication among nurses about task-relevant subjects tends to be concentrated in formal channels is related to the style of the communication employed by the superior, what effects could this have for the communicators themselves and for the hospital? Our next hypothesis, hypothesis #5 (as well as some of the hypotheses which will be examined later) was specifically designed to provide an answer to this question.

Hypothesis #5 was stated as follows: "The degree to which task-relevant communication (e.g., communication about ways to improve patient care) among nurses tends to be concentrated in formal rather than informal channels will be positively related to nursing performance (e.g., the kind of job each of the various nursing groups does)." Table 66, below, presents the results of the study that are relevant to this hypothesis. It shows a series of correlations for two topics which are task relevant: patient care and nursing supervision, and another series of corresponding correlations for two topics which are not task relevant: employee benefits and things outside the hospital. On the whole, the findings are consistent with the present hypothesis.

The first row of correlations in Table 66 shows that the more concentrated the communication about ways to improve patient care is in the formal channels the better the nursing performance. The frequency with which nonsupervisory registered nurses talk with their immediate superior, relative to talking to the most-talked-to person in the hospital, about ways to improve patient care correlates .57 with how good a job the registered nurses do, .76 with how good a job the practical nurses do, .29 with how good a job the aides do, .60 with how good a job the nursing staff as a whole does, and .43 with the overall quality of nursing care in the hospital. In other words, whether registered nurses in a hospital tend to communicate relatively more with their immediate superior than with others about patient care is associated not only with the performance of these nurses but also with the performance of practical nurses and the performance of the nursing staff as a whole. In all these cases the correlations are as predicted by hypothesis #5, being statistically significant at the .05 level or better; the correlations concerning the performance of aides and overall quality of nursing care, although not statistically significant are also positive. These relationships are not surprising, if we keep in mind the centrality of the role of the nonsupervisory registered nurse in the hospital—a fact already emphasized in this chapter.

The second row of comparable correlations in Table 66 pertains to the topic "ways to improve nursing supervision," also a task-relevant topic. Although all five correlations are again positive, in the direction predicted by hypothesis #5, none of them reaches sufficient magnitude to be statistically significant. Perhaps nursing supervision is a less salient subject among nonsupervisory registered nurses than patient care. Hence, while the findings about the latter subject produce both positive and significant relationships, as shown above, the comparable findings about nursing supervision fail to reach statistical significance. Finally, the remaining findings in this table about the two topics that are not task relevant are consistent with the hypothesis under consideration: high frequency of talking with the superior relative to the most-talked-to person about employee benefits, if anything, shows a tendency to relate negatively to nursing performance (three of the five correlations, the larger ones, are negative and the other two are practically zero, .02 and .03), although none of the correlations involved is significant; similarly, communication about things outside the hospital produces no significant correlations with the measures of nursing performance. As hypothesis #5 suggests, task-relevance is an important consideration. More importantly, however, the relative concentration of task-relevant communication in formal rather than informal channels seems to be a desirable condition from the point of view of nursing performance, according to these findings.

The findings just discussed indicate that the relative concentration of task-relevant communication in formal rather than informal channels tends to be positively associated with nursing performance in the hospital. The next question that comes to mind is whether the absolute frequency of superior-subordinate communication about task-relevant subjects bears any relationship to

TABLE 66. Relation Between the Frequency with Which Nonsupervisory Registered Nurses Talk with Their Immediate Superior Relative to Talking with the Most-talked-to Person in the Hospital and Certain Aspects of Nursing Performance *

Frequency of Talking with Superior Relative to Talking with Most-talked-to Person About:	How Good a Job R.N.'s Do	How Good a Job P.N.'s Do	How Good a Job Aides Do	How Good a Job the Nursing Staff Does	Quality of Nursing Care
Ways to improve patient care	.57	.76	.29	.60	.43
Ways to improve nursing supervision	.38	.44	.06	.18	.26
Employee wages, hours, or benefits	−.18	−.43	−.47	.02	.03
Things, people, or happenings outside the hospital	.11	.42	.13	−.04	−.08

* All figures are rank-order correlation coefficients, based on an N of 10 hospitals in each case. Coefficients larger than ±.56 are significant at the .05 level, and those ±.75 or larger are significant at the .01 level.

nursing performance. According to hypothesis #6, "the greater the amount of task-relevant communication passing through formal organizational channels . . . the better the nursing performance" should be. Table 67 presents findings relevant to this hypothesis.

The first line of correlations in Table 67 shows that the total amount of time nonsupervisory registered nurses spend, on the average, in communicating with their immediate superior correlates .73 with how good a job registered nurses do, .47 with how good a job practical nurses do, .69 with how good a job aides do, .78 with how good a job the nursing staff as a whole does, and .75 with the overall quality of nursing care. All of these correlations except one, moreover, are statistically significant at the .05 level or better. The second line shows corresponding correlations concerning the frequency of communication between nurses and their superiors about work, in general. With respect to the same performance items, the specific correlations are .40, .31, .20, .76, and .52, respectively. These correlations are all positive, i.e., in the direction predicted by hypothesis #6. From a statistical standpoint, however, only the correlation between frequency of talking about work and how good a job the nursing staff as a whole does is statistically significant. This suggests that, if the job done by the nursing staff as a whole depends on the job done by each of the specfic nursing groups (R.N.'s, P.N.'s, and Aides), which very probably is the case, an additive process operates here so that, although the specific correlations for these three groups are not significant when

TABLE 67. Relation Between the Quantity of Communication of Nonsupervisory Registered Nurses with Their Immediate Superior and Certain Aspects of Nursing Performance *

Quantity of Nurses' Communication with Immediate Superior	How Good a Job R.N.'s Do	How Good a Job P.N.'s Do	How Good a Job Aides Do	How Good a Job the Nursing Staff Does	Quality of Nursing Care
Average total amount of time spent talking to superior	.73	.47	.69	.78	.75
Frequency of talking about work, in general	.40	.31	.20	.76	.52
Frequency of talking about ways to improve patient care	.38	.47	.64	—.04	.13
Frequency of talking about ways to improve nursing supervision	.18	.48	.29	—.19	—.08

* All figures are rank-order correlation coefficients, based on an N of 10 hospitals in each case. Coefficients larger than .56 are significant at the .05 level, and those .75 or larger are significant at the .01 level.

Findings

taken one at a time, they produce a significant relationship when taken together, i.e., they produce a significant correlation between how good a job the nursing staff as a whole does and the frequency with which registered nurses talk with their superior about work.

Other correlations shown in Table 67 between frequency of talking about "ways to improve patient care" and the various nursing performance items, and between frequency of talking about "ways to improve nursing supervision" and nursing performance, fail to produce a clear-cut pattern of association between the variables involved. Most correlations regarding these two items (seven out of ten) are, as expected, positive, and one of the positive ones is statistically significant, but this pattern cannot be taken as supporting hypothesis #6 to any appreciable degree. These findings, compared with the corresponding findings involving the total amount of time nurses spend in communicating with their superiors and the frequency with which they talk about "work," suggest an interesting conclusion. It appears that the absolute frequency of talking about specific task-relevant topics, such as ways to improve patient care or nursing supervision, does not necessarily bear a relationship to nursing performance, while the total amount of time spent in communicating with the superior and the frequency of talking about work in general do. Had we asked the question in terms of patient care, or nursing supervision, in general, rather than asking in terms of "ways to improve" care and supervision, the results might have been similar to those obtained about the total amount of communication and talking about work, i.e., positive insofar as hypothesis #6 is concerned. Since we did not, we cannot be sure of what might have happened. Accordingly, in terms of all the findings shown in Table 67, the conclusion to be drawn is this: it seems that in those hospitals where channels of communication between superiors and subordinates are relatively more open, people can talk when they see a need for doing so, and problems can be readily identified and their solution can be facilitated through talking about them; this, in turn, is associated with better nursing performance rather than the mere frequency of talking about specific task-related subjects as hypothesis #6 had originally implied.

Similar to the above hypothesis is the next one to be investigated, involving the relationship between frequency of communication and commitment to the work group rather than performance. In fact, it was partly on the basis of this next hypothesis, hypothesis #7, that hypothesis #6 had been formulated. According to hypothesis #7, "the greater the amount of task-relevant communication passing through formal organizational channels (i.e., between superiors and subordinates), the higher the commitment of nurses to their work group." The results of the study concerning this hypothesis are presented in Table 68, below. Findings are presented about two kinds of "work groups"; first, about one's "immediate work group," and second about the "team that treats the patients."

On the whole, the correlations in Table 68 support the present hypothesis. The frequency of talking about ways to improve patient care correlates .61 with the degree of nurses' commitment to their immediate work group, and .66 with their commitment to the team that treats the patients. Both correlations are as predicted and statistically significant at the .05 level. Similarly, the frequency of talking about ways to improve nursing supervision correlates .71 with commitment to the work group, and .62 with commitment to the team that treats the patients. In short, in those hospitals where nurses talk more with their immediate superior about task-relevant topics, such as patient care and nursing supervision, nurses tend to be more strongly committed to their respective work group, according to the data. Incidentally, it will be recalled at this point that, commitment was defined in this study as the extent to which nurses indicate that they are "identified," or feel that they *"really* belong" to their work group.

TABLE 68. **Relation Between Certain Aspects of the Immediate Superior's Communication and Nurses' Commitment to Their Immediate Work Group, and the Team That Treats Patients** [*]

	Degree of Commitment to: [†]	
Quantitative Aspects of Immediate Superior's Communication	*The Immediate Work Group*	*The Team that Treats Patients*
Average total amount of time spent talking with the superior	.38	.35
Frequency of talking about work in general	.17	.28
Frequency of talking about ways to improve patient care	.61	.66
Frequency of talking about ways to improve nursing supervision	.71	.62

[*] All figures are rank-order correlation coefficients, based on an N of 10 hospitals in each case. Coefficients larger than .56 are significant at the .05 level.

[†] The rank-order correlation between commitment to the immediate work group and commitment to the team that treats patients is .77. Based on an N of 10 hospitals, it is statistically significant at the .01 level.

The remaining correlations in Table 68, although also positive, show no statistically significant relationship between total amount of time spent talking with the immediate superior about work in general, and nurses' commitment to their work group or team. Since hypothesis #7 predicted such a relationship only for task-relevant topics, these findings too are consistent with this hypothesis. Considered together, the correlations appearing in Table 68 show that task relevance is an important factor in connection with hypothesis #7, i.e., with respect to commitment. Apparently, nursing groups whose members feel more strongly committed to the group have members who are

Findings

likely to be more task oriented, and not particularly concerned with aspects of the work situation that are not specifically task relevant, than groups whose members feel less committed. At least this seems to be the case with respect to how nurses in the various hospitals behave toward their immediate superior in terms of communication. It is equally plausible, on the other hand, that superiors who encourage discussion about better ways of doing things may solve more task problems, thereby making the work group successful and, hence, a more likely object of identification.

The Importance of Direction of Communication

The first four hypotheses already examined involved various qualitative aspects of the immediate superior's communication to subordinates. The last three hypotheses examined involved various quantitative aspects of superior-subordinate communication among nurses. The next two hypotheses are concerned with the direction of communication among nurses. Obviously, not all communication among nurses in a hospital follows superior-subordinate lines. Nurses do a good deal of talking with their immediate superior, but they also spend a good deal of time talking to others at their own level as well as others at lower and higher levels. In addition, some nurses talk less and others talk more with people at their own level than with their immediate superior or people at other levels. The question naturally arises as to what consequences, if any, talking more to people at one level rather than another has for such things as commitment to the work group and nursing performance. Hypothesis #8 and hypothesis #9 were specifically developed to provide an answer to this question.

On the assumption that, if communication among nonsupervisory registered nurses in the hospital tends to be restricted to people at their own level—because of the rather crucial role they play in coordinating and integrating the work activities of others in the action structure of the organization—coordination and integration will be likely to suffer, hypothesis #8 was proposed. This hypothesis states that: "the extent to which nurses are likely to communicate more with people at their own level rather than across levels will be negatively related to nurses' commitment to their work group." The work group, of course, consists not only of registered nurses but also of practical nurses, aides, etc., and the registered nurse has a good deal of responsibility both for holding the group together and for coordinating the activities of its members. Hence, hypothesis #8 suggests a relationship between how nurses direct their communication and their commitment to the work group. The next hypothesis, moreover, on the further assumption that commitment to the work group is related to nursing performance, suggests a similar relationship between direction of communication and nursing performance. (Of course, there is no reason to suggest that either of these two hypotheses should also apply to practical nurses or aides—groups whose role activities are different.)

The correlational findings concerning hypothesis #8 are presented in Table 69, below. First, we find that, the higher the proportion of registered nurses who talk most with someone at their own level (i.e., other registered nurses), the less their commitment to their immediate work group and to the team that treats the patient tends to be. In both cases, we find negative correlations: a correlation of —.32 between the proportion of nurses talking most with people at their own level and their commitment to their immediate work group; and one of —.65 between the proportion of nurses talking most with people at their own level and their commitment to the team that treats the patients. Both correlations are as predicted by hypothesis #8, but only the larger one is statistically significant at the .05 level. However, since both are in the expected direction, one being significant, and since commitment to the immediate work group happens to correlate significantly with commitment to the team that treats the patients (see footnote on Table 69), we are led to conclude that the hypothesis in question receives a fair amount of support by the data. Even more importantly, the remaining findings in Table 69 provide added support for this conclusion.

The remaining correlations in Table 69 show that the higher the proportion of registered nurses talking most with someone at a lower level, e.g., with practical nurses or with aides, the stronger their commitment to the team that treats the patients, and the stronger their commitment to their immediate work group tends to be. We find a correlation of .57 with respect to commitment to the team that treats the patients, and one of .52 with respect to commitment

TABLE 69. Relation Between the Proportion of Nonsupervisory Registered Nurses Who Talk Most with Someone at a Given Organizational Level and Nurses' Commitment to Their Immediate Work Group and the Team That Treats Patients *

Organizational Level of the Person with Whom Nonsupervisory Nurses Talk Most	Degree of Commitment to: † The Immediate Work Group	The Team that Treats Patients
The same organizational level (e.g., R.N.'s talk most to other R.N.'s)	—.32	—.65
A higher organizational level (specifically, the immediate superior)	.29	.42
A higher organizational level (the immediate superior or someone else at a higher level)	.32	.55
A lower organizational level (e.g., R.N.'s talk most to aides)	.52	.57

* All figures are rank-order correlation coefficients, based on an N of 10 hospitals in each case. Coefficients larger than ±.56 are significant at the .05 level.

† The rank-order correlation between commitment to the immediate work group and commitment to the team that treats the patients is .77. Based on an N of 10 hospitals, it is statistically significant at the .01 level.

Findings

to the work group. The former correlation is statistically significant at the .05 level, the latter approaches such significance, and both are consistent with hypothesis #8. Similar positive, though smaller, correlations also obtain with respect to talking most with people at higher levels, e.g., the immediate superior or the immediate superior and others at higher organizational levels. These findings indicate that, in the hospitals studied, from the point of view of commitment to the work group, it is better when more registered nurses direct most of their communication across levels rather than when more nurses direct most of their communication to people at their own level.

Granted that direction of communication is associated with the degree of commitment to the work group, is it also significant from the standpoint of nursing performance? According to hypothesis #9, it is: "The extent to which nurses are likely to communicate more with people at their own level rather than across levels will be negatively related to nursing performance in the hospital." It will be recalled that this hypothesis was premised on the assumption that degree of commitment to the work group is related to nursing performance. According to the data, this is actually the case. For nonsupervisory registered nurses in the various hospitals, we find that strength of commitment to the immediate work group correlates .57 with how good a job registered nurses do, .70 with how good a job practical nurses do, and .79 with how good a job aides do; and strength of commitment to the team that treats the patients, similarly, correlates .49 with how good a job registered nurses do, .71 with how good a job practical nurses do, and .81 with how good a job aides do in the hospital. Based on data from ten hospitals, all these correlations, except one, are statistically significant at the .05 level or better. Let us now turn to the findings in Table 70 about direction of communication and nursing performance, which provide a test for hypothesis #9.

As far as nursing performance is concerned, the findings in Table 70 show that the best situation is for nonsupervisory registered nurses to have most of their communication with people at a lower level, e.g., practical nurses and aides, and least of their communication with people at their own level, i.e., other registered nurses. Communication directed to higher levels falls in the middle. Considering the first row of correlations in this table, we find that the higher the proportion of registered nurses in the hospital talking most with persons at their own level, the less satisfactory the performance of different nursing groups. Specifically, the proportion of nurses talking most with someone at the same level correlates —.56 with how good a job registered nurses do, —.58 with how good a job practical nurses do, —.69 with how good a job aides do, —.16 with how good a job the nursing staff as a whole does, and .—47 with overall quality of nursing care. Conversely, considering the last row of correlations in the table, we find that the proportion of registered nurses talking most with people at lower levels correlates .66 with how good a job registered nurses do, .60 with how good a job practical nurses do, .80 with how good a job aides do, .25 with how good a job the nursing staff as a whole does, and .53 with the overall quality of nursing care in the hospital. Although not all these correlations are statistically significant at the .05 level, the pattern of the findings very clearly supports hypothesis #9.

The rest of the findings in Table 70, relating the proportion of registered nurses who direct most of their communication to people at higher levels and nursing performance, suggest that it is also preferable that nurses direct their communication to higher levels rather than to persons at their own level. This is only suggestive, however, since the obtained specific correlations are not statistically significant insofar as the direction of communication upward is concerned. What emerges clearly, on the other hand, is a significant negative association between the performance of nursing groups and the proportion of registered nurses who talk most with persons at their own level, and a significant positive association between nursing performance and the proportion of nurses who talk most to persons at lower levels. These results, together with the results discussed in conjunction with Table 69, serve to emphasize the importance of the direction of communication among nurses in the hospitals studied.

TABLE 70. Relation Between the Proportion of Nonsupervisory Registered Nurses Who Talk Most with Someone at a Given Organizational Level and Certain Aspects of Nursing Performance *

Organizational Level of the Person with Whom Nonsupervisory Nurses Talk Most Frequently	How Good a Job R.N.'s Do	How Good a Job P.N.'s Do	How Good a Job Aides Do	How Good a Job the Nursing Staff Does	Quality of Nursing Care
The same organizational level (e.g., R.N.'s talk most to other R.N.'s)	−.56	−.58	−.69	−.16	−.47
A higher organizational level (specifically, the immediate superior)	.39	.44	.45	.06	.36
A higher organizational level (the immediate superior or someone else at a higher level)	.32	.43	.45	−.13	.20
A lower organizational level (e.g., R.N.'s talk most to aides)	.66	.60	.80	.25	.53

* All figures are rank-order correlation coefficients, based on an N of 10 hospitals in each case. Coefficients larger than ±.56 are significant at the .05 level, and those ±.75 or larger are significant at the .01 level.

Findings

The Importance of Communication to Other Aspects of Nursing Activity

Up to this point, we have discussed various relationships between several aspects of communication among nurses, on the one hand, and nursing role performance and commitment to the work group, on the other. In the process, we had also occasion to suggest that communication should likewise relate to the coordination of efforts within the nursing department. If, for example, superior-subordinate communication aids the articulation of interdependent activities and helps establish shared expectations among the different members of the nursing staff, it should be positively related to coordination in the nursing department and, conversely, negatively related to tension or conflict among people in the different nursing classifications. We now turn to an examination of these propositions to complete the presentation of our findings about communication among nurses in the ten hospitals participating in this research.

Hypothesis #10, the last one in the present chapter, is the specific hypothesis to be investigated here. It was stated, early in the chapter, as follows: "The extent to which task-relevant communication among registered nurses tends to be concentrated in formal rather than informal organizational channels will be positively related to nursing department coordination and negatively related to tension among people in different nursing roles." This hypothesis, like most of those which precede it, is premised on the fact of the centrality of the role of the registered nurse in the hospital and, especially, in the nursing department organization. The relevant findings are shown in Table 71, the last table in this chapter. (The measures of coordination and tension used here have been described in previous chapters.)

Table 71 shows that both the results concerning coordination and the results concerning tension are in the direction predicted by hypothesis #10. The frequency of talking with the immediate superior about ways to improve patient care, relative to talking with the most-talked-to person in the hospital, correlates .59 with the adequacy of nursing department coordination and −.21 with the extent of tension between people in the different nursing classifications. The corresponding frequency of talking about ways to improve nursing supervision correlates .58 with coordination and −.02 with tension. The comparable correlations with respect to talking about ways to improve work relations between departments are .55 and −.26, respectively; and those with respect to talking about work in general are .33 and −.25, respectively. All correlations involving coordination are positive, and all those involving tension are negative, consistent with hypothesis #10. In brief, with respect to each of the above task-relevant items, the relative concentration of registered nurses' communication in formal rather than informal organizational channels tends to be associated with better coordination in the nursing department and with less tension among people in different nursing roles.

With reference to coordination, two of the four task-relevant items studied

TABLE 71. Relation Between the Frequency with Which Nonsupervisory Registered Nurses Talk with Their Immediate Superior Relative to Talking with the Most-talked-to Person in the Hospital and Nursing Department Coordination and Tension Between Classifications *

Frequency of Talking with the Immediate Superior Relative to Talking with the Most-talked-to Person in the Hospital About:	Adequacy of Nursing Department Coordination	Tension between Nursing Classifications
Ways to improve patient care	.59	−.21
Ways to improve nursing supervision	.58	−.02
Ways to improve work relations between departments	.55	−.26
Work, in general	.33	−.25

* All figures are rank-order correlation coefficients, based on an N of 10 hospitals in each case. Coefficients larger than .56 are significant at the .05 level.

produce both positive and statistically significant relationships with communication; the correlation with a third item just misses significance at the .05 level, and that with the fourth item is positive but smaller. With reference to tension, however, only the direction of the correlations obtained is as predicted by the hypothesis; the magnitude of each of the correlations is not sufficient for statistical significance. It is likely that considerations other than communication enter the picture insofar as tension is concerned (e.g., status differences, differences in the allocation of work among various nursing roles across hospitals, and other differences among nursing roles), with the result that the relationship between communication and tension here proposed is obscured. This explanation is very plausible in view of the significant relationships obtained between level of tension and adequacy of coordination in an earlier chapter, namely Chapter 7. It is also possible, that communication plays a more significant role with respect to coordination than with respect to tension, such that better coordination through communication mitigates tension. Our findings do not permit a definitive conclusion one way or another, however. All we can say is that the overall pattern of relationships shown by Table 71 provides a good support for the association between communication and coordination, but only suggestive support with respect to tension.

SUMMARY AND CONCLUSIONS

Based on data from the ten hospitals in the study, five major aspects of communication among registered nurses—quantity, quality, concentration in formal organizational channels, task-relevance, and direction with respect to organizational levels and roles—have been related to each of several aspects

Summary and Conclusions

of nursing behavior: quality of nursing role performance, commitment to the work group, nursing department coordination, and level of tension between personnel in different nursing classifications. In all cases, the nonsupervisory registered nurses group in each hospital has served as the basis for data analysis and hypothesis testing; i.e., the hospital rather than the individual nurse across hospitals has been used as the unit of analysis.

In general, the findings indicate that in hospitals where nursing activity and performance are evaluated most favorably, the following communication patterns tend to occur: (1) nonsupervisory registered nurses are more likely to exchange a comparatively large amount of information about task-relevant topics with their immediate superior; (2) they are more likely to communicate with persons in higher and lower organizational levels than with persons at their own level; (3) they are more likely to channel their communication about task-relevant subjects in formal rather than informal channels; (4) they are more likely to evaluate the communication they receive from their immediate superior as adequate, helpful, and generally as positive or ego enhancing; and (5) the more they are likely to evaluate the communication they receive from their superior as positive, the more they tend to direct their communication about task-relevant matters to their superior relative to directing it to someone else, namely, the person with whom each talks most at the hospital.

Before summarizing the main findings in greater detail, however, it is important to note again that this part of the study has focused on the communication practices of registered nurses, and the data on which the findings are based were obtained, almost exclusively, from nonsupervisory registered nurses in each of the ten hospitals. Similarly, the various hypotheses tested by means of these data were formulated with the role of the nonsupervisory registered nurse in mind. This role has certain special characteristics that other nursing roles, such as the role of the practical nurse or of the nurse's aide, do not have. Accordingly, some of the hypotheses involved need not be applicable in the case of the latter roles. Therefore, although some of the results regarding communication among registered nurses may appropriately be generalized to other nursing groups and, indeed, to other occupational groups in different situations, the special characteristics of the group studied should be kept in mind when generalization to other groups and situations is attempted.

The role of the registered nurse in the hospital, as we have earlier indicated, is more central to nursing activity than the role of the practical nurse or that of the nurse's aide. It involves both the performance of professional-technical tasks directly relevant to patient care and the performance of coordination tasks—tasks relevant to the articulation of the work efforts of other organizational groups, such as doctors, nonprofessional nursing personnel, and personnel not directly engaged in patient-care activities. Because of her training, skills, and position in the organizational structure, the registered nurse has a good deal more responsibility than performing her own bedside functions, unlike practical nurses or aides. She is responsible for setting and maintaining nursing-care standards, for example, and for directing, supervising, or coordinating the work of nonprofessional nursing personnel. In addition, she is accountable to the individual doctor for his patients, and the doctor calls upon her rather than the practical nurses and aides involved when he wants to implement his patient-care plans or to discuss the condition, needs, and progress of his patients. She, of course, like all others in the nursing department, is also accountable to her superiors in the department for her own personal performance. Considerations such as these, therefore, should be kept in mind when attempting to generalize the results discussed here to other nursing groups. We shall now try to summarize the major results of this part of the study, following the general order in which they appeared in the findings section of the present chapter.

Considering, first, the qualitative aspects of communication among registered nurses in the ten hospitals, we have found a number of interesting relationships. First, the extent to which their immediate superior's communication is perceived by nurses as "adequate" is positively related to their satisfaction with their superior, and to the extent to which they evaluate their superior as doing a good job—being good at planning and organizing, doing the right things, being helpful, and being technically competent. Second, the extent to which their superior's communication is seen by nurses as positive, i.e., as involving such things as explanation, suggestion, or the expression of appreciation, is also positively related to the satisfaction of nurses with supervision and to how well nurses feel their superior performs her role.

Additional findings concerning style of communication show that the more adequate nurses feel the communication they receive from their superior is, the more likely they are to discuss task-relevant matters, such as ways to improve patient care or to improve nursing supervision, with their superior rather than others; in short, the more likely their communication about task-relevant topics is to be concentrated in formal rather than informal channels. The same holds also true when nurses feel that their immediate superior's communication to them is positive, i.e., it involves giving or requesting suggestions, information, or clarification, or the expression of appreciation. Finally, concerning other qualitative aspects of communication, the findings show that there is no significant relationship in this group of hospitals between the extent to which nonsupervisory registered nurses feel that the communication they receive from their superior involves unnecessary information or the expression of criticism and (1) the extent to which they are satisfied with their superior, (2) their evaluation of how well their superior performs her role, or (3) the extent to which they are likely to channel their communication about task-relevant matters in formal rather than informal channels. In all

Summary and Conclusions 537

of nursing behavior: quality of nursing role performance, commitment to the work group, nursing department coordination, and level of tension between personnel in different nursing classifications. In all cases, the nonsupervisory registered nurses group in each hospital has served as the basis for data analysis and hypothesis testing; i.e., the hospital rather than the individual nurse across hospitals has been used as the unit of analysis.

In general, the findings indicate that in hospitals where nursing activity and performance are evaluated most favorably, the following communication patterns tend to occur: (1) nonsupervisory registered nurses are more likely to exchange a comparatively large amount of information about task-relevant topics with their immediate superior; (2) they are more likely to communicate with persons in higher and lower organizational levels than with persons at their own level; (3) they are more likely to channel their communication about task-relevant subjects in formal rather than informal channels; (4) they are more likely to evaluate the communication they receive from their immediate superior as adequate, helpful, and generally as positive or ego enhancing; and (5) the more they are likely to evaluate the communication they receive from their superior as positive, the more they tend to direct their communication about task-relevant matters to their superior relative to directing it to someone else, namely, the person with whom each talks most at the hospital.

Before summarizing the main findings in greater detail, however, it is important to note again that this part of the study has focused on the communication practices of registered nurses, and the data on which the findings are based were obtained, almost exclusively, from nonsupervisory registered nurses in each of the ten hospitals. Similarly, the various hypotheses tested by means of these data were formulated with the role of the nonsupervisory registered nurse in mind. This role has certain special characteristics that other nursing roles, such as the role of the practical nurse or of the nurse's aide, do not have. Accordingly, some of the hypotheses involved need not be applicable in the case of the latter roles. Therefore, although some of the results regarding communication among registered nurses may appropriately be generalized to other nursing groups and, indeed, to other occupational groups in different situations, the special characteristics of the group studied should be kept in mind when generalization to other groups and situations is attempted.

The role of the registered nurse in the hospital, as we have earlier indicated, is more central to nursing activity than the role of the practical nurse or that of the nurse's aide. It involves both the performance of professional-technical tasks directly relevant to patient care and the performance of coordination tasks—tasks relevant to the articulation of the work efforts of other organizational groups, such as doctors, nonprofessional nursing personnel, and personnel not directly engaged in patient-care activities. Because of her training, skills, and position in the organizational structure, the registered nurse has a good deal more responsibility than performing her own bedside functions, unlike practical nurses or aides. She is responsible for setting and maintaining nursing-care standards, for example, and for directing, supervising, or coordinating the work of nonprofessional nursing personnel. In addition, she is accountable to the individual doctor for his patients, and the doctor calls upon her rather than the practical nurses and aides involved when he wants to implement his patient-care plans or to discuss the condition, needs, and progress of his patients. She, of course, like all others in the nursing department, is also accountable to her superiors in the department for her own personal performance. Considerations such as these, therefore, should be kept in mind when attempting to generalize the results discussed here to other nursing groups. We shall now try to summarize the major results of this part of the study, following the general order in which they appeared in the findings section of the present chapter.

Considering, first, the qualitative aspects of communication among registered nurses in the ten hospitals, we have found a number of interesting relationships. First, the extent to which their immediate superior's communication is perceived by nurses as "adequate" is positively related to their satisfaction with their superior, and to the extent to which they evaluate their superior as doing a good job—being good at planning and organizing, doing the right things, being helpful, and being technically competent. Second, the extent to which their superior's communication is seen by nurses as positive, i.e., as involving such things as explanation, suggestion, or the expression of appreciation, is also positively related to the satisfaction of nurses with supervision and to how well nurses feel their superior performs her role.

Additional findings concerning style of communication show that the more adequate nurses feel the communication they receive from their superior is, the more likely they are to discuss task-relevant matters, such as ways to improve patient care or to improve nursing supervision, with their superior rather than others; in short, the more likely their communication about task-relevant topics is to be concentrated in formal rather than informal channels. The same holds also true when nurses feel that their immediate superior's communication to them is positive, i.e., it involves giving or requesting suggestions, information, or clarification, or the expression of appreciation. Finally, concerning other qualitative aspects of communication, the findings show that there is no significant relationship in this group of hospitals between the extent to which nonsupervisory registered nurses feel that the communication they receive from their superior involves unnecessary information or the expression of criticism and (1) the extent to which they are satisfied with their superior, (2) their evaluation of how well their superior performs her role, or (3) the extent to which they are likely to channel their communication about task-relevant matters in formal rather than informal channels. In all

Summary and Conclusions 539

these cases, the correlations obtained vary around zero, some being negative and others positive.

With respect to the various quantitative aspects of communication studied, we find that: (1) the greater the amount of time which nonsupervisory registered nurses spend talking with their immediate superior, the better their performance, and the better the performance of practical nurses, aides, and of the nursing staff as a whole; (2) similar, but less pronounced, relationships hold between the extent to which nurses talk with their immediate superior about specific task-relevant subjects and nursing performance, as evaluated by doctors and nurses; and (3) the frequency with which nurses talk with their immediate superior about ways to improve patient care, or about ways to improve nursing supervision, relates positively to the degree to which nurses feel they are committed (extent of identification) to their immediate work group and to the team that treats the patients.

Certain relationships between the concentration of communication in formal channels and nursing activity and performance are also of interest. The extent to which professional nurses talk with their immediate superior, relative to talking with the most-talked-to person in the hospital, about ways to improve patient care relates positively and significantly to how good a job registered nurses themselves do, how good a job practical nurses do, and how good a job the nursing staff as a whole does; it also relates positively to how good a job aides do, and to the overall quality of nursing care in the hospital, but the correlations in these cases do not reach statistical significance. With respect to talking about ways to improve nursing supervision, another task-relevant subject, the corresponding correlations are all positive, as earlier hypothesized, but they are not statistically significant. Finally, the frequency with which professional nurses talk with their immediate superior, relative to talking with the most-talked-to person, about ways to improve patient care, about ways to improve nursing supervision, or about ways to improve relations between hospital departments is positively related to nursing department coordination. The higher the concentration of task-relevant communication in formal rather than informal channels, the better the coordination in the nursing department is.

Another set of findings involves the direction of communication on the part of nonsupervisory registered nurses. In this study, direction of communication has been related to the extent to which nurses feel they are committed to their group, and to nursing performance. First, the results about work group commitment will be summarized. As predicted, we find that, the extent to which nurses tend to communicate more with people at their own level rather than across levels is negatively related to their commitment to the team that treats the patients; and it also tends to be negatively related with their commitment to their immediate work group. On the other hand, the extent to which they tend to communicate more with persons at lower or higher levels, especially in the former case, tends to be positively related with their commitment to the team that treats the patients and to their immediate work group. Thus, work-group commitment on the part of nonsupervisory registered nurses is higher in hospitals where nurses direct most of their communication across levels, and lower in hospitals where they direct most of their communication to persons at their own level.

The results concerning direction of communication in relation to nursing role performance are similar. First, there is a significant negative relationship between the extent to which nurses tend to communicate more with persons at their own level rather than across levels and how good a job registered nurses themselves do, how good a job practical nurses do, and how good a job aides do. The more they confine their communication to their own level, the poorer is their performance and the performance of the other nursing groups below them. Second, the results show an opposite pattern when nurses tend to direct most of their communication to people at lower levels: there is a significant positive relationship between talking most frequently with nursing personnel at lower levels and how good a job the registered nurses themselves do, how good a job the practical nurses do, and how good a job aides do. (Incidentally, this pattern of relationships supports our earlier observation that the nonsupervisory registered nurse acts as a standard setter and task leader for nursing personnel at lower skill levels.) Finally, a similar, though less clear-cut, pattern obtains when registered nurses tend to direct most of their communication to people at higher organizational levels. In short, nursing role performance is generally better in hospitals where nonsupervisory registered nurses communicate more with persons at lower or higher levels and poorer in hospitals where they confine most of their communicative activity to their own level.

On the whole, the obtained results provide a good deal of support for the various hypotheses which we presented and discussed in detail, together with corresponding underlying assumptions, at the beginning of this chapter. In fact, subject to the limitations and modifications indicated in the findings section of the chapter, all except two of the ten hypotheses studied receive support from the data in varying degrees. The two exceptions occur in the case of hypothesis #2 and hypothesis #4. These hypotheses predicted negative relationships between the extent to which nurses feel that the communication they receive from their immediate superior involves unnecessary information or expression of criticism and the degree to which nurses are satisfied with their superior, the quality of the superior's role performance, and the concentration of communication about task-relevant matters in formal channels. In all these cases, however, the results show no relationship at all for the nonsupervisory registered nurses group of respondents, i.e., the group about which the hypotheses were formulated.

Some Further Concluding Remarks

In the ten hospitals studied, nursing role performance, satisfaction with supervision, commitment to the work group, and coordination of nursing activity are significantly associated with certain quantitative and qualitative characteristics of the communication of registered nurses. These characteristics include the amount, style, task-relevance, direction with respect to organizational levels or roles, and relative concentration of communication in formal organizational channels.

The findings demonstrate the significance and organizational utility of an unencumbered flow of task-relevant communication between nonsupervisory registered nurses and their superiors, and from nonsupervisory registered nurses to nursing personnel at lower levels, such as practical nurses and aides. The nonsupervisory registered nurse constitutes the nexus between higher and lower nursing levels, serving as a communication link between them. If this link is not firmly established, organizational coordination will suffer, and the resolution or prevention of task-related problems and of group-maintenance problems will be difficult to attain. While a certain amount of horizontal communication, i.e., communication among persons at the same level, may be necessary for the system, the data clearly show that vertical communication, both up and down, on the part of nonsupervisory registered nurses seems to be an essential requirement to effective performance by persons playing interdependent roles in the system. In hospitals where a higher proportion of professional nurses tend to confine their communication within their own level rather than across levels, nursing performance is seen as inferior.

In hospitals where task-relevant communication among nurses tends to be concentrated in formal rather than informal organizational channels, nursing performance is correspondingly satisfactory—the higher this concentration is, the better the nursing performance is likely to be. Moreover, such concentration of communication in formal channels is more likely to occur when the communication on the part of nursing supervisors toward their subordinates is perceived by the latter as being adequate and as being of a positive nature, in the sense that it is either relevant to task problems or affirms the competence and psychological security of the subordinate. Adequacy of supervisory communication, the results show, correlates positively and significantly with the extent to which the superior is seen by the subordinates as: being good at planning and organizing work, doing things that are right, being an expert, being helpful, and being likable. It also correlates positively and significantly with the frequency with which nurses are likely to talk with their immediate superior rather than the person with whom they talk most in the hospital about ways to improve patient care and ways to improve nursing supervision.

Finally, in hospitals where nonsupervisory registered nurses, on the average, spend more time communicating with their immediate superior, nursing performance is evaluated more favorably: the greater the absolute amount of time spent, the better the job done by registered nurses, by practical nurses, and by aides, the better the job done by the nursing staff as a whole, and the higher the quality of overall nursing care. The same holds true where registered nurses tend to communicate more frequently with their immediate superior rather than the person with whom they talk most in the hospital about ways to improve patient care. And the same holds true where a higher proportion of nonsupervisory registered nurses direct most of their communication to lower nursing personnel, i.e., practical nurses, aides, and orderlies. But the opposite pattern of relationships obtains, i.e., nursing performance is evaluated less favorably, where a higher proportion of registered nurses direct most of their communication to persons at their own level.

To sum up, the results of this study indicate that the communication of registered nurses in the hospitals where nursing staffs perform more effectively in part shows the following general patterns:

1. In the main, the communication of registered nurses within the nursing department is directed vertically rather than horizontally, i.e., to persons at lower and higher levels rather than persons at their own level, thus ensuring adequate coordination of activities.

2. The formal channels of communication between registered nurses and their immediate superiors are well used, thus providing continuity in work relationships and the opportunity to prevent or identify and resolve problems promptly within formal authority bounds.

3. Task-relevant communication on the part of registered nurses tends to be relatively concentrated in formal organizational channels, being encouraged by nursing supervisors who employ a positive style of communication, thus facilitating problem solving and guarding against the saturation of the communication network with irrelevant information.

4. The style and content of supervisory communication toward registered nurses suggest a concern with anticipating, preventing, and resolving problems arising in the action structure and problems affecting the maintenance of the group.

5. In hospitals where the above patterns of communication prevail, nursing role performance, satisfaction with supervision, commitment to the work group, and coordination of activity within the nursing department are likely to be superior to those in hospitals where these patterns of communication do not prevail or where they are not as evident.

The implications of these findings for nursing organization and hospital administration require no particular elaboration. One caution, however, should be repeated once more. The results here presented reveal a number of optimal communication patterns for registered nurses, with respect to nursing activity and performance. Since the data are from and about registered nurses, however, they do not specifically reveal comparable optimal patterns for the communication of other nursing groups, such as practical nurses or aides. And, although many of the findings and conclusions concerning the communication of registered nurses are undoubtedly also applicable to these other groups, generalizations should not be made without great care and without taking into account the nature of the organizational role of individuals in these groups. Apart from this limitation, the results speak for themselves.

Nursing performance is facilitated by the free flow of general information between registered nurses and their superiors, and between registered nurses and other nursing personnel at lower levels, and by the flow of specific task-relevant information along organizational channels. The communication of registered nurses in those hospitals where the nursing staff is performing most successfully reflects both the intent of the hospital organization and the function of nurses within it: it tends to be concentrated in formal channels and across levels, and to be focused on one of the nurses' greatest concerns—ways of improving patient care.

REFERENCES

1. Bales, R. F. "Some Uniformities of Behavior in Small Social Systems." In Swanson, G. E., Newcomb, T. M., and Hartley, E. L. (eds.) *Readings in Social Psychology.* New York: Holt, 1952.
2. Burling, T. "Aids and Bars to Internal Communication," *Hospitals,* 28:82–85, 1954.
3. Drucker, P. *The Practice of Management.* New York: Harper, 1954.
4. Festinger, L., Schachter, S., and Back, K. *Social Pressures in Informal Groups.* New York: Harper, 1950.
5. Jaques, E. *The Changing Culture of a Factory.* New York: Dryden, 1952.
6. Moore, W. E. *Industrial Relations and the Social Order.* New York: Macmillan, 1951.
7. Newcomb, T. M. "An Approach to the Study of Communicative Acts." In Hare, P., Borgatta, E. F., and Bales, R. F. (eds.) *Small Groups.* New York: Knopf, 1955.

11 COMMENTARY ON SELECTED PROBLEMS AND ISSUES

In discussing the main problem areas of the study in the preceding chapters, we frequently presented data touching on a variety of other topics about the hospital or its different groups. Most of these special topics are only tangential to the main interests of our research. Several of them, however, reflect problems or issues that are frequently of concern not only to researchers in this field but also to hospital practitioners. Accordingly, it would be worth while to comment upon these special topics somewhat more systematically, before concluding the book. Secondly, it would be likewise appropriate to discuss briefly a few additional available data which, being of little interest to this study and having only indirect or secondary relevance to its main objectives, were reported only partially in previous chapters. And, finally, it might also be well to reiterate and further highlight some of the descriptive results which were presented in Chapters 3 and 4, because of the apparent concrete implications of these results for those interested in the action and practical aspects of hospital functioning. The present chapter is, therefore, a supplementary chapter to all chapters that preceded it and is intended to serve these three secondary, and largely overlapping aims, in the interests of complete reporting.

As might be expected, the data available for most of the topics to be discussed here are admittedly limited. In a sense, they are "surplus" data from the standpoint of the objectives and design of the present research. However, they are often quite interesting and illuminating—and perhaps even challenging in some instances—apart from their potential usefulness in serving to guide future research efforts in the areas involved. The specific topics with which we shall be concerned are: (1) the external image of the community general hospital, (2) the hospital as a place to work, (3) certain problems pertaining to the nursing staff, (4) certain problems and issues pertaining to the medical staff, (5) the value orientations of the top echelon groups in hospital organization, (6) the influence of key groups on hospital functioning, and (7) or-

The External Image of the Hospital

ganizational change and its accommodation in the hospitals studied. In each case, the main concern will be with problems and issues rather than with variables and their interrelationships, with the result that we shall frequently deviate here from our custom of using the total hospital as the unit of analysis.

THE EXTERNAL IMAGE OF THE HOSPITAL

Even though we obtained no data about the external image of the hospital, or about hospital-community relations, from sources outside the hospitals studied, certain data from our respondents in the various hospitals are relevant to the question of what the external image of the typical participating hospital is like.

The community's image of a hospital presumably depends upon, and would be reflected in, such things as the information or misinformation that the community has about the hospital, the extent to which the hospital satisfies the expectations and health needs of its community, the appeals or demands of the hospital to the community for financial support, the relations between the hospital and other community institutions, including other hospitals, and generally the acceptance and prestige which the hospital is enjoying in its community. Moreover, the external image of a hospital is undoubtedly affected and shaped by what the patients (and those close to them) and former patients have to say about their experience in the hospital, by what the trustees, the doctors, the administrator, and other hospital personnel (all of whom inevitably represent the hospital in the eyes of the public) do or say outside the hospital, by the public relations program of the hospital, and similar other factors. This being the case, it is possible to make some statements about the external image of the "typical" hospital in this study (for a description of the typical hospital see Chap. 4), using information from people within the hospital.

On the whole, the available data indicate that the external image of the typical participating hospital is a favorable one but, at the same time, there is considerable room for improvement. For example, we find that half of the medical and professional nurse respondents in the study, and about two-thirds of the trustees, administrators, and department heads feel that "nearly all" or all the patients in their respective hospital speak "very well" of the hospital. And, in each case, even a higher proportion of the respondents feel that the "majority" of the patients speak very well of the hospital. Similarly, in the typical hospital, about 75 percent of the professional nursing staff, 80 percent of the medical staff, and 90 percent of the trustees and top administrative staff say that their hospital enjoys a "very good" or "excellent" reputation in the community. (Of course, individual hospitals vary somewhat from these specific percentages which are based on averaged data from all ten participating hospitals combined.)

Many other data presented in previous chapters, particularly the data about patient care in Chapter 5, and the data concerning the facilities available in the typical hospital in the study, discussed in Chapter 4 and Chapter 8, also suggest a predominantly favorable external image for the typical participating hospital. With respect to facilities, the data showed that most, if not all, of the hospitals in the study apparently have adequate physical facilities and equipment, with the exception of space difficulties, which are experienced by nearly all of them (rather seriously by six of the ten institutions). This is not to say that facilities are completely adequate in these hospitals, or that all the hospitals studied have equally adequate facilities; some have generally superior facilities than others. Nevertheless, none of these hospitals complains seriously about inadequate physical facilities or lack of equipment. Interestingly enough, any complaints raised in this area have to do more with the use rather than the lack of facilities. For example, we have seen in Chapter 4 that four of the hospitals are concerned with the extent to which their facilities are being increasingly used by low socioeconomic groups in the community (perhaps suggesting a possibility for future hospital-community problems in this connection). This concern is most often centered on the use of the emergency service and constitutes only one side of the issue—the other side being a concern that some doctors abuse or misuse the emergency service by bringing patients there instead of to their office. Apart from some difficulties such as these, the preponderance of the evidence about facilities, patient care, patient reaction toward the hospital, and public reputation indicates a very favorable external image for the average hospital.

Certain other data, on the other hand, indicate that problems that may require the active attention of hospital people also exist in relation to the external image of the hospital. First, at a very general level, as shown in Chapter 4, some concern for improving hospital-community relations is expressed in the majority of the hospitals. Second, in response to the question "How adequate, would you say, is the community's knowledge of this hospital and its problems?" only one-fifth of the hospital administrators and trustees in the study, one-fourth of the doctors, and one-third of the non-medical department heads answered that the community's knowledge is "very adequate" or "completely adequate." Third, when asked to indicate "How well is this hospital doing in the area of public relations?", less than half of the administrators and trustees in the study said that their hospital is doing a "very good" (or better than very good) job. All these findings suggest that the external image of the hospitals involved could be improved.

Finally, of relevance here are also the answers of both medical and nonmedical respondents to the following question: "Considering the kind of service this hospital gives to its patients, how do you feel about what it charges for patient care?" The data from this question, if not outright alarming because of the great discrepancy of opinion they show to prevail among various groups within the hospital itself, are certainly such as to warrant a good deal of concern on the part of hospital authorities. Specifically, the data show that while only 7 percent of the trustees, administrators, and nonmedical department heads in the study feel that charges for patient care in their hospital are "quite high" or "too high," 31 percent (more than four times as many) of the doctors and the professional nurses feel that this is the case. And conversely, while only 6 percent of the doctors and professional nurses feel that the charges are "low," 24 percent of the trustees, administrators, and department heads express this belief. Some discussion or explaining within the hospital itself would probably be very much in order in this connection. Internal lack of consensus on such a sensitive matter as charges for patient care can hardly be expected to aid or enhance the external image of the hospital.

THE HOSPITAL AS A PLACE TO WORK

The way people feel about working in the hospital, among other things, tells us something about the internal image of the hospital. In discussing the people around the patient, in Chapter 3, we presented considerable data about the occupational-career patterns, the job status and outlook, and other characteristics of the different groups in the hospital. Most of these data have some bearing on the question of what the internal image of the hospital is like, shedding some light on the hospital as a place to work. By and large, the data again indicate an overall favorable image. However, they also point to some difficulties. Without repeating data already reported, let us look briefly at some of the problems.

In the typical hospital, six out of every ten professional nurses feel that the hospital is a "very good" or an "excellent" place in which to work. But, at the same time, only about half the professional nurses report that they would like to stay in the hospital for as long as they can work. Of the practical nurses, eight out of every ten feel that the hospital is a very good or excellent place to work, but only about five out of every ten would like to stay in the hospital for as long as they can work. The case of laboratory and x-ray technicians, and of aides, is similar. In both cases a higher proportion of group members view the hospital as a good place to work than the proportion who would like to stay in the hospital for as long as they can work. These results suggest that the long-run commitment of these groups to the organization is not as high as it should be, particularly in view of the high proportions of personnel in each case who are favorably viewing the hospital as a place to work. That commitment to the organization leaves much to be desired is also supported by earlier reported findings showing that nonsupervisory registered nurses, practical nurses, and technicians feel most strongly identified with their profession-occupation, next most strongly identified with the team that treats the patients and/or their immediate work group, and least strongly identified with the hospital and with the outside community.

The strong professional commitment that nurses and technicians report, of course, implies that they view their job as intrinsically rewarding. In turn, this implies that their relatively low commitment to the hospital must be due not to lack of sufficient liking for their work, but rather to considerations related to the nature of other rewards and satisfactions that they derive, or do not derive, from working in their particular hospital. In this connection, pertinent data show that the situation is not very comforting. For example, while about three out of every ten professional nurses and technicians express high satisfaction with their salary, between 20 and 25 percent of all nurses and technicians say that they are "somewhat" to "completely" dissatisfied with their salary—and this is a substantial figure. In the case of practical nurses and aides the situation is somewhat worse, for the proportion who are clearly dissatisfied exceeds the proportion who are highly satisfied with their salary (33 percent vs. 23 percent for practical nurses, and 44 percent vs. 17 percent for aides).

These facts assume even greater significance, moreover, when one recalls that: (1) nonsupervisory registered nurses most frequently mention that the single main reason for working in the hospital is "to supplement my family's income"—this also being the second most frequently mentioned reason by all other nursing groups (see Chap. 3); (2) nonsupervisory registered nurses and technicians constitute the most unstable, from an organizational point of view (in terms of turnover, length of service, etc.), of all groups in the community general hospital (see Chap. 3); and (3) hospitals are experiencing problems of recruitment, staff shortages, and turnover among professional nurses and other personnel. Prevailing salary levels in the participating hospitals (see Chap. 3 for details) are neither conducive to high organizational commitment on the part of nurses and other nonmedical employees, nor effective in alleviating shortages and turnover. However, fortunately for the hospital, most of these people are highly motivated by the content and nature of the work itself, otherwise hospitals would be facing even a more serious problem in their efforts to maintain an adequate and stable staff.

The nonmedical department heads, as a group, by comparison with the nursing groups and the technicians, are considerably more satisfied with their salary, as well as with their chances for advancement in the hospital. They are also more likely to be satisfied with their respective immediate superiors, and generally consider the hospital as a better place to work than the other nonmedical groups. In other words, they have a more favorable overall image of the hospital as a place to work. This is consistent with the relatively high organizational stability of the department heads group, which was pointed out in Chapter 3.

The hospital administrators are very much like the department heads—their immediate subordinates—insofar as having very favorable attitudes toward the hospital as a place to work, from the point of view of job satisfaction, and in terms of organizational stability. The trustees are not employees of the hospital and do not work at the hospital on any regular basis. However, they are the most stable of all groups in the study, and their appraisal of different aspects of the hospital situation tends to be extremely favorable, according to the data.

Finally, the doctors who, like the trustees, are not employees of the hospital, but who, unlike the trustees, work regularly at the hospital appear to be considerably more interested in the hospital and considerably more identified with it than frequently prevailing assertions among hospital people and in the literature would lead one to believe. While, along with other members of the organization, they view the hospital as their place of work, doctors are not as prone as is frequently believed to consider the hospital merely as a "workshop" at the service of their self-interest. The majority indicate that they consider the hospital as an organization whose primary objective is service to the patients. And although some doctors may "misuse" certain hospital facilities, such as the emergency service, the majority are clear about the purpose of the organization. Moreover, in their general attitude toward the hospital and their appraisal of different aspects of the hospital situation, the doctors are less critical than the nonsupervisory registered nurses and the technicians, about as critical as the supervisory nurses, but more critical, or less favorable, than the trustees, administrators, and department heads. Doctors are neither the most nor the least critical group in the hospital. Nor are they as "individualistic" or "selfish" in their relations with the hospital as is often alleged.

PROBLEMS PERTAINING TO THE NURSING STAFF

It is clear from our discussions in previous chapters that the community general hospital faces a number of problems concerning the nursing staff—the largest of all its groups. Here we shall comment on the more prevalent of these problems. One major problem is that of attracting and retaining a sufficient professional nursing staff, especially nonsupervisory registered nurses. Part of this problem lies in the fact that the number of professional nurses being trained in nursing schools is much too low to meet an ever-increasing demand for professional nurses by hospitals and other sources. Part of the problem lies in the fact that, as shown in Chapter 3, nonsupervisory registered nurses are very likely to be, or get, married and to have family responsibilities (more so than any of the other nursing groups in the hospital), with the result that a good proportion of them cease to view nursing practice as a career, move to other communities in order to accompany their husbands when the latter change place of employment, or find that activities other than nursing are equally or more important and rewarding, thus eliminating themselves from the active nursing work force. Over these forces, individual hospitals have, of course, little direct or immediate control.

On the other hand, individual hospitals could do a great deal to alleviate the problems of shortages and turnover among their nonsupervisory registered nurses. In the first place, the prevailing low salaries for this personnel (particularly in the absence of other tangible rewards of any significance, and in view of the fact that these nurses consider supplementing their family's income as the single most important reason for working in the hospital) constitute a great handicap in the efforts of the hospital to attract nurses and then minimize their turnover. The high organizational instability of nonsupervisory registered nurses, so forcefully demonstrated by the data in Chapter 3, might be reduced with increased financial return.

In the second place, it must be remembered that, unlike other groups in the hospital, the nonsupervisory nurses group is, to a high degree, a part-time professional group (and this is a most interesting and unusual characteristic for a professional group) for, according to the data, an impressive 45 percent of all nonsupervisory registered nurses in the hospitals studied are working part time, this figure ranging across hospitals between a low of 33 and a high of 58 percent. Since hospitals obviously depend so greatly on part-time registered nurses, they should make part-time employment for them as attractive as possible, both from the financial standpoint, and psychologically in terms of choice of shifts, choice of specific job assignments, and the like. It is our impression that, instead of actively encouraging part-time employment, some hospitals fail to recognize the significance of utilizing part-time professional nurses to the fullest.

In the third place, the fact that hospitals are ordinarily understaffed in the nonsupervisory registered nurses category generates forces which, in effect, make the solution of the problem of attracting and maintaining an adequate staff very difficult. Being understaffed, hospitals often assign to the professional nurse a rather heavy workload that is not seen as normal or reasonable by many nurses. Other things being equal, this is not a satisfactory experience to the nurse. Furthermore, as we have earlier shown, pressure for performance that is considered unreasonable by the individuals involved is negatively related to nursing performance. Understaffing is also likely to create tensions among nursing personnel in various roles, and to be associated with miscellaneous additional difficulties (e.g., professional nurses often find that they have to spend substantial time in supervising and coordinating the activities of the nonprofessional nursing staff, in doing paper work, in activities requiring little or no personal contact with the patient, or in functions they do not consider a legitimate part of their professional-organizational role), the net effect of which is to make working in the hospital less attractive, less rewarding, and less meaningful for the nonsupervisory registered nurse. Some of the difficulties resulting from understaffing could be mitigated to an extent by careful planning, effective supervision, adequate communication, and, generally, by fostering psychologically satisfying work relations and interactions among nurses and between nurses and other groups in the organization.

Another important problem, closely related to the preceding, involves the composition of the total nursing staff, and the question of optimum balance in the proportions of staff members who are registered nurses, practical nurses, and aides. Because of the difficulty of acquiring and maintaining a sufficient number of professional nurses, and in their eagerness to operate with maximum economy, hospitals frequently fall into a dangerous trap. They tend to employ more untrained staff than they would normally do, on the assumption that having more aides, for example, would somehow compensate for an insufficient number of practical nurses, or having more practical nurses would be a substitute for an insufficient number of professional nurses. This is indeed a very risky assumption in the light of the findings of this study. Yet, hospitals are tempted to make it and to act upon it, because the acquisition of untrained nursing staff is much easier than the acquisition of trained staff, and because it is substantially less expensive to have to pay aides instead of practical or registered nurses, and perceptibly less expensive to have to pay practical nurses instead of registered nurses. Besides, it is implicitly argued, employing more staff (regardless of its training) would result in a high ratio of personnel to patients (and this is presumably good). As the data have shown, however, it is not the total number of nursing personnel per patient that makes a difference in relation to such things as the quality of patient care, coordination, etc. What counts is the availability of skilled and trained, in relation to or as against untrained, nursing talent, rather than total staff size in relation to patient load.

The findings have shown that: (1) the higher the proportion of nursing staff members who are registered nurses, the better the nursing care and the better the medical care in the hospital; (2) the higher the proportion of staff members who are practical nurses, the better the nursing care and the better the coordination (probably due to the relatively high organizational stability of the practical nurses group), but the proportion of practical nurses is not related to the quality of medical care; and (3) the higher the proportion of staff members who are aides, the poorer the nursing care and the poorer the coordination in the hospital. The implications of these and similar other findings for hospital effectiveness are clear and forceful. High proportions of untrained nursing personnel on the staff make for poorer patient care. According to the findings, registered nurses constitute the backbone of the nursing staff and should be preferred over practical nurses, and practical nurses should be preferred over aides, from the point of view of the overall composition of the total nursing staff. However, while having more practical nurses would compensate for having fewer aides, it would not compensate for having fewer registered nurses. Improvement of the quality of patient care is, in large measure, contingent upon the willingness and ability of the hospitals to cease overloading their nursing staff with aides, while simultaneously intensifying their efforts to employ more registered nurses and more practical nurses, or at least employ more practical nurses and fewer aides. Trained nursing skill may be costly and difficult to find, but it is indispensable to high-quality care.

A final problem that we wish to comment upon here has to do with the relationships among nursing personnel in different roles. While not unrelated to the problems of staff shortages and imbalances (which serve to accentuate it), this problem is more directly associated with difficulties arising out of status differences, role ambiguities, and nonlegitimate role performances among nursing personnel in different classifications. But, whatever its specific source, the problem in question has serious repercussions for effective hospital functioning. Specifically, the data show that a considerable proportion of the nonsupervisory registered nurses in the typical hospital feel that personnel in one nursing role are prone (more than to "a small extent") to attempt to do things that personnel in some other nursing role should be doing: 53 percent of these respondents indicate that registered nurses (i.e., themselves) are prone to try to do things that practical nurses should be doing, 51 percent report that practical nurses are prone to do things that registered nurses should be doing, 35 percent report that aides are prone to do things that practical or registered nurses should be doing, and 31 percent report that supervisory nurses are prone to do things that nonsupervisory nurses should be doing. Data from other nursing groups, moreover, confirm that nonlegitimate attempts of this kind occur in the hospitals studied with some frequency—much more in some than others. The problem may not be too great, but it is of sufficient proportions to warrant attention in many of the hospitals.

Apparently there is some need here for greater definitional clarity for the different nursing roles and, more importantly, for developing greater consensus and conformity among nursing personnel in the different roles regarding their proper spheres of activity in relation to each other. The extent to which attempts of the above kind prevail in the various hospitals is, according to previously reported results, negatively related to organizational coordination, and is likely to create tensions within the nursing staff. In this connection, we find that from two to three out of every ten members of each nursing group in the average hospital report more than "a little" tension between nursing personnel in one classification and nursing personnel in another classification. Some of this tension is undoubtedly due to attempts at nonlegitimate role performance.

ISSUES AND PROBLEMS CONCERNING THE MEDICAL STAFF

A frequently raised issue among doctors and other hospital people is that of the relationship between members of the medical staff who are "specialists" (whether "board-certified" or not) and those who engage in general practice—the "general practitioners." Specialization—one of the hallmarks of the community general hospital, as well as of most modern large-scale organizations—has given rise to a great many medical specialties and, over the years, has resulted in a continuous decrease in the proportion of doctors who are engaged

Issues and Problems Concerning Medical Staff

in general practice. In the ten hospitals participating in this study, those members of the active-attending medical staff who are classified as general practitioners amount to an average of only 29 percent of the total staff—the figure ranging across individual hospitals from a high of 41 percent to a low of 19 percent. In other words, general practitioners are the minority group in relation to the specialists.

While several different problems may be connected with the issue of specialists vs. general practitioners, the most acute and most frequently raised problems in this connection revolve around the question of what privileges should general practitioners have in the hospital (which is a touchy issue because it concerns the definition of the role and functions of general practitioners), what limits or restrictions there should be in their practice of medicine, how are privileges and restrictions to be decided upon, how are they to be assigned to individual staff members, and ultimately how are they to be enforced. Obviously, these are important questions both for the medical staff and the hospital, and indirectly also for the patient. The generality of the issue in question is clearly suggested by the fact that, in all but one of the hospitals in the study, the relationships between specialists and general practitioners received some comments by doctors and others, who perceived such relationships as more or less problematic—and as considerably problematic in three hospitals (see Chap. 4).

Interestingly enough, however, in its totality, our evidence indicates that the specialists–general-practitioners issue is not actually a big issue in the hospitals studied. In large measure, the issue is spuriously inflated on the part of some of those affected by it, while in fact it has been practically resolved in most of the participating hospitals. Part of the problem here seems to be due to lack of accurate information or pluralistic ignorance, to emotionalism, and to beliefs and attitudes among people within the hospital that are lagging behind actual practice in the hospitals themselves. In any event, there are good reasons to believe that the present issue is not a sharp issue in the hospitals studied.

The most direct evidence in support of the above conclusions has its source in the answers that medical respondents gave to this question: "In your opinion, are the general practitioners in this hospital given as many privileges and opportunities as they should have?" In answering this question, an overall average of 49 percent of the doctors indicated that general practitioners in their hospital have "exactly as many privileges as they should have;" another 19 percent indicated that general practitioners have "somewhat fewer" privileges but, at the same time, an additional 20 percent indicated that general practitioners have "somewhat more" privileges than they should have (i.e., the proportion of doctors who felt that general practitioners have somewhat fewer privileges is almost identical with the proportion who felt that general practitioners have somewhat more privileges than they should have). The above figures account for 88 percent of the medical staff. And only the remaining 12 percent of the doctors from the hospitals studied felt that general practitioners are given "too few" (9 percent) or "too many" (3 percent) privileges in their respective hospitals. It should also be noted in this connection that the above respondents included both specialists and general practitioners, and that the proportion of general practitioners on the staff of the various hospitals, as well as in our sample, is higher than 9 percent, i.e., it is higher than the percentage of all doctors who felt that general practitioners are given too few privileges.

Other, less direct evidence, reported in previous chapters, also supports the conclusion that the alleged cleavage between specialists and general practitioners is neither as sharp nor as wide as it is often believed to be. For one thing, as we have pointed out in Chapter 4, relatively acute problems between these two groups exist in only three of the ten participating hospitals. For another thing, as we have pointed out in Chapter 5, a rather wide variety of data shows that in their evaluations of different aspects of the hospital situation (including their evaluations of the quality of patient care) specialists as a group do not differ significantly from general practitioners, and vice versa. It seems, then, that in the hospitals studied the issue of specialists vs. general practitioners has been largely resolved and, judging from the above data regarding the privileges of the latter, it has been resolved rather satisfactorily for most of those concerned.

By contrast, a problem which is seldom discussed in the literature, and which is rarely seen as salient by hospital people, even though it is not unrelated to the above issue, is quite evident in the data as a problem of major proportions. We refer to the fact that, as we have seen in Chapter 4, relationships among the members of the medical staff (not confined to specialists vis-à-vis general practitioners) in many of the hospitals in the study are problematic, as well as to the relatively high degree of tension which prevails among doctors in the various hospitals. This was documented in Chapter 7. In that chapter we commented upon the remarkably high agreement on the part of doctors, trustees, administrators, and professional nurses to the effect that a good deal of tension prevails among the members of the medical staff in their respective hospitals. In fact, the data showed that, on the average, all these groups agree that there is greater tension in their hospital between doctors and other doctors, *than* between doctors and nurses, *than* between doctors and the administrator, *than* between doctors and trustees, in that order. We have also seen, of course, that tension among interacting groups in the hospital is negatively related to organizational coordination and to the quality of patient care. Consequently, hospital people can ill afford to be either ignorant or complacent about this problem of tension and its potential adverse effects for hospital functioning.

Some of the tension between doctors and other doctors in the hospital may have its source in the specialist–general-practitioner controversy, but most of the tension must be attributed to other causes, if the preceding analysis is

Issues and Problems Concerning Medical Staff

correct. One obvious source of tension is the frequent professional competition among doctors for patients in the community which cannot be divorced from what happens in the hospital. Another source of tension is the competition among doctors for hospital beds for their patients. This is no small problem in view of the fact that nearly all the hospitals are concerned with the problem of space and expansion, and in view of the fact that hospitals are frequently too short of beds to accommodate all the patients of all doctors at a particular time. A related source of tension is competition among doctors for priority, and sometimes also favoritism, in such things as the operating-room schedules, securing a particular or desirable time for the performance of surgery, etc. The presence of different "factions" or "cliques" among doctors in some hospitals, status differences, feelings by some doctors that other doctors are not as interested in the hospital as they are or that they are not doing as good a job as they are, and similar other factors also constitute potential sources of tension among the members of the medical staff and must be taken into account.

On the other hand, it is noteworthy that the formal organization of the medical staff does not appear to be a major source of tension among doctors in the hospitals studied. This conclusion is supported by two pieces of evidence. First, in response to a question about the things with which doctors were most concerned at the time of data collection, in only one or two of the participating hospitals was there much preference expressed by any sizable proportion of the doctors for changes in the medical staff organization, even though the question explicitly asked about possible concern with this matter. (We shall return to this question in the next section.) Second, when asked to indicate if any subgroups of the medical staff were not represented on the medical executive committee in their respective hospitals, 75 percent of all the doctors in the study said that there are no subgroups in their hospital which are underrepresented on the executive committee. (Of the remaining, 7 percent said that the "younger" members of the staff are underrepresented, 10 percent said that the general practitioners are underrepresented, and the other 8 percent mentioned various other subgroups as not being represented on the medical executive committee.)

Another problem pertaining to the medical staff that is raised with some regularity by hospital people, especially administrators and nonmedical personnel, has to do with the interest that the medical staff shows toward the hospital. It is often said that doctors take little interest or that they should be more interested in the hospital than they are. The data actually show that, in the hospitals studied, the medical staff does take a great deal of interest in the hospital. In response to the question "Except for medical aspects, how much interest does the medical staff take in this hospital as an institution?," 80 percent of the professional nurses, 83 percent of the trustees, administrators, and nonmedical department heads, and 85 percent of the doctors from the ten participating hospitals answered that the medical staff in their respective hospitals is "quite a bit interested" or "extremely interested in this hospital as an institution." Other, less direct, data also confirm these findings. For example, in one of the hospitals the medical staff, on its own initiative, had set up a fund to which doctors made voluntary contributions and then turned the money over to the hospital for the purchase of equipment. Similarly, it is not an uncommon practice for doctors to contribute to expansion or building funds for the hospital and occasionally also to be "assessed" for this purpose by the hospital. Doctors may be relatively uninformed or naïve about different aspects of organizational behavior, or about some of the nonmedical problems of hospital functioning, but certainly they are not disinterested or uninterested in the hospital.

The data do show that doctors do not generally have as good an understanding of the problems and needs of other groups in the hospital as these other groups have of the problems and needs of the medical staff. But this is a different matter from the alleged lack of interest in the hospital on the part of the doctors. The problem is more one of insufficient understanding, which may be due to lack of enough information, deficient communication between doctors and other relevant members of the organization (in which case the problem could not be attributed only to the doctors), and reasons other than lack of sufficient interest in the hospital. Incidentally, one should note that trustees are also not particularly well informed about many aspects of the day-to-day situation in the hospital. This is reflected in the fact that they consistently evaluate most aspects of hospital functioning more favorably, or less critically, than most of the other groups of respondents in the study.

That doctors have a relatively poorer understanding of the problems of other groups than the latter have of the problems of doctors is both admitted by the doctors and concurred to by others in the organization. The data show, for example, that 58 percent of the doctors and 67 percent of the trustees, but only 30 percent of the administrators, feel that trustees have a "very good" or "excellent" understanding of the problems and needs of the medical staff. By contrast, only 41 percent of the doctors, 61 percent of the trustees, and 20 percent of the administrators feel that the doctors have a very good or excellent understanding of the problems of the board of trustees. A greater proportion of the members of each group, in other words, indicate that trustees have a better understanding of the problems of doctors than the latter have of the problems of the former. It is also interesting to observe that, while administrators underestimate, trustees overestimate the understanding doctors have of the problems of trustees (shown by comparing the responses of doctors with those of the administrators and trustees cited above). And the proportion of doctors who feel that trustees have a high degree of understanding of the problems of doctors is considerably larger than the proportion of doctors who feel that doctors have a high degree of understanding of the problems of trustees.

Similar additional findings, moreover, show that doctors have a poorer understanding of the problems of nurses than nurses have of the problems of doctors. Specifically, while only 25 percent of the professional nurses (supervisory and nonsupervisory), 30 percent of the administrators, and 47 percent of the doctors in the study say that the medical staff has a "very good" or "excellent" understanding of the problems and needs of the nursing staff, 49 percent of the professional nurses, 70 percent of the administrators, and 66 percent of the doctors say that the nursing staff has a very good or excellent understanding of the problems and needs of the medical staff. Again, all groups are agreeing. Furthermore, according to these data, it is evident that, while doctors overestimate their own understanding of the problems of nurses, nurses do not overestimate their understanding of the problems of doctors. The administrators, on the other hand, tend to overestimate the understanding nurses have of the problems of doctors.

The relatively inadequate understanding doctors have of the problems and needs of the nursing staff, one might add, is in part responsible for, and helps explain, the earlier cited finding that, except for the tension prevailing among doctors and other doctors in the hospitals studied, there is more tension between doctors and nurses than between doctors and any of the other major groups in the hospital, including the trustees and the administrative group. Deficient understanding of the problems of nurses on the part of the medical staff, moreover, is probably a more serious problem for hospital functioning than deficient understanding of the problems of trustees on the part of the medical staff, principally because doctors and nurses are constantly and directly interacting and their work is highly interdependent, unlike the case of doctors and trustees.

Another frequently raised issue concerning the medical staff has to do with the doctors' appreciation of hospital costs and financial problems. One familiar with the hospital scene often hears comments to the effect that doctors are prone to insist that the hospital spend money for certain purposes without appreciating the financial difficulties which may be involved, or that doctors are apt to make excessive or wasteful use of tests and similar other materials or, more generally, that doctors are not as "cost-conscious" as they should be. Our data about this issue are rather meager. Nevertheless, in their entirety, they indicate that the issue is exaggerated, even though a certain lack of cost-consciousness on the part of the doctors actually exists.

For example, the data show no serious excesses by the doctors in their use of tests. In answering the question, "What is your opinion about the number and quantity of laboratory and x-ray tests and other similar items of this type that the medical staff uses for diagnostic purposes?", seven of the ten hospital administrators in the study, and 46 percent of the doctors said that "in general, the medical staff uses the right number and quantity" of these items. The remaining three administrators, and an additional 39 percent of the doctors said that "the staff uses perhaps a little more than what it should." Only 8 percent of the doctors, and none of the administrators, felt that the staff makes excessive use of tests and test materials for diagnostic purposes. (Many of these respondents attribute most such excesses to the "younger" members of the medical staff.)

The tendency on the part of doctors to use "perhaps a little more" than what they should is, of course, understandable, for there is little or no margin for error when the life of patients may be at stake. The patient takes precedence over financial considerations. Furthermore, because there is no room for error, tests, materials, and facilities, which may be used only infrequently or rarely, must still be available, and this results in some "inherent inefficiency"—as one of our doctor respondents put it—from the standpoint of operating economy and financial outlay.

It should also be added, at this point, that several of the doctors in the study spontaneously commented on the issue of cost-consciousness. The majority of those who commented, moreover, in effect argued that administrators and trustees often underestimate the doctors' concern over the financial problems of the hospital. And, after a rather lengthy commentary on the matter, one doctor concluded by suggesting that doctors are also "businessmen, and pretty good ones." On the other hand, there is little argument that doctors are not as cost-conscious as the trustees. In response to a question about how "business-minded or cost-conscious" the doctors and the trustees are, seven of the ten administrators and 43 percent of the doctors indicated that the medical staff in their respective hospitals is less cost-conscious "than they should be;" in addition, only 9 percent of the doctors and none of the administrators felt that the medical staff is more cost-conscious than it should be. By contrast, all the administrators and 85 percent of the doctors said that the trustees are as much cost-conscious as "they should be" (with another 14 percent of the doctors saying that trustees are more cost-conscious than they should be, and 1 percent saying that trustees are less cost-conscious than they should be). These differences are completely consistent with what one might have anticipated on the basis of the division of labor prevailing in the community general hospital—the division of labor makes it the primary institutional function of trustees to mind the purse, and the corresponding function of doctors to mind the patient. Still, the concern of doctors with the financial problems of the hospital might in fact be greater than these differences suggest, however, for while 76 percent of the trustees and 70 percent of the administrators characterized the general financial condition of their respective hospitals as "completely adequate" or "very adequate," only 56 percent of the doctors so characterized it.

Finally, regarding the professional conduct of doctors, their competence, and their practice of medicine, our data do not show any acute or widespread problems in the ten participating hospitals (see Chap. 4, for example). On the whole, the data—mostly interview data—suggest some problems in this area, but no flagrant violations on the part of doctors were reported with any regularity in any of the hospitals. On occasion, some doctor respondents accused some of their colleagues of questionable professional judgment, mistakes or negligence, or practices they did not consider ethical (e.g., "fee-splitting"), but comments of this kind were rather rare. The most frequently mentioned problems regarding matters of professional conduct were: (1) that it is difficult to "discipline" members of the medical staff, or that medical discipline is lax in some hospitals, primarily because doctors have to be disciplined by their colleagues when the occasion arises and, more generally, because it is difficult to discipline professionals; (2) that some doctors habitually fail to be prompt or, less frequently, thorough in processing the records of their patients; (3) that the medical staff organization is weak, could be improved, or should be revised in some hospitals; and (4) that medical staff rules and regulations are inadequate, not sufficiently strict, or poorly implemented, in the opinion of a number of doctors from some of the hospitals. Individual hospitals vary a good deal with respect to which of these problems they are experiencing at a given time, and with respect to the relative magnitude of each problem being experienced. However, these problems do not seem to be too serious or too salient for the majority of the hospitals studied, according to the data.

THE VALUE ORIENTATIONS OF THE TOP-ECHELON GROUPS IN THE HOSPITAL

Many specific problems and issues about the community general hospital are frequently attributed by the literature to more basic underlying considerations having to do with an alleged wide divergence, and associated incompatibilities, in the philosophies, values, and interests of the top groups in the organization. They are attributed to presumed basic differences in point of view and conviction among the trustees, the administrator and his staff, and the medical staff, which constitute the top three groups in the community general hospital (and which are followed, at some distance, by the nursing group in fourth place). It is alleged that a sharp cleavage exists between the orientations of the professionals (primarily the doctors, but perhaps also the nurses) and the orientations of the top lay authorities in the organization (the trustees and the administrator). Furthermore, this cleavage is frequently translated into an issue of "service vs. finances," with the professionals overemphasizing the service aspects without commensurate appreciation of the financial aspects, and the trustees and administrators overemphasizing the financial aspects without commensurate appreciation of the service aspects. The cleavage itself is primarily attributed to the business background of trustees and administrators, on the one hand, and the professional-nonbusiness background of doctors, on the other—the two presumably being incompatible in one way or another. Further, it is hypothesized that this cleavage in value orientations leads to tensions and conflicts, to difficulties in power and authority relations in the organization, to inadequate coordination, to lack of consensus on issues of common concern, and to differential emphasis on problems and their means of resolution—all of these tending to undermine a unified point of view and unified action by the total organizational system.

Certainly, if and where basic cleavages in the value orientations of the top groups in the hospital (or any other organization, for that matter) exist and operate unrestrained, one can expect serious problems and undesirable consequences. Actually, however, the quantitative evidence available to date in this area does not permit any definitive conclusions regarding the prevalence of sharp cleavages of this kind in community general hospitals. The evidence adduced in support of the value-cleavage hypothesis is generally meager and statistically nongeneralizable, and the methodology on which some of the evidence is based is highly questionable. Our own evidence, even though it cannot be indiscriminately generalized to hospitals other than those studied, shows neither sharp cleavages in the value orientations of doctors and trustees, nor widespread serious problems that could be accounted for in any substantial degree by invoking the notions of divergent and incompatible orientations among the key groups in the hospital. Differences, of course, exist but no sharp differences.

What evidence is there for questioning the hypothesis of sharp cleavage among the orientations of doctors, trustees, and administrators? (Here we shall be primarily dealing with the question of differences between doctors and trustees, because most of the issues raised concern these two groups and because, as we have shown in previous chapters, administrators are employed by the trustees and share the points of view of trustees in the great majority of issues or items about which data are available.) First, we have already seen that, contrary to popular assertions, there is relatively little tension between doctors and trustees in the hospitals studied. There is *less* tension between doctors and trustees than between doctors and any other major group in the hospital. Sixty-one percent of all doctors and 52 percent of all trustees in the study report "no tension at all" between doctors and trustees; and of the remaining group members in each case most report only a little or some tension, with very few reporting "considerable" tension. Interestingly enough, the administrators overestimate the tension between doctors and trustees, only three of the ten reporting no tension at all. Nevertheless, the data from doctors, trustees, nurses, and even the administrators are in agreement to the

Value Orientations of Top-Echelon Groups 561

effect that there is more tension between doctors and other doctors in the various hospitals, than between doctors and nurses, doctors and the administrators, and doctors and trustees, in this order. In short, we find more tension among the professionals than between the professionals and the top lay people in the hospital—something which has received little attention by researchers. In fact, as we have pointed out in Chapter 4, in only two of the ten hospitals do we find much evidence for problems in the relations between doctors and trustees. In most hospitals, each group's sphere of competence is recognized and accepted by the other.

Second, concerning the degree of interest doctors and trustees show in the hospital as an institution, we find very little difference. Specifically, the data show that 84 percent of all the doctors in the study (and 100 percent of the trustees) feel that, apart from their interest in financial matters, the trustees are "quite a bit" or "extremely" interested in the operations and problems of the hospital. Similarly, 87 percent of the trustees (and 85 percent of the doctors) feel that, apart from their interest in medical matters, doctors are "quite a bit" or "extremely" interested in the hospital as an institution. Relevant data from the administrators and the department heads, moreover, also confirm the finding that both doctors and trustees show a high degree of interest in the hospital as an institution, and that doctors and trustees do not differ in this respect. Exceptions, of course, occur, for it should be remembered that individual hospitals differ to a certain extent from these average patterns (for specific deviations, see Chap. 4), but these exceptions are minor compared to the prevailing average pattern.

Third, when asked to indicate how adequate several major hospital facilities are in their respective hospitals, doctors, trustees, and administrators all agreed as to which of the various facilities were most inadequate. Each group indicated that "space and beds" was the least adequate of seven different facilities, and all chose "the physical plant and layout of the hospital" as the next least adequate facility. For each of the remaining five facilities (equipment, supplies, x-ray and laboratory facilities, medical records organization and facilities, and the general financial condition of the hospital), however, proportionately more trustees than doctors felt that each item was "completely adequate" or "very adequate." And the same is true for the proportion of administrators who felt each item was adequate, except that a higher proportion of doctors than administrators felt that x-ray and laboratory facilities were very adequate or completely adequate. These differential proportions, however, are not as important as the agreement among the three groups regarding the least adequate facilities, insofar as the issue of cleavage with which we are dealing here is concerned.

A fourth set of relevant findings has to do with problems of the hospital with which doctors, trustees, and administrators were most concerned at the time of data collection. In each hospital, the administrator and all the doctors and trustees who participated in the study as respondents were asked the following question:

> In the life history of a hospital different issues assume particular importance at different times. On the following list, please check the *three* items with which you are *most concerned* at present:
>
> _____ Improvements in nursing care
> _____ Improvements or expansion of the hospital building or equipment
> _____ Improvements in wages, hours, working conditions, or employee benefits for hospital personnel
> _____ Changes in the organization of the board of trustees
> _____ Changes in the organization of the medical staff
> _____ Improvements in the quality or completion rate for medical records
> _____ Changes in the qualifications, rights, or responsibilities expected for members of the medical staff
> _____ Improvements in the economy or efficiency of operation in offices or departments
> _____ Improvements in training programs

On the whole, the results show rather high agreement among doctors, trustees, and administrators, although agreement is higher between the two subgroups of doctors in the study (general medical staff and selected medical staff), and between trustees and administrators, than between any other possible pair of groups. When the items listed above are ranked according to the frequency with which they were checked by each group of respondents, using data from all participating hospitals combined, we find considerable agreement among the different groups. First, the single most frequently chosen item among the above nine items by the trustees, by the administrators, *and* by the selected medical staff was "improvements or expansion;" for the general medical staff, this was the second most frequently chosen item (the first being improvements in nursing care). Second, the item "improvements in training programs" was checked as a problem of great concern by all the respondent groups: it was the third most frequently chosen item by the selected and general medical staff, and the fourth most frequently chosen item by the trustees and by the administrators. Third, none of these four groups of respondents selected "changes in the organization of the board of trustees" among the four items that each group chose most frequently as items of most concern. And the same is true for the item "changes in the organization of the medical staff." Among other things, these latter results would also imply that, on the average, both the organization of the board of trustees and the organization of the medical staff were basically satisfactory to the top groups in the hospitals studied.

The above findings show almost perfect consensus among the top groups in the hospital, both medical and lay, on the problems and issues of the hospital that these groups consider to be among those problems with which they are most concerned. However, it would have been a most remarkable coincidence had each of the four groups involved made completely identical choices among the nine items presented to them. Of course, no such thing happened. As expected, some differences among the four groups were also found. The main differences were as follows: (1) while both of the medical groups chose the item "improvements in nursing care" among the two most frequently selected items of great concern to them, the administrators gave it fourth place (a tie with the item "improvements in training programs," which is not unrelated to improvements in nursing care), and the trustees gave it fifth place; and (2) while the trustees and the administrators selected "improvements in economy" and "improvements in employee benefits" among the four most frequently selected items from the list of nine items, the doctors did not.[1]

These differences are, of course, quite understandable, if one takes into consideration that nursing care is more of a medical-professional matter, while economy and concern with employee benefits are less of a medical matter and more of a lay matter. It is part of the legitimate and expected organizational role of trustees to be particularly concerned with the latter items, as it is part of the legitimate organizational role of the medical staff to be particularly concerned with problems of nursing care. In short, the differences shown by the above data are entirely congruent with the differential requirements of the role of doctors and of the role of trustees in the hospital, and can be probably attributed to these requirements, i.e., in effect, the doctors and the trustees accept and do what is organizationally expected of them. In any event, there is no reason for one to attribute the obtained differences to any schisms in the value orientations of doctors and trustees, particularly since the evidence available does not show any sharp cleavages between the two groups. Moreover, it should be remembered that, apart from occupational-professional differences or differences in the background characteristics of the two groups, ideologically doctors and trustees are very much alike—they are both predominantly conservative groups. Above all, the obtained differences should not be allowed to obscure the total pattern of the findings in the present series. The pattern indicates a good deal of agreement among doctors, trustees, and administrators as to the problems and issues (from the list presented to them) which are of the greatest concern to each group. Some differences also exist, but the agreement and similarities are much greater than the differences in

[1] As a matter of interest, we might also mention here the rather unexpected finding that the selected medical staff group, but not the general medical staff, the trustees, or the administrators, selected the item "improvements in the quality or completion rate for medical records" among the four items which this group chose most frequently as the items of greatest concern. Ordinarily, it is the administrators and trustees, rather than the doctors, who complain (or are "most concerned") that doctors are not prompt with their patient records.

this connection—certainly sufficient to show lack of sharp disagreements among the groups involved.

A fifth set of findings, closely related to the preceding set, serves to confirm and reinforce the above conclusions regarding consensus on important problems or issues among doctors, trustees, and administrators. These findings were obtained from the answers given by administrators, doctors, and trustees in the various hospitals to the following question:

> How would *you* rank the importance of the following items? (Please number the items listed in order of their importance, by putting 1 in front of the most important item, 2 in front of the next most important item, etc.)
> _____ How satisfied patients are
> _____ Balancing the budget
> _____ What the community thinks of the hospital
> _____ How satisfied hospital employees are
> _____ How adequate the hospital plant, layout, and equipment are
> _____ How high the standards of patient care are

The question was answered completely, i.e., all six items were ranked as required by over 90 percent of the doctors, trustees, and administrators in the study, indicating that the respondents had little difficulty in judging the relative importance of the items involved. More significantly, the consensus among the three groups of respondents shown by the results is very high. We find that both the doctor group and the trustee group ranked the six items in exactly the same order of importance. Specifically, in order of decreasing importance, the two groups ranked the six items as follows: how high the standards of patient care are (1.39, 1.29); how satisfied patients are (2.29, 2.49); how adequate the hospital plant, layout, and equipment are (3.32, 3.50); what the community thinks of the hospital (4.31, 4.07); how satisfied hospital employees are (4.44, 4.23); and balancing the budget (5.10, 4.69), in last place. The figures in the parentheses show the mean-rank for each item, computed from the ranks given to each item by the doctors and by the trustees, respectively. Theoretically, the mean-rank of a given item could vary from 1.00, if all respondents had ranked the item in first place, to 6.00, if all respondents had ranked the item in last place of importance.

These results show virtually complete agreement between doctors and trustees as to the relative importance of the organizational values reflected in the above six items. Even the mean-rank received by each item from the doctors does not differ much from the mean-rank received by the same item from the trustees. The highest difference between the two mean-ranks for any of the six items is .41 of one scale point (theoretically, it could be as high as five scale points), and it occurs in connection with the item "balancing the budget," which is ranked slightly more highly in importance by the trustees.

The corresponding data from the hospital administrators show that administrators, like the doctors and the trustees, ranked "how high the standards of patient care are" (1.50) in first place, and "how satisfied patients are" (2.00) in second place. Similarly, like the doctors and the trustees, they ranked "what the community thinks of the hospital" (4.10) in fourth place, and "balancing the budget" (4.90) in sixth or last place. But, the administrators ranked "how satisfied hospital employees are" (3.60) in third place, while the doctors and the trustees ranked this item in fifth place; and, conversely, the administrators ranked "how adequate the hospital plant, layout, and equipment are" (4.90) in last place (for a tie with "balancing the budget"), while the doctors and the trustees ranked this item in third place among the six items involved. Obviously, it is the administrators among the top three groups in the hospital who constitute the "deviant" group in relation to the matter in question. However, even the administrators agree much more than they deviate from the positions of the doctors and trustees (which are identical) regarding the relative importance of the six organizational values contained in the items ranked.[2] Considering the results in their totality, one cannot fail to be impressed by the remarkably high degree of consensus, and implied value co-orientation, which prevails among the top three groups in the community general hospitals studied with respect to the six values examined.

Finally, the preceding conclusions receive indirect confirmation from still another source. In response to the question "To what extent has this hospital been able to achieve singleness of direction in the efforts of its many groups, departments, and individuals?" a substantial proportion of the doctors, trustees, administrators, and administrative department heads in the study answered "to a considerable extent" or "to a very great extent." More specifically, 72 percent of the doctors from all hospitals in the study, 75 percent of the administrative-nonmedical department heads, 96 percent of the trustees, and 100 percent of the administrators gave one of these two answers. If sharp cleavages in the basic value orientations of the top groups were actually operative in the various hospitals, these percentages would have been considerably smaller. Furthermore, the answers of nursing personnel and laboratory and x-ray technicians to the same question suggest that there is a good deal more consensus at the top levels in the hospital than in the lower levels regarding the degree to which the organization has achieved singleness of direction. By comparison with the above percentages, the data show that a smaller percentage of the supervisory nurses (55 percent), nonsupervisory registered nurses (57 percent), practical nurses (61 percent), and technicians (63 percent) in the study felt that their respective hospital had achieved singleness of direction to "a considerable" or "very great" extent.

[2] Incidentally, the slight deviance of the administrators concerning the importance of these values may be a "good" thing rather than disruptive, for it may be serving to focus attention on some areas that otherwise might be neglected, or to de-emphasize some areas that might otherwise receive disproportionately too much attention by the top groups in the organization.

On the basis of all the evidence in this section, as well as auxiliary evidence presented in the foregoing sections and in previous chapters (especially Chap. 4), and notwithstanding the fact that certain differences among the top groups in hospital organization exist (including differential emphasis on financial matters by doctors and trustees, and other differences that are both recognized and accepted as legitimate on the part of those directly concerned), it must be concluded that there are no serious or disruptive cleavages in the basic value orientations of the top echelon groups in the hospitals studied. This conclusion, of course, does not apply to each and every one of the ten participating hospitals, since in some individual hospitals there are problems which have some bearing on one or another of the issues here discussed (e.g., in Chap. 4, we have seen that in two of the hospitals studied there is evidence of problems between doctors and trustees). But, it applies to the "typical" participating hospital and to most of the hospitals studied.

THE INFLUENCE OF KEY GROUPS IN THE HOSPITAL

In the hospital, as in any complex organization, some groups and individuals have more influence on the operations of the organization than others. And the part each group or person plays in the organization depends, among other things, on the relative amount of influence that it has. Moreover, a particular group may be perceived by its members, and/or others in the organization, as wielding more, or less, influence than it should insofar as organizational functioning is concerned. The prevailing distribution of influence in the organization may or may not coincide with the distribution that is preferred by those concerned. Imbalances of influence may be present in the organization. More importantly for our purposes, such imbalances, or discrepancies between prevailing and desired patterns of influence in the system, when large enough and unmitigated, could result in power conflicts, intraorganizational strains, and dissatisfactions among organizational members, ultimately affecting the performance of the organization adversely.

It is, therefore, important to know something about the distribution and balance of influence in the hospital, especially about the influence of key groups in the organization. This is a particularly intriguing area, moreover, when one considers the multiple seats of power and multiple lines of authority characteristic of hospital organization—the overall institutional authority line originating from the board of trustees, the lay authority line through the hospital administrator, the professional authority line originating from the medical staff, and the mixed lay-professional authority to which nonmedical personnel, such as nurses and technicians, are subject. In the community general hospital, the locus and origins of authority are considerably different from the situation in industrial and other organizations, which depend on a single line of command.

The principal areas of interest on which the present research was focused

Influence of Key Groups in the Hospital

do not include the area of influence. However, because of the obvious importance of this area, we did obtain certain data which help us explore the distribution of influence among the top groups in the hospital—the board of trustees, the administrator, the medical staff, and the nursing staff. In this section, we will be mainly discussing these data, which were obtained from the doctors, trustees, and administrators in the study. However, several of the findings presented in previous sections of this chapter, as well as the results about the relationships among the key groups in the hospital presented in earlier chapters, also have some relevance to the question of influence, thus permitting us to make some general observations on the topic, before discussing the more specific and more directly relevant data.

First, it can be surmised from our previous discussions that the most influential groups in the hospital organization are the trustees, the administrator (and his department heads), and the doctors, followed in fourth place—but at some distance—by the nurses. (The patients and the community also exert a good deal of influence on the community general hospital, but their influence is indirect and of a different kind, and we shall not be concerned with it here.) Second, while the administrators, the trustees, and the doctors constitute the most influential groups in community voluntary hospitals, each group exercises more influence than the others within its own sphere of jurisdiction. The administrator, within the limits set for him by the board of trustees, is most influential with respect to the day-to-day operations of the hospital and in all nonmedical areas; the doctors are most influential in purely medical matters; and the trustees are most influential with respect to long-range institutional policies, financial matters, and hospital-community relations. The influence of the nursing staff is much more circumscribed than the influence of doctors, trustees, and administrators. It is usually confined to matters and issues affecting the nursing staff directly rather than to organization-wide matters, and is often expressed through other groups, such as the medical staff, rather than directly.

Third, it should be noted that doctors derive their influence primarily from professional expertness and the high prestige, status, and power which they enjoy among patients and in the larger community outside the hospital. The influence of trustees, on the other hand, is primarily based on the fact that they constitute the highest legal authority in hospital organization and on the fact that most trustees are usually prominent men in community affairs. In other words, both groups derive additional influence from their respective prestige and power in the community, but the influence of trustees is mainly based on institutional-constitutional legitimacy, while the influence of doctors is mainly based on professional expertness. The influence of the administrator derives from the authority granted to him by the board of trustees, by which he is employed and to which he is ultimately responsible. The influence of the nursing staff has its source in professional expertness.

In theory, and consistent with the above considerations, the board of trustees constitutes the ultimate overall authority in the community general hospital, having authority over all other groups in the organization, including both medical and nonmedical groups. In practice, however, the authority of trustees over the medical staff is quite limited. As we have pointed out in earlier chapters, the doctors are not employees of the hospital and, consequently, the hospital (represented by the trustees as a corporate entity) does not have direct control over them on the basis of conventional employer-employee considerations. In fact, it is a most interesting, if not entirely unique, organizational feature of the community general hospital that the organization has little direct *de facto* control over two of its most central components —the doctors and the patients.

In practice, doctors are more responsible to their own staff organization, rules, and standards than they are to the total hospital organization. Medical rules and regulations are established by the medical staff itself, according to professional-medical considerations and the requirements of the Joint Commission on Accreditation of Hospitals. Furthermore, medical rules and standards are subject to few restrictions by the hospital constitution and/or the board of trustees, although they must not trespass very broadly defined organizational boundaries and must be approved or ratified by the board of trustees. Not only are the medical rules and regulations established by the medical staff, but their very implementation and enforcement are largely under the control of the medical staff. Even the matter of appointments to the medical staff in practice falls under the control of doctors, although the trustees must approve the staff recommended appointments—something which they do, with only rare exceptions.

When one adds to these considerations the extremely high prestige and extrainstitutional influence which doctors ordinarily enjoy, one can readily see why the medical staff in the community general hospital is subject to little lay authority, or why it enjoys exceedingly high autonomy in that organization (autonomy within the limits posed by its functional-professional interdependence with other groups, however, as well as within the limits which may be imposed by informal pressures or informal influence relations between doctors and others). For the same reasons, one can also readily see why the hospital depends more on medical staff self-discipline than on formal superordinate authority for exercising some organizational control over the doctors. Medical self-discipline, of course, itself is not an easy matter. Disciplining professionals is difficult for any organization, especially when it must be left in the hands of the professionals themselves.

In spite of these considerations, the influence of the medical staff upon the organizational-nonmedical aspects of hospital functioning is rather limited, as we are about to see. In fact, according to the data, neither the trustees, nor the administrator, nor the doctors can "run the hospital" unilaterally or determine the fate of the organization as a whole. Certainly, the trustees and the administrator cannot act arbitrarily or unrestrained, in view of the power of the medical staff. But, the converse is also true. The medical staff cannot take any sustained or effective action without at least the consent of trustees and the administrator.

The factors that keep the power of the medical staff "in check" are many and varied. In the first place, the doctors, along with the trustees and the administrator, accept the basic objectives of the organization, i.e., the objectives of patient care and service to the community, more than just superficially. This acceptance generates a good deal of consensus among doctors, trustees, and administrators regarding the organization, with the result that the three power centers cooperate to a substantial degree. In the second place, the organizational division of labor among the three is sufficiently clear and unambiguous to make readily apparent any attempts on the part of one of them to usurp authority or to act in ways that are inconsistent with its functions, authority, and responsibility. Furthermore, the prevailing division of labor among the three—which, incidentally, resembles the familiar separation of powers characteristic of our federal government organization—is more than nominally accepted by the great majority of all concerned in the hospitals studied. In the third place, the trustees, the administrator, and the doctors are all very influential, each having sufficient power to facilitate or obstruct the interests of the others. Each can, therefore, act as a mechanism of "checks and balances" in relation to the other two. Last, but not least, because of the relatively high functional interdependence among the three, cooperation among them is practically inevitable—at least, other things being equal, cooperation is much more likely than lack of cooperation. The elaborate system of committees, conferences, mutual consultations, and joint committees for coordination and joint decision making among the three power centers in the hospital is partly designed to ensure minimum cooperation, while also serving to promote and reinforce cooperation and coordination among them. And the role of the administrator, being primarily a coordinative role, also serves the same functions.

Actually, as we have pointed out, the cooperation among trustees, administrators, and doctors in the participating hospitals is quite high—especially when viewed in conjunction with the relatively sharp division of labor among them, and in the context of their different professional-occupational origins and backgrounds (see Chaps. 3 and 4). According to the data, in only two of the ten hospitals do we find much evidence for poor relations between doctors and trustees, for example (see Chap. 4). Similarly, the results about the tension which prevails among different groups in the hospital, and the results concerning the value orientations of the top groups in the organization, lead to the same conclusion. Generally speaking, no serious tension exists between the doctors and the trustees, the trustees and the administrator, or the administrator and the doctors in most of the hospitals studied, although individual hospitals vary from one another on the specific degree of tension prevailing among these top groups. The degree of tension is higher between doctors and the administrator than between doctors and trustees or between trustees and the administrator, however, probably because the administrator serves as a liaison between doctors and trustees; being a main point of contact, or a "middleman," between these two groups, he probably absorbs the initial impact of many problems, thus minimizing some of the potential tensions that could otherwise develop between doctors and trustees. We have also seen that doctors and trustees are in substantial agreement about the main objectives of the hospital, in their concern over important problems that the hospital faces, and about what particular issues are the important or crucial ones in the organization. Finally, one does not have to be reminded that both doctors and trustees are essentially conservative groups, having no fundamental ideological conflicts separating them.

Certain differences of opinion and interest, of course, exist among the top groups in the hospital (e.g., trustees are more cost-conscious than doctors—but they are not seen as more cost-conscious than "they should be"), as do differences in emphasis or approach in relation to particular organizational problems or specific aspects of hospital functioning. But, such differences are generally considered "legitimate" by the three groups and do not impair satisfactory symbiosis among them, although they probably set limits to the level of cooperation that may be feasible. They are differences which are both expected and accepted (or, at least, tolerated) by all of the key groups and which apparently do not result in open conflicts, sustained feuds, or excessive intergroup tensions that would undermine the effectiveness and integration of the organization. In the hospitals studied, we find no evidence of large-scale power conflicts among doctors, trustees, and administrators, or of overt attempts on the part of one of these groups to usurp authority from another. Each group is fully aware of the power of the others, and each group's jurisdiction is recognized and basically accepted by the others. However, the three groups are watchful of their respective prerogatives and frankly sensitive about their authority and power relations—no group would like its influence reduced. And, the fact that they are power-conscious suggests that the balance of power among them is very delicate and potentially subject to change.

In summary, then, within its own defined sphere of competence, each of the top groups in the hospital exercises more influence than the others, without being seriously challenged in this respect. The overall influence that each group has over the functioning of the hospital as a total organization, however, is another matter. The several top groups differ in their overall influence on hospital operations, and the influence that each group has in this connection is not necessarily the same as the influence that it would like to have, or the influence that other groups would like it to have. In other words, the distribution of prevailing influence among the top groups is not necessarily the same as the distribution of desired influence.

Prevailing and Desired Influence Patterns

To assess the distribution of both prevailing and desired influence upon the functioning of the hospital on the part of the top groups in the organization, the doctors, the trustees, and the administrators from the participating hospitals were asked a series of questions. Two questions were asked about the influence of each group, one about the influence which the group actually has (prevailing influence), the other about the influence which the same group should have (desired influence). In all cases, the latter question was asked immediately after the former. All questions in the series offered five response alternatives, ranging from "little or no influence" to "a very great deal of influence." The groups about which the influence questions were asked include the medical staff, the nursing staff, the board of trustees, and the hospital administrator(s). The format of the two questions about the influence of each group was as follows:

> In general, how much influence do you think [the medical staff] *has* on how this hospital as a total organization functions—on how it is run and how it operates?

> In general, how much influence do you think [the medical staff] *should have* on how this hospital as a total organization functions—on how it is run and how it operates?

Considering first the data about prevailing influence, we find that on the average the administrators, the trustees, and the doctors agree in attributing more overall influence to the administrator than to the trustees, than to the medical staff, than to the nursing staff, in that order. For example, 100 percent of the administrators in the study indicate that the administrator has a "very great deal" or a "great deal" of influence on the functioning of their respective hospital, 80 percent feel that the board of trustees has that much influence, 30 percent feel that the medical staff has that much influence, and also 30 percent feel that the nursing staff has that much influence. The corresponding percentages based on data from the trustees in the study are 96 percent, 80 percent, 58 percent, and 44 percent, respectively. And those based on data from the doctors are 77 percent, 73 percent, 58 percent, and 27 percent, respectively. Thus, the hospital administrator is seen by each of the three groups of respondents as the most influential among the top four groups in the organization followed, in order of decreasing influence, by the trustees, the doctors, and the nurses. It is also obvious, of course, that the two lay-authority groups are seen as more influential than the two professional groups.

Considering next the data about desired influence, or the amount of influence that each group "should have" according to the respondents, we find that: (1) 100 percent of the administrators feel that the hospital administrator should have a great or very great deal of influence on how the hospital operates, 80 percent feel that the board of trustees should have that much influence,

30 percent feel that the medical staff should have that much influence, and also 30 percent feel that the nursing staff should have that much influence; (2) the corresponding percentage figures based on data from the trustees are 98 percent, 87 percent, 67 percent, and 60 percent, respectively; and the corresponding figures based on data from the doctors in the study are 69 percent, 69 percent, 80 percent, and 39 percent, respectively. We shall return to these data shortly.

A closer examination of the data on prevailing influence reveals a number of interesting results. First, it is clear that proportionately more administrators (100 percent) than trustees (96 percent), than doctors (77 percent) see the hospital administrator as having a great or very great deal of influence on hospital functioning (although the difference between administrators and trustees is not statistically significant). Second, an identical proportion (80 percent) of trustees and administrators see the board of trustees as having a great or very great deal of influence, this proportion being greater than the proportion of doctors (73 percent) who attribute that much influence to the board of trustees. Third, an identical proportion (58 percent) of doctors and trustees see the medical staff as having a great or very great deal in influence, this proportion being greater than the proportion of administrators (30 percent) who attribute that much influence to the medical staff. And fourth, a higher proportion of trustees (44 percent) than either administrators (30 percent) or doctors (27 percent) see the nursing staff as having a great or very great deal of influence on hospital functioning. (These are, of course, average figures which are based on data from all participating hospitals combined; the specific situation in individual hospitals need not follow exactly these patterns of influence.)

It is also evident from the data on prevailing influence that administrators perceive a greater gap between the influence of the administrator and that of the medical staff (100 vs. 30 percent) than do the trustees (96 vs. 58 percent) or the doctors (77 vs. 58 percent); the doctors see the smallest gap, i.e., they tend to minimize the difference between the influence of the administrator and their own influence. Similarly, administrators perceive a greater gap between the influence of trustees and that of doctors than either the trustees or the doctors do. Moreover, it is interesting to note that only 30 percent of the administrators in the study see the medical staff as having a great or very great deal of influence in their respective hospitals—suggesting an amount of influence for the medical staff which is much smaller than the amount of influence administrators attribute to the trustees or to themselves and which, surprisingly, is equal to the amount of influence administrators attribute to the nursing staff. Parenthetically, not shown in the above data, those of the administrators (three of the ten in the study) who see the medical staff as very influential are the same as those who also see the nursing staff as very influential, i.e., in hospitals where the medical staff is seen as very influential by the administrator, the nursing staff is also seen by him as very influential.

Briefly, then, although the administrators, doctors, and trustees agree as to the relative influence position of the four top groups in the hospital, the gap in the amount of prevailing influence which separates any two of the four groups is smaller or greater depending on the source of the data, i.e., on whether the administrators, the trustees, or the doctors are judging the influence of the various groups. On the average, administrators attribute much less influence to the medical and nursing staffs than do the trustees; trustees attribute much more influence to the nursing staff than either the doctors or the administrators do; and doctors see a smaller gap between their own influence and that of the trustees or that of the administrator than the latter two see. This last finding indicates that, in effect, doctors see a more balanced distribution of prevailing influence among the top groups in the hospital than the composite picture from all of the available data would indicate. And the fact that they do see a more balanced distribution than the administrator and trustees probably mitigates any problems which could arise from the existing gaps in influence that are shown by the data.

The gaps in prevailing influence which separate the top groups in the hospital are not merely interesting. They are of sufficient magnitude to warrant more detailed studies aimed at ascertaining the precise significance and consequences of such gaps. On the other hand, the observed gaps are not so great as to suggest any active power struggles or conflicts among the top groups in the hospitals studied—and, as we have observed, no such conflicts were detected in these organizations. It must be remembered in this connection that: administrators, doctors, and trustees are in agreement as to the relative position of each group in the hierarchy of prevailing influence; doctors perceive a more balanced distribution of influence among the top groups than is actually the case; and the degree of tension between doctors and trustees, and between doctors and the administrator, is in fact rather small in the majority of the hospitals involved.

Still, one could not conclude from the available evidence that the existing distribution of influence among the top groups in the participating hospitals is optimal, or even free of problems, from the standpoint of hospital effectiveness, or from the standpoint of each of the several groups concerned. We have already shown in Chapter 4, for example, that in three of the ten participating hospitals the president of the board of trustees (though not the entire board) is seen by doctors and others as a powerful and dominating individual who, allegedly, has disproportionately too much influence in determining hospital policies. Similarly, we have earlier suggested that the top groups in the different hospitals are very sensitive to their power relations, this being indicative of a balance of power-influence among them that is delicate and potentially subject to change. More importantly, when the data about prevailing influence are compared with the data about influence desired (the two sets of data that were presented above), certain discrepancies between the actual and desired influence of each group are evident (and the greater these discrepancies, the greater the potential problems concerning the distribution of influence among the top groups in the organization). All of these discrepancies occur when comparing prevailing with desired influence, as appraised by doctors or by trustees, but not by administrators.

It is apparent from the data presented earlier that, as a group, the hospital administrators feel that the trustees, the medical staff, and the nursing staff in their respective hospitals should each have exactly the same amount of influence that now prevails. In other words, the distribution of desired influence for the four top groups in the organization should be identical with the distribution of prevailing influence, according to the administrators. For example, 30 percent of the administrators said that the medical staff has a great or very great deal of influence on how the hospital operates, and the same identical proportion, i.e., again 30 percent, of them said that the medical staff should have that much influence; the remaining administrators would give the medical staff less than a "great deal" of influence. The administrators would, therefore, prefer no changes in the relative influence position of the four top groups in the organization.

The trustees, on the other hand, feel that each and every one of the four groups should have somewhat more influence on hospital functioning than they now have. But, while they would increase the influence of every group, they would not change the rank-order of influence, i.e., they would not change the relative position of the four groups on the influence hierarchy—the administrator would still be the most influential, followed by the trustees, then the medical staff, and finally the nursing staff. However, the trustees would increase the influence of each group disproportionately, increasing most the influence of the nursing staff, and then the influence of the medical staff. In effect, this would result in a more equalitarian balance of influence among the four groups by comparison to the balance of influence that now prevails. More specifically, the data show that: (1) 96 percent of the trustees feel that the administrator has a great or very great deal of influence, and 98 percent feel that the administrator should have a great or very great deal of influence; (2) 80 percent of the trustees feel that they themselves, as a group, have a great or very great deal of influence, and 87 percent feel that they should have that much influence; (3) 58 percent of the trustees feel that the medical staff has a great or very great deal of influence, and 67 percent feel that the medical staff should have a great or very great deal of influence; and (4) 44 percent of the trustees feel that the nursing staff in their respective hospitals has a great or very great deal of influence on hospital functioning, and 60 percent feel that the nursing staff should have a great or very great deal of influence on hospital functioning.

Thus, the trustees would increase the influence of each group, increasing more the influence of the two professional groups, and they would minimize the discrepancies in the amounts of influence exercised by the four groups involved, but without changing the relative influence position that each group now holds. The administrators would make no changes at all, as we have seen. Essentially, then, neither the administrators nor the trustees from the participating hospitals would like to see much change in the balance of influence which is prevailing among the top four groups in the organization, even though the trustees would be willing to make some modifications in the direction of a more equalitarian distribution of influence.

By contrast, the doctors would prefer to alter the current balance of influence. They would give more influence to the medical staff and to the nursing staff, while decreasing somewhat the influence of the administrator and the influence of trustees. Specifically, while 77 percent, 73 percent, 58 percent, and 27 percent of the doctors feel that the administrator, the trustees, the medical staff, and the nursing staff, respectively, have a great or very great deal of influence, the corresponding proportion of doctors who feel that each of these should have that much influence is 69 percent, 69 percent, 80 percent, and 39 percent, respectively. The greatest gap between prevailing and desired influence occurs in the case of doctors with reference to their own influence: 58 percent of the doctors feel that the medical staff in their respective hospital has a great or very great deal of influence on hospital functioning, but 80 percent feel that the medical staff should have a great or very great deal of influence.

The net result of the changes in the distribution of prevailing influence preferred by the doctors would be an altered hierarchy of influence wherein the medical staff would be the most influential group, followed by the administrator and by the trustees at about the same level (and not too far behind), followed by the nursing staff in last place. It is also clear that the changes in influence preferred by the medical staff would mean departing much more from the distribution of influence envisioned by the administrators than that envisioned by the trustees. Whether the distribution and balance of influence desired by the doctors would be feasible, or whether it would have positive, negative, or neutral effects on the functioning of the hospital, if implemented, are questions that cannot be answered on the basis of available data. It is safe to assume, however, that substantial change in the power relations of the top groups in the hospital—in fact, substantial change in any important parameter of an organization—would be neither easy nor free of difficulties.

ORGANIZATIONAL CHANGE AND ITS ACCOMMODATION

The last topic to be commented upon in this chapter is that of organizational change. Fulfillment of organizational goals requires, among other things, that the organization be able to respond successfully to important alterations in its external environment and its internal situation. While stability and continuity are indispensable to effective organizational functioning, ability to introduce and assimilate change is no less essential in the long run. Organizations are dynamic, developing systems; they are not static or "closed" systems. They are expected to change over time, and the adequacy with which they can meet new conditions is a sign of organizational strength. Consequently, how successfully an organization can adapt to environmental changes and adjust to internal changes, and whether it is sufficiently flexible to accommodate necessary changes when they arise are vital questions for all organizations.

In the case of hospitals, such things as medical and technological advances, the development and increasing utilization of hospitalization plans, community growth, and other external factors make certain demands upon the organization, requiring corresponding adaptation on its part. Similarly, internal changes in professional and administrative practices, changes in personnel, changes in equipment, modification of routines, etc., require organizational adjustments. Furthermore, in addition to having to adapt to relatively gradual, long-term changes in its environment, and adjust to more or less frequent internal changes, the hospital must also be able to cope with sudden changes that are necessitated by crises or emergencies, e.g., changes necessitated by an occasional disaster, a major accident in the community, and the like. These relatively unusual and unpredictable situations place additional strain upon the organization.

Without attempting to specify the changes which may occur in a community general hospital, it is clear that many and varied changes are frequently introduced by the organization, in an effort to handle existing problems or to avoid future difficulties. Success does not always or automatically accompany the change, however. New problems attending a change may rival those which it was intended to eliminate if the organization is not prepared to incorporate it, or if those of its members who are affected by the altered situation resist it, fail to accept it, or fail to adjust to it promptly. If, on the other hand, the members of the organization are "accustomed" to the phenomenon of change, if their experience with similar previous changes has been satisfactory, and if their perception of the consequences of the proposed change is not a negative one, then the introduction of change and the adjustments it may require will be correspondingly facilitated.

For these reasons, it is as important to know something about the attitudes and reactions of organizational members to change as it is to know the kinds of change that are most likely in the hospital, as well as their respective rates. An understanding of the social-psychological aspects of change is all the more important in the case of hospitals, moreover, for hospitals are among those organizations which are experiencing, or are apt to experience, a great many changes (only a few of which are likely to be mainly technological

Organizational Change and its Accommodation

in character). In the present research, we have not investigated the question of organizational change and its accommodation in any detail, since change was not one of our major objectives. However, because of the obvious practical and theoretical significance of this subject for the community general hospital, we obtained certain data which help illuminate some of its many aspects.

Internal Changes in the Hospital

Information concerning internally induced changes and related adjustment to change in the participating hospitals was obtained by means of the following set of questions:

> From time to time changes in policies, procedures, and equipment are introduced by the hospital. How often do these changes lead to better ways of doing things? (Check one.)
>
> _____(1) Changes of this kind are always an improvement
> _____(2) Most of the time they are an improvement
> _____(3) About half of the time they are an improvement
> _____(4) They seldom improve things
> _____(5) Changes of this kind never improve things
>
> How well do the various people in the hospital who are affected by these changes accept the change? (Check one.)
>
> _____(1) Practically all of the people involved accept the changes and adjust to them
> _____(2) The majority of the people involved accept the changes and adjust to them
> _____(3) About half of the people involved accept the changes and adjust to them
> _____(4) Less than half of the people involved accept the changes and adjust to them
> _____(5) Very few of the people involved accept the changes and adjust to them
>
> How quickly, would you say, do the various people (or groups) that are affected by the introduction of these changes come to adjust to the new situations? (Check one.)
>
> _____(1) Most of the people involved adjust to the new situation immediately
> _____(2) They adjust very rapidly but not immediately
> _____(3) They adjust fairly rapidly
> _____(4) They adjust fairly slowly
> _____(5) They adjust slowly
> _____(6) They adjust very slowly
> _____(7) Most of the people involved never adjust to the new situation

These three questions were asked consecutively, and in the order shown, of the following groups of respondents: the administrator and the administrative department heads, the general medical staff, the professional nurses, the practical nurses, and the laboratory and x-ray technicians from each hospital.

Considering the data from all hospitals combined, we first find that the vast majority of the respondents have a very favorable attitude toward internal changes in their respective hospitals. Specifically, in answering the first of the three questions, no less than 85 percent of the members of each respondent group report that changes in policies, procedures, and equipment, most of the time lead to better ways of doing things ("always" or "most of the time are an improvement"). The percentage of group members who report this to be the case varies between 85 and 96 percent, depending on the particular group involved (85 percent of the technicians, 87 percent of the doctors, 89 percent of the practical nurses, 90 percent of the administrators, 91 percent of the professional nurses, and 96 percent of the department heads). Judging from these data, the internal organizational changes with which the respondents are familiar have apparently produced satisfactory results in practically all of the hospitals. Not only do we find a high overall percentage of respondents indicating that changes of the specified kind lead to improvements most of the time, we also find that the several groups of respondents are in remarkable agreement on this point, while the individual hospitals themselves (not shown by the above figures) vary little from one another or from the average percentages cited above.

Next, in connection with the second of the above three questions, we find that no less than 90 percent of the members of each group of respondents involved feel that "practically all" or "the majority" of those affected by the various changes in hospital policies, procedures, and equipment accept these changes and adjust to them. All ten of the administrators, 97 percent of the department heads, 95 percent of the doctors, 94 percent of the practical nurses, 93 percent of the professional nurses, and 90 percent of the technicians in the study feel that, in their respective hospitals, the majority of the people affected accept the changes and adjust to them. Interhospital differences are again small, while agreement among the several respondent groups is very high.

Regarding the question about promptness of adjustment to the same internal changes, we find that an average of between 54 and 80 percent of the members of each respondent group feel that most of the people in their hospital who are affected by the various changes adjust to the new situation "immediately" or "very rapidly" (80 percent of the administrators, 62 percent of the department heads, 61 percent of the technicians, 61 percent of the doctors, 55 percent of the practical nurses, and 54 percent of the professional nurses are of this opinion). Of the remaining members of each group, moreover, approximately nine out of every ten feel that those affected by the changes adjust to the new situation "fairly rapidly." Thus, only a very small proportion (less than 5 percent on the aggregate) of all respondents from all participating hospitals say that those affected by the various internal changes in their respective hospitals adjust to the new situation slowly.

These results about promptness of adjustment, however, also suggest that in some of the hospitals adjustment to change is more rapid than in others. And an actual comparison of the data from the different individual hospitals (not shown here) confirms the existence of considerable interhospital differences in promptness of adjustment to internal change. These differences, further analysis shows, are due to a number of specific factors, several of which indicate that good communication in the organization greatly facilitates adjustment on the part of organizational members. Promptness of adjustment in the hospitals studied correlates positively and significantly with: (1) the extent to which doctors feel that the communication which they receive from the administrator is adequate (.69); (2) the extent to which the department heads feel that the communication which they receive from the administrator is adequate (.79); (3) the degree to which the administrator is aware of problems faced by other members of the organization (.61); and (4) the degree to which the administrator is effective in solving conflicts that arise in the organization (.78). These relationships also indicate, of course, that the role of the hospital administrator is particularly crucial in facilitating prompt adjustment to changes introduced by the hospital.

Promptness of adjustment also correlates positively and significantly with the extent to which the board of trustees understands the problems and needs of the medical staff (.67), and the extent to which the medical staff understands the problems and needs of the board of trustees. On the other hand, promptness of adjustment is impaired by (correlates negatively with) the prevalence of intraorganizational strain in the hospital.[3] (All of the independent variables mentioned here have been introduced and discussed in detail in previous chapters.)

Other findings from the study, reported elsewhere by Mott (1), indicate that, when we take into account both the promptness with which hospital people adjust to changes in policies, procedures, and equipment, and the total proportion of organizational members who accept these changes and adjust to them (i.e., when we take into account the overall success of adjustment to change), successful overall adjustment is maximized, or facilitated, in hospitals where:

1. Communication among the top levels (administrator, doctors, and trustees) is perceived as adequate by those concerned;

[3] For a detailed elaboration of various problems and issues relevant to the question of adjustment to internal change in the community general hospital, see Mott's doctoral dissertation, titled "Sources of Adaptation and Flexibility in Large Organizations" (1). Dr. Mott had an active part in the present research, as an assistant study director, and wrote his dissertation using data from the same ten hospitals which participated in the study.

2. Organizational members in different, but related, postions have a good understanding of each other's problems and needs;

3. There is little tension among interacting groups in the organization, and organizational pressure upon members for better performance is not perceived as unreasonable or excessive;

4. The hospital administrator has a high awareness of the problems of others in the organization and effectively solves conflicts;

5. Nonsupervisory, nonmedical personnel feel that their respective immediate superiors understand their point of view, and evaluate their superiors highly on technical skill;

6. Hospital policies, rules, and regulations are clearly defined in the opinion of organizational members; and

7. Coordination of the preventive type is relatively good.

In other words, the data show that overall adjustment to internal organizational change is most successful in those of the hospitals where these conditions prevail. It is also evident from the foregoing discussion, however, that, although individual hospitals differ with respect to promptness of adjustment, overall adjustment to internal change is generally quite good in most of the hospitals. The data show little resistance to internal change on the part of the different members of the organization. Since hospitals constantly face the prospect of introducing and assimilating many and varied changes, these results should be encouraging to those concerned with the problem of change in these organizations.

Finally, certain additional data provide us with a clue as to the frequency or rate of internal change in the participating hospitals. These data were obtained from nonsupervisory registered nurses, laboratory and x-ray technicians, and practical nurses in each hospital, about (1) changes recently introduced by the hospital, and (2) anticipated changes for the near future. Concerning the former kind of changes, these groups were asked the following question: "During the last two years, have you noticed any changes in hospital policy, personnel, procedures, or equipment that have improved hospital operations?" The results show that 43 percent of the registered nurses, 51 percent of the technicians, and 55 percent of the practical nurses felt that "many good changes were introduced during the last two years" in their respective hospitals. In addition, 47 percent of the registered nurses, 37 percent of the technicians, and 37 percent of the practical nurses indicated that "some good changes" were introduced. Stated differently, about nine out of every ten nurses and technicians felt that at least "some" beneficial changes had occurred. If one would also add changes that were not seen as beneficial by the respondents involved, one could surmise that considerable changes had taken place in the hospitals studied during that two-year period.

That the rate of internal change in the community general hospital is probably rather high is further suggested by the data concerning anticipated changes for the near future. The same groups of respondents which were asked the question about recent changes were also asked this question about anticipated change: "Considering the various changes that have taken place in the hospital while you have worked here, how much change would you expect in the next couple of years?" In answering this question, 47 percent of the registered nurses, 59 percent of the technicians, and 65 percent of the practical nurses (the group which also happens to be the longest-service group in the hospital among the three) said that "there are likely to be a great many important changes" or that "many important changes will be made," in their respective hospitals. Furthermore, another 46 percent of the registered nurses, 23 percent of the technicians, and 26 percent of the practical nurses indicated that "some important changes will be made." Thus, the large majority of the members of each of the three groups predict not only numerous changes in their hospitals for the near future, but they also expect quite a few "important" changes to occur.

Organizational Adaptation to Externally Induced Change

Organizations in general and hospitals in particular face not only problems of introducing and assimilating internal change, but also problems of accommodating exogenous changes, i.e., problems of coping with relevant stimuli from their environment. Problems of this latter type are potentially more difficult, more dangerous, and more disruptive, moreover, because their magnitude, significance, and impact upon the organization are difficult to predict and evaluate. Ordinarily, an organization has little or no control over externally imposed changes. Furthermore, the organization may not be sufficiently flexible to respond to such changes, it may lack the required mechanisms to handle specific changes, or it may be unable to respond to the new situation as promptly as needed.

Therefore, organizational accommodation of exogenous change is at best a rather difficult matter, and it cannot be accomplished without creating some strain for the organization and its members in the process. And, the more sudden or unpredictable the change, the greater the difficulty, the strain, and risk of serious disruption for the organization are likely to be. Yet, no organization can escape from, or can afford to disregard, the problems posed by the demands of its environment. Hospitals must be particularly vulnerable in this connection, moreover, because they are continuously dealing with their environment. Their main objective is service to the outside community. They are expected to meet the relatively normal health needs of their community, to be responsive to the general and specific demands of their community, and also to be capable of handling any emergencies or crises that may arise from time to time in the community. In addition, they are expected to keep up with any and all advancements in the fields of medicine and health and, in fact, to handle "successfully" any relevant problems that may result from changes in their environment. We need hardly add, of course, that there is no guarantee that an organization which is successful in adjusting to changes that itself introduces will also be successful in accommodating those changes which are imposed upon it by its environment. The problems of exogenous change require separate examination from the problems of internal change.

Although the problem of accommodating exogenous change is undoubtedly a very important organizational problem for the community general hospital —and a problem whose understanding would require substantial research efforts, both in hospitals and other types of organizations—in the present study we could do no more than examine one or two of its many facets. Our specific interest in this area was purely exploratory and was confined to examining two questions: (1) how successfully do the participating hospitals meet certain temporarily unpredictable changes that are necessitated by extraorganizational conditions, and (2) how much strain do these changes create for the organization and its members. Corresponding to these two aims, we asked the following pair of questions:

> Occasionally, a major accident (e.g., a bus accident) happens in the community or too many patients are admitted at the same time and the *patient load suddenly increases* beyond the normal census. In general, how well does this hospital handle these unusual situations? (Check one.)
>
> _____(1) The hospital handles unusual situations of this kind completely adequately
> _____(2) Quite adequately
> _____(3) Fairly adequately
> _____(4) Not so adequately
> _____(5) The hospital handles unusual situations of this kind inadequately
>
> How much strain (or stress) do these unusual situations create for the various people who work in the hospital? (Check one.)
>
> _____(1) These unusual situations result in extremely high strain for the people who work in the hospital
> _____(2) Result in very high strain
> _____(3) Result in fairly high strain
> _____(4) Result in some strain
> _____(5) These unusual situations result in little or no strain

These questions were asked of the administrator, the department heads, the trustees, the doctors, the professional nurses, the practical nurses, and the technicians from each participating hospital. The average nonresponse rate, as might be expected, was somewhat higher for these questions than for the great majority of questions that the respondents were called upon to answer, because some of the respondents had not experienced any of the "unusual" situations referred to in the present two questions. Still, the

Organizational Change and its Accommodation

overall nonresponse rate for either of the two questions averaged a little less than 10 percent of all respondents from all hospitals combined, and did not exceed 15 percent for any single group of respondents. Accordingly, the data are not subject to serious nonresponse error, and can be treated as most other data from the study have been treated.

The large majority of respondents believe that their respective hospitals handle change situations of the kind described by the above questions adequately. Seventy-six percent of the professional nurses from the hospitals in the study, 78 percent of the doctors, 80 percent of the administrators, 84 percent of the technicians and of the practical nurses, 91 percent of the trustees, and 99 percent of the department heads report that their hospital handles these externally induced changes "quite adequately" or "completely adequately." Therefore, as a group of organizations, the participating hospitals are very successful in adapting to temporarily unanticipated changes (almost as successful as they are in adjusting to internal changes) which, while having their origin outside the organization, occasion a sudden, abnormal rise in the patient load of the hospital.

But, while the hospitals may be ultimately successful in adapting to these exogenous changes, accommodating the change generates a good deal of stress in the organization—success comes at a price. The data show that the above unusual situations, which the typical hospital handles quite adequately, create considerable strain for the members of the organization. Specifically, less than 10 percent of the trustees, the doctors, and the professional nurses in the study report that these situations result only in "little" or no strain. Conversely, 29 percent of the trustees, 26 percent of the doctors, and 17 percent of the professional nurses report that these situations create "very high" or "extremely high" strain in their respective hospitals. On the average, or based on data from all hospitals combined, 32 percent of the administrators and department heads, 36 percent of the practical nurses, 42 percent of the technicians, 45 percent of the professional nurses, 60 percent of the doctors, and 69 percent of the trustees feel that the change situations under consideration result in "fairly high" to "extremely high" strain for the people working in the hospital.[4]

Individual hospitals, of course, differ from the above average figures (which depict the situation for the typical participating hospital), some experiencing more and others less strain than the specific percentages might imply. In general, however, those of the hospitals which, in the view of our respondents,

---

[4] One interesting issue that might be raised at this point is that the data just cited indicate considerable differences among the various groups of respondents involved, suggesting lack of high consensus as to the amount of strain experienced by organizational members. Why is it that the administrators and department heads, for example, report much less strain than the doctors and the trustees? Or, why do the doctors report more strain than the nurses? Unfortunately, the reasons underlying these differences cannot be determined from the available data.

adapt better to the exogenous changes in question also happen to experience a greater amount of strain in the process, according to the data. More specifically, we find a correlation of .59 between how adequately the hospitals studied accommodate the externally induced changes that we have been discussing and the amount of strain that these temporarily unpredictable changes create in the organization. That is, the more successful a hospital is in handling the change, the more likely it is to experience higher strain. Successful accommodation of the change often requires prompt and unusual response by the organization, and a prompt or novel reaction to a stimulus which has not been anticipated is likely to disturb the normal equilibrium of the organization (at least temporarily), thus resulting in intraorganizational strain. Alternately, it is also possible that, in its efforts to accommodate the change, an organization may neglect temporarily some of its normal problems and routines, and this too may result in strain.

In spite of the moderate positive relationship between the adequacy of handling exogenous changes and the amount of strain that is likely to be generated in the process, however, it is still possible for an organization to be able to accommodate such changes successfully and with relatively little strain. An examination of the data for individual hospitals reveals, for example, that some of the hospitals in the study (Hospitals #1, #8, and #9) are apparently able to handle external changes both more adequately and with less strain than most of the remaining seven hospitals. (On the other hand, another two of the hospitals, Hospitals #0 and #2, handle these changes both less adequately and with considerably more strain than most of the remaining hospitals.) But, under what specific conditions it would be possible for a given hospital to adapt to externally induced changes satisfactorily and with little strain, or minimal disruption, is a very interesting question that cannot be answered in the present study.

Disregarding the matter of strain, however, it is possible, on the basis of the available data, to make some statements about the conditions under which hospitals are likely to accommodate externally induced changes (of the kind specified above) most adequately. In this connection, a correlational analysis of the data shows that exogenous changes are likely to be handled more adequately by those of the hospitals where: (1) tension between nursing personnel in the different shifts is at a minimum—intershift tension correlates —.69 with the relative adequacy with which the hospitals handle such changes; (2) each shift is able to take over from the preceding shift without confusion—how well shifts can take over from one another without confusion correlates .74 with the relative adequacy of handling the changes; (3) cooperation among the different shifts is high—how well the various shifts work together correlates .85 with the relative adequacy of handling the changes; and (4) interdepartmental problems in the hospital tend to be settled without delay—how rapidly interdepartmental problems are usually settled correlates

.50 with the relative adequacy with which the organization handles exogenous changes.

On the whole, these findings, elaborated elsewhere in greater detail by Mott (1), suggest that cooperation among nursing personnel and coordination within the nursing department are important facilitating factors, insofar as organizational adaptation to externally induced change is concerned. The underlying explanation for this may be that the nursing staff has to absorb the initial impact (or a good part of it) of such change, if not indeed handle the change (remember that the changes examined had to do with sudden-abnormal increases in the patient load of the hospital). These findings also suggest that the absence of internal organizational problems, as reflected in the habit of resolving such problems without delay, may likewise facilitate organizational adaptation to exogenous change. These results—interesting as they may be—are, admittedly, quite meager compared to the magnitude of the problem to which they refer; they are only tentative, and the product of a small exploratory effort. More definitive answers must, therefore, come from future research.

Before concluding this section, we might raise one more question. What relationship is there, if any, between adjustment to internal changes, as discussed earlier in the section, and adaptation to externally induced change in the hospitals studied? We have already suggested, it may be recalled, that there is no guarantee that an organization which is successful in adjusting to changes which it itself introduces will also be successful in accommodating changes imposed upon it by its environment. But, what do the data acutally show? The data, though far from being conclusive, suggest an answer to our question that dispels any expectations for a positive relationship. Specifically, we find that, in the hospitals studied, successful adjustment to internal changes (as measured by the relative proportion of organizational members who accept the change and adjust to it) correlates —.43 with how well the hospital handles exogenous changes (as measured by the relative adequacy with which the hospital accommodates unusual situations resulting from such things as major accidents in the community).

In other words, those of the hospitals which are most successful in adjusting to internal changes are not the same as those which are most successful in adapting to changes originating from their environment. In fact, the negative, though not statistically significant, correlation between these two variables is mildly suggestive of a possible opposite tendency—hospitals which do relatively well with reference to endogenous changes, if anything, may be somewhat less likely also to do well with reference to exogenous changes, or vice versa. This rather intriguing and unorthodox hypothesis, tenuous and unexpected as it may be, is emerging from the data. Accordingly, it deserves thoughtful, but cautious, consideration by those interested in the area of organizational change, for it implies that adjustment to internal organizational changes may be relatively incompatible (or incapable of simultaneous maximization) with organizational adaptation to changes originating in the external environment of the community general hospital. It may turn out that some of the major factors and conditions which facilitate, or impede, adjustment to internal change are very different from those which facilitate, or impede, adaptation to exogenous change by the hospital, thus accounting for the absence of a positive relationship between adjustment and adaptation.

SUMMARY

This chapter was primarily devoted to a discussion of certain topics which are generally considered important by both researchers and practitioners in the hospital field, but which being outside the central scope of the present investigation were only explored here. The topics discussed included: the external and internal image of the "typical" hospital in the study, certain problems and issues pertaining to the nursing staff and the medical staff, the value orientations of the top echelon groups in the community general hospital, the relative influence of administrators, trustees, doctors, and nurses on the overall functioning of the hospital, and certain aspects of organizational change.

The emphasis in this chapter—which might be best viewed as complementing previous chapters, especially Chapters 3 and 4—was more on descriptive exposition than on relational analysis. For the most part, special attention was given to the characteristics of the typical hospital in the study, and not to testing specific hypothesized relationships among particular variables. The objective was to comment, on the basis of whatever data we had in each case, upon problems and issues which have apparent practical implications for those concerned with the action aspects of hospital functioning and administration, problems and issues which most directly concern particular groups within the hospital, and problems and issues which have received little systematic attention by previous studies.

The data discussed in connection with each of the several topics covered by the chapter are rather meager in many cases, for the study did not focus on these topics. Accordingly, many of the conclusions drawn from these data are tentative rather than definitive, and must be viewed with some caution. Most of the results are, nevertheless, consistent with our findings about the main problem areas with which the study was concerned, serving to supplement and, often, make more meaningful some of the principal findings and their significance. A good many of the results clearly point to specific directions that future research in the hospital field must take, if we are to increase our knowledge of the structure and functioning of community general hospitals. The results also help clarify various aspects of the topics discussed, demonstrating in the process that some so-called problems or issues concerning the hospital situation are often exaggerated, while certain other important problems and issues actually escape the attention of hospital people. In effect, important standing issues faced by the community general hospital are highlighted by the data, while some alleged issues are recast in a form which more closely corresponds to the organizational realities which prevail in the hospitals studied.

REFERENCES

1. Mott, P. E. "Sources of Adaptation and Flexibility in Large Organizations." Doctoral Dissertation. University of Michigan, 1961.

12 SUMMARY AND CONCLUSIONS

The community general hospital could easily claim the dubious honor of being one of the least researched modern large-scale organizations. In spite of its crucial function of aiding the integration and stability of society, through the maintenance of a level of health that permits other social institutions to accomplish their objectives, and in spite of its far-reaching impact upon nearly every facet of everyday life—particularly our economy, standards of living, and community welfare—the community general hospital has not received more than a fraction of the scientific attention that its importance as an organization would warrant. As yet, our understanding of its functioning, problems, and characteristics is extremely limited.

Research in the field of health has, of course, had a rather long standing, especially in the areas of diagnosis, treatment, and prevention of disease. But research viewing the hospital as a complex social system, or as an organization with its own character, problems, and needs, has just begun to make its appearance. It is true that certain problems of the hospital, such as those involving specific technical and medical matters, economic-financial aspects, and professional considerations, have been studied with some regularity, as have some of the individual components of the hospital and their respective circumscribed problems. For example, there have been studies of nursing and about nurses and their training, functions, hospital role, and professional status; studies of the accounting, financial, and records systems of the hospital; and even studies of its dietary and architectural problems. Some studies of hospital administrators and their profession, of doctor-patient, doctor-nurse, and doctor-hospital relations, as well as of the medical profession itself, have also been conducted. It is also true that hospitals have been studied from the standpoint of their historical development. But, studies of the structure and functioning of the community general hospital as an organizational system, similar to those by Smith (6), Wessen (7), and Burling, Lentz, and Wilson (2), are both very recent and very sparse, and the same is true—only more so—regarding comparative studies of hospitals.

Summary and Conclusions

At this stage, we know very little, for example, about how hospitals can operate most effectively, given certain resources and facilities, or how they can best allocate their resources, facilities, and personnel in order to attain their objectives successfully and economically. Similarly, we know very little about the measurement and evaluation of patient care provided in hospitals, about the criteria and determinants of hospital effectiveness, or about why some hospitals are able to render better patient care than others even though their financial status, technical equipment, and other facilities may not be superior. We also know too little both about the important differences among hospitals of the same type, such as community general hospitals, and about the organizational problems and characteristics these organizations share in common. The same is true regarding the question of how hospitals compare with, or differ from, other complex organizations.

Similarly, we have only a vague understanding of how the hospital manages to adapt to changes in medicine, nursing, pharmacology, pathology, and other relevant fields, as well as to changes in the community which it serves, or of the factors which facilitate or hinder adaptation of this kind. The same may be said regarding the question of how the hospital as an organization can maintain sufficient flexibility to meet emergencies successfully and without strain, considering that its workflow is too variable, irregular, and unstandardized to permit extensive and intensive advance planning of the kind one finds in more automated organizations.

There are many other important unanswered questions. Considering the high degree of specialization and heterogeneity, but also interdependence, which characterizes the various roles and positions in the organization, how does the hospital manage to articulate, channel, and concentrate the diverse efforts of its many organizational groups and members toward the attainment of its institutional purposes? What are the requirements for coordinating the activities of the diverse professional-occupational groups in the hospital, and how does the organization achieve singleness of direction, stability, unity, and coherence in its structure and functioning? What are the determinants and effects of adequate organizational coordination, and why are some hospitals better able than others to attain and maintain good coordination? What styles or practices of supervision and administration are most effective in hospitals? What aspects and patterns of communication facilitate performance? What is the relationship between particular supervisory skills or practices and communication, between supervision—communication and coordination, and between coordination and patient care or hospital effectiveness? What are the sources of intraorganizational strain in the hospital, and what are its consequences for communication, supervision, coordination, and patient care?

These apparently crucial problems and questions about the community general hospital remain largely untackled and unanswered, and the list is only illustrative of pressing current needs for organizational research in hospitals such as those in the present study. And, although it could be argued rather forcefully that, as yet, we do not even have answers to most of the above questions in the case of other kinds of organizations, the fact remains that much more empirical research of the kind here suggested has been conducted in industrial and other settings than in hospitals. The fact is that systematic social-psychological studies of the hospital are still rare, while comparative studies involving several individual hospitals simultaneously are even more rare, and systematic comparative studies utilizing quantitative techniques of research are lacking.[1]

It is in this context that the present study was undertaken, in the hope of contributing some answers—even partial ones—to some of the above questions, and in the hope that it may be followed by a series of similar studies. The slow but steady accumulation of pertinent research, the interest of social scientists and people in the hospital field alike, an increasing sensitivity to the potentialities of utilizing the results of research to improve hospital functioning, general theoretical advances regarding the behavior of complex organizations, and specific methodological advances in survey, interview, and other techniques of research in recent years make the prospects for systematic quantitative research in the hospital field very promising. There are many indications that research efforts in this area will be intensified, and studies of the community general hospital as an organization will be initiated at an increasing rate. For the moment, however, let us return to review the objectives of the present study.

THE AIMS AND STRATEGY OF THE STUDY

The thinking underlying both the aims and strategy of the present research could be summed up rather well by quoting from a recent speech by R. W. Revans, Professor of Industrial Administration, The Manchester College of Science and Technology. Professor Revans delivered this speech on the subject of "How Should a Hospital be Judged," at the Annual Conference of Chief Financial Officers in the Hospital Service in England and Wales, in November 1960—four years after our own study was initiated. Here is, in part, what he had to say:

> As we have looked at these [many] different aspects of the hospital, we have gradually come round more and more to realize the need for taking a synoptic view of the whole hospital, of studying, not the efficiency of some particular department but the efficiency of the whole hospital as a system.
> I believe we need some quite new thinking upon the totality of hospitals. They are organic unities which have admission systems, diagnostic systems, treatment systems, control systems, discharge systems, supply systems, communication

---

[1] For the kinds of research that are currently most prevalent in the hospital field, see the last annual issue of "An Inventory of Social and Economic Research in Health" (3).

The Aims and Strategy of the Study

systems, and so forth, all integrated just like the various systems of the human being are integrated into the total personality. All the researches we have been doing have been aimed at leading more and more towards this concept of the synoptic view of the hospital. What success we are meeting, goodness knows, because the longer one studies the problem of the hospital the more clearly one sees that one knows very little about it.

What has all that to do with efficiency? In my opinion, you cannot study the efficiency of any particular branch of the hospital unless you are prepared to study the hospital as a total entity. (4, p. 36).

Our study may be viewed as one which has attempted to investigate certain problems of the community general hospital from a "synoptic" point of view, to use Professor Revans' term. Both theoretically and methodologically, it has tried to capture the image of the total hospital as a complex organizational system, and to examine some of the problems and characteristics of hospital organization that are system-wide in nature, or at least have direct system-wide implications. Without denying that there is also room, even need, for investigating the more circumscribed problems of particular units or groups within the hospital, this study has dealt with problems of this latter kind only, or mainly, from the standpoint of their relevance to the total system. Most of the concepts and variables with which it is concerned were defined and measured at the organizational or group level, and not at the individual level, the primary interest being in the behavior of hospitals as organizations, and in phenomena having organization-wide significance. The details of our approach and procedure have been discussed fully in Chapter 2.

The research strategy employed was, of course, dictated by the main objectives of the study and related theoretical and methodological considerations. The general aim of the study was to obtain information about a number of different aspects of the structure and functioning of the community general hospital and, more importantly, to provide some answers to certain specific questions regarding the following problem areas: the assessment and criteria of hospital patient care (Chap. 5); social-psychological factors affecting the quality of patient care (Chap. 8); the problem of organizational coordination (Chap. 6); social-psychological factors affecting organizational coordination (Chap. 7); the problem of supervision and related administrative activities at different organizational levels, with emphasis on superior-subordinate relationships (Chap. 9); and certain aspects of communication in the nursing department, as they relate to nursing activity and performance (Chap. 10). In addition, the study was designed to provide information highlighting the major background characteristics and problems of the principal groups (doctors, nurses, trustees, administrators and department heads, and laboratory and x-ray technicians) in the hospitals studied (Chap. 3), as well as the organizational characteristics of the hospitals themselves, including important similarities and differences among them, and a number of issues and problems which are considered salient by members of these organizations (Chap. 4).

In conjunction with the major problem areas with which the research is concerned, moreover, certain other aspects of the hospital situation were also investigated, but not as intensively. Included among these were: intraorganizational strain, in the form of intergroup tensions and pressures; certain financial matters; various personnel-related aspects, such as the composition of professional staffs, salaries and rewards, commitment to the organization, absenteeism and turnover, and the organizational stability of different groups in the hospital; and a number of special issues and problems pertaining to the hospital or to some of its major components, e.g., the medical and nursing staffs. Various special issues were introduced in Chapters 3 and 4, with the more important of them being further elaborated in Chapter 11, along with certain questions about the influence and value orientations of the key groups in the hospital. Questions regarding such other topics as the historical development of community general hospitals, utilization of services, hospital economics, and hospital-community relationships were not investigated in this research.

In every problem area examined, with the exception of some of the issues treated in Chapters 3, 4, and 11, the emphasis was on organizational variables and characteristics, rather than on the behavior and attitudes of particular groups or individuals in the hospitals involved. The research design called for the measurement of a relatively large number of variables in each of the major study areas, and for relating variables from one area to variables representing the other areas studied. The objective of our analysis was to answer a number of specific questions, or test certain social-psychological hypotheses, concerning the behavior of the ten hospitals which participated in the research (and, to an extent, also of other hospitals which happen to be similar to the participating hospitals).

Among the principal questions and issues examined were the following: How is the quality of hospital patient care to be assessed? In what specific respects are the hospitals which provide superior nursing, medical, and overall care to their patients different from those where care is of relatively lower quality? Stated differently, what are some of the main factors which influence or determine the quality of patient care rendered by the various hospitals, or what accounts for the fact that some hospitals are more effective organizations than others? Moreover, is the quality of nursing care related to the same, or some of the same, variables to which the quality of medical care is related, and are the better medical care hospitals the same as the better nursing care hospitals?

What is the relationship between patient care, or hospital effectiveness, and internal coordination of activities in the organization? Why is coordination crucial to effective hospital functioning, and what kinds of coordination are necessary or most important? What are the factors which affect the adequacy

The Aims and Strategy of the Study

of overall organizational coordination, and the quality of specific kinds of coordination, in the hospital? Similarly, what are the prevailing patterns of supervision in the hospitals studied, and how do different supervisory skills and practices relate to the satisfaction and behavior of subordinates, to patient care, and to coordination? What are some of the effects of intraorganizational strain in the hospital? What is the relationship between performance and personnel absenteeism and turnover? What kinds of communication, and what specific aspects of communication, facilitate or hinder organizational functioning in the hospital? What is the relationship between the adequacy of facilities, equipment, and finances, on the one hand, and the quality of patient care on the other? Does the composition of the medical and nursing staffs affect the quality of patient care or coordination? And, generally, what particular aspects of intergroup relations, organizational coordination, supervision and administrative behavior, and communication are crucial or significant in relation to the effectiveness of the community general hospital?

Obviously, not all of these questions could be investigated thoroughly, be given all of the attention that they may deserve, or be given equal emphasis, in a single study. For one thing, this would have been impossible because the present stage of our theoretical, empirical, and methodological knowledge permits us to do a great deal in certain areas (e.g., in the areas of supervision and communication) and less in others (e.g., the development of uniform and standard criteria evaluating the quality of patient care). Second, although most of the questions and problems investigated have organization-wide significance, some questions pertain to more delimited problems. And third, in this research, we deliberately chose to investigate in greater detail those problems of the hospital which, in our opinion, are of great importance to the hospital—and in some cases to many other organizations as well—but which have not yet been studied sufficiently or systematically (e.g., the problem of organizational coordination was given a good deal of emphasis).

In short, technical limitations, the decision to confine the study to the examination of certain problems and not others, the fact that some problems are more important than others, and research preference resulted in paying differential attention to the problems and questions with which we have been concerned. Nevertheless, we attempted to examine systematically, or at least explore, each of the questions raised above, as well as a number of more specific hypotheses, in addition to obtaining descriptive information about many of the characteristics and problems of the people around the patient and the hospitals themselves. In this connection, it should be noted that the present inquiry was partly exploratory and descriptive, and partly analytical and hypothesis-testing (see Chap. 1 and Chap. 2). With reference to the analytical and explanatory aspects of the study, we attempted to provide at least a partial, and more or less satisfactory, answer to each question and hypothesis involved, even though some of the questions were undoubtedly answered more successfully than others (while some may still have remained unanswered), and even though several new issues may have emerged in the process to be added to old ones.

Empirical data for the measurement of several different aspects of each problem area studied, and for testing specific hypotheses in relation to each of the objectives and questions listed above, were collected during the last two months of 1957, following more than a year's exploratory field work and preparatory research activities. Twelve community general hospitals, all in Michigan, were included in the study. Two of these served as sites for a considerable amount of exploration, and for pretesting the research instruments, preceding the full-scale collection of data. The remaining ten hospitals participated in the research proper, comprising the "sample" of the study.

In selecting the hospitals, an attempt was made to "control" through the research design several important factors which may have a direct influence upon the variables investigated, but which, being of no special interest to the research, were not themselves measured. Control was partly attained by including in the study only hospitals which met the following criteria: (1) were short-stay, community general hospitals, not affiliated with religious or governmental institutions; (2) were of "medium" size, having between 100 and 350 beds; (3) were fully accredited by the Joint Commission on Accreditation of Hospitals; (4) were administered by a nonmedical, male administrator, under a lay board of trustees; and (5) were located in Michigan cities whose population was larger than 10,000. One of the main reasons for imposing these restrictions, apart from reasons of practicality and economy, was the great variability which hospitals exhibit on numerous characteristics. We wanted to restrict this variability by means of the research design, so that we might more systematically compare and contrast the hospitals studied on the specific aspects of organizational structure and functioning with which we are primarily concerned.

The necessary data were obtained from several sources. Standardized paper-and-pencil questionnaires and semistructured personal interviews administered to certain people in each participating hospital constitute the main source of the data. These data were supplemented by frequent comments, or spontaneous observations, volunteered by many of the respondents. Organizational documents and administrative and medical records from each hospital constitute a second source. A group of outside doctors, who were familiar with the medical situation prevailing in the participating hospitals, but who were not on the staff of any of these hospitals, constitute the last source of data. These outside doctors provided certain data about the quality of medical care in the hospitals studied, supplementing comparable data collected from the medical staff of each hospital.

Several forms of questionnaires and interviews were used, each tailored for a particular group of respondents, but with identical instruments being used for each particular respondent group across hospitals. The questionnaires and interviews were administered, on location, to over 100 individuals from each hospital who were selected to represent their respective hospitals and groups. The respondents who furnished the required data about each hospital were: the hospital administrator; the members of the executive committee of the board of trustees (about 5); members of the medical staff (about 25); all administrative, nonmedical department heads (about 10); all supervisory nurses (about 18); a sample of nonsupervisory registered nurses (about 20), practical nurses (about 14), and aides and orderlies (about 20); and the technicians from the laboratory and x-ray (about 13). In all, 1265 individual respondents from the ten hospitals participated in the study. Thus, on the average, each hospital is represented by about 127 persons belonging to the above groups of respondents.

For some of the respondent groups, all of the members of the group were asked to furnish data; for other groups, only a sample, or a fraction, of the total group membership were asked to participate. When groups were sampled, every member of the group (separately in each hospital) was given an equal and known chance of being selected into the sample. Most respondents were required to complete appropriate questionnaires, but certain key respondents were asked for a personal interview in addition. In either case, respondents were treated both as "subjects," i.e., provided data about their own attitudes, feelings, etc., and as "observers," i.e., provided their observations about different aspects of the situation in their respective hospitals (in this sense, respondents served as "measuring instruments"). For the details of the research design, the selection of respondents, the research instruments, and the methods and procedures of data collection, see Chapter 2; for the characteristics of the respondents, see Chapter 3; and for the characteristics of the hospitals studied, as well as a profile of the "typical" participating hospital, see Chapter 4.

Apart from specific methodological issues or weaknesses regarding the measurement of particular variables, some of which concern the assessment of the quality of patient care (see Chap. 5), the principal methodological limitation of the study stems from the deliberate decision to restrict the population of hospitals covered to a particular class of community general hospitals, as described above in conjunction with the problem of variability. This decision, which in effect limits the statistical generalizability of the findings, was necessary primarily because too little was known, either theoretically or empirically, about the phenomena with which the research deals to argue in favor of a broader coverage at that time. In view of this limitation, to the extent that other community general hospitals deviate in their characteristics from the hospitals here studied, one becomes increasingly uncertain about the applicability or generality of the obtained results. Caution is, therefore, required against indiscriminate overgeneralization of specific findings to all hospitals or to particular hospitals without taking into account the degree to which such hospitals are similar to, or different from, those in the study.[2] It must also be remembered that the present study represents partly an exploratory and partly an explanatory effort. It does not claim to have answered all questions about all hospitals, or even about the few hospitals which it actually covered.

In summary, this study of the short-stay, community general hospital focuses on the total hospital as a complex organizational system. Organizational coordination, patient care, superior-subordinate relations and administrative problems, communication practices among nursing personnel, and certain other related aspects of hospital structure and functioning, as specified above, are the main problem areas investigated. Apart from the exploratory and descriptive aspects of the study, a number of hypotheses regarding the interrelationship of different variables from the several areas of interest constitute the analytical and explanatory aspects of the research. The study is a comparative study of hospitals. That is, the research design basically involves the comparison and contrast of the ten participating hospitals with one another on each of the variables, or characteristics, contained in the hypotheses that were investigated. With only a few exceptions, the emphasis is on organizational phenomena, and not on the more delimited problems and characteristics of particular groups or individuals within the hospital. For the most part, the theoretical interest is in social-psychological concepts and, correspondingly, the unit of measurement, analysis, and hypothesis-testing is the total hospital or some major component of the hospital, such as the nursing department.

With this brief review of the aims and strategy of the research, we next turn to summarize the principal findings obtained for each major area investigated, and reiterate some of the important problems and issues that the community general hospital faces, as indicated by the empirical results.

ORGANIZATIONAL COORDINATION

Of all areas studied, except that of patient care or hospital effectiveness with which it is intimately associated, the area of organizational coordination received the greatest attention in this research, both as an independent variable in relation to patient care, and as a dependent variable, i.e., as an important organizational phenomenon in its own right. Internal coordination constitutes one of the principal and most difficult problems faced by all complex organizations and especially by hospitals, due to the great heterogeneity, specializa-

[2] Very limited evidence is available about the question of differences-similarities between the hospitals here studied and other community general hospitals in the nation. According to this evidence, as pointed out in Chapter 4, the "typical" hospital in our study is very similar in many of its gross characteristics to the "average" 200-bed hospital in the United States, as described in Block's "prototype" study (1). Yet, important differences undoubtedly also exist between the two.

tion, and interdependence which characterize the membership and action structure of these organizations. Because the specialized roles and activities within the hospital (or any other large-scale organization) are interrelated and not independent of each other, the organization constantly faces the problem of coordinating the activities of its many different parts and members. Without coordination, effective concerted action and organizational integration are impossible.

The significance of coordination for organizational functioning is, of course, widely acknowledged, and it has been recognized for some time by both scientists and practitioners. Yet, empirical quantitative research into the nature and determinants of coordination, and about the relationship of coordination to other social-psychological phenomena, is virtually completely lacking. Previous studies in hospitals and industrial organizations have often paid lip service to coordination as an organizational problem, among many such problems, but it is other problems on which they have focused their attention. For these reasons, the investigation of coordination was one of the central objectives of the present research.

For hospitals and other organizations, the problem of coordination is the problem of articulating and interrelating the diversified, but interacting and interdependent, parts of the organizational system, and the specialized activities of these parts, so that the total system can attain structural coherence and functional unity. It is the problem of how best to fit together the different elements and activities of the organization, and how to gear available resources and facilities in a direction that enables the organization to respond as a unified system. In Chapters 6 and 7, where it was discussed in detail, coordination was viewed as representing the processes of articulation and the state of adjustment among the different elements of an organization, and was defined as the extent to which the interdependent parts of the organization function each according to the needs and requirements of the other parts and of the total organizational system.

All of the coordinative activities of organizations were considered as falling into two broad categories, *programed* and *nonprogramed*. Programed coordination revolves around a special set of means of coordination, the most important of which is organizational planning of different kinds. It involves an approach which relies very heavily on the specification of functions to be associated with the various roles in the organization, and on ways of regulating prescribed interaction within the system. Programed coordination is attained through such things as the establishment of appropriate departmental routines, the timing and sequencing of activities, and the planning of work, and is indicative of the extent to which the organization functions as a well-regulated machine. Nonprogramed coordination, on the other hand, relies on informal coordinative efforts on the part of all the different groups and members of the organization, and on voluntary rather than prescribed adjustment among them which is ultimately based on their own motives and efforts. Nonprogramed coordination (also referred to as general coordination, coordination by "feedback," or informal coordination) is particularly important in organizations where activity is not or cannot be completely routinized, mechanized, or automated, for it makes allowance for adjustments required to meet organizational needs which arise in the day-to-day operations of the system, but which cannot be satisfied through formal programing or advance planning. It is attained and maintained through the development of reciprocal understandings, shared attitudes and complementary expectations, and common frames of reference among organizational members—through powerful social-psychological forces which facilitate voluntary and spontaneous adjustment.

In addition to the two basic coordination categories, programed and nonprogramed, a distinction was made among different major types of organizational coordination. These were: *preventive, promotive, corrective,* and *regulatory coordination*. If the objective of a set of coordinative activities is to correct a dysfunction in the system after it has occurred, the type of coordination involved is corrective. If coordinative activity is initiated in anticipation of a problem or difficulty, the type of coordination involved is preventive. When coordinative activity is aimed at the preservation of existing organizational arrangements, i.e., at the maintenance of the *status quo,* not involving the cognizance of any particular problems or malfunctions, whether in retrospect or anticipation, the type of coordination involved is regulatory. When positive attempts are made to improve the articulation of the system or existing organizational arrangements without regard for specific problems, or when attempts are made on the assumption that the system is imperfectly coordinated and capable of being better coordinated rather than for the purpose of correcting or preventing particular difficulties, the type of coordination involved is promotive. (There is probably a fifth type of coordination which might be called *representational* coordination—involving activities wherein different organizational parts or members interact for the specific purpose of representing themselves to one another, but this could probably be better treated as an aspect of the communication system of the organization.)

In the present study, we dealt both with programed and nonprogramed coordination in the community general hospital. Moreover, apart from examining overall hospital coordination, or the coordination of the total organizational system, we also studied coordination within the nursing department, or nursing department coordination. Of the different major types of coordination, we investigated preventive and promotive coordination. In Chapter 6, we discussed the nature of coordination and its importance for organizational functioning, the different bases and mechanisms of coordination, the different categories and types of coordination, and certain related theoretical and con-

Organizational Coordination

ceptual issues. In that same chapter, we presented several measures of hospital coordination—two measures of overall organizational coordination, an overall measure of programed coordination and an overall measure of nonprogramed or general coordination, as well as seven specific measures of coordination from which the overall measures were derived. Interrelationships among the different measures and types of coordination were also shown in Chapter 6. The measures of nursing department coordination were introduced and discussed in Chapter 7, along with related empirical findings.

In Chapter 6, we finally specified several sets of factors representing different aspects of organizational structure and functioning that were hypothesized to affect coordination in large-scale organizations in general, and in community general hospitals in particular. These sets of independent variables, which were further elaborated in Chapter 7, in conjunction with specific findings, are: (1) certain aspects of organizational planning; (2) certain aspects of sharedness and complementarity of work-related expectations among organizational members, and certain aspects of cooperation; (3) intraorganizational strain; (4) problem awareness and problem solving on the part of members in key organizational roles; (5) certain aspects of communication; and (6) certain structural features of hospital organization, including size and size-related variables, and the composition of its work force.

The results which show the relationship between different variables in each of these sets and the various measures and types of hospital coordination were presented and discussed in Chapter 7. In that same chapter, findings were presented about nursing department coordination, showing the relationship between nursing department coordination and various aspects of the structure and functioning of the nursing department (including the composition of the nursing staff, absenteeism and turnover among nursing personnel, tensions and pressures among different shifts and groups, and performance relations between different nursing classifications). A profile of the best coordinated hospital and the poorest coordinated hospital, among the ten studied, was also presented in Chapter 7 to show certain important differences between the two organizations. The chapter concluded with the discussion of certain practical and theoretical implications emerging from the findings about coordination.

Factors Related to Overall Hospital Coordination

The results, simply stated, show that overall organizational coordination is better, or more adequate, in those hospitals where:

1. Organizational rules and regulations are more clearly defined.
2. The extent of conformity to rules, regulations, and policies on the part of the different members of the organization is greater.

3. There is greater sharedness and complementarity of work-related expectations among organizational members: people see more eye-to-eye about the daily operations of the hospital, and the medical and nursing staff have a better understanding of each other's work problems and needs.

4. There is more willingness on the part of people in related jobs to assist each other when needed.

5. There is less tension or conflict among the different interacting groups in the organization, there is less tension among key groups, and less "unreasonable" pressure for better performance is experienced by nursing and nonmedical personnel.

6. Problems of working together that arise in the organization are handled more satisfactorily for all concerned, and are handled more promptly.

7. The administrator and the director of nursing, considered together, are more likely to be aware of problems that arise in the organization, and are more effective in solving conflicts. However, it is their combined problem awareness and problem-solving effectiveness, rather than their individual performance in these respects, which is positively and significantly related to coordination.

8. The extent to which organizational members feel that decisions which affect their work are explained to them adequately is greater, and people in related jobs find it easier to meet and exchange information and ideas about the work.

9. The patient charts (records) at the nursing stations are evaluated as more complete or more adequate by registered nurses.

10. The proportion of nursing staff members who are practical nurses is higher, and the proportion who are aides is lower.

11. Certain supervisory and administrative practices which foster superior-subordinate communication on work-relevant matters are more prevalent: Superiors more frequently ask subordinates their opinion about work problems; superiors express appreciation to subordinates for their work more often; and subordinates find it easier to get their ideas and suggestions about work changes or improvements across to their superiors.

12. Organizational size, in terms of number of beds, average daily census of patients, or total number of paid personnel in the hospital, tends to be smaller. Smaller hospitals seem to have the advantage, for size tends to be negatively related to coordination. However, only a few of the correlations between size and coordination are statistically significant, and the evidence must be considered as tentative and suggestive rather than conclusive. It is also important to remember here that only medium-sized hospitals were studied.

13. Nursing department coordination is better.

Findings Concerning Nursing Department Coordination

Nursing department coordination, measured by such things as the extent to which one shift can take over from another smoothly or without confusion, the ease with which the nursing staff can find out what happened on the job since last at work, and the degree to which the previous shift did not leave for the succeeding shift problems or work that it should have handled, is generally superior in nursing departments (or hospitals) where:

Organizational Coordination

1. There is less tension among nursing personnel in the different roles, or classifications.
2. There is less tension among nursing personnel in the different shifts.
3. There is less tension between the nursing staff and the hospital administrator.
4. Less "unreasonable" pressure for better performance is experienced by the nursing staff.
5. The proportion of nursing staff members who are aides is smaller, and the proportion who are practical, or practical and registered, nurses is greater.
6. There is less unexcused absenteeism among registered nurses.
7. There is higher turnover among aides.
8. Registered nurses are more likely to talk to their immediate superior than others in the hospital about work-related matters (e.g., about ways to improve patient care, ways to improve nursing supervision, ways to improve work relations between departments). That is, professional nurses are more likely to channel their work-relevant communication through formal rather than informal organizational channels.
9. Registered nurses are less prone to try to do things that head nurses should be doing, or practical nurses should be doing, and practical nurses are less prone to attempt things that professional nurses should be doing.
10. And, generally, most of the factors which relate positively to overall hospital coordination, as summarized above, also relate to coordination in the nursing department alone, in an analogous fashion. Essentially, the variables which make for better hospital coordination also seem to facilitate nursing department coordination (or vice versa).

Programed and Nonprogramed Coordination

Programed coordination was measured by the extent to which activities in the hospital are well timed, the extent to which departmental routines are well established, and the extent to which work assignments are well planned. Of these three aspects of programed coordination, the timing of activities is the most crucial in the hospital situation, according to the data.

As might be expected, since it is a part of overall hospital coordination, programed coordination is better in hospitals having better overall coordination. In addition, programed coordination is positively and significantly associated with nonprogramed coordination; hospitals having better programed coordination are significantly more likely than other hospitals also to have better nonprogramed coordination, and conversely. In view of these relationships, it is not surprising that most of the different aspects of hospital structure and functioning which were found to facilitate overall organizational coordination are also positively related to programed coordination, and the same is true for most of the variables which were found to relate significantly to nonprogramed or general coordination. However, certain particular independent variables relate better to programed than nonprogramed coordination, and vice versa.

The following variables correlate especially well with programed coordination, i.e., programed coordination, by comparison to nonprogramed coordination, is particularly better in hospitals where:

1. The proportion of nursing staff members who are aides is lower, and the proportion who are practical nurses is higher.
2. The extent to which organizational members follow established rules and regulations is greater.
3. Complementarity of work-related expectations among organizational members, and particularly between medical and nursing staff, is higher.
4. The combined problem awareness of the administrator and the director of nursing is greater.
5. The combined effectiveness of the administrator and the director of nursing in solving conflicts that arise in the organization is higher.

On the other hand, by comparison to programed coordination, nonprogramed coordination relates more closely to certain other aspects of the hospital situation. Specifically, nonprogramed coordination is especially better in hospitals where:

1. There is greater willingness among organizational members to cooperate where appropriate, particularly to assist each other when needed.
2. Decisions which affect their work are explained to organizational members more adequately.
3. Other "good" communication practices, such as those mentioned in the preceding pages, are also more prevalent.
4. Coordination in the nursing department is better.
5. Organizational size tends to be smaller. (It will be remembered, however, that only some of the correlations between size or size-related variables and coordination are statistically significant.)

Preventive and Promotive Coordination

Promotive and preventive coordination, as measured in the present study, both represent the basic category of general or nonprogramed coordination, as against the category of programed coordination. The preventive type of coordination was measured in terms of the extent to which organizational members make an effort to avoid creating problems or interference in their work relationships, and the extent to which they perform their work without getting in each other's way. The promotive type was also measured using two items—how well the different related jobs and activities in the hospital fit together, and the extent to which patients feel (according to medical, nursing, and other respondents) that hospital personnel around them work together smoothly. The findings show that, as in the case of programed vs. nonprogramed coordination, some of the independent variables which are significantly related to organizational coordination relate more strongly to the preventive than the promotive type of coordination, and conversely. In other words, certain aspects of hospital structure and functioning are more

Organizational Coordination

important to preventive than to promotive coordination, the reverse also being true.

The major independent variables which were found to be especially well related to preventive coordination are:

1. The clarity of hospital rules, regulations, and policies.
2. The extent of conformity with hospital rules and regulations by organizational members.
3. The degree to which the hospital administrator is aware of problems faced by other organizational members.
4. The effectiveness of the director of nursing in solving conflicts that arise in the organization.
5. The skill of supervisory personnel in planning and scheduling the work.
6. The adequacy with which decisions that affect their work are explained to organizational members.
7. The frequency with which organizational members meet to exchange ideas and discuss problems which arise in their work relations.

Each of these variables is positively and significantly related to preventive coordination, at the same time being more highly related to preventive than to promotive coordination.

On the other hand, the independent variables which were found to relate especially well to promotive coordination are:

1. Hospital size, which is negatively related to promotive coordination.
2. The degree of prevailing tension among interdependent groups in the hospital, which is also negatively related to promotive coordination.
3. The adequacy of patient charts at the nursing stations, as appraised by registered nurses, which is positively related to promotive coordination.

Promotive coordination is also significantly related to many other factors, but these three variables are the ones which appear to be more important with respect to promotive than to preventive coordination.

Summary

In all complex organizations where there is detailed division of labor, extensive departmentalization, specialization of functions, and a high degree of interdependence among the different parts and members of the organization, there is also a critical need for coordinating the various roles and activities in the system. Concerted effort, unified action, and orderly organizational functioning depend upon coordination, and coordination itself frequently tends to become one of the most important specialized activities of the organization. The community general hospital belongs among organizations of this kind. The great emphasis on rules, regulations, and schedules, the alleged importance of "teamwork," the fact that the role of the hospital administrator is seen primarily as a coordinative role both by himself and others in the organization, the proliferation of joint meetings, committees, and conferences, and the fact that department heads and supervisory nurses consider their job as involving a great many coordinative activities (see Chap. 3) are not accidental. They all point to the importance of coordination and the necessity for coordination—a necessity of which organizational members are often and explicitly quite conscious (see Chap. 4).

Large-scale organizations typically depend for the attainment and maintenance of good coordination upon such things as standardized workflows, routinization of functions, explicitly defined statuses and roles, formal rules and procedures, advance planning, and precise regulation of activities in the system. In short, they depend upon an elaborate system of programed coordination. The hospital presents no exception in this respect. However, as we have pointed out, the features of hospital organization are such that the system cannot rely exclusively, or even mainly, upon programed coordination. The results show that the adequacy of overall coordination in the hospital also depends, to a very great extent, upon such things as the degree to which interacting members understand and appreciate each other's work problems and needs, the willingness of members in related jobs to assist each other when needed, the minimization of intergroup tensions and excessive organizational pressures upon members, the extent to which members adhere to established rules and procedures, the problem awareness and problem-solving effectiveness of key organizational members, communication that facilitates the transmission and exchange of work-relevant information and, generally, the presence of a system of well-shared frames of reference and complementary expectations about the work among interacting organizational members. Therefore, the hospital must rely rather heavily upon nonprogramed or general coordination—coordination that is possible through the day-to-day voluntary and spontaneous adjustments which organizational members can make, and which cannot be automatically assured through planning and programing alone.

Good programed coordination facilitates nonprogramed coordination, and vice versa, as the findings indicate. But, the findings also show that the set of specific factors which are associated with good programed coordination is not the same as the set of factors which are associated with good nonprogramed coordination, even though the two sets overlap. Hospitals, in company with many other organizations, will have to realize that nonprogramed coordination is as important, if not more important, as programed coordination, and then act accordingly, if they are to achieve and maintain adequate overall organizational coordination. All too often, programed coordination is emphasized almost to the point that nonprogramed coordination receives little, if any, attention, with the net result that overall coordination, and even programed coordination, is considerably poorer than it might be. The results summarized in the present section suggest many specific ways in which hospitals might improve both their programed and nonprogramed coordination, thereby attaining better overall coordination.

Another risk that organizations often run in the area of coordination is to over-rely upon some one specific type of coordination, while neglecting other types. Too much dependence on preventive or corrective coordination, for example, can easily lead to too little effort toward promotive coordination with the consequence that, in the long run, good overall coordination becomes extremely difficult to attain. It is our impression that many hospitals tend to resolve most of their coordinative difficulties mainly through corrective coordination, thus missing the opportunity to improve their overall coordination through promotive or preventive efforts. In any event, organizations cannot expect to attain good overall coordination by merely emphasizing a particular type of coordination while failing to exploit the other types which we have discussed. The findings show, for example, that certain factors in the hospital situation relate more strongly to preventive than to promotive coordination, while some factors which are significantly associated with one of these two types of coordination are not associated with the other. Even though promotive and preventive coordination are interrelated, their particular requirements and consequences for organizational functioning are not necessarily the same.

The specific results which show how different aspects of hospital structure and functioning relate to organizational coordination—overall hospital coordination, nursing department coordination, programed and nonprogramed coordination, and promotive and preventive coordination—have already been summarized, and are sufficiently clear to require no further comment. We might indicate, however, that, thus far, coordination has been treated as a dependent variable, in an attempt (1) to identify important factors in the hospital situation which are significantly associated with coordination, whether they facilitate or impede good coordination, and (2) to show how the better coordinated hospitals differ from the less adequately coordinated hospitals. But coordination was also treated as an independent variable in relation to patient care. The results showing the relationship of coordination to patient care, or hospital effectiveness, will be summarized in the next section, which is concerned with factors associated with the quality of patient care in the hospitals studied.

PATIENT CARE

Findings concerning the quality of patient care were obtained separately with respect to: (1) the quality of nursing care that on the average patients receive in the participating hospitals; (2) the quality of medical care, including surgical care, patients receive; (3) the quality of overall or total patient care (including both medical and nursing care) that on the average patients receive; and (4) the quality of comparative overall care, or the quality of total patient care in the hospital as compared to the quality of total care rendered in other similar community general hospitals. The several measures of patient care used in the study have been presented and discussed in detail in Chapter 5, along with data about their validity and reliability.

Factors Related to the Quality of Nursing Care

The principal results in this area, presented here in their simplest form, show that the quality of nursing care is generally higher in hospitals (or the better nursing care hospitals are those) where:

1. The quality of medical care is higher.
2. The proportion of nursing staff members who are registered nurses (and/or practical nurses) is higher, and the proportion who are aides is lower.
3. The number of registered nurses (and/or practical nurses) per patient, or average daily census, is higher, and the number of aides is lower.
4. The rates of unexcused absenteeism among registered nurses are lower.
5. Turnover among aides is higher.
6. The admissions department is seen as doing a better job.
7. Tension among the various interacting groups (and among the key groups) in the hospital is lower.
8. "Unreasonable" organizational pressure for better performance, as experienced by nursing and nonmedical personnel, is lower.
9. The medical staff have a better understanding of the work problems and needs of the nursing staff, as seen by nurses or by nurses and doctors combined, i.e., complementarity of work-related expectations on the part of these key groups is higher.
10. The nursing staff have a better understanding of the work problems and needs of the medical staff, as seen by doctors or by doctors and nurses combined.
11. The following communication patterns tend to prevail among professional nurses: (1) nonsupervisory registered nurses evaluate the communication which they receive from their superiors as more adequate, helpful, and positive, or ego enhancing; (2) on the average, they spend more time communicating with their superiors and are likely to exchange a comparatively large amount of information about task-relevant matters with them; (3) they are more likely to direct their communication to persons at lower, or higher, organizational levels rather than to persons at their own level; and (4) they are more likely to channel their communication about task-relevant subjects through formal rather than informal channels.
12. Coordination of activities within the nursing department is better, and overall hospital coordination is also better.

Coordination emerges as one of the most crucial variables, from among all the variables examined, in relation to nursing care. The results show that the quality of nursing care is higher in hospitals where nursing department coordination is more adequate, and in hospitals having better overall organizational coordination. Programed coordination in the hospital correlates highly and significantly with the quality of nursing care, and the same is true for nonprogramed or general coordination, according to the data. Furthermore, coordination of the promotive type is positively related to the quality of nursing care, as is coordination of the preventive type. However, promotive coordination produces a stronger relationship to the quality of nursing care, and also to the quality of overall patient care, than does preventive coordination, indicating that effective hospital functioning requires not only preventive but also, and very probably more importantly, promotive efforts toward the attainment and maintenance of good coordination.

Factors Related to the Quality of Medical Care

The principal findings concerning medical care show that the quality of medical care is higher in hospitals where:

1. The quality of nursing care is higher.
2. The nursing department and the nursing staff, as a whole, are doing a better job.
3. The proportion of nursing staff members who are registered nurses is greater.
4. The number of registered nurses per patient, or per average daily census, is greater.
5. Unexcused absenteeism rates among nonsupervisory registered nurses are lower.
6. Turnover among aides is higher.
7. The extent to which the medical staff as a whole uses the "right" number and quantity of laboratory and x-ray tests and other items of this type for diagnostic purposes (or the "right" volume and "a little more than they should"), according to the opinion of the doctors themselves, is higher.
8. The nursing staff have a better understanding of the work problems and needs of the medical staff, as seen by doctors or by doctors and nurses combined.
9. The percentage of all hospital expenses going into payroll is higher. (This particular finding should be viewed with caution, however, for it is likely to be due to chance rather than represent a genuine relationship, as indicated in Chap. 8.)

A number of additional results are probably also indicative of a possible relationship between the quality of medical care and certain other variables, but the specific correlations do not quite reach statistical significance in these cases. Included among these variables, all of which tend to relate positively to the quality of medical care, are: (1) the proportion of medical staff members in the hospital who are specialty "board certified" men; (2) the extent to which the hospital surpasses minimum accreditation requirements, according to medical and administrative respondents; (3) how active the tissue committee of the medical staff is, according to medical respondents; (4) how good a job the medical executive committee does, according to medical respondents; (5) the adequacy of coordination within the nursing department, and certain aspects of overall hospital coordination; and (6) the extent to which doctors feel that the communication which they receive from the hospital administrator is adequate.

Factors Related to the Quality of Overall Patient Care (Noncomparative and Comparative Care)

As might be expected, the quality of overall patient care is generally related to the same variables to which the quality of nursing care and the quality of medical care were found to relate, as summarized above. In other words, the hospitals where overall patient care is of higher quality are those which have better nursing care and better medical care, and the factors associated with better nursing care and better medical care are also associated with better overall care. Certain particular variables, however, are more strongly related to the quality of overall patient care than either to the quality of medical care or the quality of nursing care. And, similarly, certain factors relate better to the comparative measure of overall care (the quality of overall care in the hospital as compared to the quality of overall care in other similar hospitals) than to the noncomparative measure. These differential relationships have been discussed in Chapter 8. Finally, it is worth noting that the quality of overall patient care in the participating hospitals also correlates significantly with two variables, which were used in Chapter 5 for the purpose of "validating" the measure of overall care. These variables are: the kind of reputation which the hospital enjoys in its community (according to both medical and administrative-nonmedical respondents), and the extent to which patients speak well of the hospital (according to doctors, nurses, and other respondents). The better-care hospitals have a better reputation in their community, as well as a greater proportion of patients who express satisfaction with the hospital.

Other Findings Concerning the Quality of Patient Care

Certain additional aspects of hospital structure and functioning were also examined in relation to the four measures of patient care. These include: (1) hospital size and size-related variables; (2) the adequacy of available physical facilities, as evaluated by different groups of respondents; (3) the financial status of the hospitals; (4) the performance of individual paramedical departments; and (5) certain aspects of supervision. In these cases, the results are not as clear-cut as those presented above, at least from the standpoint of statistical significance. However, the direction and total pattern of results in each case are relatively unambiguous, interesting, and illuminating—and perhaps even surprising in some instances. Let us briefly summarize these results.

1. Hospital Size and the Quality of Patient Care. A number of findings suggest that, for medium-sized hospitals (i.e., hospitals having between 100 and 350 beds), the relationship between organizational size and the quality of patient care may be a negative one. As measured by number of beds, average daily census of patients, and total number of patient admissions, size produces generally small but consistently negative correlations with the measures of patient care. However, since none of the specific correlations is statistically significant, the only conclusion that may be properly drawn from these results is that, for medium-sized hospitals (it is important to remember here that only hospitals of a certain size range were studied), the quality of patient care rendered by the larger institutions is *not* superior to the care provided by the smaller ones. If anything, the advantage appears to be on the side of the smaller hospitals.

The number of hospital-paid personnel, the number of paid personnel per patient, and the average number of (full-time) paid personnel per bed in the hospitals studied are not related to the quality of patient care—unlike the several other aspects of the composition of the professional staff which were earlier reported to be positively related to the quality of patient care. By themselves, numbers of staff are not important; it is staff training and skill that count in relation to the quality of care. Another interesting finding in this area is that, while the number of total patient admissions (which correlates very highly with hospital size or number of beds) produces small negative correlations with the measures of patient care, the number of patient admissions per bed does not. This indicates that the quality of patient care is not poorer in hospitals where the patient load is greater; nor is it appreciably better, however, for the correlations involved are not statistically significant.

2. Physical Facilities and the Quality of Patient Care. The adequacy of several material facilities, as evaluated by doctors, the administrator and executive trustees, and the laboratory and x-ray technicians in each participating hospital, shows very little relationship to the quality of patient care. The correlations between the patient care measures, on the one hand, and the relative adequacy of such hospital facilities as the physical plant and layout of the hospital, space and beds available, equipment, supplies, and the general financial condition of the hospital, on the other, are generally positive but not large enough to be statistically significant. Only the adequacy of equipment, as evaluated by technicians, but not as evaluated by doctors or by trustees and the administrator, is significantly related to the quality of nursing care and overall care (but not to the quality of medical care or the comparative measure of overall care).

It, therefore, seems that, even though considerable differences exist among the ten participating hospitals as to the perceived adequacy of their various facilities, hospitals having superior facilities are not significantly more likely to provide superior care to their patients than hospitals having relatively less adequate facilities. Nor do the former hospitals provide poorer care than the latter, of course. Perhaps all of the hospitals in the study have at least "minimally adequate" material facilities (relevant data in Chapter 8 and in Chapter

4 support this contention), so that superiority in physical facilities beyond this minimum adequacy point has no appreciable effect upon the quality of care in the hospitals involved. In any event, the available data show that having more adequate material facilities does not necessarily assure better patient care. The manner in which facilities are being utilized is probably a more important factor.

3. *Financial Considerations and the Quality of Patient Care.* As a group, the findings from relating eleven different income and expenditure items to the measures of patient care support the conclusion that the better-care hospitals are also the more economical (and probably better managed) organizations, from a financial standpoint. The results show that the quality of nursing care, medical care, and overall patient care is not higher in the higher-income, higher-cost, or more expensive hospitals. On balance, the evidence suggests the opposite. The better-care hospitals tend to be the ones with relatively lower income (total hospital income, total income per bed, total income per patient), lower expenses (total expenses, total expenses per bed, total expenses per patient, total payroll expenses, total expenses per paid employee), and lower costs (average hospital costs per patient day). However, patient care appears to be better in those of the hospitals where a higher proportion of the institution's total expenses are assigned to payroll, but the reasons for this relationship are not clear, and the relationship itself could possibly be due to chance. Apart from this exception, and although most of the specific correlations involved are not statistically significant, the total pattern and direction of the results clearly point to the above general conclusion that the better-care hospitals are also the more economical, rather than the more affluent, institutions. Financial well-being *per se* does not make for greater hospital effectiveness or better patient care.

4. *The Performance of Individual Paramedical Departments and the Quality of Patient Care.* In each hospital, the doctors, the trustees and the administrator, the supervisory nurses, and the laboratory and x-ray technicians evaluated the overall performance of the nursing, records, admissions, laboratory, and x-ray departments by answering this question: "On the whole, what kind of a job would you say each of [these departments] does for this hospital?" These measures of the individual performance of each of the five paramedical departments were examined in relation to our measures of the quality of patient care.

While the results are a good deal more complex than the brief summary here given might imply, they generally show that one should not expect the performance of every individual department, when considered independently of the performance of other departments, to be directly related to the quality of patient care in the hospital. More specifically, the results show that only the performance of the nursing department and of the admissions department correlates positively and significantly with the quality of nursing care and the quality of overall patient care rendered in the hospitals studied. On the other hand, hospitals having better performing records departments, laboratories, or x-ray departments are not significantly more likely to have better patient care than hospitals where each of these departments is seen to perform less well. In Chapter 8, we have proposed certain interpretations for these differential relationships between individual departmental performance and patient care, including an explanation based on the fact that the nursing department occupies a central place in hospital organization in relation to patient care. In general, it seems that the quality of patient care in the community general hospital is a function of the joint performance of all departments considered together, rather than a matter of how good a job the several departments do individually. (Furthermore, when the performance of individual hospital and medical committees is considered in relation to the quality of patient care, the results lead to the same conclusion.) It is the concerted action of all the departments, and not their individual performance, that makes the difference.

5. *Supervision and the Quality of Patient Care.* Certain measures of the technical, administrative, and human relations skills of supervisory and administrative personnel at different levels in the hospital organization were also studied in relation to the quality of patient care, and the same is true with respect to certain more specific supervisory practices and characteristics (see Chap. 9). The results of the analyses showed no direct significant relationships between supervisory skills or behavior and the quality of nursing, medical, and overall patient care in the participating hospitals. (These same measures of supervision, however, were found to relate significantly to the satisfaction of subordinates with their respective immediate superiors in the various hospitals and, more importantly, to certain aspects of communication and organizational coordination as well.)

Further analysis of the data revealed, however, that the relationship between supervision and patient care in the hospitals studied is complex and indirect rather than simple or direct. The pertinent findings suggest that certain supervisory practices (e.g., superiors ask subordinates their opinion about work problems, express appreciation to subordinates for their work, make it easy for subordinates to get their ideas and suggestions about work changes and improvements across to their superiors) may be indirectly related to the quality of patient care, through making for better organizational coordination (particularly coordination of the preventive type). In other words, certain supervisory practices seemingly contribute to coordination and, in turn, coordination contributes to organizational effectiveness. These supervisory practices are those that foster work-relevant communication between supervisory and nonsupervisory personnel at various levels, thus facilitating coordination, and coordination allows the hospital as an organization to accomplish its objectives effectively.

Summary

In this study, many different aspects of hospital structure and functioning were examined as independent variables, and their relationship to the quality of nursing, medical, and overall care given to patients in the participating hospitals was ascertained. A number of these variables were found to be highly and significantly related to the quality of patient care, while others yielded only suggestive relationships, and some were found to be completely unrelated to patient care, as indicated above. On the whole, the results showed stronger relationships between the measures of patient care and those of the independent variables which represent either aspects of the composition, skill, and behavior of the therapeutic staff in the hospital, or certain social-psychological aspects of the hospital situation, such as interdepartmental relations and coordination, rather than with those variables which represent the adequacy of physical facilities, financial matters, the performance of individual organizational units, and hospital size and size-related factors. Of the four measures of the quality of patient care—nursing care, medical care, overall care, and comparative overall care—used in the analyses, the measure of the quality of medical care was found to relate to a smaller cluster of variables than the other measures, suggesting the need for additional research in this area. Moreover, some of the independent variables were found to be more closely related to the quality of nursing care than to the quality of medical care, or overall care, and vice versa, as might be expected.

Considered as a group, the principal results about patient care show, among other things, that patient care is of relatively higher quality in hospitals which:

1. Have nursing staffs consisting predominantly of trained professional nurses, and practical nurses, and proportionately fewer aides.
2. Have more registered nurses per patient.
3. Have less unexcused absenteeism among their registered nurses.
4. Have better overall organizational coordination, programed as well as nonprogramed, and better nursing department coordination.
5. Have less intraorganizational strain, in the form of tension among key groups, tension among interacting groups and departments in general, or perceived "unreasonable" pressure for better performance on the part of nonmedical personnel.
6. Have communication and supervisory-administrative practices which facilitate and promote organizational coordination.
7. Have better shared expectations about work and work problems on the part of their many diverse, but interacting and interdependent, groups, and have attained greater complementarity of work-related expectations between their medical and nursing staffs.
8. Do not have significantly superior physical facilities, greater financial affluence, or fewer economic problems than the poorer-care hospitals, but they are probably better managed organizations from the financial point of view.

Supervision 613

9. Do not have lighter patient loads than hospitals where care is of relatively poorer quality.
10. Are not the larger of the institutions studied.

Several major conclusions, with a good deal of both practical and theoretical significance, emerge from these findings. First, it is clear that, consistent with common sense, the role of the registered nurse is a very central one in relation to patient care. Registered nurse skill, and its availability, are essential requirements for high quality care (nursing as well as medical care) in the community general hospital. Second, organizational bigness (size), financial superiority, and superiority in physical-material facilities, contrary to frequently encountered beliefs in the hospital field, do not assure superior patient care. Among the medium-sized hospitals studied, the better-care institutions are not the larger ones, the ones that have a better financial standing, or the ones which, in the judgment of doctors, trustees, administrators, and technicians, have the more adequate facilities; nor are the most expensive institutions. At the same time, the more affluent hospitals are not necessarily the poorer-care hospitals. Finances and facilities undoubtedly help up to a certain point, but beyond this point it is the management of finances, or the manner in which income and expenditures are allocated and disposed, and the kind of use which is made of the available facilities, among other things, that count. Third, consistent with the results of previous research cited earlier in this volume, the prevalence of high intraorganizational strain undermines effective hospital functioning. The degree of tension among interdependent groups in the hospital is strongly and negatively related to the quality of patient care, and the same is true of the degree of "unreasonable" pressure for better performance experienced by nonmedical personnel. Excessive organizational pressure upon members not only fails to improve performance, but it works in the opposite direction. Fourth, it is necessary that the nursing staff have a good understanding of the work problems and needs of the medical staff, and that the medical staff have a good understanding of the problems and needs of the nursing staff. Complementarity of work-related expectations on the part of the two major therapeutic groups in the hospital is an important correlate of the quality of patient care. And fifth, consistent with theoretical expectations, good organizational coordination, both programed and nonprogramed, emerges as another *sine qua non* in relation to patient care and organizational effectiveness in the community general hospital.

SUPERVISION

Supervisors, administrators, and other formal leaders in the hospital perform several important organizational functions. Among other things, they are expected to plan, coordinate, and regulate organizational activities. These functions require administrative skill. Second, they are expected to perform various specific tasks that their position demands, including the direction of the work of their subordinates, and the task of training subordinates so that they learn to follow procedures, handle equipment, and do their work properly. These activities require technical skill. Third, supervisors are also expected to translate organizational requirements in terms that are meaningful and acceptable to the subordinates, to reconcile the impersonal demands of the organization with the personal needs and goals of their subordinates, and generally to motivate the subordinates toward their job and the organization. These activities require an understanding of human behavior and interpersonal relations—they require human relations skill.

All supervisors and administrators must have some minimum administrative skill, some minimum technical skill, and some minimum skill in human relations in order to be able to perform their various functions. However, these basic supervisory skills are not all equally important for all supervisory personnel in an organization, for all levels of supervision, or at all times. The particular combination of the three skills which is required, or which is most effective, in a particular situation will depend on a number of considerations, including the type of organization involved, the stage of development of the organization, supervisory level within the organization, the kind of task to be accomplished, and similar other factors. When viewed in this context, the question of what kind of supervision is most desirable or most appropriate for an organization, such as the community general hospital, is a highly relative one, and must be answered by taking into account these important considerations as they apply to the situation involved.

The effects of particular supervisory practices, like the case of supervisory skills, will also differ depending upon the organization, the organizational levels, and organizational tasks involved. Supervisory practices and superior-subordinate relationships that may be effective at a given organizational level, for example, are not necessarily effective at other levels. The problem of effective supervision, then, becomes one of specifying the combination of supervisory skills, and the set of particular supervisory practices, which are most effective at particular organizational levels, in particular types of organizations, and with reference to particular criteria of "effectiveness" (such as the performance and satisfaction of subordinates). Effective supervision would require matching the demands of the organizational setting with the skills of available supervisory personnel, or placing supervisors with particular combinations of skills in organizational positions demanding such combinations, and supervisory practices that maximize given criteria of effectiveness. It follows, of course, that the kind or style of supervision that may be effective in other organizational settings, with reference to some particular criteria, need not necessarily be effective in the community general hospital. There are many limiting factors and conditions which may intervene to affect the relationship between supervision and effectiveness in an organization.

Within this framework, we attempted to explore the role of supervision in the community general hospital, in the hope of securing results which would facilitate answering the general question of what kind of supervision is most appropriate for effective hospital functioning. Relevant data about the skills, practices, and characteristics of supervisory personnel at each of several organizational levels in the participating hospitals were obtained from administrative department heads, supervisory nurses, nonsupervisory registered nurses, practical nurses, aides, and laboratory and x-ray technicians. Respondents at each of these levels were asked both to evaluate the technical, administrative, and human relations skills of their respective immediate superiors, and to provide information for the measurement of nine specific supervisory practices and characteristics as they apply to their immediate superior. The measures of supervisory skills and practices, as discussed in Chapter 9, were then studied in relation to each other and, more importantly, in relation to the following criteria: the satisfaction of subordinates with their immediate superior at each level of supervision; the quality of patient care rendered in the participating hospitals; and organizational coordination. The principal findings from these analyses are summarized below.

Results Concerning Supervisory Skills and Practices

With reference to the three supervisory skills, the data show that, at every level of supervision studied, respondents evaluate their immediate superiors higher on technical skill than on administrative skill or human relations skill, on which they evaluate their superiors least highly. This is consistent with the relatively high task-orientation that prevails in hospitals and the corresponding emphasis on technical competence at almost every level in the organization. The differences among the three skills are not extremely great, however, although their size varies from one level of supervision to another, and from one hospital to another.

Across hospitals, we find that the three skills are interrelated at every level of supervision, so that those hospitals whose supervisory personnel are evaluated highly on one skill are also more likely to have supervisory personnel evaluated highly on each of the other two skills. The size of the relationship between any two of the three skills, however, varies a great deal with level of supervision, indicating that different combinations of skills may be expected for different levels, as was hypothesized.

Considering the nine specific supervisory practices studied, we again find that different levels of supervision show different patterns of supervisory practices, as expected. And, similarly, different levels of supervision have different patterns of supervisory practices associated with each of the major supervisory skills. Each supervisory skill relates only to some of the specific supervisory practices and not to others. For most levels of supervision, technical skill correlates significantly only with two of the nine items measuring supervisory practices and characteristics—with how good the supervisor is in planning, organizing, and scheduling the work, and with how well he understands the viewpoint of his subordinates. Administrative skill relates significantly to these two items and, in addition, to the extent to which subordinates are sure of what their superiors expect of them, and the ease with which subordinates can get their ideas and suggestions about work changes or improvements across to superiors. And human relations skill correlates significantly with how good the supervisor is in dealing with people, how good an understanding he has of the viewpoint of his subordinates, and how free subordinates feel to discuss personal problems with him. Of the nine supervisory practices examined, only one relates significantly to all three supervisory skills at most levels of supervision—how well the superior understands the viewpoint of his subordinates.

Results Concerning Satisfaction with Supervision

At every level of supervision, except one (the level responsible for the supervision of practical nurses), subordinates are more satisfied with their immediate superior in those hospitals where supervisors are evaluated more highly on technical, administrative, and human relations skill. In other words, each of the three skills is positively related to subordinate satisfaction with supervision, indicating that all three skills are important insofar as satisfaction with supervision is concerned. The particular degree to which each skill contributes to satisfaction with supervision, however, varies across organizational levels. The satisfaction of department heads with their immediate superior (the hospital administrator), for example, is primarily determined by the administrative skill of their superior, according to the findings, while the satisfaction of supervisory nurses with their immediate superior (the director of nursing, or some top nursing supervisor) is primarily determined by the human relations skill of their superior.

Similarly, we find that the various specific supervisory practices and characteristics contribute differentially to the satisfaction of subordinates with supervision, depending upon the supervisory level considered. In general, however, we find that: (1) The extent to which supervisors are seen as good in dealing with people, and their ability to plan, organize, and schedule the work, are more important to the satisfaction of subordinates at the lower, rather than the higher, levels of supervision in the hospitals studied. (2) How good an understanding supervisors have of the viewpoint of their subordinates, and the ease with which subordinates can get their ideas and suggestions across to their superiors, are most important to the satisfaction of subordinates with supervision at the higher levels. And (3) such practices as the extent to which the superior informs subordinates in advance of changes that affect their work, the frequency with which he asks subordinates their opinion about work problems, and how free subordinates feel to discuss personal problems with their superior, are most important at the middle levels of supervision. (The remaining two of the nine items studied—how often the superior expresses appreciation to subordinates for their work, and how sure subordinates are of what he thinks of them and their work—yield no consistent results in relation to subordinate satisfaction with supervision.)

The higher levels of supervision referred to here are those charged with the responsibility of supervising the administrative department heads and the supervisory nurses. The middle levels are those supervising the nonsupervisory registered nurses and the laboratory and x-ray technicians. And the lower levels are those supervising the practical nurses and the aides in the participating hospitals.

Supervision and Organizational Coordination

In summarizing the various aspects of hospital structure and functioning that were found to relate to coordination, earlier in this chapter, we pointed out that certain aspects of supervision are also positively related to coordination in the hospital. That such a relationship should exist is almost obvious for, as we have shown in Chapter 3, many coordinative functions in the hospital are carried out by department heads, supervisory nurses, and others in supervisory or administrative positions. It is also obvious because of the high organizational reliance on formal rules and procedures, and formal authority and hierarchical relationships in the hospital. However, the kinds of supervisory practices which facilitate coordination in the hospital, and the type of coordination which relates most strongly to these practices, are not obvious without consulting the specific findings.

While the technical, administrative, and human relations skills of supervisory personnel, and most of the nine supervisory practices and characteristics studied, were found to be positively related to the satisfaction of subordinates with supervision, as already indicated, only some of the specific supervisory practices were found to be significantly related to coordination. More specifically, the results show that overall hospital coordination is better in hospitals where supervisory personnel (1) ask subordinates their opinion about work problems more frequently, and (2) express appreciation to subordinates for their work more often. (It is also worth reiterating here that expressing appreciation is one of the two supervisory practices, among the nine examined, that produced no consistent relationship to subordinate satisfaction with supervision.) In addition, hospital coordination tends to be better in hospitals where subordinates find it easier to get their ideas and suggestions about the work across to their superiors, and where subordinates are more sure of what their superiors expect of them or think about them and their work.

These supervisory practices which are positively related to coordination share in common the fact that they all pertain to some aspect of superior-subordinate communication which is work-relevant. (The importance of communication for hospital coordination has already been pointed out, and will be further commented upon in the next section of this chapter.) Moreover, according to the findings, these supervisory practices contribute to hospital coordination by facilitating the preventive type of coordination.

Supervision and Patient Care

That "good" supervision is important to organizational functioning in large-scale organizations has been amply demonstrated in previous research and cannot be doubted. However, as we concluded in Chapter 9 (following our review of numerous studies concerned with the relationship between supervision and organizational effectiveness), the consequences of particular supervisory behaviors and skills, or of particular styles of supervision, for organizational performance may be more or less pronounced or direct, depending on the type of organizations being studied and on the particular criteria of effectiveness being used.

In the present study, for example, we have seen that certain supervisory skills and practices contribute to the satisfaction of subordinates with supervision at different levels in the participating hospitals. Similarly, we have seen that some, but not all, of the specific supervisory practices and characteristics facilitate organizational coordination. These results, however, cannot be indiscriminately generalized to criteria other than those of satisfaction and coordination. They do not automatically entitle us, for example, to expect a similar relationship between these supervisory practices and the quality of patient care—which is a more direct and more important criterion of organizational effectiveness in this case than either satisfaction with supervision or organizational coordination—in the hospitals studied. In fact, from our earlier summary in this chapter, concerning the factors associated with patient care, it may be recalled that no significant relationship was found between supervision and the quality of patient care in the present research.

As a group, the relevant findings show that the hospitals where supervisory personnel are evaluated more highly on administrative, technical, or human relations skill are not necessarily the better-care hospitals. None of the three supervisory skills is significantly related to the quality of nursing, medical, and overall patient care. Similarly, no such relationship exists between any of the nine supervisory practices studied and any of the measures of patient care. Whether a particular supervisory skill or practice is examined in relation to patient care using data about all supervisory levels in the hospital combined, or whether it is examined using data separately for each level involved, moreover, the results lead to the same conclusion. In the hospitals studied, and in contrast to the results concerning the relationship between supervision and subordinate satisfaction or between supervision and coordination, there is no direct significant relationship between the quality of nursing, medical,

Supervision

and overall patient care, on the one hand, and the several supervisory skills and practices, on the other.

This lack of a direct significant relationship between supervisory behavior and patient care or hospital effectiveness, while not anticipated, is not too surprising. As we have argued in Chapter 9, the relationship of supervisory behavior to organizational effectiveness is not invariant across social organizations. It depends upon the kinds of criteria of effectiveness employed; it is affected, and even suppressed, by a variety of intervening factors and conditions; it may be more or less marked; it may be direct or indirect; and it is generally very complex rather than simple or constant. Furthermore, in connection with this issue of limiting conditions and intervening factors, we have presented evidence which suggests that certain of the supervisory practices studied are very probably related to the quality of patient care in the participating hospitals, but indirectly rather than directly, through facilitating organizational coordination.

The evidence shows that supervisory practices which facilitate work-relevant communication between superiors and subordinates contribute to coordination, and coordination allows the hospital to function effectively. For example, the frequency with which superiors ask subordinates their opinion about work problems relates positively and significantly to various aspects of organizational coordination, and particularly to preventive coordination. In turn, as we have already seen, patient care is of higher quality in the better coordinated hospitals. In other words, supervisory practices which promote the exchange of work-relevant information are directly related to coordination and, through coordination, indirectly related to the quality of patient care in the hospitals studied.

Summary

In composite, the data concerning the relationship between supervision and organizational effectiveness lead to the conclusion that neither the traditional directive-autocratic style of supervision nor the more recently emphasized equalitarian-democratic "human relations" approach would be most appropriate for the community general hospital. An alternative approach, incorporating some elements from both of these approaches, would be required. In part, this approach would be such that results in good organizational coordination by fostering supervisory practices of the kind that we have specified, with no predominant emphasis on directive leadership or one-sided dependence on human relations practices.

The failure of the autocratic approach with its almost exclusive reliance on formal authority and hierarchical relationships has, of course, been widely documented and well established by research in many different organizational settings, and requires no special comment here. The success of the human relations approach has likewise been documented in a great many cases but, as we have shown in Chapter 9, this approach does not always "work" as expected. With respect to the criterion of performance, human relations practices would work, in the sense of directly influencing performance, only to the extent that they affect, or are directly relevant to, the motivation to produce among organizational members. The relative failure of the human relations approach in particular situations should be neither surprising nor disturbing. It could be satisfactorily explained if researchers and practitioners would do what they usually fail to do, namely, take into account the limiting conditions and intervening variables which may be influencing the expected relationship between a given style of supervision and given criteria of organizational effectiveness.

The results obtained in the present study clearly suggest that considerable additional research will be necessary, before we are in a position to unravel all of the complexities that seem to surround the question of what type of supervision would best enable the community general hospital to provide the highest quality of patient care possible. Nevertheless, according to our findings, it is highly unlikely that a single particular type of supervision will be shown to provide an answer that is applicable to all or most hospitals, or even to all levels within a hospital, without important qualifications. What we will probably get will be a number of principles and partial, but useful, answers, which are similar to those here reported, and which indicate the kinds of supervisory practices that are more or less likely to be successful, under specified conditions, in relation to the quality of patient care or some other specific criteria of hospital effectiveness.

In conclusion, the relative importance of particular supervisory skills and practices for hospital functioning varies according to organizational-supervisory level. In general, however, we find that purely emotional-supportive behavior (which is an integral part of the human relations approach) on the part of supervisory and administrative personnel in the hospitals studied does not affect the quality of patient care directly and significantly. Most of the human relations skills and practices of supervisors at different levels in the hospital (e.g., superior is good in dealing with people, is receptive so that subordinates can discuss their personal problems with him, and the like) are much more important to the criterion of subordinate satisfaction with supervision than to the criterion of patient care or the criterion of organizational coordination. The supervisory practices which are important to the latter two criteria are those fostering work-relevant communication between superiors and subordinates. And although such communication does not necessarily contradict the practice of human relations principles, it is highly selective and not merely the same as informal communication or communication that is mainly supportive of the emotional aspects of the superior-subordinate relationship.

Communication

The limitations of the human relations approach in the hospital setting—where there is great emphasis on task-orientation and little mechanical routinization in the work structure—vary by organizational level involved, and they are perfectly understandable, if we remember the heavy and serious responsibilities which patient care places upon nursing and other personnel. Professional nurses, for example, even though handicapped with frequent or continuous staff shortages, must be able both to perform their functions promptly, accurately, and efficiently, and to adjust their behavior so as to accommodate crises and emergencies while still having to follow rather strict formal rules and procedures. Under these circumstances, they are expected to, and in fact they themselves expect to, submit to some regimentation (but only to as much regimentation as is consistent with their organizational roles and professional norms, otherwise the result would be dissatisfaction with supervision, tension, and inadequate motivation), for they cannot tolerate ambiguities arising from lack of sufficient supervisory direction or from coordinative malfunctions, as they cannot tolerate errors, whatever their origin. In today's community general hospitals, professional nurses are both unable and reluctant to operate either in an autocratic atmosphere or in a purely laissez-faire atmosphere.

COMMUNICATION

Communication is intimately related to the other areas with which the study is concerned. We already had the opportunity to comment on its significance for supervision, coordination, and patient care. However, both because of the importance of communication for hospital functioning and because of the strategic position that professional nurses occupy in the communication network—in fact, in the entire work structure—of hospital organization, an effort was made to examine rather closely certain aspects of communication on the part of professional nurses, particularly communication variables that are often overlooked. The results of this examination were reported in Chapter 10, under the title of "The Communication Patterns of Registered Nurses in Relation to Nursing Activity and Performance," which reflects the focus of our interest in the area of communication.

In hospitals, as well as other organizations, the principal organizational function of communication is to transmit sufficient relevant information, accurately and efficiently, so as to enable people to make decisions, regulate their behavior and, ultimately, to reduce or prevent unwanted diversity, irrationality, and incompatibility in the attitudes and behavior of organizational members. Through communication, members can be informed about organizational goals and standards, about the rules, procedures, and conditions that govern their jobs and work relations with others, about departmental routines and schedules, etc. Moreover, communication is essential for the development of consensus about the work situation on the part of a large and heterogeneous organizational membership, and for the development of shared and complementary points of view among members who are expected to work in relation to one another. Communication is also needed to coordinate the different roles and activities in the organization, and to ensure the continuity of the organizational system. Performance can be generally facilitated, or hindered, depending on the flow of relevant information among the different parts of the organization.

The consequences of particular communication practices for organizational behavior will depend on such specific considerations as who talks with whom, about what, under what conditions, in what manner, how frequently, and how long. Both the quantitative and the qualitative characteristics of communication are important. Similarly, both the formal and informal channels of communication in the organization, and their relative availability and use are important. How much relevant, and/or irrelevant, information is passing through the various formal and informal channels will affect the detection and solution of problems, decision making, and successful role performance on the part of organizational members. It is clear, however, that not all communication in a hospital, or any other organization, is functional. Too little communication or, less frequently, too much communication, communication of the wrong kind or with the wrong people, may well be dysfunctional for the organization and the performance of its members. It is, therefore, important to ascertain the communication practices and patterns which facilitate or impede performance in the organization.

In the present study of communication patterns among registered nurses in the community general hospital, the following aspects of communication were examined in relation to various measures of nursing activity and performance: the quality and adequacy of communication; the quantity and frequency of communication; the direction of communication with respect to organizational levels and roles; and the relative concentration of task-relevant communication in formal, as against informal, channels. The measures of nursing activity and performance used in the analysis included: the performance of nursing personnel in different roles; nursing department coordination; and commitment to, or identification with, the work group and with the team that treats the patients. In all cases, the nonsupervisory registered nurses group from each of the ten participating hospitals served as the basis for analysis. A total of ten specific hypotheses concerning the relationship between communication on the part of registered nurses and nursing activity and performance were tested (for a full statement of the particular hypotheses, see Chap. 10).

Importance of the Adequacy and Quality of Communication

The findings show that, in hospitals where registered nurses consider the communication which they receive from their immediate superior as more adequate, nurses: (1) are more satisfied with their superior, (2) evaluate their superior as doing a better job (with respect to being good in planning and organizing the work, being technically competent, doing the "right" things, being helpful), and (3) are more likely to discuss task-relevant matters, such as ways of improving patient care, with their superior rather than some one else in the hospital with whom they communicate frequently—they are more likely to concentrate their task-relevant communication in formal rather than informal channels.

Similarly, in hospitals where registered nurses evaluate the communication which they receive from their superior as more positive or facilitative (e.g., as involving clarification, requests for explanation or suggestions, the expression of appreciation), nurses: (1) are more satisfied with their superior, (2) feel that their superior performs her role better, and (3) are more apt to discuss task-relevant topics with their superior rather than the person with whom they talk the most in the hospital (who is someone other than their immediate superior, for the great majority of nonsupervisory registered nurses).

On the other hand, in hospitals where nurses perceive the communication which they receive from their immediate superior as more negative or non-facilitative (specifically, as involving unnecessary information, or the expression of criticism), nurses: (1) are neither more nor less likely to be satisfied with their superior, (2) are neither more nor less likely to feel that their superior is doing a good job, and (3) are neither more nor less likely to concentrate their task-relevant communication in formal rather than informal channels. These results are consistent with some of the findings in the area of supervision, and can be explained by: (1) the lack of great status differences and psychological distance between the nonsupervisory registered nurses and their superiors (the supervisory registered nurses); (2) the many similarities characteristic of supervisory and nonsupervisory professional nurses (see Chap. 3); (3) the fact that the extent of negative communication reported by the nurses was not particularly great in any of the hospitals studied; (4) the fact that professional peers are probably more receptive to mutual criticism; and (5) the fact that, as we have already shown, the importance of purely emotional-supportive behavior on the part of supervisory personnel toward their subordinates in the community general hospital is very limited.

Importance of the Quantity and Frequency of Communication

In hospitals where nonsupervisory registered nurses spend a greater amount of time in communicating with their immediate superior: (1) the nurses themselves, as a group, do a better job, (2) the practical nurses and the aides also do a better job, and (3) the nursing staff as a whole is doing a better job. Furthermore, the results indicate a similar relationship between nursing performance, as evaluated by doctors, and the extent to which nurses talk with their immediate superior about specific task-relevant matters.

Other findings show that in hospitals where nurses talk with their immediate superior about ways to improve patient care and ways to improve nursing supervision, more frequently, nurses are more strongly committed to, or identified with, their immediate work group and the team that treats the patients.

Results Involving the Direction of Communication

In hospitals where the nonsupervisory nurses tend to direct their communication to people at lower levels (practical nurses and aides) or higher levels (supervisory nurses), especially the former: (1) the nurses are more strongly committed to the team that treats the patients and to their immediate work group, (2) they are doing a better job, and (3) the practical nurses and the aides are also doing a better job.

By contrast, in hospitals where the nonsupervisory registered nurses communicate more with people at their own level (other registered nurses) rather than across levels: (1) the nurses are less committed to the team that treats the patients, (2) they are performing less well, and (3) the practical nurses and the aides are also performing less well. Confining most of their communication to their own level results, among other things, in inadequate coordination, thus impeding nursing performance.

Importance of the Concentration of Task-Relevant Communication in Formal Channels

Another interesting set of findings in this area shows that in hospitals where the nonsupervisory registered nurses talk more often with their immediate superior, relative to talking to the person with whom they talk most in the hospital (usually a person having no supervisory role), about (1) ways to improve patient care, (2) ways to improve nursing supervision, and (3) ways to improve relations among hospital departments, there is better nursing department coordination. In other words, the higher the concentration of task-relevant communication in formal rather than informal channels, the better the coordination in the nursing department.

Moreover, the extent to which professional nurses talk with their immediate superior, relative to talking to the most-talked-to person in the hospital, about ways to improve patient care relates positively and significantly to how good a job the registered nurses themselves do, to how good a job the practical nurses do, and to how good a job the nursing staff as a whole does. It also tends to relate positively to how good a job the aides do, and to the overall quality of nursing care in the hospital, but in these cases the correlations do not quite reach statistical significance.

Summary

Of ten specific hypotheses stating certain relationships between different aspects of communication among professional nurses and various measures of nursing activity and performance in the community general hospital, only two were not supported by the data (see Chap. 10). Both of these hypotheses contained qualitative variables of communication—the extent to which professional nurses perceive the communication which they receive from their immediate superior either as involving unnecessary information or as involving the expression of criticism. The lack of support in these two cases can be readily accounted for in terms of the specific explanations which we have proposed in Chapter 10.

On the positive side, the findings demonstrate the organizational utility for nursing activity and performance of an unencumbered flow of task-relevant information between nonsupervisory registered nurses and their superiors. And, similarly, they demonstrate the importance of communication from the nonsupervisory registered nurses to personnel at lower levels—the practical nurses, and the aides. Good vertical communication is necessary for the understanding and acceptance of organizational rules and standards. In addition, it facilitates the detection and solution of work problems, contributes to organizational coordination, and generally aids the development of shared and complementary expectations about the work on the part of people at different levels in the organization.

In conclusion, according to the findings, in hospitals where the nursing staff is performing most satisfactorily, the communication of professional nurses exhibits the following important characteristics: (1) the communication of nonsupervisory registered nurses is mainly directed vertically rather than horizontally, i.e., nurses tend to communicate more with people in lower and/or higher levels rather than with other nurses at the same level; (2) the communication channels between supervisory and nonsupervisory registered nurses, judging from the frequency and amount of communication passing through them, are apparently open and well used; (3) the nonsupervisory registered nurses evaluate the communication which they receive from their respective immediate superiors, i.e., from supervisory nurses, as adequate; (4) task-relevant communication on the part of nonsupervisory registered nurses tends to be concentrated in formal rather than informal channels; and (5) the content and quality of supervisory communication indicate an active concern with task-relevant matters, as well as a concern on the part of supervisory nurses for positive-facilitative communication toward their subordinates.[3]

---

[3] Additional findings from the present study regarding the importance of communication patterns such as the above for the social integration of the hospital, and the communication practices of nonprofessional nursing personnel, are discussed by Dr. Ruth E. Searles in her doctoral dissertation, titled "The Relation Between Communication and Social Integration in the Community Hospital" (5). Dr. Searles had an active part in the research, as an assistant study director, and wrote her dissertation using data from the same hospitals which participated in the study.

SUPPLEMENTARY DATA AND FINDINGS

While the study has been mainly concerned with problems in the areas of organizational coordination, patient care, supervision, and communication, it has also explored various other aspects of the structure and functioning of the community general hospital. This exploration, too, yielded many useful data and interesting findings, some of which suggest specific directions for future research. A good many of these findings were presented in conjunction with our analyses of patient care, coordination, supervision, and communication. The results about intraorganizational strain, for example, fall in this category. But, most of the data and findings pertaining to secondary areas of interest were reported separately in the several descriptive chapters, Chapters 3, 4, and 11. And, it is these that will briefly occupy our attention here.

In Chapter 3 we showed the major characteristics of the different people who, directly or indirectly, serve the patient in the community general hospital. We discussed and compared their personal-demographic characteristics; their professional or occupational career patterns; their job status and outlook, including earnings and job satisfaction and commitment; and certain other aspects of their work, including type of employment, turnover and absenteeism, and organizational stability. The objective was both to describe the main characteristics of each major group of people working in the hospital—doctors, trustees, administrators, nonmedical department heads, supervisory nurses, nonsupervisory registered nurses, practical nurses, aides, and laboratory and x-ray technicians—and to show the important differences and similarities among several of these groups. The data were organized in a manner that makes it possible both to follow a particular group through the many specific items covered by the chapter, and to compare and contrast the various groups with one another on each particular item. In composite, the results from this part of the study supply a basic understanding of the background and outlook of the different people who make up the organizations with which the study is concerned while, at the same time, providing useful insights into some of the problems these people and their hospitals face.

In Chapter 4 we presented data from hospital documents and records, and qualitative data from interviews with various respondents, showing some of the major features of the hospitals themselves, and describing many of the organizational characteristics of the "average" or "typical" participating hospital. Information from records about such things as the distribution of beds and patients among medical services, patient admissions, daily census, length of stay, and mortality rates, special facilities and personnel available, income and expenses, etc., was averaged for the ten hospitals and then used to provide a descriptive sketch of the typical institution. And information from interviews and certain organizational documents was used to construct a short

Supplementary Data and Findings

profile for each individual hospital. The hospital profiles covered, in overview form, a rather wide range of subjects that respondents felt were of importance to them or their respective organizations, and indicated some of the problems, weaknesses, and strengths of each hospital. These data make it possible for one both to view each particular hospital as a separate and distinct organization with its own character and uniquenesses, and to compare the ten hospitals on a variety of basic characteristics. In effect, these background data serve as an introduction to the general question of what kind of organizations these community general hospitals are and how they operate, while also focusing attention on interhospital differences and similarities, and on particular difficulties in the areas of patient care, coordination, supervision and administration, and communication.

Some of the contents of Chapters 3 and 4 were examined further in Chapter 11 where, based on empirical evidence, we discussed a number of special problems and issues that are relevant to the total hospital or to particular groups within the hospital. These had to do with the community image and internal image of the typical hospital in the study, the medical and the nursing staff, the influence of key groups on hospital functioning, the value orientations of doctors, trustees, and administrators, and the question of organizational change. Most of the problems and issues treated in Chapter 11 were not studied intensively, however, because they were of secondary interest to the principal objectives of the research. Yet, they were explored rather systematically for one or more of these reasons: (1) they are generally considered to be important by researchers and hospital people; (2) they have obvious practical implications for hospital functicning and administration, in addition to being theoretically interesting; (3) they are shown to be important by findings obtained in connection with the major problem areas of the study; (4) they help clarify and augment some of the findings concerning the more intensively studied areas; and (5) they provide certain information about a number of seemingly important aspects of the hospital situation that have heretofore received little or no scientific attention. As a result of this exploration, several conclusions reached in earlier chapters about the behavior of the community general hospital are amplified, various traditionally raised issues are placed into proper perspective, while some other unsuspected issues emerge, and attention is directed to a number of research questions that must be eventually answered.

Some Illustrative Findings and Conclusions

Without attempting to summarize here all of the results from the various exploratory and supplementary analyses of the study, we would like, in the remaining few pages, to deal with a few illustrative results. First, we shall mention some findings of methodological interest, and then continue with substantive findings and conclusions.

Many of the results obtained in the secondary as well as the principal areas of the research have a direct bearing on the question of interhospital differences, or heterogeneity, and the analogous question of differences among the groups representing the hospitals. As expected, the results show numerous specific differences among the various groups in the study, including differences in attitudes and evaluations of the hospital situation. In most cases, these differences are more pronounced between more and less professionalized groups, and among nonmedical-nonsupervisory groups than among administrative and nonmedical-supervisory groups. Interestingly, however, the results show very few differences in attitudes and evaluations between the two medical groups in the study—the selected medical staff, which consists of doctors having administrative and other organizational responsibilities, and the general medical staff whose members have no other than medical functions—and the same tends to hold true when the trustees, administrators, and nonmedical department heads are compared with each other. Considering all groups, we generally find that, in terms of attitudes and evaluations, the nonsupervisory registered nurses and the laboratory and x-ray technicians are the most critical groups, while trustees, administrators, department heads, and practical nurses are the least critical, with the doctors and the supervisory nurses occupying the intermediate position.

In spite of certain differences among particular groups, however, it is clear that some of the hospitals are consistently seen and evaluated more favorably than others by any given hospital group, or set of groups, on nearly every aspect of patient care, organizational coordination, etc., examined in the study. There are more striking differences among the hospitals themselves than among the evaluations of the hospitals by different groups, in spite of the fact that the ten participating hospitals had been selected for study because they shared a number of basic characteristics in common (see criteria of selection in Chap. 2). Interhospital variation was, of course, anticipated for every area studied, but the magnitude and extensiveness of obtained differences were not expected to be as great as they actually turned out to be for numerous variables.

Turning now to more substantive matters, we would first like to direct attention to an interesting cluster of results having to do with the relative organizational stability-instability of various groups in the hospital. Here, we shall confine discussion to the nonsupervisory registered nurses group, which best exemplifies many of the ramifications of the problem of stability. Organizationally speaking, according to a variety of secondary findings, the nonsupervisory registered nurses in the community general hospital constitute a highly unstable group. Specifically, they and the technicians, of all the groups in the study, are the two most unstable groups in the hospital, judging from such things as length of service, turnover, job history, strength of commitment to the organization, desire to remain in the present hospital indefinitely, and the like. The relative instability of the nonsupervisory professional nurses is, of

Supplementary Data and Findings

course, a very important factor from the standpoint of hospital functioning, for it is intimately and directly associated with a host of practical questions concerning staff and organizational maintenance. But, the full significance of the organizational instability of this group can be best appreciated if one recalls that this is a very crucial group, judging from our findings on patient care and coordination, and if one also recalls that hospitals are experiencing frequent and rather serious shortages of professional nurses.

In relation to the question of shortages, the findings suggest that a hospital cannot possibly rely on recruiting many nonsupervisory professional nurses from other hospitals or from among older-retired nurses. Fewer than three out of every ten of the nonsupervisory registered nurses in the hospitals studied have held the same or a similar job at another hospital prior to joining their present hospital, and only one out of every ten are as old as 50 or older. For its supply of nurses in this category, a hospital must apparently rely heavily on: (1) recruiting nurses who are graduating from nursing schools, (2) enticing more nurses who are willing to work only part-time, and (3) keeping the nurses who are already on the staff, by minimizing their turnover and deferring their retirement. The first of these sources cannot possibly supply more than a fraction of the professional nurses who will be needed in the foreseeable future, unless substantially more people are attracted by nursing schools and the nursing profession than currently is the case.

The second source of supply must be cultivated to the fullest, by making part-time employment financially and psychologically rewarding for all nurses who would be potentially able and willing to enter part-time employment. (Incidentally, as a group, the part-time professional nurses do not differ significantly from the full-time nurses, either in their attitudes and evaluations of the hospital situation or in terms of the quality of their work—a high proportion of full-time R.N.'s on the staff is associated with high-quality care, and so is a high proportion of part-time R.N.'s.) That part-time employment is potentially a very important source of supply becomes quite obvious when one remembers (1) that fully 45 percent of all the nonsupervisory registered nurses in the hospitals studied are working part-time, and (2) that part-time employment is consistent with the family pressures and responsibilities of the nonsupervisory professional nurses (who, among all nursing groups, are most likely to be married, are more likely than any other nursing group except practical nurses to have children, and who are also one of the youngest groups in the hospital). Whether a hospital is successful in attracting and retaining part-time R.N.'s, however, will partly depend on some of the same factors which help the hospital maintain the R.N.'s who are presently on its staff.

The last major source of supply, keeping the nurses who are already on the staff, also deserves serious attention. In view of the relatively high turnover of nonsupervisory registered nurses which prevails in the participating hospitals —a turnover which is twice as high as that of aides, who are also a high turnover group—a hospital can hardly afford not to take all possible measures that would reduce the turnover and prolong the stay of these nurses. But this would by no means be an easy task for a hospital to accomplish. In the first place, as already pointed out, the nonsupervisory registered nurses are subject to family pressures which tend to eliminate many of them from the active work force. Second, only one in four of these nurses feels very strongly committed to (identified with) her present hospital, and only one in two would like to stay in the hospital for as long as she can work. Third, among all nursing groups and the technicians, they are most likely to consider supplementing their family's income (44 percent of them do), rather than career (30 percent) or some other reason, as their main reason for working in the hospital. But, as is common knowledge, the salaries of nonsupervisory registered nurses in hospitals are too low to act as a potent incentive in this connection.[4] Fourth, because of frequent understaffing, these nurses often have to carry correspondingly heavier than normal work loads, in addition to carrying out various coordinative and quasi-supervisory activities which leave them less and less time to spend on direct contacts with the patient. (Professional nurses spend less time in direct contact with the patient than the practical nurses or the untrained aides do.) If one also recalls that the nonsupervisory registered nurses and the technicians are the most critical groups in the community general hospital, one can more fully understand the difficulties of hospitals in attracting and maintaining a sufficient number of professional nurses in the nonsupervisory category.

It appears that, unless they take strong action along lines suggested by the considerations given above, hospitals will not be able, at least in the short-run, to solve the problems of shortages and turnover among their nonsupervisory registered nurses. As a last resort, a hospital might consider the possibility of training and employing more practical nurses—not as a substitute for professional nurses, but rather as a substitute for, and antidote against, utilizing too many untrained aides. In this connection, we have seen that the higher the proportion of nursing staff members who are aides, the poorer the patient care and the poorer the coordination in the hospital are likely to be, but the higher the proportion of registered and practical nurses, the better the nursing care and the better the coordination. However, only a high proportion of registered (and not practical) nurses on the staff is associated with both better nursing and better medical care, according to the findings. In this respect, aides and practical nurses are a poor substitute for highly trained professional nursing skill.

Other findings concerning the nursing staff show that a certain amount of tension exists among different nursing groups in the hospital. Generally, this

[4] Based on rates prevailing during the last quarter of 1957 in the ten participating hospitals, for example, the average annual salary for a full-time nurse in this category was only $3,700.00, with virtually no other financial rewards available to her.

Supplementary Data and Findings

tension is greater between different shifts than between personnel in different positions or classifications. In either case, the level of tension varies considerably from hospital to hospital. Coordinative difficulties probably account for a large part of the tension between shifts, while defects in the clarity of organizational rules and regulations, and defects in the understanding which personnel in the different nursing positions have of their own organizational role and of each other's role, along with coordinative difficulties, contribute to tensions among personnel in the different classifications. The incidence of some attempts on the part of nursing personnel in one classification to engage in activities that are more legitimately considered to fall in the province of personnel in another nursing classification is also a contributory factor, as are a number of other things such as poor supervision, poor communication, and the like.

A number of conclusions concerning the medical staff in the hospital are also worth reiterating. Included among these are the following:

1. The majority of doctors in the hospitals studied are not prone to view the hospital merely as their "workshop"; they do take a high degree of interest in the hospital as an institution, over and above their interest in purely medical matters, and consider service to the patient as the main objective of the organization.

2. Doctors are, on the whole, less "cost-conscious" than either trustees or administrators, but they are not as unconcerned about costs as it is often assumed, they are not prone to make excessive-wasteful use of diagnostic test materials, and they do not feel that the greater cost-consciousness of administrators and trustees is improper or unreasonable.

3. However, doctors as well as the nurses tend to feel that hospital charges for patient care are high, while trustees, administrators, and department heads tend to feel that they are low—an interesting and relatively unusual instance of lack of substantial consensus on important hospital matters on the part of these groups.

4. In their attitudes and evaluations of the hospital situation, doctors are not the most critical group.

5. The general level of understanding which doctors have of the problems and needs of other principal groups, e.g., the nursing staff or the trustees, is lower than the level of understanding which these other groups have of the problems and needs of the medical staff.

6. In the majority of the hospitals, doctors are largely satisfied with their own medical staff organization, as well as with the organization of the board of trustees.

7. Problems in the relations among different members of the medical staff exist in most of the hospitals, as is evidenced by the finding that there is more tension between doctors and other doctors in the hospitals studied, than between doctors and any other major group in the organization, or between any other two major groups or subgroups. However, as we have pointed out in Chapter 11, not much of this tension could be attributed to difficulties between members of the medical staff who are specialists and those who are general practitioners. The specialist vs. general practitioner issue has been largely resolved, and apparently resolved satisfactorily, in the hospitals studied. In that same chapter we discussed several

factors which contribute to tensions among members of the medical staff, but more research will be necessary to ascertain and evaluate the sources of tension.

Many other statements and observations could be made about the medical staff based on the data in Chapter 3 concerning the background and work characteristics of doctors, based on the evaluations of patient care by doctors shown in Chapter 5, or based on the findings in Chapters 4 and 11 regarding different aspects of the relationship between doctors and other groups in the organization. Here, however, we shall confine ourselves to a few illustrative conclusions which derive from data about the relationship of the medical staff to other key groups in the hospital. First, and perhaps most significantly, a cluster of findings presented in Chapter 11 shows that, in the hospitals studied, there are no sharp cleavages between the value orientations of doctors, on the one hand, and those of trustees or administrators, on the other. In fact, there are no serious or widespread problems of divergence in value orientation or in ideology among these top three groups. On the contrary, the results demonstrate a high degree of consensus among them about the objectives of the hospital, about important problems and issues pertaining to the hospital or being of concern to the top groups of the organization, and about the relative importance or priority of several specific organizational values that were examined in this research. In short, doctors, trustees, and administrators exhibit substantial value co-orientation. Certain differences of opinion and interest, of course, exist among the three top groups, as might be expected, but such differences are generally recognized and accepted by all concerned as legitimate. In any event, no schisms or serious conflicts exist among them in the large majority of the hospitals. Relationships among doctors, trustees, and administrators, and especially between doctors and trustees, are on the whole cordial and unproblematic.

Another cluster of findings from secondary analyses, also discussed in Chapter 11, has to do with the relative influence which doctors, nurses, trustees, and administrators have, and "should have" (in their own view), on hospital functioning. Several interesting conclusions emerge from these findings. First, it is clear that within its own sphere of activity and competence, which is recognized by all concerned, each of these four groups is the most influential (excepting perhaps the nursing staff), i.e., each exercises more influence in its own province than any of the other groups, without being seriously challenged in this respect. Second, although legally and in theory the board of trustees has ultimate authority over all hospital affairs, and over all other groups in the organization, including the medical staff, in practice the authority and power of trustees over the doctors is quite limited. On the other hand, the relatively great power of the medical staff is effectively held in check by a variety of existing mechanisms and organizational conditions, as discussed in Chapter 11. Third, the balance of organizational power in the hospitals studied is such that

Supplementary Data and Findings 633

neither the doctors, nor the trustees, nor the administrator can actually "run" the hospital unilaterally, or even pursue their respective objectives independently.

Still, doctors, nurses, trustees, and administrators differ in their respective influence on the overall functioning of the hospital. In this connection, doctors, trustees, and administrators all agree that the hospital administrator is the most influential, followed by the board of trustees, then the medical staff, and the nursing staff in last place. This distribution of prevailing influence, however, does not coincide completely with the distribution of desired influence for each group, or the relative influence that each of these groups "should have" on hospital functioning, in the judgment of trustees or of doctors.

According to the administrators, each of the four groups in question should have the same amount of overall influence that it now has—the distribution of desired influence for each group should be the same as the distribution of prevailing influence. According to the trustees, every group should have somewhat more influence than it now has. But, the new distribution of influence would not actually change the relative influence position now held by the four groups, although it would be more symmetrical than it now is because the trustees would increase the influence of doctors and nurses more than the influence of administrators and trustees. According to the doctors, however, the medical staff and the nursing staff should have more influence than they now do, while the administrator and the trustees should have somewhat less influence than they now do. In effect, doctors would prefer a distribution of influence such that the medical staff would become the most influential group, followed by the administrator and the trustees at approximately the same level and at a rather close distance, with the nursing staff being the least influential of the four. The consequences of such a distribution of influence for hospital functioning could not possibly be ascertained in the present research, however, since none of the hospitals in the study actually exhibits an influence distribution of this kind.

As a concluding illustration of results obtained from our exploration of various areas which were of secondary interest to the study, we might briefly consider the subject of organizational change. The community general hospital can be classed among large-scale organizations which experience a good deal of change over time. Many changes are often initiated by the hospital itself, while others have their origins in the external environment of the organization. The question of how successful a hospital, or any other organization, is in adjusting to internal changes and in adapting to externally induced changes is, of course, a very important one, for it concerns the continuity, effectiveness, and survival of the organization.

Our data on organizational change are rather limited. Nevertheless, they do suggest a number of interesting things which should, at least, stimulate further research. They indicate, for example, that hospitals which are relatively successful in adjusting to changes that they themselves initiate are not, by extension, also likely to be successful in adapting to externally induced change. Moreover, those of the hospitals which are more successful in adapting to changes originating in their environment also appear to experience a good deal of strain in the process of accommodating the change, at least in the early stages. They, in fact, experience more strain than the relatively less successful hospitals. The data also show that the large majority of organizational members who are affected by the changes which the hospital initiates generally accept the new situation and adjust to it rather rapidly. Successful overall adjustment on their part is aided by adequate communication at the top levels of the organization, by clearly defined policies, rules, and regulations, and by good organizational coordination of the preventive type. The promptness of adjustment is facilitated if doctors and trustees have a good understanding of each other's problems, and is impaired by the existence of tensions among different groups in the hospital. Finally, organizational adaptation to externally induced change appears to be more successful in hospitals where interdepartmental problems tend to be settled without delay, in hospitals where cooperation among nursing personnel in different shifts is high and tension is low, and in hospitals having good nursing department coordination.

CONCLUDING REMARKS

The present study represents an effort toward our understanding of the behavior and problems of an important and largely unexplored social organization—the voluntary, community general hospital. The research began in a general, exploratory way, and then developed into a more rigorous and quantitative investigation of certain aspects of the structure and functioning of the hospital, in an attempt to specify and evaluate some of the factors and conditions which affect or relate to the overall effectiveness of this organization. The study was particularly concerned with problems in the areas of patient care, organizational coordination, supervision and administration, and communication, but it also examined a number of questions in areas of secondary interest, including questions about intraorganizational strain, organizational change and its accommodation, the influence and value orientations of key groups in the hospital, the background and work characteristics of different organizational groups, and certain problems and issues regarding the hospital or particular groups in the hospital.

The study was a comparative one, utilizing both qualitative and quantitative data from ten hospitals. The research design fundamentally involved a systematic comparison and contrast of the ten participating hospitals, in relation to one another, on each of a large number of variables or characteristics in the above problem areas. The approach was a wholistic one, in the sense that the study deliberately attempted to take a synoptic view of the hospital, i.e., to view the hospital as a total organization, and to investigate variables, problems, and phenomena of organization-wide significance. Correspondingly, for most aspects of the hospital situation examined, the total hospital served as the unit of description, analysis, and hypothesis testing. The analysis was mainly relational and comparative or cross-organizational. The theoretical emphasis, for the most part, was on social-psychological variables and concepts, since the main interest was in the behavior of the hospital as an organization. The aims were partly exploratory and partly analytical and explanatory. The study sought both to provide descriptive information about the community general hospital and its different people, and to make statements about the factors and conditions which distinguish the more from the less effective hospitals in terms of quality of care, adequacy of organizational coordination, and other criteria of organizational effectiveness.

Large-scale organizations are both very rewarding and very frustrating sites in which to study phenomena of organized human behavior. And, among complex organizations, the community general hospital with its intricate structure and delicate division of labor is probably unexcelled on both counts. It offers almost unlimited opportunities for the investigation of practically any major organizational problem in all of its social-psychological complexity and ramifications, while it can easily demonstrate to us all how little we really know about it and about organizations, more generally. A serious study of as complicated an organization as the hospital cannot but raise many questions and issues—perhaps more than it may help resolve—in its attempts to tackle a few problems of organizational behavior. Moreover, however systematic it might be, a single study cannot, in its inevitably limited scope, supply answers to more than a relatively few questions regarding the phenomena with which it is concerned. This is true of both comparative and noncomparative research. Yet, by answering a few basic questions and stimulating new ones, a well-designed and carefully executed comparative study of community general hospitals can contribute not only to our knowledge of the problems and characteristics which hospitals of this type share, or do not share, among themselves or with hospitals of a different type, but also to our general knowledge of human organizations. The present research was conceived and carried out in the context of this conviction. How successful it has been in accomplishing the objectives to which it was addressed will be settled partly by the judgment of our colleagues, critics, and readers, and partly by the future research efforts which it may aid or stimulate.

REFERENCES

1. Block, L. "Prototype Study: 200 Bed Hospital," *Mod. Hosp.*, 82:76–80, (Jan.) 1954.
2. Burling, T., Lentz, E. M., and Wilson, R. N. *The Give and Take in Hospitals*. New York: Putnam, 1956.

3. Health Information Foundation. *An Inventory of Social and Economic Research in Health.* New York: Annual publication of the Health Information Foundation.

4. Revans, R. W. "How Should a Hospital be Judged?" *Hospital Service Finance,* 9:34–48, (Nov.–Dec.) 1960.

5. Searles, R. E. "The Relation Between Communication and Social Integration in the Community Hospital." Doctoral Dissertation. University of Michigan, 1961.

6. Smith, H. L. "The Sociological Study of Hospitals." Doctoral Dissertation. University of Chicago, 1949.

7. Wessen, A. F. "The Social Structure of a Modern Hospital." Doctoral Dissertation. Yale University, 1951.

APPENDIX A QUESTIONNAIRE ADMINISTERED TO NONSUPERVISORY NURSES: A SAMPLE QUESTIONNAIRE

Form 2

UNIVERSITY OF MICHIGAN
SURVEY RESEARCH CENTER
ANN ARBOR, MICHIGAN

A Division of the
Institute for Social Research

Study 243
Fall 1957

This is a study about community general hospitals. It is one of many similar studies made by research teams from the University of Michigan. The main purpose of these studies is to learn how different types of organizations operate and what makes an organization a good place in which to work.

Your hospital is one of many similar hospitals which have been selected to participate in the present study. It is cooperating with us in this research along with these other Michigan hospitals. In each hospital, we need the cooperation of many people like yourself, and the success of the study will depend on the information that you give us. We will need to know your ideas and opinions about the hospital, your work, and various aspects of hospital functioning.

To get the information on how you think and feel about the hospital and the people who work in it, we would like you to fill out this questionnaire. Your individual answers are *completely confidential*. No one in the hospital will ever see or know the answers given by you or any other person.

The final value of our study will depend upon the frankness and care with which you answer the questions. *This is not a test.* There are no right or wrong answers. The main idea is for you to answer the questions the way you really feel—the way things seem to you personally. Your answers will be combined with those of other people and only summarized results will be returned when the research is completed.

Thank you very much for your cooperation.

Survey Research Center
University of Michigan

INSTRUCTIONS

1. Please answer the questions in order. Do not skip around.
2. Most questions can be answered by checking (√) one of the answers provided. If you do not find the exact answer that fits your case, check the one that comes closest to it, or write your own answer.
3. If you wish to write an explanation or comment about an answer, feel free to do so. Make your comments right on the questionnaire.
4. Please use the space on the back of the questionnaire to make as many additional comments and suggestions as you like.

SOME THINGS ABOUT YOURSELF

The way people feel and the ideas they have may be different because of the years they have worked, the amount of money they make, or the kind of job they have, etc. We, therefore, need some background information about you, such as length of service with the hospital, age, education, and other things. Let us remind you again about the confidential nature of our research. *No one in the hospital will ever see your answers.*

Now for the questions

1. What is the total length of time you have worked at this hospital? (Check one.)
I:10
   ___(1) Six months or less
   ___(2) Between six months and one year
   ___(3) Between one and two years
   ___(4) Between two and five years
   ___(5) Between five and ten years
   ___(6) Ten years or more

2. Did you have a regular job before you joined this hospital? (Check one.)
I:11
   ___(1) Yes, I had the same job in another hospital
   ___(2) Yes, I had a similar job in another hospital
   ___(3) Yes, I had another job in the hospital field or in the field of health
   ___(4) Yes, I had another job but not related to hospital work (another job in some other type of organization or business)
   ___(5) No, I had no other regular job

3. What is your present job at this hospital? (Check one.)
I:12
   ___(1) Assistant head nurse
   ___(2) Registered nurse
   ___(3) Licensed practical nurse
   ___(4) Practical nurse
   ___(5) Student nurse
   ___(6) Secretary, floor secretary, or ward clerk
   ___(7) Other

4. Here at this hospital, how long have you been doing the job you are now on? (Check one.)
I:13
   ___(1) Six months or less
   ___(2) Between six months and one year
   ___(3) Between one and two years
   ___(4) Between two and five years
   ___(5) Five years or more

5. In what major division, or section, of the hospital are you now working? (Check *only* one.)
I:14
   ___(1) Operating room
   ___(2) Medical section
   ___(3) Surgical section
   ___(4) Pediatrics
   ___(5) Obstetrics and gynecology
   ___(6) Central supply
   ___(7) Emergency
   ___(8) Outpatient
   ___(9) No special area or section
   ___(0) Other

6. How long have you been working in your present division (or section) at this hospital? (Check one.)
I:15
   ___(1) Six months or less
   ___(2) Between six months and one year
   ___(3) Between one and two years
   ___(4) Between two and five years
   ___(5) Five years or more

7. Have you ever worked in any other division (or section) of this hospital other than your present division? (Check one.)
I:16
   ___(1) Yes
   ___(2) No

8. What shift are you now on? (Check one.)
I:17
   ___(1) Day shift
   ___(2) Afternoon shift
   ___(3) Night shift

9. Do you usually work on this shift? (Check one.)
I:18
   ___(1) Yes, I always work on this shift
   ___(2) Yes, I work on this shift most of the time
   ___(3) Yes, I work on this shift regularly but I rotate sometimes
   ___(4) No, I usually work on another shift

10. Here at the hospital, are you working full-time? (Check one.)
I:19
   ___(1) Yes
   ___(2) No, I am working part-time

11. What is your sex? (Check one.)
I:20
   ___(1) Male
   ___(2) Female

12. What is your marital status? (Check one.)
I:21
   ___(1) Married
   ___(2) Single
   ___(3) Widowed, divorced, or separated

Questionnaire—Nonsupervisory Nurses

13. Do you have children? (Check
I:22 one.)
    ___(1) Yes
    ___(2) No

14. How old are you? (Check
I:23 one.)
    ___(1) Under 20 years
    ___(2) Between 20 and 30
    ___(3) Between 30 and 40
    ___(4) Between 40 and 50
    ___(5) Between 50 and 60
    ___(6) 60 years or over

15. How much formal education
I:24 have you had? (Check the *highest* completed.)
    ___(1) Grade school
    ___(2) Some high school
    ___(3) Completed high school
    ___(4) Some college
    ___(5) Completed college

16. Of the following, which one
I:25 would you say is your main reason for working here? (Check *only* one.)
    ___(1) To be financially independent
    ___(2) To maintain myself temporarily until I get married or get another job
    ___(3) It is my career—my profession
    ___(4) To supplement my family's income
    ___(5) I just like my job and want to keep it
    ___(6) I live here
    ___(7) Other reasons

17. How much *professional school-*
I:26 *ing* have you had? (Check one.)
    ___(1) Less than one year of professional schooling
    ___(2) One year
    ___(3) Two years
    ___(4) Three years
    ___(5) Four years
    ___(6) Five years
    ___(7) Over five years of professional schooling

ABOUT YOUR JOB

18. How satisfied are you with the training you have had for this job? (Check one.)
I:27
    ___(1) Completely dissatisfied
    ___(2) Very dissatisfied
    ___(3) Somewhat dissatisfied
    ___(4) A little satisfied
    ___(5) Fairly satisfied
    ___(6) Very well satisfied
    ___(7) Completely satisfied

19. How satisfied are you with your present salary or wages? (Check one.)
I:28
    ___(1) Completely satisfied
    ___(2) Very well satisfied
    ___(3) Fairly satisfied
    ___(4) A little satisfied
    ___(5) Somewhat dissatisfied
    ___(6) Very dissatisfied
    ___(7) Completely dissatisfied

20. How much does your job give you a chance to do the things you are best at? (Check one.)
I:29
    ___(1) An excellent chance to do the things I am best at
    ___(2) A very good chance
    ___(3) A good chance
    ___(4) A fair chance
    ___(5) Little chance
    ___(6) Very little chance
    ___(7) No chance at all to do the things I am best at

21. On the job, do you feel any pressure for better performance *over and above what you think is reasonable?* (Check one.)
I:30
    ___(1) I feel a great deal of pressure over and above what is reasonable
    ___(2) Considerable pressure
    ___(3) Some pressure
    ___(4) A little pressure
    ___(5) Very little pressure
    ___(0) I feel no pressure at all over and above what is reasonable

22. If you feel any pressure at all, what is the *main source* of this pressure? (Check *only* one.)
I:31
    ___(0) I feel no pressure at all
    ___(1) The main source of the pressure is the people I usually work with
    ___(2) The kind of work I do
    ___(3) My superiors in our department
    ___(4) People from other departments
    ___(5) The patients
    ___(6) Patients' relatives or visitors
    ___(7) Myself
    ___(8) The doctors
    ___(9) The main source of the pressure is something else other than the above (write in): _____

23. How satisfied do you feel about your chances for advancement or for promotion in this hospital? (Check one.)
I:32
- ___(1) Completely dissatisfied
- ___(2) Very dissatisfied
- ___(3) Somewhat dissatisfied
- ___(4) A little satisfied
- ___(5) Fairly satisfied
- ___(6) Very well satisfied
- ___(7) Completely satisfied

24. How long would you like to stay with this hospital? (Check one.)
I:33
- ___(1) I would like to stay for as long as I can work
- ___(2) I would like to stay for as long as I can work, unless things around here change too much
- ___(3) I would like to stay, but I would leave for a better job
- ___(4) I would like to leave (I am planning to leave)
- ___(5) I will definitely leave as soon as I can

25. On the job, how free do you feel to set your own work pace? (Check one.)
I:34
- ___(1) I feel completely free to set my own work pace
- ___(2) Quite a bit of freedom to do so
- ___(3) Some freedom
- ___(4) Little freedom
- ___(5) I have no freedom at all to set my own work pace

26. To what extent does your work here help you learn more about your profession or occupation? (Check one.)
I:35
- ___(1) To a very great extent
- ___(2) To a great extent
- ___(3) To some extent
- ___(4) To a small extent
- ___(5) Not at all

27. To what extent does your work here help you develop more confidence in yourself? (Check one.)
I:36
- ___(1) To a very great extent
- ___(2) To a great extent
- ___(3) To some extent
- ___(4) To a small extent
- ___(5) Not at all

28. On the whole, what do you think of this hospital as a place to work? (Check one.)
I:37
- ___(1) It is an excellent place to work
- ___(2) A very good place
- ___(3) A good place
- ___(4) A fair place
- ___(5) A rather poor place
- ___(6) A poor place
- ___(7) It is a very poor place to work

ABOUT LEADERSHIP AND SUPERVISION

29. What is the name of the person who is your *immediate superior* (the
I:38 person who usually directs your work)?
-39
    The name of my immediate superior is: _____
                                             (Please name one person only)

THE FOLLOWING QUESTIONS ARE ABOUT THE PERSON YOU HAVE JUST NAMED AS YOUR *IMMEDIATE SUPERIOR*

30. On the whole, how does your immediate superior handle the *human rela-*
I:40 *tions side* of the job? (This includes such things as getting people to work together, getting them to do the best they can, giving recognition and expressing appreciation for good work done, letting people know where they stand, and the like.) (Check one.)
    ___(1) My immediate superior handles the human relations side of the job extremely well
    ___(2) Very well
    ___(3) Fairly well
    ___(4) Not so well
    ___(5) Not at all well

31. On the whole, how well does your immediate superior handle the *adminis-*
I:41 *trative side* of the job? (This includes such things as assigning the right job to the right people, indicating clearly when work is to be finished or what is to be done first, giving people the right amount of responsibility and authority they need to do their job, inspecting and following up the work, organizing, making overall plans about the work, and the like.) (Check one.)
    ___(1) My immediate superior handles the administrative side of the job extremely well
    ___(2) Very well
    ___(3) Fairly well
    ___(4) Not so well
    ___(5) Not at all well

32. On the whole, how well does your immediate superior handle the *purely*
I:42 *technical side* of the job? (This includes *other than* "human relations" and "administrative" aspects of the job; for example, it includes such things as knowledge of the job, technical skills needed by his profession, the operation of equipment, and the like.) (Check one.)
    ___(1) My immediate superior handles the technical side of the job extremely well
    ___(2) Very well
    ___(3) Fairly well
    ___(4) Not so well
    ___(5) Not at all well

Questionnaire—Nonsupervisory Nurses

33. How do you feel about what
I:43 your immediate superior expects you to do? (Check one.)
   ___(1) What my immediate superior expects is far too much
   ___(2) It is too much
   ___(3) It is a little too much
   ___(4) It is about right
   ___(5) It is exactly right
   ___(9) I don't know what my immediate superior expects

34. How well do you think your
I:44 immediate superior understands the employees' viewpoint? (Check one.)
   ___(1) Has complete understanding of how employees think and feel
   ___(2) A very good understanding
   ___(3) A good understanding
   ___(4) A fair understanding
   ___(5) Has a rather poor understanding of how employees think and feel

35. How often does your imme-
I:45 diate superior tell you in advance about any changes that affect you or your work? (Check one.)
   ___(1) Always or nearly always tells me in advance about any changes that affect me or my work
   ___(2) More often than not
   ___(3) Sometimes
   ___(4) Seldom
   ___(5) Never tells me in advance about any changes that affect me or my work

36. How sure are you of what
I:46 your immediate superior thinks of you and your work? (Check one.)
   ___(1) I am very sure of what my immediate superior thinks of me and my work
   ___(2) Quite sure
   ___(3) Fairly sure
   ___(4) Not too sure
   ___(5) I am not sure at all of what my immediate superior thinks of me and my work

37. Does your immediate superior
I:47 ask your opinion when a problem comes up that involves your work? (Check one.)
   ___(1) Always or nearly always asks my opinion
   ___(2) Very often
   ___(3) Often
   ___(4) Sometimes
   ___(5) Seldom or never asks my opinion

38. How often does your imme-
I:48 diate superior express appreciation for your work? (Check one.)
   ___(1) Always or nearly always expresses appreciation for my work
   ___(2) Very often
   ___(3) Often
   ___(4) Sometimes
   ___(5) Seldom or never expresses appreciation for my work

39. How free do you feel to discuss personal problems with your immediate superior? (Check one.)
I:49
- ___(1) I always feel free to discuss personal problems with my immediate superior
- ___(2) I usually feel free
- ___(3) Sometimes I feel free
- ___(4) Only once in a while I feel free
- ___(5) I never feel free to discuss personal problems with my immediate superior

40. How good is your immediate superior in planning, organizing, and scheduling the work? (Check one.)
I:50
- ___(1) Excellent in planning, organizing, and scheduling the work
- ___(2) Very good
- ___(3) Good
- ___(4) Fair
- ___(5) Rather poor
- ___(6) Poor
- ___(7) Very poor in planning, organizing, and scheduling the work

41. How good is your immediate superior in dealing with people? (Check one.)
I:51
- ___(1) Excellent in dealing with people
- ___(2) Very good
- ___(3) Good
- ___(4) Fair
- ___(5) Rather poor
- ___(6) Poor
- ___(7) Very poor in dealing with people

42. Taking all things into consideration, how satisfied are you with your *immediate superior?* (Check one)
I:52
- ___(1) I am completely satisfied with my immediate superior
- ___(2) I am very well satisfied
- ___(3) I am fairly well satisfied
- ___(4) I am somewhat dissatisfied
- ___(5) I am dissatisfied with my immediate superior

ABOUT OVERALL SUPERVISION

43. If you have a suggestion for improving the job or changing the setup in some way, how easy is it for you to get your ideas across to your superiors? (Check one.)
I:53
- ___(1) It is very difficult to to get my ideas across to my superior
- ___(2) It is rather difficult
- ___(3) It is not too easy
- ___(4) It is fairly easy
- ___(5) It is very easy to get my ideas across to my superior

44. On the whole, to what extent do the *key people* in this hospital make an effort to make you feel that you are an important part of the team? (Check one.)
I:54
- ___(1) To a very great extent
- ___(2) To a great extent
- ___(3) To a fair extent
- ___(4) To a small extent
- ___(5) Not at all

45. Are there any group meetings in which you and the people you work with can discuss things with your superiors? (Check one.)
   ___(0) No, we never have such group meetings
   ___(1) Yes, we have such group meetings and they are always worth while
   ___(2) Yes, and they are usually worth while
   ___(3) Yes, but only sometimes they are worth while
   ___(4) Yes, but usually nothing much is accomplished
   ___(5) Yes, but they are just a waste of time

46. If you have these group meetings, how much opportunity do you have to express your own ideas and opinions during the meetings? (Check one.)
   ___(0) We never have such group meetings
   ___(1) I have full opportunity to express my ideas and opinions during these meetings
   ___(2) Quite a bit of opportunity to do so
   ___(3) Some opportunity
   ___(4) Very little opportunity
   ___(5) I have no opportunity to express my ideas and opinions during these group meetings

47. If you have these group meetings, how often are they held? (Check one.)
   ___(0) Such group meetings are never held
   ___(1) These group meetings are held about once every three months or less often
   ___(2) About once every two months
   ___(3) About once a month
   ___(4) About once every three weeks
   ___(5) Every two weeks
   ___(6) Once a week
   ___(7) About twice a week or more often

WORKING WITH EACH OTHER

48. Here is a list of major hospital departments. Check the *three* departments with which you usually have the most contacts in connection with your work:
I:58
-59
-60
   ___(1) Dietetics
   ___(2) X-ray
   ___(3) Housekeeping
   ___(4) Laboratory
   ___(5) Maintenance
   ___(6) Front office (business office)
   ___(7) Personnel
   ___(8) Admissions
   ___(9) Records
   ___(0) Pharmacy

49. In your opinion, to what extent has this hospital been able to achieve *singleness of direction* in the efforts of its many groups, departments, and individuals? (Check one.)
I:61
   ___(1) To a very great extent
   ___(2) To a considerable extent
   ___(3) To a fair extent
   ___(4) To a small extent
   ___(5) To a very small extent

50. To what degree do people from different departments see the other person's viewpoint in connection with their mutual working relationships? (Check one.)
I:62
   ___(1) To a very great degree
   ___(2) To a considerable degree
   ___(3) To a fair degree
   ___(4) To a small degree
   ___(5) To a very small degree

51. Do the people from different departments who have to work together do their full share so that each contributes to making the other person's work a little easier? (Check one.)
I:63
   ___(1) They all do their full share
   ___(2) Nearly all of them do their full share
   ___(3) The majority do their full share
   ___(4) About half do their full share
   ___(5) Less than half do their full share

52. In general, do your various work contacts with people in other departments produce satisfactory results (i.e., do they help your mutual working relationships)? (Check one.)
I:64
   ___(1) All of my work contacts with people in other departments produce satisfactory results
   ___(2) Nearly all of my work contacts produce satisfactory results
   ___(3) Most of my work contacts produce satisfactory results
   ___(4) About half of my work contacts produce satisfactory results
   ___(5) Less than half of my work contacts with people in other departments produce satisfactory results

Questionnaire—Nonsupervisory Nurses

53. How easy is it for you to get
I:65 together and exchange information and ideas about the work with people from other departments whose jobs are related to yours? (Check one.)

___(1) It is very easy
___(2) It is fairly easy
___(3) Not as easy as it could be
___(4) It is rather difficult
___(5) It is very difficult

54. In general, *how prompt* is each of the following departments in filling out your various requests for supplies, information, or services? (Check one for each department or office.)

		It is only occasionally prompt (1)	Sometimes it is prompt (2)	Most of the time it is prompt (3)	It is always prompt (4)
I:66	Admissions	☐	☐	☐	☐
I:67	Records	☐	☐	☐	☐
I:68	X-ray	☐	☐	☐	☐
I:69	Laboratory	☐	☐	☐	☐
I:70	Pharmacy	☐	☐	☐	☐
I:71	Business office (front office)	☐	☐	☐	☐
I:72	Personnel	☐	☐	☐	☐
I:73	Dietetics	☐	☐	☐	☐
I:74	Housekeeping	☐	☐	☐	☐
I:75	Maintenance	☐	☐	☐	☐

55. To what extent do the people
I:76 from the various interrelated departments make an effort to avoid creating problems or interference with each other's duties and responsibilities? (Check one.)

___(1) To a very great extent
___(2) To a great extent
___(3) To a fair extent
___(4) To a small extent
___(5) To a very little extent

56. In general, how well established
I:77 are the routines of the different departments that have to work with one another? (Check one.)

___(1) Their routines are extremely well established
___(2) Very well established
___(3) Fairly well established
___(4) Not too well established
___(5) Their routines are not well established

57. To what extent do people from different departments who have to work together do their job properly and efficiently without getting in each other's way? (Check one.)
II:21
___(1) To a very great extent
___(2) To a great extent
___(3) To a fair extent
___(4) To a small extent
___(5) To a very little extent

58. In general, to what extent do people in the different jobs and departments follow policies and the various rules and regulations set up by the hospital? (Check one.)
II:22
___(1) Everyone, without exception, follows the policy and the rules and regulations of the hospital
___(2) Almost everyone does
___(3) The large majority of the people do
___(4) A little over half of the people do
___(5) About half or less than half of the people follow the policy and the rules and regulations of the hospital

59. How often do people from different jobs and departments get together when needed to discuss and try to do something about problems and differences arising in their working relationships with one another? (Check one.)
II:23
___(1) Always they get together for this purpose when needed
___(2) Nearly always
___(3) Most of the time
___(4) About half of the time
___(5) Less than half of the time they get together when needed

Questionnaire—Nonsupervisory Nurses

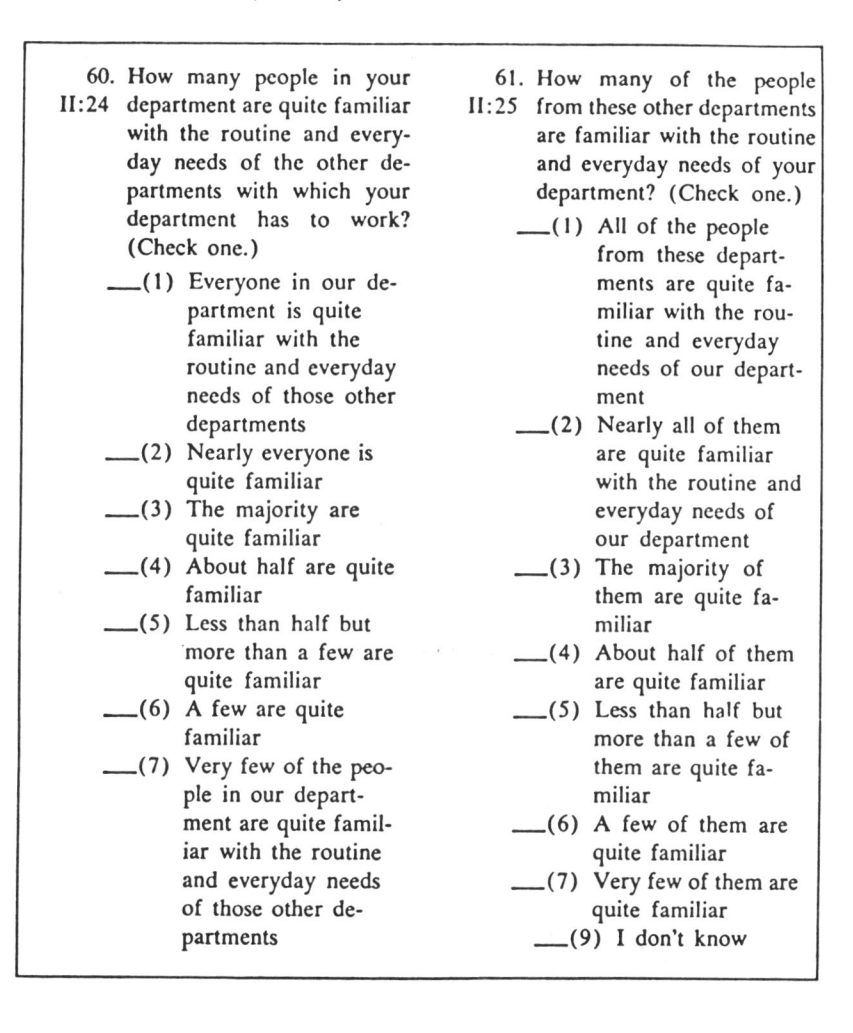

60.
II:24 How many people in your department are quite familiar with the routine and everyday needs of the other departments with which your department has to work? (Check one.)

___(1) Everyone in our department is quite familiar with the routine and everyday needs of those other departments
___(2) Nearly everyone is quite familiar
___(3) The majority are quite familiar
___(4) About half are quite familiar
___(5) Less than half but more than a few are quite familiar
___(6) A few are quite familiar
___(7) Very few of the people in our department are quite familiar with the routine and everyday needs of those other departments

61.
II:25 How many of the people from these other departments are familiar with the routine and everyday needs of your department? (Check one.)

___(1) All of the people from these departments are quite familiar with the routine and everyday needs of our department
___(2) Nearly all of them are quite familiar with the routine and everyday needs of our department
___(3) The majority of them are quite familiar
___(4) About half of them are quite familiar
___(5) Less than half but more than a few of them are quite familiar
___(6) A few of them are quite familiar
___(7) Very few of them are quite familiar
___(9) I don't know

62. How strongly identified do you feel (how much do you feel that you *really belong*) with each of the following? Or, how committed do you feel you are to each of the following? (Check one for each line.)

		Very strongly (1)	Quite strongly (2)	Fairly strongly (3)	A little (4)
II:26	My immediate work group	☐	☐	☐	☐
II:27	This hospital and its goals	☐	☐	☐	☐
II:28	My profession or occupation	☐	☐	☐	☐
II:29	The team that treats the patients	☐	☐	☐	☐
II:30	The community outside	☐	☐	☐	☐

63. To what extent are all related
II:31 things and activities well timed in the everyday routine of the hospital? (Check one.)
  ___(1) All related things and activities in the everyday routine are perfectly timed
  ___(2) They are very well timed
  ___(3) They are fairly well timed
  ___(4) They are not so well timed
  ___(5) They are rather poorly timed

64. How well planned are the work
II:32 assignments of the people from the different departments who work together? (Check one.)
  ___(1) Extremely well planned
  ___(2) Very well planned
  ___(3) Fairly well planned
  ___(4) Not so well planned
  ___(5) Not well planned at all

Questionnaire—Nonsupervisory Nurses

65.
II:33 When people from different departments have to work together in order to accomplish something in common, various problems are likely to arise. In your experience while working here, how are such problems of working together and fitting into the overall pattern handled? (Check one.)
___(1) These kinds of problems are handled completely satisfactorily for all concerned
___(2) They are handled very satisfactorily
___(3) They are handled fairly satisfactorily
___(4) They are handled rather unsatisfactorily
___(5) These kinds of problems are handled unsatisfactorily

66.
II:34 When problems of this kind arise, how quickly are they generally settled? (Check one.)
___(1) Usually they are settled immediately
___(2) Usually they are settled very quickly
___(3) Usually they are settled rather quickly
___(4) Usually they are settled after some delay
___(5) Usually they are settled after a good deal of delay
___(0) Usually they are not settled at all

67.
II:35 How well do the different jobs and work activities around the patient fit together, or how well are all things geared in the direction of giving good patient care? (Check one.)
___(1) Perfectly
___(2) Very well
___(3) Fairly well
___(4) Not so well
___(5) Not at all well

68.
II:36 In general, how do the patients feel about how smoothly the various personnel around them work together? (Check one.)
___(1) The patients feel that the personnel work together completely smoothly
___(2) The patients feel that the personnel work together very smoothly
___(3) The patients feel that the personnel work together fairly smoothly
___(4) The patients feel that the personnel do not work together smoothly
___(5) The patients feel that the personnel do not work together smoothly at all

69. How do you feel about how
II:37 your working time is divided among the different things that you usually do on the job? (Check one.)
    __(1) My working time is divided exactly right
    __(2) My working time is divided about right
    __(3) My working time is divided fairly close to the way it should be divided
    __(4) My working time should be divided somewhat differently
    __(5) My working time should be divided much differently

70. How clearly defined are the
II:38 policies and the various rules and regulations of the hospital that affect your job? (Check one.)
    __(1) They are defined as clearly as they should be defined
    __(2) They are defined almost as clearly as they should be defined
    __(3) They should be defined somewhat more clearly
    __(4) They should be defined more clearly
    __(5) They should be defined much more clearly

71. How much agreement is there
II:39 among people in the various related jobs and departments about the everyday operations of the hospital (or to what extent do these people see eye-to-eye on things about the everyday operations of the hospital)? (Check one.)
    __(1) There is complete agreement; people see eye-to-eye very fully
    __(2) A good deal of agreement
    __(3) Some agreement (a fair amount of agreement)
    __(4) Little agreement
    __(5) There is no agreement; people do not see eye-to-eye at all

72. How many of the people you
II:40 work with would agree with your answer to the question you have just answered? (Check one.)
    __(1) Almost all of them would agree with my answer
    __(2) Most of them would agree
    __(3) About half of them would agree
    __(4) Less than half but more than a few would agree
    __(5) A few of them would agree with my answer
    __(9) I can't judge

Questionnaire—Nonsupervisory Nurses

73. In your opinion how smoothly are the patients admitted to the hospital and discharged from the hospital? (Check one.)
II:41
___(1) In general, patients are admitted and discharged without any confusion
___(2) With no confusion to speak of
___(3) With only occasional confusion
___(4) With some confusion
___(5) In general, patients are admitted and discharged with quite a bit of confusion

74. On the whole, how good, would you say, are your various dealings with people from other departments in connection with your working relationships with these people? (Check one.)
II:42
___(1) Excellent
___(2) Very good
___(3) Good
___(4) Fair
___(5) Rather poor

75. How willing are people in the different related jobs to assist each other when needed? (Check one.)
II:43
___(1) The great majority are more than willing to assist each other
___(2) The great majority are very willing
___(3) The great majority are fairly willing
___(4) The great majority are not too willing
___(5) The great majority are not willing to assist each other

76. In general, how adequately do the doctors explain things to the nursing personnel about the condition and needs of the patients? (Check one.)
II:44
___(1) Completely adequately
___(2) Very adequately
___(3) Fairly adequately
___(4) Rather inadequately
___(5) Inadequately

77. How complete, or how adequate, are the patients' charts (records) at the nurses' stations? (Check one.)
II:45
___(1) They are completely adequate
___(2) They are very adequate
___(3) They are fairly adequate
___(4) They are somewhat inadequate
___(5) They are inadequate

78. On the whole, to what extent does the nursing staff understand and appreciate the work problems and needs of the medical staff? (Check one.)
II:46
___(1) They have an excellent understanding
___(2) A very good understanding
___(3) A good understanding
___(4) A fair understanding
___(5) They have a rather poor understanding

79. To what extent does the medical staff understand and appreciate the work problems and needs of the nursing staff? (Check one.)
II:47
- ___(1) They have an excellent understanding
- ___(2) A very good understanding
- ___(3) A good understanding
- ___(4) A fair understanding
- ___(5) They have a rather poor understanding

80. How well do you feel the different shifts work together with one another? (Check one.)
II:48
- ___(1) Extremely well
- ___(2) Very well
- ___(3) Fairly well
- ___(4) Not so well
- ___(5) Not well at all

81. How easy is it for one shift to take over without confusion from where the previous shift left off? (Check one.)
II:49
- ___(1) It is extremely easy
- ___(2) It is very easy
- ___(3) It is fairly easy
- ___(4) It is not so easy
- ___(5) It is hard or difficult

82. When you come to work, how hard is it for you to find out what went on on the job since you last were there? (Check one.)
II:50
- ___(1) It is extremely hard
- ___(2) It is very hard
- ___(3) It is fairly hard
- ___(4) It is not so hard
- ___(5) It is rather easy
- ___(6) It is very easy
- ___(7) It is extremely easy

83. How often do you feel that people from the previous shift left you with unfinished work or with problems that they should have handled during their own shift? (Check one.)
II:51
- ___(1) I always feel this way
- ___(2) Nearly always I feel this way
- ___(3) Most of the time I feel this way
- ___(4) About half of the time I feel this way
- ___(5) Sometimes I feel this way
- ___(6) Only occasionally I feel this way
- ___(7) I never feel this way

84. How promptly, would you say, do the nursing personnel answer the calls of the patients? (Check one.)
II:52
- ___(1) They answer more promptly than they should
- ___(2) They answer as promptly as they should
- ___(3) They should answer a little more promptly
- ___(4) They should answer quite a bit more promptly
- ___(5) They should answer a great deal more promptly

Questionnaire—Nonsupervisory Nurses

85. To what extent are head nurses and nursing supervisors prone to try to do things that R.N.'s or P.N.'s should be doing? (Check one.)
II:53
___(1) To a very great extent
___(2) To a considerable extent
___(3) To some extent
___(4) To a small extent
___(5) Not at all

86. To what extent are aides prone to try to do things that R.N.'s or P.N.'s should be doing? (Check one.)
II:54
___(1) To a very great extent
___(2) To a considerable extent
___(3) To some extent
___(4) To a small extent
___(5) Not at all

87. To what extent are P.N.'s prone to try to do things that R.N.'s should be doing? (Check one.)
II:55
___(1) To a very great extent
___(2) To a considerable extent
___(3) To some extent
___(4) To a small extent
___(5) Not at all

88. To what extent are R.N.'s prone to try to do things that P.N.'s should be doing? (Check one.)
II:56
___(1) To a very great extent
___(2) To a considerable extent
___(3) To some extent
___(4) To a small extent
___(5) Not at all

89. To what extent are R.N.'s prone to try to do things that head nurses should be doing? (Check one.)
II:57
___(1) To a very great extent
___(2) To a considerable extent
___(3) To some extent
___(4) To a small extent
___(5) Not at all

HOSPITAL FUNCTIONING

90. Occasionally, a major accident (e.g., a bus accident) happens in the community or too many patients are admitted at the same time and the *patient load suddenly increases* beyond the normal census. In general, how well does this hospital handle these unusual situations? (Check one.)
II:58
___(1) The hospital handles unusual situations of this kind completely adequately
___(2) Quite adequately
___(3) Fairly adequately
___(4) Not so adequately
___(5) The hospital handles unusual situations of this kind inadequately

91. How much strain (or stress) do these unusual situations create for the various people who work in the hospital? (Check one.)
II:59
___(1) These unusual situations result in extremely high strain for the people who work in the hospital
___(2) Result in very high strain
___(3) Result in fairly high strain
___(4) Result in some strain
___(5) These unusual situations result in little or no strain

92. In your opinion, how well is this hospital doing in making the patients comfortable? (Check one.)
II:60
___(1) Patient comfort in this hospital is excellent
___(2) Good
___(3) Fair
___(4) Rather poor
___(5) Patient comfort in this hospital is poor

93. How would you rate the quality of *overall patient care* in this hospital as compared to similar community general hospitals? (Check one.)
II:61
___(1) Overall patient care in this hospital is outstanding compared to most other hospitals of this kind
___(2) Much better
___(3) Generally better
___(4) About the same
___(5) Somewhat poorer
___(6) Generally poorer
___(7) Overall patient care in this hospital is much poorer than in most other hospitals of this kind

94. In your opinion, how well is this hospital doing in providing its patients with adequate personal attention? (Check one.)
II:62
___(1) Patients do not receive any personal attention
___(2) Patients do not receive enough personal attention
___(3) Patients receive almost enough personal attention
___(4) Patients receive enough personal attention
___(5) Patients receive more than enough personal attention

95. How well, would you say, is the nursing department doing in relation to what it should be accomplishing? (Check one.)
II:63
___(1) It is doing extremely well in relation to what it should be accomplishing
___(2) Very well
___(3) Fairly well
___(4) Not so well
___(5) It is not doing well at all considering what it should be accomplishing

96. On the basis of your experience and information, how would you rate the quality of the *overall care* that the patients generally receive from this hospital? (Check one.)
II:64
___(1) Overall patient care in this hospital is outstanding
___(2) Excellent
___(3) Very good
___(4) Good
___(5) Fair
___(6) Rather poor
___(7) Overall patient care in this hospital is poor

97. How good, would you say, is the *nursing care* given to patients in this hospital? (Check one.)
II:65
___(1) Nursing care in this hospital is outstanding
___(2) Excellent
___(3) Very good
___(4) Good
___(5) Fair
___(6) Rather poor
___(7) Nursing care in this hospital is poor

98. How good, would you say, is the *medical care (including surgical work)* given to patients in this hospital? (Check one.)
II:66
___(1) Medical care in this hospital is outstanding
___(2) Excellent
___(3) Very good
___(4) Good
___(5) Fair
___(6) Rather poor
___(7) Medical care in this hospital is poor

99. Except for medical aspects how much interest does the medical staff take in this hospital as an institution? (Check one.)
II:67
- ___(1) Aside from medical work, the medical staff is extremely interested in this hospital as an institution
- ___(2) The medical staff is quite a bit interested
- ___(3) The medical staff takes some interest
- ___(4) The medical staff is only slightly interested
- ___(5) Aside from medical work, the medical staff takes no interest in this hospital as an institution

100. Except for financial aspects, how much interest does the board of trustees take in the operation and problems of this hospital? (Check one.)
II:68
- ___(1) Aside from financial aspects, the board of trustees is extremely interested in the operation and problems of the hospital
- ___(2) The board is quite a bit interested
- ___(3) The board takes some interest
- ___(4) The board is only slightly interested
- ___(5) Aside from financial aspects, the board takes no interest in the operation and problems of this hospital
- ___(9) I don't know

101. On the whole, would you say that in this hospital there is some tension or conflict (friction) between the two groups in each of the following pairs? (Check one for every pair of groups.)

Between:	A very great deal of tension (1)	A great deal of tension (2)	Some tension (3)	A little tension (4)	No tension at all (5)
II:69 Nursing personnel in one shift *and* nursing personnel in another shift	☐	☐	☐	☐	☐
II:70 Nursing personnel in one division (section) *and* nursing personnel in some other division (section)	☐	☐	☐	☐	☐
II:71 Nursing personnel in one classification *and* nursing personnel in another classification	☐	☐	☐	☐	☐
II:72 Nursing personnel *and* patients	☐	☐	☐	☐	☐
II:73 Nursing personnel *and* patients' visitors	☐	☐	☐	☐	☐
II:74 Nursing personnel *and* hospital administrator	☐	☐	☐	☐	☐

Questionnaire—Nonsupervisory Nurses

II:75 102. What kind of reputation does this hospital have in the community? (Check one.)
  ___(1) This hospital has an excellent reputation in the community
  ___(2) A very good reputation
  ___(3) A good reputation
  ___(4) A fair reputation
  ___(5) This hospital has a rather poor reputation in the community
  ___(9) I can't judge

II:76 103. On the basis of your experience and information, how do the patients feel about this hospital? (Check one.)
  ___(1) All patients without exception speak very well of this hospital
  ___(2) Nearly all of the patients speak very well of this hospital
  ___(3) The large majority of the patients speak very well of this hospital
  ___(4) A little over half of the patients speak very well of this hospital
  ___(5) About half of the patients speak very well of this hospital
  ___(6) Less than half of the patients speak very well of this hospital
  ___(7) Only a few of the patients speak very well of this hospital

III:21 104. From time to time changes in policies, procedures, and equipment are introduced by the hospital. How often do these changes lead to better ways of doing things? (Check one.)
  ___(1) Changes of this kind are always an improvement
  ___(2) Most of the time they are an improvement
  ___(3) About half of the time they are an improvement
  ___(4) They seldom improve things
  ___(5) Changes of this kind never improve things

III:22 105. How well do the various people in the hospital who are affected by these changes accept the change? (Check one.)
  ___(1) Practically all of the people involved accept the changes and adjust to them
  ___(2) The majority of the people involved accept the changes and adjust to them
  ___(3) About half of the people involved accept the changes and adjust to them
  ___(4) Less than half of the people involved accept the changes and adjust to them
  ___(5) Very few of the people involved accept the changes and adjust to them

106. How quickly, would you say, do the various people (or groups) that are affected by the introduction of these changes come to adjust to the new situations? (Check one.)

___(1) Most of the people involved adjust to the new situation immediately
___(2) They adjust very rapidly but not immediately
___(3) They adjust fairly rapidly
___(4) They adjust rather slowly
___(5) They adjust slowly
___(6) They adjust very slowly
___(7) Most of the people involved never adjust to to the new situation

107. During the last two years, have you noticed any changes in hospital policy, personnel, procedures, or equipment that have improved hospital operations? (Check one.)

___(1) Many good changes in these areas were introduced during the last two years
___(2) Some good changes were introduced in these areas
___(3) Few good changes were introduced in these areas during the last two years

108. Considering the various changes that have taken place in the hospital while you have worked here, how much change would you expect in the next couple of years? (Check one.)

___(1) There are likely to be a great many important changes in the hospital in the next couple of years
___(2) Many important changes will be made
___(3) Some important changes will be made
___(4) Few important changes will be made
___(5) Very few or no important changes will be made in the next couple of years

Questionnaire—Nonsupervisory Nurses

109. On the whole, would you say that in this hospital there is some tension or conflict (friction) between the two groups in each of the following pairs? (Check one for every pair of groups.)

Between:	A very great deal of tension (1)	A great deal of tension (2)	Some tension (3)	A little tension (4)	No tension at all (5)
III:26 X-ray *and* nursing	☐	☐	☐	☐	☐
III:27 Admissions *and* nursing	☐	☐	☐	☐	☐
III:28 Maintenance *and* housekeeping	☐	☐	☐	☐	☐
III:29 Laboratory *and* nursing	☐	☐	☐	☐	☐
III:30 Laboratory *and* x-ray	☐	☐	☐	☐	☐
III:31 Dietetics *and* nursing	☐	☐	☐	☐	☐
III:32 Front office *and* nursing (business office)	☐	☐	☐	☐	☐
III:33 Housekeeping *and* nursing	☐	☐	☐	☐	☐
III:34 Maintenance *and* nursing	☐	☐	☐	☐	☐
III:35 The hospital *and* the community	☐	☐	☐	☐	☐

110. On the whole, what kind of a job would you say each of the following does for this hospital? (Check one for each line.)

	An excellent job (1)	A very good job (2)	A good job (3)	A fair job (4)	A rather poor job (5)
III:36 The director of nursing	☐	☐	☐	☐	☐
III:37 The associate director of nursing	☐	☐	☐	☐	☐
III:38 The nursing supervisors	☐	☐	☐	☐	☐
III:39 The head nurses	☐	☐	☐	☐	☐
III:40 The R.N.'s	☐	☐	☐	☐	☐
III:41 The P.N.'s	☐	☐	☐	☐	☐
III:42 The aides	☐	☐	☐	☐	☐

111. On the whole, how "business-minded" or "cost-conscious" is each of the following? (Check one for each line.)

	More than they should be (1)	As much as they should be (2)	Less than they should be (3)
III:43 The nursing staff	☐	☐	☐
III:44 The medical staff	☐	☐	☐
III:45 The administrator	☐	☐	☐
III:46 The director of nursing	☐	☐	☐
III:47 The nonprofessional personnel of the hospital	☐	☐	☐

112. Considering the kind of service this hospital gives to its patients, how do you feel about what it charges for patient care? (Check one.)
III:48
   ___(1) Considering the service it provides, this hospital's charges for patient care are far too high
   ___(2) Too high
   ___(3) Quite high
   ___(4) Somewhat high
   ___(5) Just right
   ___(6) Low
   ___(7) Considering the service, this hospital's charges for patient care are too low

113. On the following list, please check the *two* departments that you find most difficult (least easy) to work with or deal with:
III:49
−50
   ___(1) Dietetics
   ___(2) Maintenance
   ___(3) X-ray
   ___(4) Housekeeping
   ___(5) Laboratory
   ___(6) Admissions
   ___(7) Personnel
   ___(8) Front office (business office)
   ___(9) Records
   ___(0) Pharmacy

ABOUT COMMUNICATIONS

114. When people work together they talk about work, their personal interests, and other things which may or may not be related to the job. And, usually people talk more with certain persons than with others. Think of that person in this hospital *with whom you usually talk the most*. Then check the average amount of time *per week* you talk with this person while at the hospital. (Check one.)
III:51
   ___(1) I usually talk with this person less than ½ hour per week
   ___(2) Between ½ and 1 hour per week
   ___(3) Between 1 and 2 hours per week
   ___(4) Between 2 and 4 hours per week
   ___(5) Between 4 and 6 hours per week
   ___(6) I usually talk with this person more than 6 hours per week

Questionnaire—Nonsupervisory Nurses

115. How often do you usually talk with this person about each of the following things? (Check one for each item.)

		Once a month or less often (1)	Two or three times a month (2)	About once a week (3)	Several times a week (4)	Once a day or more often (5)
III:52	About ways in which patient care could be improved	☐	☐	☐	☐	☐
III:53	About ways in which nursing supervision could be improved	☐	☐	☐	☐	☐
III:54	About work	☐	☐	☐	☐	☐
III:55	About employee wages, hours, or benefits	☐	☐	☐	☐	☐
III:56	About ways in which working relations between departments could be improved	☐	☐	☐	☐	☐
III:57	About ways in which satisfaction or morale among nursing personnel could be improved	☐	☐	☐	☐	☐
III:58	About things, people, or happenings outside the hospital	☐	☐	☐	☐	☐

116. What position in the hospital does this person with whom you talk most
III:59 frequently have? (Check one.)

___(1) This person has a position lower than mine
___(2) This person has a position at the same level as mine
___(3) This person is my immediate superior
___(4) This person has a position higher than mine (but is not my immediate superior)

117. On the whole, what is the average amount of time per week you talk
III:60 with your *immediate superior* in the hospital? (Check one.)
  ___(1) I usually talk with my immediate superior less than ¼ hour per week
  ___(2) Between ¼ and ½ hour per week
  ___(3) Between ½ and 1 hour per week
  ___(4) Between 1 and 2 hours per week
  ___(5) Between 2 and 4 hours per week
  ___(6) I usually talk with my immediate superior more than 4 hours per week

118. How much variation is there
III:61 in the *length of time* or in *how often* you talk with your immediate superior? (Check one.)
  ___(1) There is an extremely large amount of variation
  ___(2) A very large amount of variation
  ___(3) A large amount of variation
  ___(4) A moderate amount of variation
  ___(5) A small amount of variation
  ___(6) An extremely small amount of variation

119. In general, how do you feel
III:62 about the kind of communication which you receive from your *immediate superior?* (Check one.)
  ___(1) The kind of communication I receive from my immediate superior is completely adequate
  ___(2) Very adequate
  ___(3) Fairly adequate
  ___(4) Rather inadequate
  ___(5) The kind of communication I receive from my immediate superior is inadequate

Questionnaire—Nonsupervisory Nurses

120. How often do you usually talk with your *immediate superior* about each of the following things? (Check one for each item.)

		Once a month or less often (1)	Two or three times a month (2)	About once a week (3)	Several times a week (4)	Once a day or more often (5)
III:63	About ways in which patient care could be improved	☐	☐	☐	☐	☐
III:64	About ways in which nursing supervision could be improved	☐	☐	☐	☐	☐
III:65	About work	☐	☐	☐	☐	☐
III:66	About employee wages, hours, or benefits	☐	☐	☐	☐	☐
III:67	About ways in which working relations between departments could be improved	☐	☐	☐	☐	☐
III:68	About ways in which satisfaction or morale among nursing personnel could be improved	☐	☐	☐	☐	☐
III:69	About things, people, or happenings outside the hospital	☐	☐	☐	☐	☐

121. Check the *two* most important reasons why you follow the directions or
III:70 orders of your immediate superior:
−71

___(1) She might give me a better recommendation if I followed her directions or orders

___(2) She might make it difficult for me or give me a bad recommendation if I failed to follow her directions or orders

___(3) It is my duty to follow her directions or orders because I am under her supervision

___(4) I like her, so I want to follow her directions or orders

___(5) She is very competent in her field, so she knows the right orders to give

122. Check in the appropriate column below how often your *immediate superior* talks to you in the following ways: (Check one for each item.)

		Always or nearly always (1)	Most of the time (2)	Some- times (3)	A few times (4)	Seldom or never (5)
IV:21	Shows appreciation for your work, shows confidence in you	☐	☐	☐	☐	☐
IV:22	Gives you directions or orders	☐	☐	☐	☐	☐
IV:23	Explains things or gives information and suggestions	☐	☐	☐	☐	☐
IV:24	Asks you for suggestions or opinions	☐	☐	☐	☐	☐
IV:25	Asks you for information, explanation, or clarification	☐	☐	☐	☐	☐
IV:26	Criticizes you, refuses to help, or is unnecessarily formal	☐	☐	☐	☐	☐
IV:27	Gives excess, unnecessary information or comments	☐	☐	☐	☐	☐

123. Check in the appropriate column below how much you agree with each statement as it applies to your *immediate superior*. (Check one for each item.)

		Strongly agree (1)	Agree (2)	I cannot decide (3)	Dis- agree (4)	Strongly disagree (5)
IV:28	Represents the sort of person I would like to be myself	☐	☐	☐	☐	☐
IV:29	Is helpful; is a person whom I can usually count on to take action which is useful or helpful to me in the hospital	☐	☐	☐	☐	☐
IV:30	Does the things which are right for someone in her position	☐	☐	☐	☐	☐
IV:31	Is personally likable; is someone I enjoy being with	☐	☐	☐	☐	☐
IV:32	Is an expert in her field; is exceptionally competent in her field	☐	☐	☐	☐	☐
IV:33	Has the power to make changes in my job title or my income	☐	☐	☐	☐	☐

Questionnaire—Nonsupervisory Nurses 669

A FEW FINAL QUESTIONS

124. When decisions that affect your
IV:34 work are made, how adequately are such decisions explained to you? (Check one.)
 ___(1) Completely adequately
 ___(2) Very adequately
 ___(3) Fairly adequately
 ___(4) Somewhat inadequately
 ___(5) Inadequately

125. When decisions that affect your
IV:35 work are made, from whom do you normally *first* learn of such decisions? (Check one *only*.)
 ___(1) From my colleagues or co-workers
 ___(2) My friends
 ___(3) The "grapevine"
 ___(4) In meetings or conferences
 ___(5) From bulletins, memos, or other written materials
 ___(6) From my immediate superior
 ___(7) From people in higher positions
 ___(8) From sources other than the above

126. Which of the following persons
IV:36 is *especially effective* in setting high standards of nursing care? (Check one *only*.)
 ___(0) Nobody is especially effective
 ___(1) The director of nurses
 ___(2) The associate director of nurses
 ___(3) The nursing supervisor of your section
 ___(4) Someone else

127. Which of the following persons
IV:37 is *especially effective* in trying to improve wages, hours, working conditions, or employee benefits? (Check one *only*.)
 ___(0) Nobody is especially effective
 ___(1) The director of nurses
 ___(2) The associate director of nurses
 ___(3) The nursing supervisor of your section
 ___(4) Someone else

128. Which of the following persons
IV:38 is *especially effective* in improving relations between doctors and nurses? (Check one *only*.)
 ___(0) Nobody is especially effective
 ___(1) The director of nurses
 ___(2) The associate director of nurses
 ___(3) The nursing supervisor of your section
 ___(4) Someone else

129. Which of the following persons
IV:39 is *especially effective* in seeing that your department saves time and money? (Check one *only*.)
 ___(0) Nobody is especially effective
 ___(1) The director of nurses
 ___(2) The associate director of nurses
 ___(3) The nursing supervisor of your section
 ___(4) Someone else

130. Which of the following persons
IV:40 is *especially effective* in improving your work relations with other departments on which your work depends? (Check one *only*.)
- ___(0) Nobody is especially effective
- ___(1) The director of nurses
- ___(2) The associate director of nurses
- ___(3) The nursing supervisor of your section
- ___(4) Someone else

131. Which of the following persons
IV:41 is *especially effective* in ironing out problems that arise between different people in your department? (Check one *only*.)
- ___(0) Nobody is especially effective
- ___(1) The director of nurses
- ___(2) The associate director of nurses
- ___(3) The nursing supervisor of your section
- ___(4) Someone else

132. Now that you have filled it out,
IV:42 how do you feel about this questionnaire? (Check one.)
- ___(1) Excellent; it covers everything that I feel is important
- ___(2) Very good; it covers almost everything that I feel is important
- ___(3) Good; it covers most things that I feel are important
- ___(4) Fair; it covers some important things, but misses others
- ___(5) Poor; it misses the things that I feel are important

THANK YOU VERY MUCH FOR YOUR COOPERATION

APPENDIX B **INTERVIEW WITH HOSPITAL ADMINISTRATORS: A SAMPLE INTERVIEW**

Form 9A

ADMINISTRATORS' INTERVIEW, PART A

1. What, would you say, are some of the most important problems this hospital faces at present?

2. Has this hospital undergone any major changes in the last two or three years? (If *yes*, what changes?)

3. Is there anything about the community which, in your opinion, tends to create problems or be a burden to this hospital? (If *yes*, what?)

4. What are the two or three most important ways in which you feel hospitals of this kind are *most different* from other large organizations such as industry?

5. What are the two or three most important ways in which you feel hospitals of this kind are *most similar* to other large organizations such as industry?

6. What are some of the things or areas in which you consider this hospital to be particularly *strong or especially outstanding?*

7. What are some of the things or areas in which you consider this hospital to be particularly *weak or most wanting?*

8. How difficult do you find it to fill any vacancies that may occur among the nonmedical personnel? (For what classes of personnel do you find this *most difficult?*)

9. Does the size of this hospital create any handicaps regarding the accomplishment of the hospital's objective? (If *yes*, what are these handicaps?)

10. What do you see to be the main differences in the way the board of trustees usually looks at problems in comparison to the way the medical staff see the same problems?

Interview—Hospital Administrators

11. Can a doctor be dropped from the staff? (If *yes*, how?)

12. Can a trustee be dropped from the board? (If *yes*, how?)

13. Which *two* hospital departments do you find most difficult to work with? (Why do you feel so?)

14. Considering the president of the board, the chief of staff, and the director of nursing, which one of the three do you feel has the least understanding of your position in the hospital? (Why do you feel so?)

15. In general, which five persons associated with this hospital (whether or not they hold formal positions) do you believe to have the *greatest influence in determining its overall, long-range policies*? (You should also include yourself if you feel that you are among these five persons.)
    a. _____   c. _____
    b. _____   d. _____
        e. _____

16. If you felt that some changes were needed in the organization of the medical staff or its committees, what person's backing would you most need to have in order to get those changes made?
    a. _____

17. If you felt that some changes were needed in the organization of the board of trustees or its committees, what person's backing would you most need to have in order to get those changes made?

   a. _____
   _____
   _____

18. If you felt that some changes were needed in the hospital plant which would require both a major expenditure and rearrangement of facilities, what person's backing would you most need to have in order to get these changes made?

   a. _____
   _____
   _____
   _____

19. Now we would like you to name one or two members of the board of trustees whom you consider to be *particularly outstanding* with respect to each of five areas:

   Names

   First, "devoting a great deal of time to the hospital as an organization"
   a. _____
   b. _____

   Next, "being very well informed about hospital affairs"
   a. _____
   b. _____

   "Being personally popular among his associates"
   a. _____
   b. _____

   "Having a good deal of influence in business or professional circles, e.g., in the Chamber of Commerce, the County Bar Association, etc."
   a. _____
   b. _____

   "Being particularly outstanding in his occupational or professional field—an 'expert' businessman or attorney, etc."
   a. _____
   b. _____

Interview—Hospital Administrators

20. Now we would like you to name one or two members of the medical staff whom you consider to be *particularly outstanding* with respect to each of five areas?

	Names
First, "devoting a great deal of time to the hospital as an organization"	a. _____ b. _____
Next, "being very well informed about hospital affairs"	a. _____ b. _____
"Being personally popular among his professional associates"	a. _____ b. _____
"Having a good deal of influence in professional circles, the County Medical Society or the A.M.A., etc."	a. _____ b. _____
"Being particularly outstanding in his professional field—an expert or a 'doctor's' doctor"	a. _____ b. _____

INTERVIEWER: GIVE PART B (Questionnaire)

INDEX

[The letter *n* as a superscript indicates a footnote.]

Absenteeism among nursing personnel, incidence and rates of, 114–18
  aides, 117
  practical nurses, 117
  registered nurses, 117
  measures of, 114–16
  and nursing department coordination, 350–51
    Table 40, 346–47
  and patient care, 383–86
    Table 46, 385
  and turnover, 116–17
Accreditation, 50, 162, 201–2
Adaptation. *See* Organizational adaptation to exogenous change
Administration. *See* Administrators; Department heads; Profiles, of participating hospitals; Supervision and administrative behavior; specific topics
Administrative skill. *See* Supervisory skills and practices
Administrators, age distribution, 95
  comparative overview in ten hospitals, 194–95
  comparative profile, 144
  family status, 95
  formal education, 96
  length of association with hospital, 104
  organizational stability, 628–30
  sex distribution, 92
  training, 100
  type of, as a criterion of hospital selection, 50
  See also Hospital groups in the study; Hospitals in the study; Influence of key groups; Intraorganizational strain; Organizational coordination; Problem awareness and problem solving; Profiles, of participating hospitals; Respondents; Supervision and administrative behavior; Value orientations of top groups; specific topics
Admissions. *See* Size and size-related variables
Age distribution, of medical, administrative, and trustee groups, *Table 8*, 94. *See also* specific groups
  of nursing staff and technicians, *Table 7*, 93. *See also* specific groups
Aides, nurse's. *See* Nursing staff
Aims of the research, 591–93. *See also* Objectives of the research
American Nurses' Association, 148, 154
Analysis and interpretation, statistical significance, 80
  techniques of, 78–82
  See also Methodological considerations; Research design
Andrews, R. E., 388, 421
Appendix A, 64, 66, 637–70
Appendix B, 64, 671–75
Apple, D., 22, 29
Argyris, C., 22, 29, 148[n], 154, 432, 473, 498
Assessment of patient care, 201–7. *See also* Patient care
Assumptions. *See* specific topics
Authority, 11–13. *See also* Influence of key groups
Average daily census of patients. *See* Size and size-related variables
"Average" hospital. *See* "Typical" hospital in the study

Babcock, K. B., 29, 162[n], 197, 202, 225, 262, 263
Bachrach, C. A., 203, 262
Back, K., 501, 543
Background of hospital personnel. *See* specific groups
Backmayer, A. C., 21, 29

Bailey, N. D., 21, 29
Bales, R. F., 502, 543
Barnard, C. I., 272, 304
Bases and means of coordination, 274–77. *See also* Organizational coordination
Bauer, H., 150ⁿ, 154
Belknap, I., 21, 29
Bennis, W. G., 421
Berger, D. G., 203, 263
Berkowitz, N. H., 421
Block, L., 83ⁿ, 87, 162, 197, 596ⁿ, 635
"Board men." *See* Medical staff
Boards of trustees, 190–91. *See also* Trustees
Brayfield, A. H., 384, 421, 477, 498
Broom, L., 364
Brown, E. L., 22, 29
Budget, balancing, 564–65. *See also* Financial considerations; Hospitals in the study; Profiles, of participating hospitals
Bullock, R. P., 22, 29, 148ⁿ, 154
Bureaucratic aspects of the hospital. *See* Characteristics and problems of the community general hospital; Hospital, as an organization; Hospital structure; Hospitals in the study; Large-scale organizations; Profiles, of participating hospitals; "Typical" hospital in the study
Burling, T., 20, 29, 31, 89ⁿ, 148ⁿ, 150ⁿ, 154, 274ⁿ, 304, 349, 364, 500, 543, 588, 635

Carmelita, Sister Mary, 150ⁿ, 155
Cartwright, D., 474, 498
Caudill, W., 22, 29
Change. *See* Organizational change and its accommodation
Characteristics and problems of the community general hospital, authoritarian character, 7–9
 authority, lines of, 11–13
 coordination, 10
 efficiency, 9–10
 general properties, 1–3
 organizational effectiveness, 4
 predictability of performance, 8–9
 professionalization, 10–11
 specialization and departmentalization, 10–11
 vs. those of other large-scale organizations, 13–15
 See also Hospital, as an organization; Hospital groups in the study; Hospital structure; Hospitals in the study; Profiles, of participating hospitals; "Typical" hospital in the study; and more specific problems and topics
Charges for patient care, 546–47. *See also* Financial considerations
Chiefs of staff. *See* Medical staff; Problem awareness and problem solving; Profiles, of participating hospitals
Chronology of the research, 37–46
Cleven, W. A., 475, 498
Commission on Professional and Hospital Activities, 202ⁿ, 204, 262
Communication, adequacy, administrator to medical staff, 332–33
 of explanation of decisions, 331–32
 medical and nursing staff, 333
 of patient charts, 333–35
 and coordination, 328–36
 Table 37, 330
 frequency of, 330–31
 importance, 500–504
 of adequacy and quality, 622–23
 of concentration of task-relevant information in formal channels, 624
 of direction, 624
 of quantity and frequency, 623–24
 in supervision—patient care, 497–98
 major findings summarized, 624–25
 among nurses, concentration of task-relevant communication in formal channels and nursing department coordination, 535–36
 Table 71, 536
 direction of, 531–35
 and nurse commitment or identification with work groups, 531–32
 Table 69, 532
 and nursing performance, 533–34
 Table 70, 534
 hypotheses involving communication variables, 509
 measures of, 512–16
 qualitative aspects of, 519–25
 and frequency of superior-subordinate communication, 523–25
 Table 65, 524
 and superior's role performance, 523
 Table 64, 521
 quantitative aspects of, 525–31
 nurse commitment or identification with work groups, 529–31

Index

Table 68, 530
and nursing performance, 526–29
Table 66, 527
Table 67, 528
openness of channels, 329–30
theoretical considerations, 504–10
See also Nursing department coordination; Organizational coordination; Supervision and administrative behavior
Community's knowledge of the hospital, 546. *See also* External image of "typical" hospital in the study; Hospital-community relations; Profiles, of participating hospitals
Comparative group profiles of hospital personnel, 142–52
Comparative measure of patient care, 249–57
consistency and stability of, 253–56
derivation, 251–54
Table 25, 253
Table 26, 254
validation of, 256–57
See also Medical care; Medical staff; Nursing care; Overall patient care; Patient care; Profiles, of participating hospitals
Complementarity of work-related expectations among organizational members, 294–95
and coordination, 308–12
Table 34, 310
measures of, 309–14
and patient care, 399–402
Table 51, 400
Composition and distribution of therapeutic staff, and coordination, 338–41
Table 38, 338
measures of, 379–81
and patient care, 379–83
Table 45, 381
Comrey, A. L., 474, 498
Concluding remarks, 634–35
Context of the research, 15–23
"Control" factors, 594. *See also* Methodological considerations; Research design
Coons, A. E., 499
Cooperation among hospital personnel, and coordination, 311–12
Table 34, 310
distinct from coordination, 272–73
general comments, 294–95
measures of, 311–12

See also Sharedness of expectations among organizational members
Coordination. *See* Organizational coordination
within the nursing department. *See* Nursing department coordination
Corrective coordination. *See* Organizational coordination
Corwin, E. H. L., 21, 29
Costs and expenses. *See* Facilities in hospitals studied; Financial considerations
Cottrell, L. S., Jr., 364
Criteria used in selecting hospitals, 3, 50–51. *See also* Hospitals in the study; Research design; Respondents; Sampling; Selection of hospitals and respondents
Criterion measures. *See* specific topics.
Crockett, W. H., 384, 421, 477, 498
Cumming, E., 294, 304
Cumming, J., 294, 304

Danhorst, H. E., 262
Data collection, 61–72. *See also* Hospital groups in the study; Hospitals in the study; Pretest of research instruments; Questionnaires and interviews; Research design; Respondents; Response and nonresponse rates; Sampling; Sources, of data
Davis, J. W., 262
Davis, M. M., 21, 29, 200, 262
Dent, J. K., 429ª, 474, 499
Department heads (nonmedical, administrative), age distribution, 95
comparative profile, 144–45
family status, 95
formal education, 96
job history, 101–2
length of association with hospital, 104
organizational stability, 628–30
sex distribution, 92
training, 100
See also Administrators; Hospital, as an organization; Hospital groups in the study; Paramedical departments; Profiles, of participating hospitals; Supervision and administrative behavior; "Typical" hospital in the study; specific topics
Departmentalization. *See* Characteristics and problems of the community general hospital; Department

Departmentalization [*Cont.*] heads; Hospital, as an organization; Hospital structure; Hospitals in the study; Paramedical departments; Profiles, of participating hospitals; Supervision and administrative behavior; specific topics
Dependent variables, 36–37. *See also* specific topics
Description, forms of, 72–82
  qualitative mode, 74
  quantitative mode, 74
Descriptive data. *See* specific topics
Deutsch, M., 295[a], 304, 388, 421
Deutscher, I., 22, 29, 148[a], 154
Diagnostic test materials, 557–58
Dichter, E., 201, 205, 262
Diebold, J., 267[a], 304
Directors of nursing. *See* Department heads; Hospital groups in the study; Nursing staff; Respondents; Supervision and administrative behavior
Doctors. *See* Medical staff
Drucker, P., 500, 543
Dunham, W., 21, 29

Earnings of nonmedical personnel, 132–37
  average annual, selected groups, 134
    Table 17, 134
  concern for improvements in wages, hours, working conditions, or employee benefits, 562–64
  satisfaction with salaries, 135–37
  See also Facilities in hospitals studied; Financial considerations; specific groups
Economy of operation, improvements, 561–64. *See also* Financial considerations; Profiles, of participating hospitals
Education of nonmedical personnel, formal, 96–98
  Table 9, 97
  See also professional training of nonmedical groups; specific groups
Emergency service, 195, 546, 549. *See also* Patient care; Profiles, of participating hospitals
Equipment. *See* Facilities in hospitals studied
Executive trustees. *See* Boards of trustees; Trustees
Explanatory studies. *See* Research design

External image of "typical" hospital in the study, 545–47. *See also* Community's knowledge of the hospital; Hospital-community relations; Hospitals in the study; Profiles, of participating hospitals

Facilities in hospitals studied, adequacy, 366–70
  evaluated by key hospital groups, 561–64
  interrelationships among, 367–69
  and patient care, 366–70
    Table 42, 368
  "typical" hospital, 159–61
  See also Financial considerations; Hospital groups in the study; Hospitals in the study; Profiles, of participating hospitals; "Typical" hospital in the study
Factors, affecting coordination. *See* Organizational coordination
  affecting patient care. *See* Patient care
Faxon, N. W., 21, 29
Fayol, H., 302, 304
Feibleman, J., 272, 304
Festinger, L., 501, 543
Fiedler, F. E., 475, 498
Financial considerations, charges for patient care, 546–47
  general financial condition, 367–69
  income and expenditure data, 370–76
  and hospital size, 371
  interrelationships among, 371
  and patient care, 370–76
    Table 43, 373
  salaries—earnings of nonmedical personnel, 130–36
  service vs. finances, 559–60
  See also Facilities in hospitals studied; Hospital groups in the study; Hospitals in the study; Profiles, of participating hospitals; "Typical" hospital in the study; Value orientations of top groups
Fleishman, E. A., 476, 498
Floor, L. G., 16, 30
Follett, Mary Parker, 273[a], 302, 304
Ford, T. R., 148[a], 154
Formal organizations. *See* Large-scale organizations
Friend, J. W., 272, 304
Full- vs. part-time work in the hospital, 106–8
  administrators, 107
  department heads, 107

Index

medical staff, 107
nursing staff, 107–8
technicians, 107
trustees, 106–7
See also specific groups
Functional interdependence, 274, 403. See also Organizational coordination
Furstenberg, F. F., 205[a], 262

General coordination. See Organizational coordination
General medical staff, 57. See also Medical staff
General practitioners. See Medical staff
Georgopoulos, B. S., 16, 29, 87, 88, 251, 262, 271[a], 272, 295[a], 304, 384, 397, 421, 474, 477, 499
Ginzberg, E., 22, 29
Goldberg, H., 262
Goldwater, S. S., 21, 29, 204, 262, 271, 304, 377, 421
"Good-care" hospitals, 200–201. See also Patient care
Gordon, H. P., 148[a], 154
Greenblatt, M., 21, 29
Groups studied. See Hospital groups in the study; Respondents
Gulick, L. H., 302, 304
Gurin, G., 16, 30

Hall, O., 22, 29
Halpin, A. W., 433, 476, 499
Hanson, H. C., 148[a], 154
Hartman, G., 21, 29
Hawley, A. H., 274, 275, 304
Hawley, P. R., 201, 203, 204, 206, 262
Head nurses. See Hospital groups in the study; Nursing staff; Respondents
Health Information Foundation, 1, 29, 148, 154, 636
Health Insurance Institute, 11, 29
Heinemann, R. I., 150[a], 154
Hemphill, J. K., 433, 475, 476, 499
High, W. S., 474, 498
Hill, F. T., 203, 262
Hoffman, L. R., 16, 30, 267[a], 304, 429[a], 441, 499
Hospital, as an organization, 5–15
as a place to work, 547–49
See also Characteristics and problems of the community general hospital; Hospital groups in the study; Hospital structure; Hospitals in the study; Organizational adaptation to exogenous change; Organizational change and its accommodation; Organizational coordination; Patient care; Profiles, of participating hospitals; "Typical" hospital in the study; specific topics
Hospital building, concern for improvements or expansion of, 562–64. See also Facilities in hospitals studied; Hospital plant; Profiles, of participating hospitals
Hospital-community relations, 189–90, 546, 564–65
what the community thinks of the hospital, 564–65
See also Community's knowledge of the hospital; External image of the "typical" hospital in the study; Profiles, of participating hospitals
Hospital coordination. See Organizational coordination
Hospital groups in the study, comparative profiles of, 142–52
administrators, 144
aides and orderlies, 149–50
department heads, 144–45
laboratory and x-ray technicians, 150
medical staff, 143–44
nonsupervisory registered nurses, 147
supervisory nurses, 146–47
trustees, 144
interaction patterns of, 120–23
organizational stability of, 628–30
satisfaction of employees, 564–65
selection of individual groups and respondents, 53–61
See also Hospitals in the study; Respondents; specific groups
Hospital personnel. See Hospital groups in the study; Respondents; specific groups
Hospital plant, importance of, 564–65
See also Facilities in hospitals studied; Hospital building; Profiles, of participating hospitals
Hospital profiles. See Hospitals in the study; Profiles, of participating hospitals
Hospital size. See Composition and distribution of therapeutic staff; Facilities in hospitals studied; Hospital groups in the study; Hospital structure; Hospitals in the study; Respondents; Size and size-related variables; "Typical" hospital in the study

Hospital structure, and coordination, 336–41
  Table 38, 338
  and patient care, 379–83
  Table 45, 381
  size and size-related features, 336–38
    average daily census, 337
    number, of beds, 337
    of personnel, 337
  work force composition and distribution,
    aides, 340–41
    board-certified specialists, 338–39
    general practitioners, 338–39
    practical nurses, 339–40
    registered nurses, 339
  See also Characteristics and problems of the community general hospital; Composition and distribution of therapeutic staff; Hospital, as an organization; Hospital groups in the study; Hospitals in the study; Size and size-related variables; "Typical" hospital in the study
Hospitals, "Guide Issue," 1, 2, 29, 88, 160, 197
Hospitals in the study, comparative overview, 189–96
  administration and related aspects, 194–96
  boards of trustees, 190–91
  local setting, 188–89
  medical and nursing care, 193–94
  medical staffs, 191–94
  relations between doctors and trustees, 192–93
  relations with the community, 189–90
  criteria for inclusion in the research, 3, 50–51
    accreditation, 50
    administration, 50
    length of patient stay, 50
    location, 50
    religious affiliation, 50
    service, 50
    size, 50, 52
  pilot hospital sites, 39–41, 51–52
  profiles, 162–87
  selection of, 46–53
  size of, 52
  See also Hospital groups in the study; Research design; Respondents; specific topics
Howland, D., 206[a], 263
Human relations. *See* Supervision and administrative behavior
  skill. *See* Supervisory skills at different levels

Hyman, H. H., 47, 81, 88
Hypotheses. *See* specific topics

Income and expenditures. *See* Facilities in hospitals studied; Financial considerations; "Typical" hospital in the study
Independent variables, 36–37. *See also* specific topics
Indik, B. P., 384, 421, 477, 499
Influence of key groups, desired, on hospital affairs, 574–75
  distribution of prevailing and desired influence on hospital functioning among administrators, doctors, nurses, trustees, 571–73
  gaps in prevailing, 572–73
  general considerations regarding, 566–70
  selected conclusions, 632–33
  See also Intraorganizational strain; Issues and problems concerning medical staff; Profiles, of participating hospitals; Value orientations of top groups; specific groups
Interaction patterns of hospital groups, and coordination functions, 122–23
  Table 16, 123
  hospital departments, most difficult to deal with, 120–21
  of most frequent contact, 119–20
  See also Hospital groups in the study; specific groups
Interest, of medical staff in nonmedical affairs of hospital, 555–56, 561
  of trustees in nonfinancial affairs of hospital, 561
Interhospital differences, 628. *See also* specific topics
Interjob shifting of nonmedical personnel, 105–6. *See also* specific groups
Interview with hospital administrators, 671–75
Intraorganizational strain, and coordination, 295–96, 312–20
  Table 35, 318
  and patient care, 396–99
  Table 50, 398
  tension between interacting groups, 312–20, 630–31
    measure #1, 314
    measure #2, 314–15
    unreasonable pressure for better per-

Index

formance, on nonmedical personnel, 316–20
measure #1, 316
measure #2, 316–17
See also Hospital groups in the study; Influence of key groups; Medical staff; Nursing staff; Profiles, of participating hospitals; Value orientations of top groups
Issues and problems concerning medical staff, formal organization, 555
hospital costs and financial problems, 557–58
importance of selected aspects of hospital functioning, 564–65
nonmedical hospital affairs, 555–56, 561
professional conduct and discipline, 559
relationships among members, 554
relative concern with each of nine issues, 561–64
representation by its executive committee, 555
specialists vs. general practitioners, 552–54
staff privileges, 553
tension within medical staff and between staff and other groups, 554–55
understanding of the problems of other groups, 556–57
use of diagnostic materials, 557–58
See also Influence of key groups; Intraorganizational strain; Medical care; Medical committee activity and performance; Medical staff; Profiles, of participating hospitals; Value orientations of top groups; specific topics

Jaco, E. G., 22, 29
Jacobson, E., 16, 19
Jaques, E., 503, 543
Job characteristics of hospital personnel. See specific groups
Job history of nonmedical personnel, 101–3
Table 11, 102
See also specific groups
Johnson, L. W., 203, 263
Joint Commission on Accreditation of Hospitals, 50, 162, 201–2
Jones, E. W., 263
Jones, W. N., Jr., 16, 19, 477, 499

Kahn, R. L., 16, 29, 30, 31, 250, 263, 433, 474, 499
Katz, D., 16, 30, 250, 263, 433, 474

Katz, R. L., 429[*], 430, 499
King, F., 202, 263
Klein, M. W., 388, 421
Kossack, C. F., 202, 212[*], 251, 263
Kundsen, H. L., 150[*], 154

Laboratory. See Hospital groups in the study; Paramedical departments; Technicians
and x-ray facilities. See Facilities in hospitals studied
Laboratory technicians. See Profiles, of groups in the hospital; Respondents; Supervisory and administrative behavior; Technicians
Lancet, 200, 263
Large-scale organizations, 13–15. See also Characteristics and problems of the community general hospital; Departmentalization; Hospital, as an organization; Hospital groups in the study; Hospital structure; Hospitals in the study; Profiles, of participating hospitals; "Typical" hospital in the study; specific topics
Leadership. See Supervision and administrative behavior
Lederer, H. D., 205, 263
Lembcke, P. A., 204, 263
Length of association with hospital, 103–5
Table 12, 103
See also specific groups
Lentz, E. M., 8, 20, 21, 29, 30, 31, 89[*], 148[*], 150[*], 154, 274[*], 304, 364, 588, 635
Levinson, D. J., 21, 29
Lieberman, S., 16, 30
Likert, R., 16, 30, 432, 473, 499
Limitations of the study. See Methodological considerations
Literature, review of, 38
Low, J., 269[*], 304

Maccoby, N., 16, 30
MacEachern, M. T., 21, 30, 203, 263
Mahoney, G. M., 16, 29, 477, 499
Malone, M. F., 421
Mann, F. C., 16, 19, 30, 87, 88, 267[*], 304, 429[*], 430, 441, 474, 475, 499
March, J. G., 278, 302, 304
Matthews, B. P., 22, 30
McGibony, J. R., 21, 30, 203, 263
McNerney, W. J., 21, 30

Measurement—forms of, arithmetic means (averages), 75–77
hospital means, 77
percentages, 74
proportions, 74
rank-orders, 74–75
See also Analysis and interpretation; Comparative measure of patient care; Description; Medical care measure; Methodological considerations; Nursing care measure; Overall patient care; Research design; Research instruments; Respondents; specific topics
Medical care, comparative overview in ten hospitals, 193–94
  measure of, 223–42
    consistency and stability, 228–32
    derivation, 225–28
    Table 23, 228
    theoretical bases for, 225–27
    validation, 232–42
    rated by outside doctors, 234–36
    See also Medical committee activity and performance; Medical staff; Patient care; Profiles, of participating hospitals
Medical committee activity and performance, measures of, 403–4
  interrelationships, 404–5
  and patient care, 402–7
  Table 52, 406
Medical records, adequacy of, 333–35
  concern for improvements of, 562–64
  See also Facilities in hospitals studied; Issues and problems concerning medical staff; Medical staff
Medical staff, age distribution, 94–95
  comparative group profile, 143–44
  comparative overview in ten hospitals, 191–92
  composition and distribution, 338–41, 379–83
  concern for changes, in organization of, 562–64
    in rights and responsibilities of, 562–64
  family status, 95
  "general medical staff," 57
  issues and problems concerning, 552–59
  length of association with hospital, 104
  organizational stability, 628–30
  relations with trustees, 192–93
  selected conclusions about, 631–32
  "selected medical staff," 56
  service and divisional characteristics, 110–12

sex distribution, 92
specialists vs. general practitioners, 552–54
training, 98
See also Hospital groups in the study; Influence of key groups; Intra-organizational strain; Issues and problems concerning medical staff; Medical care; Medical committee activity and performance; Patient care; Profiles, of participating hospitals; Respondents; Value orientations of top groups; more specific headings
Medicine. *See* Medical care; Medical staff; Patient care
Merton, R. K., 364
Metcalf, H. C., 304
Methodological considerations, factor analysis, 299–302
  limitations of the research, 82–85
  pretest of research instruments, 41–42
  "response set," 299–302
  See also Analysis and interpretation; Data collection; Description; Measurement—forms of; Objectives of the research; Research design; Research instruments; Respondents; Response and nonresponse rates; specific headings (e.g., Medical care, measure of)
Metzner, H., 474, 499
Michigan Hospital Association, 39, 44–45
Michigan Nurses' Association, 39
Michigan State Medical Society, 39
Moench, L. G., 205, 263
Mooi, H. R., 263
Moore, W. E., 500, 543
Morse, N. C., 16, 29, 30
Mortality rates, gross, 238–39
  infant, 238–39
Mott, P. E., 265[a], 579, 587
Mudd, M. C., 204, 263
Murray, M., 103, 155
Myers, R. S., 202, 204, 206, 225, 263

Neff, F. W., 162[a]
New England Journal of Medicine, 1, 30
Newcomb, T. M., 501, 543
Number, of beds. *See* Size and size-related variables
  of paid personnel. *See* Size and size-related variables
Nurses. *See* Nursing staff
Nursing care, comparative overview in ten hospitals, 193–94

Index 685

concern for improvements in, 562–64
measure of, 209–23
  consistency and stability of, 216–19
  reasons for adopting, 216
  Table 20, 211
  Table 21, 214
  Table 22, 217
  validation of, 219–23
See also Communication, among nurses; Nursing staff; Patient care; Performance, of paramedical departments; Problems, pertaining to nursing staff; Profiles, of participating hospitals; Role performance of nursing personnel

Nursing department coordination, measures of, 342–44
  and hospital-organizational coordination, 344–52
  Table 39, 345
  and patient care, 392–94
  Table 49, 393
  and various independent variables, 345–52
    absenteeism and turnover among nursing staff, 350–51
    intraorganizational strain, 348–49
    nursing staff composition, 348
    overlap among nursing roles, 349–50
  Table 40, 346–47

Nursing staff, absenteeism, 114–18, 350–51, 383–86
  age distribution, 93–94
  comparative profiles, 146–50
  composition and distribution, 338–41, 379–83
  divisional and service characteristics, 110–12
  earnings and satisfaction with salary, 132–37
  family status, 95–96
  formal education, 97–98
  full- vs. part-time work, 107–8
  interaction patterns with others, 119–23
  job history, 101–3
  length of association with hospital, 104
  opportunities for advancement, 130–32
  organizational commitment, 139–42
  organizational stability, 628–30
  problems pertaining to, 549–52
  role performance, 516–19
  satisfaction with supervision, 128–30
  sex distribution, 91–92
  shift-work patterns, 108–10
  shortages and supply sources, 103, 629–30
  skill utilization and improvement, 127–29
  tension among different nursing roles, 630–31
  time on present job, 105–6
  training and professional schooling, 99–101
  turnover, 113–17, 383–87
  work motivation, 136–39
  work pace and pressure, 125–27
See also Communication, among nurses; Hospital groups in the study; Influence of key groups; Intraorganizational strain; Nursing care; Nursing department coordination; Patient care; Performance, of paramedical departments; Profiles, of participating hospitals; Respondents; Response and nonresponse rates; Supervision and administrative behavior; specific headings

Objectives of the research, 15–21, 33–37, 85. *See also* Aims of the research; Research design; Strategy of the study
O'Malley, M., 212[*], 263
Opportunities for advancement of nonmedical personnel, 130–32. *See also* specific groups
Orderlies. *See* Nursing staff
Organizational adaptation to exogenous change, and adjustment to internal changes, 585–86
  conditions facilitating, 584–85
  coping with temporarily unpredictable changes, 582–83
  strain created by unusual changes, 582–84
See also Organizational change and its accommodation
Organizational change and its accommodation, acceptance of and adjustment to internal changes, 578
  and adaptation to exogenous change, 585–86
  factors maximizing adjustment, 579–80
  frequency or rate of internal changes, 580–81
  general considerations, 575–77
  internal changes, 577–81
    promptness of adjustment to, 578–79
  results summarized, 633–34

Organizational change [Cont.]
  See also Organizational adaptation to exogenous change
Organizational commitment of nonmedical personnel, identification with selected referent groups, 139–42
  Table 19, 140
  See also specific groups
Organizational coordination, and administrative expertise, 271–72
  bases of, 274–75
  "best" vs. "poorest" coordination hospital, 352–55
    Table 41, 353–54
  categories and types, 277–79, 358–59, 596–605
    nonprogramed (by feedback, informal) or general, 278, 358–59, 597–98
      corrective, 277, 598
      preventive, 277, 598
      promotive, 277, 598
      regulatory, 277, 598
      representational, 598
    programed (by plan, formal), 278, 358–59, 597–98
  concept of, 269–73
  defined, 273
  and cooperation, 272
  and effectiveness, 271
  factors affecting, communication, 297, 328–36
    complementarity of work-related expectations, 294–96, 309–11
    cooperation, 294–96, 312
    intraorganizational strain, 295–96, 312–20
    organizational planning, 293–94, 306–8
    problem awareness and problem solving, 296, 320–28
    sharedness of member expectations, 294–96, 308–9
    structural features of organization, 297–98, 336–41
  means for achieving, 275–78
  measures of, 279–93
    consistency and stability of, 284–93
    interrelationships among overall measures, 289
      Table 31, 289
    related to singleness of direction of efforts, 291
      Table 32, 291
    Table 28, 285
    Table 29, 286
    Table 30, 288
  and patient care, 387–96
    Table 48, 390
  principal findings, 355–63
    categories and types, 358–59
    implications, 359–63
    nursing department coordination, 600–601
    overall hospital coordination, 599–600
    summary, 603–5
    variables highly related, to nonprogramed coordination, 601–2
      to preventive coordination, 603
      to programed coordination, 601–2
      to promotive coordination, 603
    See also Nursing department coordination
Organizational effectiveness. See Characteristics and problems of the community general hospital; Patient care; Performance, of paramedical departments; Role performance of nursing personnel; and more specific variables regarding such things as absenteeism among nursing personnel, communication, intraorganizational strain, medical care, medical committee activity and performance, nursing care, organizational adaptation, organizational change, organizational coordination, supervision and administrative behavior, turnover among nursing staff, etc.
Organizational flexibility. See Organizational adaptation to exogenous change; Organizational change and its accommodation
Organizational planning, adherence to plans, policies, regulations, rules, 307
  and coordination, 306–8
    Table 33, 307
  definitional clarity of rules, 306–7
  general considerations, 293–94
  work planning and scheduling, 307–8
Organizational problems. See Characteristics and problems of the community general hospital; Hospital, as an organization; Hospital groups in the study; Hospitals in the study; Influence of key groups; Intraorganizational strain; Issues and problems concerning the medical staff; Organizational adaptation to exogenous change;

Index

Organizational coordination; Patient care; Problem awareness and problem solving; Problems, of the nursing staff; Profiles, of participating hospitals; Value orientations of top groups; specific headings
Organizational stability of groups, 628–30. See also specific groups
Overall coordination. See Organizational coordination
Overall patient care, and hospital's reputation in the community, 247–49
measure (noncomparative) of, 242–49
derivation, 243
Table 24, 244
validation of, 246–49
See also Comparative measure of patient care; Medical care; Nursing care; Patient care; Profiles, of participating hospitals

Paramedical departments, 408–12. See also Department heads; Hospital, as an organization; Hospital groups in the study; Supervision and administrative behavior
Parsons, T., 13, 30, 268, 304, 360, 364
Partial tau-correlations, 83
Participating hospitals. See Hospitals in the study; Profiles, of participating hospitals
Patient admissions. See Size and size-related variables
Patient care, assessment of, 201–7
accreditation approach, 201–2
clinical approach, 205–7
"satisfied customer" approach, 204–5
statistical approach, 202–4
charges for, 546–47
and coordination, of hospital, 387–96
Table 48, 390
of nursing department, 392–94
Table 49, 393
measures of, 257–60
Table 27, 258
principal results, 601–13
quality, of medical care, 607–8
of nursing care, 606–7
of overall patient care, 608
selected variables and the quality of, absenteeism and turnover among nursing personnel, 383–86
complementary of work-related expectations, 399–402
financial items, 370–76, 610

hospital size, 376–83, 608–9
intraorganizational strain, 396–99
medical committee activity and performance, 402–7
organizational coordination, 387–96
performance of paramedical departments, 407–12, 610–11
physical and material facilities, 366–70, 609–10
supervision, 611
summary of major findings about, 612–13
See also Absenteeism among nursing personnel; Communication, among nurses; Comparative measure of patient care; Composition and distribution of therapeutic staff; Intraorganizational strain; Medical care; Medical staff; Nursing care; Nursing department coordination; Nursing staff; Organizational coordination; Overall patient care; Profiles, of participating hospitals; Supervision and administrative behavior; Turnover among nursing staff; specific variables
Patients, admissions, 376–79
average daily census, 376–79
how feel about hospital, 545
as possible respondents, 204–5
satisfaction of, 564–65
See also External image of "typical" hospital; Hospital-community relations; Patient care; Profiles, of participating hospitals
Pelz, D. C., 16, 30
Performance. See Medical committee activity and performance; Organizational effectiveness; Patient care; Performance, of paramedical departments; Role performance of nursing personnel
of paramedical departments, measures of 408–9
interhospital range on, 409
interrelationships among, 409
and patient care, 409–12, 610–11
Table 53, 410
Personal characteristics of hospital personnel. See specific groups
Personnel. See Hospital groups in the study; Respondents
shortages. See Organizational stability of groups; Professional nurse shortages; Profiles, of participating hospitals; Sources, of supply

Personnel [Cont.]
  of professional nurses; Turnover among nursing staff; specific groups
Phenix, F. L., 204, 263, 274*, 304
Physical plant and layout. See Facilities in hospitals studied
Ponton, T. R., 22, 30
Practical nurses. See Nursing staff
Pratt, L., 204, 263
Pressure at work. See Intraorganizational strain
Pretest of research instruments, 41–42
Preventive coordination. See Organizational coordination
Problem awareness and problem solving, degree of awareness, 322–24
  administrators, 323–24
  directors of nursing, 323–24
  effectiveness in solving problems, 324–27
  administrators, 324–25
  chiefs of staff, 325–27
  directors of nursing, 324
  presidents of trustees, 325–26
  how promptly problems are settled, 321–22
  how satisfactorily problems are handled, 321
  in relation to coordination, 321–28
  Table 36, 322
Problems, of the hospital. See Characteristics and problems of the community general hospital; Hospital, as an organization; Hospital groups in the study; Hospital structure; Influence of key groups; Intraorganizational strain; Issues and problems concerning medical staff; Organizational adaptation to exogenous change; Organizational coordination; Problems, pertaining to nursing staff; Profiles, of participating hospitals; Value orientations of top groups; specific topics
  of the medical staff. See Issues and problems concerning medical staff; Medical care; Profiles, of participating hospitals; Value orientations of top groups
  of the nursing staff, attracting and retaining professional nurses, 549
  composition and distribution of nursing staff, 379–83
  composition of nursing staff in relation to employment, 550–51
  improvement of patient care, 551
  part-time employment, 550
  relationships among nursing personnel in different roles, 552
  salaries and rewards, 549–50
  shortages of professional nurses, 103
  sources of supply of professional nurses, 629–30
  tension between nursing personnel in different classifications, 552
  See also Communication, among nurses; Interaction patterns of hospital groups; Intraorganizational strain; Nursing care; Nursing department coordination; Nursing staff; Patient care; Profiles, of participating hospitals; Supervision and administrative behavior; specific topics
Professional and occupational characteristics of hospital personnel. See specific groups
Professional conduct and discipline, medical staff, 559
Professional nurse shortages, 103. See also Nursing staff, turnover
Professional nurses. See Nursing staff
Professional training of nonmedical groups, different aspects of, 98–101
  satisfaction with, 100–101
  Table 10, 99
  See also specific groups
Professionalization, 10–11
Profiles, of groups in the hospital, 142–52. See also Hospital groups in the study; Respondents
  of participating hospitals, 163–87
Programed coordination. See Organizational coordination
Promotive coordination. See Organizational coordination
Public relations. See Community's knowledge of the hospital; External image of "typical" hospital; Hospital-community relations; Profiles, of participating hospitals

Qualitative data. See Data collection; Profiles, of participating hospitals; specific topics
Quality of care. See Comparative measure of patient care; Medical care; Medical staff; Nursing care; Nursing staff; Overall patient care; Profiles, of participating hospitals

Index

Quantitative data. *See* Data collection; specific topics
Questionnaires and interviews, administered to nonsupervisory nurses, 637–70
 different forms used, 62–64
 pretest of, 41–42
 See also Data collection; Hospital groups in the study; Interview with hospital administrators; Research design; Research instruments; Respondents; Response and nonresponse rates; Sources, of data; measures under specific topics

Rating of medical care by outside doctors, 234–36
Reader, G. G., 204, 263
Registered nurses. *See* Nursing staff
Regulatory coordination. *See* Organizational coordination
Reimer, E., 16, 30
Reissman, L., 22, 30
Relations among groups in the hospital. *See* specific groups and topics
Relationships among variables. *See* specific topics
Reports to participating hospitals, Report I, 44–45
 Report II, 44–45
Representational coordination. *See* Organizational coordination
Research design, forms of description, measurement, and analysis, 72–82
 methodological limitations, 82–85
 overview of, 33–37
 research instruments and data collection, 61–72
 sampling, 55–61
 selection, of participating hospitals, 50–52
  of respondents, 53–61
 summary, 85–87
 See also Aims of the research; Data collection; Hospital groups in the study; Hospitals in the study; Methodological considerations; Objectives of the research; Research instruments; Respondents; Response and nonresponse rates; Sources, of data; Strategy of the study; measures under specific topics
Research instruments, interview with hospital administrators, 671–75
 pretest of, 41–42
 questionnaire, administered to nonsupervisory nurses, 637–70
 and interview forms, 62–64
 rating of quality of medical care by outside doctors, 234–36
 sampling, 55–61
 sources of data, 86–87
 See also Data collection; Methodological considerations; Research design; Respondents; measures under specific topics
Respondents, attitude toward hospital charges, 546–47
 final number, by category, 70–71
  Table 5, 71
 groups and individuals selected, 56–57
 reaction to the study, 70–73
  Table 6, 72
 selection of, 53–61
  number of individuals initially selected, 60–61
  Table 2, 61
 specification of, 55–59
 See also Data collection; Hospital groups in the study; Methodological considerations; Profiles, of groups in the hospital; Profiles, of participating hospitals; Research design; Response and nonresponse rates; Sampling; specific groups
Response and nonresponse rates, attained rates, 67–71
 gross and net, 68–69
  Table 3, 68
  Table 4, 69
 See also Respondents
Revans, R. W., 590, 591, 636
Richardson, H. B., 22, 30
Roberts, M. M., 22, 30, 148*, 155
Roethlisberger, F. J., 433, 499
Rohrer, J. H., 22, 30
Role performance of nursing personnel, selected aspects, 516–19
 See also Absenteeism among nursing personnel; Communication, among nurses; Intraorganizational strain; Nursing care; Nursing department coordination; Nursing staff; Performance, of paramedical departments; Supervision and administrative behavior; Turnover among nursing staff; specific topics
Rourke, A. J. J., 202, 263

Salaries of nonmedical personnel. *See* Earnings of nonmedical personnel
Sampling, different aspects of, 55–61
 rates and ratios used, 58–60
 Table 1, 60
 "representativeness," 48–49
 See also Hospital groups in the study; Hospitals in the study; Methodological considerations; Research design; Respondents; Response and nonresponse rates; Statistical aspects; measures under specific topics
"Satisfied customer" approach, 204–5
Schachter, S., 501, 543
Schwartz, M. S., 21, 31
Searles, R. E., 87, 500ⁿ, 625ⁿ, 636
Seashore, S. E., 16, 30, 384, 421, 474, 477, 499
Selected medical staff, 56. *See also* Medical staff
Selected problems and issues, 544
Selection of hospitals and respondents, participating hospitals, 46–53
 groups and individuals, 53–61
Service and divisional characteristics of therapeutic staff, distribution of medical and nursing staff, 110–12
 Table 15, 111
Service vs. finances, 559–60. *See also* Facilities; Financial considerations; Value orientations of top groups
Sewall, L. G., 203, 263
Sharedness of expectations among organizational members, attitudinal sharedness, 309
 and coordination, 308–12
 Table 34, 310
 generalized consensus, 309
 measures of, 311–12
 See also Complementarity of work-related expectations; Cooperation among hospital personnel
Sheps, M. C., 204, 206, 207, 251, 263
Shift work patterns in the hospital, administrative personnel, 109
 distribution of nursing personnel, according to shift, 108–10
 Table 13, 109
 according to work regularity on present shift, 109–10
 Table 14, 110
 medical staff, 109
Shils, E. A., 304
Siegel, S., 442, 444ⁿ, 499
Simmons, L. W., 22, 30

Simon, H. A., 271, 273, 278, 302, 304, 388, 421
Size and size-related variables, aspects of, 376–79
 average daily census of patients, 376–79
 number, of beds, 376–79
 of paid personnel, 376–79
 patient admissions, 376–79
 and coordination, 336–41
 Table 38, 338
 and patient care, 376–79
 Table 44, 377
 See also Composition and distribution of therapeutic staff; Hospital structure; Respondents; "Typical" hospital in the study
Skill utilization and improvement for nonmedical personnel, 127–29
Skills (administrative, human relations, technical). *See* Supervisory skills at different levels
Slee, V. N., 263
Smith, A. W., 203, 263
Smith, G., 21, 30
Smith, H. L., 11, 19, 20, 30, 361, 364, 588, 636
Sofer, C., 22, 30
Sources, of data, 86–87. *See also* Data collection; Hospital groups in the study; Hospitals in the study; Profiles, of participating hospitals; Rating of medical care by outside doctors; Research design; Research instruments; Respondents; "Typical" hospital in the study
 of supply of professional nurses, 629–30
Southmayd, H. J., 21, 30
Space and beds available. *See* Facilities in hospitals studied
Specialists vs. general practitioners, 552–54. *See also* Issues and problems concerning medical staff; Medical staff
Specialization, 10–11. *See also* Hospital, as an organization; Large-scale organizations; Organizational coordination
Staff nurses. *See* Nursing staff
Standards of care, importance of, 564–65
 See also Patient care; Profiles, of participating hospitals; Value orientations of top groups
Stanton, A. H., 21, 31

Index

Statistical aspects, miscellaneous statistics, 1–4, 33–34, 159–62
  See also Methodological considerations; Research design; Response and nonresponse rates; Sampling
Stecklein, J. E., 148[n], 154
Stephenson, D. D., 148[n], 154
Stewart, D. D., 148[n], 155
Stogdill, R. M., 475, 499
Stouffer, S. A., 91, 155
Strategy of the study, 590–96. See also Aims of the research; Objectives of the research; Research design
Supervision and administrative behavior,
  "effective" supervision, 432–33
  general observations, 422–25
  and organizational effectiveness, 472–78
  principal findings, 613–21
  relationship of supervision, to organizational coordination, 617–18
    to patient care, 618–19
  satisfaction of subordinates with supervision, 616–17
  summary, 619–21
  supervisory skills and practices, 615–16
  satisfaction with supervision, 129–30
  theoretical considerations, 425–33
  See also Administrators; Communication, among nurses; Department heads; Supervisory practices and characteristics; Supervisory skills and practices; Supervisory skills at different levels
Supervisory nurses. See Communication, among nurses; Nursing staff; Supervision and administrative behavior
Supervisory practices and characteristics, and satisfaction with supervision at various levels, 456–71
  department heads, 456–58
  nonsupervisory registered nurses, 461–64
  practical nurses and aides, 464–65
  supervisory nurses, 458–61
  technicians, 465–68
  and supervisory skills at various levels, 456–68
  department heads, 456–58
  Table 57, 457
  nonsupervisory registered nurses, 461–64
  Table 59, 462
  supervisory nurses, 458–61
  Table 58, 459

  technicians, 465–68
  Table 60, 466
  measures of, 452–56
  their relative importance to satisfaction of subordinates with supervision at different levels, 468–71
  See also Communication, among nurses; Supervision and administrative behavior; Supervisory skills and practices; Supervisory skills at different levels
Supervisory skills and practices, and organizational coordination, 483–91
  Table 62, 484
  and organizational effectiveness, 472–78
  and patient care, 478–83
  Table 61, 480–81
    through the mediation of coordination variables, 486–90
  Table 63, 487
  See also Communication, among nurses; Supervision and administrative behavior; Supervisory practices and characteristics; Supervisory skills at different levels
Supervisory skills at different levels, as determinants of subordinate satisfaction at various levels, 449–52
  department heads, 449
  nonsupervisory registered nurses, 450
  practical nurses, 450
  supervisory nurses, 450
  technicians, 451
  different skills, 427–32
  administrative, 428
  human relations, 428
  technical, 427
  measures of, 434–38
  interrelationships among, 437–40
  Table 54, 437
  Table 55, 439
  respondent discrimination, 440–44
  and satisfaction of subordinates with supervision, 444–49
  Table 56, 447
  "supervisory skill-mix," 429–32
  Figure 1, 431
  See also Communication, among nurses; Supervision and administrative behavior; Supervisory practices and characteristics; Supervisory skills and practices
Supplies. See Facilities in hospitals studied
Surgery. See Medical care; Medical staff; Patient care

Survey Research Center, coding, 43
field section, 64
studies by, 15–16
tabulating, 43

Taback, M., 262
Tables. See specific topics
Technical skill. See Supervisory skills at different levels
Technicians (laboratory and x-ray), age distribution, 94
comparative profile, 150–52
earnings and satisfaction with salary, 132–37
family status, 96
formal education, 97–98
full- vs. part-time work, 107–8
job history, 101–2
length of association with hospital, 104–5
organizational stability, 628–30
professional training, 100–101
satisfaction with supervision, 128–30
sex distribution, 92
time on present job, 105–6
See also Hospital groups in the study; Intraorganizational strain; Profiles, of participating hospitals; Respondents; Supervision and administrative behavior; specific topics
Tension among different groups. See Intraorganizational strain
Thruelson, R., 150*, 155
Time on present job for nursing personnel and technicians, 105–6
Timing of activities in the hospital. See Organizational coordination categories and types, programed
Torrence, E. P., 388, 421
Training of nonmedical personnel. See Professional training of nonmedical groups
Training programs, concern for improvements in, 562–64
See also Profiles, of participating hospitals
Trustees, age distribution, 94
comparative overview in ten hospitals, 190–91
comparative profile, 144
concern for changes in organization of, 562–64
family status, 95
formal education, 96
interest of trustees in nonfinancial hospital affairs, 561
length of association with hospital, 104
organizational stability, 628–30
relations with medical staff, 192–93
sex distribution, 92
training (occupational), 98–99
See also Hospital groups in the study; Influence of key groups; Intraorganizational strain; Profiles, of participating hospitals; Respondents; Supervision and administrative behavior; Value orientations of top groups
Turner, J. G., 274*, 304
Turnover among nursing staff, and absenteeism, 116–17
measures and rates, 113–14
aides, 113–14
registered nurses, 113–14
and nursing department coordination, 350–51
Table 40, 346–47
and patient care, 383–87
Table 47, 386
See also Absenteeism among nursing personnel; Professional nurse shortages; Sources, of supply of professional nurses
"Typical" hospital in the study (sketch of), 158–62
See also External image of "typical" hospital; Profiles, of participating hospitals

Unanswered questions, 589
Urwick, L., 302, 304

Value orientations of top groups (administrators, doctors, trustees), adequacy of major hospital facilities, 561
charges for patient care, 546–47
interest of doctors in nonmedical hospital affairs, 555–56, 561
interest of trustees in nonfinancial hospital affairs, 561
issues and problems of great concern, 561–63
relative importance of selected aspects of hospital functioning, 564–65
service vs. finances, 559–60
tension among doctors, trustees, administrators, 560–61

Index

See also Administrators; Hospital, as an organization; Influence of key groups in the hospital; Intraorganizational strain; Issues and problems concerning medical staff; Medical staff; Patient care; Profiles, of participating hospitals; Trustees; specific organizational problems

Veterans Administration, Department of Medicine and Surgery, 206*, 264

Warner, W. L., 269*, 304
Weinberg, S. K., 21, 29
Weiss, R. S., 16, 31, 290, 304
Wessen, A. F., 20, 31, 268, 304, 361, 364, 588, 636
Whyte, W. F., 296, 304
Williams, L. K., 429*, 430, 441, 475, 499
Williams, R. H., 21, 29
Wilson, A. T. M., 22, 31
Wilson, R. C., 474, 498
Wilson, R. N., 20, 29, 31, 89*, 148*, 150, 154, 274*, 304, 364, 588, 635
Wolff, H. G., 22, 30
Work characteristics of hospital personnel. See specific groups
Work force characteristics of hospital personnel. See specific groups

Work motivation of nonmedical personnel, 136–39
Table 18, 138
See also specific groups
Work pace of nonmedical personnel, 125–26. See also specific groups
Work pressure for nonmedical personnel, 126–27
amount experienced, 126
origins of, 126–27
See also Intraorganizational strain; specific groups
Wright, M. G., 21, 31

X-ray. See Departments; Hospital groups in the study; Performance, of paramedical departments; Profiles, of participating hospitals; Technicians
X-ray technicians. See Profiles, of different groups in the hospital; Respondents; Supervision and administrative behavior; Technicians

Zander, A., 474, 498
Zugich, J. J., 30, 31, 39, 361, 364

TITLES IN THIS SERIES

1. Chris Argyris, *Personality and Organization*, New York, 1957
2. Chris Argyris et al., *Social Science Approaches to Business Behavior*, Homewood, 1962
3. Timothy W. Costello and Sheldon S. Zalkind, *Psychology in Administration*, Englewood Cliffs, 1963
4. Melville Dalton, *Men Who Manage*, New York, 1959
5. Robert Dubin, *The World of Work*, Englewood Cliffs, 1958
6. M. P. Follett, *Freedom and Coordination*, London, 1949
7. Basil Georgopoulos and Floyd C. Mann, *The Community General Hospital*, New York, 1962
8. Alvin W. Gouldner, editor, *Studies in Leadership*, New York, 1950
9. Luther Gulick and L. Urwick, editors, *Papers on the Science of Administration*, New York, 1937
10. Robert Aaron Gordon and James Edwin Howell, *Higher Education for Business*, New York, 1959
11. Mason Haire, editor, *Modern Organization Theory*, New York, 1959
12. John K. Hemphill, *Dimensions of Executive Positions*, Columbus, 1960
13. Frederick Herzberg et al., *Job Attitudes: Review of Research and Opinion*, Pittsburgh, 1957
14. Elliot Jaques, *The Changing Culture of a Factory*, London, 1951
15. Daniel Katz, Nathan Maccoby, and Nancy C. Morse, *Productivity, Supervision, and Morale in an Office Situation*, Ann Arbor, 1950
16. Harold J. Leavitt, editor, *The Social Science of Organization*, Englewood Cliffs, 1963
17. Rensis Likert, *New Patterns of Management*, New York, 1961
18. James G. March, editor, *Handbook of Organizations*, Chicago, 1965 (2 volumes)
19. A. K. Rice, *Productivity and Social Organization: The Ahmedebad Experiment*, London, 1958
20. Herbert A. Simon, *Models of Man*, New York, 1957
21. Ross Stagner, *Psychology of Industrial Conflict*, New York, 1956
22. Robert Tannenbaum, Irving R. Weschler, and Fred Massarik, *Leadership and Organization, A Behavioral Science Approach*, New York, 1961
23. James D. Thompson et al., editors, *Comparative Studies in Administration*, Pittsburgh, 1959
    bound with
    Joan Woodward, *Management and Technology*, London, 1958
24. Joseph Tiffin, *Industrial Psychology*, Englewood Cliffs, 1942
25. E. L. Trist, et al., *Organizational Choice*, London, 1963
26. L. Urwick, *The Golden Book of Management*, London, 1956
27. Morris S. Viteles, *Industrial Psychology*, New York, 1932
28. Victor H. Vroom, *Some Personality Determinants of the Effects of Participation*, Englewood Cliffs, 1960
29. Charles R. Walker, Robert H. Guest, and Arthur N. Turner, *The Foreman on the Assembly Line*, Cambridge, 1956
30. William Foote Whyte, *Pattern for Industrial Peace*, New York, 1951